Drug Design and Medicinal Chemistry

Drug Design and Medicinal Chemistry

Edited by **Erica Helmer**

Callisto Reference

New York

Published by Callisto Reference,
106 Park Avenue, Suite 200,
New York, NY 10016, USA
www.callistoreference.com

Drug Design and Medicinal Chemistry
Edited by Erica Helmer

International Standard Book Number: 978-1-63239-154-4 (Hardback)

Printed in China.

Contents

	Preface	**VII**
Chapter 1	**Analysis of Protein Interaction Networks to Prioritize Drug Targets of Neglected-Diseases Pathogens** Aldo Segura-Cabrera, Carlos A. García-Pérez, Mario A. Rodríguez-Pérez, Xianwu Guo, Gildardo Rivera and Virgilio Bocanegra-García	**1**
Chapter 2	**Kojic Acid Derivatives** Mutlu D. Aytemir and G. Karakaya	**29**
Chapter 3	**Recent Applications of Quantitative Structure-Activity Relationships in Drug Design** Omar Deeb	**55**
Chapter 4	**Inhibitors of Serine Proteinase – Application in Agriculture and Medicine** Rinat Islamov, Tatyana Kustova and Alexander Ilin	**83**
Chapter 5	**Atherosclerosis and Antihyperlipidemic Agents** Laila Mahmoud Mohamed Gad	**99**
Chapter 6	**Pyrrolobenzodiazepines as Sequence Selective DNA Binding Agents** Ahmed Kamal, M. Kashi Reddy, Ajay Kumar Srivastava and Y. V. V. Srikanth	**119**
Chapter 7	**Regulation of EC-SOD in Hypoxic Adipocytes** Tetsuro Kamiya, Hirokazu Hara, Naoki Inagaki and Tetsuo Adachi	**143**
Chapter 8	**Pattern Recognition Receptors Based Immune Adjuvants: Their Role and Importance in Vaccine Design** Halmuthur M. Sampath Kumar, Irfan Hyder and Parvinder Pal Singh	**159**

Chapter 9 **Development of an Ultrasensitive CRP Latex Agglutination Reagent by Using Amino Acid Spacers** **185**
Tomoe Komoriya, Kazuaki Yoshimune, Masahiro Ogawa, Mitsuhiko Moriyama and Hideki Kohno

Chapter 10 **Microarray Analysis in Drug Discovery and Biomarker Identification** **203**
Yushi Liu and Joseph S. Verducci

Chapter 11 **Effective Kinetic Methods and Tools in Investigating the Mechanism of Action of Specific Hydrolases** **227**
Emmanuel M. Papamichael, Panagiota-Yiolanda Stergiou, Athanasios Foukis, Marina Kokkinou and Leonidas G. Theodorou

Chapter 12 **Supraventricular Tachycardia Due to Dopamine Infused Through Epidural Catheter Accidentally (A Case Report and Review)** **267**
Demet Coskun and Ahmet Mahli

Chapter 13 **Aluminium – Non-Essential Activator of Pepsin: Kinetics and Thermodynamics** **275**
Vesna Pavelkic, Tanja Brdaric and Kristina Gopcevic

Chapter 14 **Peptides and Peptidomimetics in Medicinal Chemistry** **297**
Paolo Ruzza

Chapter 15 **Carbonic Anhydrase Inhibitors and Activators: Small Organic Molecules as Drugs and Prodrugs** **315**
Murat Şentürk, Hüseyin Çavdar, Oktay Talaz and Claudiu T. Supuran

Chapter 16 **Stochastic Simulation for Biochemical Reaction Networks in Infectious Disease** **329**
Shailza Singh and Sonali Shinde

Chapter 17 **Molecular Modeling and Simulation of Membrane Transport Proteins** **357**
Andreas Jurik, Freya Klepsch and Barbara Zdrazil

Chapter 18 **Alternative Perspectives of Enzyme Kinetic Modeling** **391**
Ryan Walsh

Permissions

List of Contributors

Preface

It is often said that books are a boon to mankind. They document every progress and pass on the knowledge from one generation to the other. They play a crucial role in our lives. Thus I was both excited and nervous while editing this book. I was pleased by the thought of being able to make a mark but I was also nervous to do it right because the future of students depends upon it. Hence, I took a few months to research further into the discipline, revise my knowledge and also explore some more aspects. Post this process, I begun with the editing of this book.

This book covers the different aspects of drug design and medicinal chemistry. Recently, medicinal chemistry has become accountable for clarifying interactions of chemical molecules procedures, such that many experts in life sciences, from agronomy to medication, are occupied in medicinal study. This book comprises of researches centering on molecular features of drug metabolism, pro-drug production, in silico and chemical compounds used in applicable methods. It even deals with fundamental issues and developments in medicinal chemistry and drug design. Particular significance is given to both conjectural and investigational features of contemporary drug design. This book intends to provide some useful knowledge to students and even experts working on the above stated topic. This book is a compilation of data provided by some of the renowned experts working in this field of science for years.

I thank my publisher with all my heart for considering me worthy of this unparalleled opportunity and for showing unwavering faith in my skills. I would also like to thank the editorial team who worked closely with me at every step and contributed immensely towards the successful completion of this book. Last but not the least, I wish to thank my friends and colleagues for their support.

Editor

1

Analysis of Protein Interaction Networks to Prioritize Drug Targets of Neglected-Diseases Pathogens

Aldo Segura-Cabrera[1,5], Carlos A. García-Pérez[1], Mario A. Rodríguez-Pérez[2], Xianwu Guo[2], Gildardo Rivera[3] and Virgilio Bocanegra-García[4]
[1]*Laboratorio de Bioinformática*
[2]*Laboratorio de Biomedicina Molecular*
[3]*Laboratorio de Biotecnología Ambiental*
[4] *Laboratorio de Medicina de Conservación*
Centro de Biotecnología Genómica, Instituto Politécnico Nacional
[5]*U.A.M. Reynosa Aztlán, Universidad Autónoma de Tamaulipas, Reynosa*
México

1. Introduction

Many technological, social and biological systems have been modeled in terms of large networks providing invaluable insight in the understanding of such systems. Systems biology is an emerging and multi-disciplinary discipline that studies the interactions of cellular components by treating them as part of an integrated system. Thus, systems biology has shown that functional molecules are involved in complex networks of inter-relationships, and that most of the cellular processes depend on functional modules rather than isolated components. Large amounts of biological network data of different types are available, e.g., protein-protein interaction, transcriptional regulatory, signal transduction, and metabolic networks. Since proteins carry out most biological processes, the protein interaction networks (PINs) are of particular importance. The advancement of the functional genomics and systems biology of model organisms such as *Saccharomyces cerevisiae*, *Caenorhabditis elegans*, and *Drosophila melanogaster* has contributed to the development of experimental and computational methods, and also to the understanding of human complex diseases. The availability of these methods has facilitated systematic efforts at creating large-scale data sets of protein interactions, which are modeled as PINs.

Usually, a PIN is represented as a graph where the proteins are the nodes and the interactions are the edges. According to the complex network theory, PINs are scale-free networks characterized by a power-law degree distribution. In scale-free networks, most nodes have a small number of links between them; whereas, a small percentage of nodes interact with a disproportionately large number of others. The nodes with a large number of links in PINs are called hub proteins. Functional genomics studies showed that in PINs, the deletion of a hub protein is lethal to the organism, a phenomenon known as the centrality-lethality rule. This rule is widely believed to reflect the special importance of hubs in organizing the network, which in turn suggests the biological significance of network topology. Several well-known studied proteins that are implicated in human diseases are hub proteins. Examples include p53, p21, p27, BRCA1, ubiquitin, calmodulin, and others which play central roles in various cellular mechanisms.

Despite recent advances in systems biology of model organisms, the systems biology of human pathogenic organisms such as those that cause the so-called "neglected-diseases" has not received much attention. Neglected-diseases are chronic or related disabling infections affecting more than 1 billion people worldwide, mainly in Africa. Pathogens of neglected-diseases include: Protozoan parasites (e.g., *Leishmania* spp., *Plasmodium* spp., and *Trypanosoma* spp.), vector-borne helminthes (e.g., *Schistosoma* spp., *Brugia malayi*, and *Onchocerca volvulus*), soil-transmitted helminthes (e.g., *Ascaris lumbricoides* and *Trichuris trichura*), bacteria (e.g., *Mycobacterium tuberculosis* and *M. leprae*), and viruses (e.g., dengue and yellow fever virus). A number of factors limit the utility of existing drugs in neglected-diseases such as high cost, poor compliance, drug resistance, low efficacy, and poor safety. Since the evolution of drug resistance is likely to compromise every drug over time, the demand for new drugs and targets is continuous. The drug target identification is the first step in the drug discovery flow-through process. This step is complicated because a drug target must satisfy a variety of criteria. The important factors in this context are mainly related to the toxicity to host, and the essentiality of the target to the pathogen's physiology for growth and survival. Thus, the topological and functional analysis of neglected-disease pathogen PINs offers a potentially effective strategy for identifying and prioritizing new drug targets.

This chapter will introduce the reader to the basic concepts of network analyses and outline why it is important in terms of predicting protein function and essentiality. Work involving PINs of neglected-disease pathogens will be explained so that the reader will understand the current state in terms of its application to prioritize drug targets. The experimental and computational methods most likely to be used to identify and predict PINs, and the strategies for identifying multiple potential drug targets in neglected-disease pathogens will be also outlined using several biological databases in an integrated way.

To achieve this goal, the chapter includes three sections. Firstly, we present an outline of the conceptual development of network biology. The applied functional genomics involving the analysis of PINs of model organisms has led to developing methods and principles for elucidating protein function. We will also explain how these concepts are connected with protein essentiality to identify their “weak” points on the PINs of neglected-disease pathogens and its use for prioritizing drug targets. In the second section, we outline the experimental and computational methods that are most extensively to be used to identify and predict PINs. Some new approaches for predicting PINs are also introduced. These include the probabilistic integrated network methods which have shown the capability to increase the accuracy and coverage of the PINs. These primary research articles will be reviewed and the potential applications for the future be explained. This section mainly focused on analyzing the PINs of most prevalent neglected-disease pathogens in which the use of drugs is often limited by factors including high cost, low efficacy, toxicity, and the emergence of drug resistance. The potential use as an integrated strategy aimed at prioritizing and identifying drug targets of neglected-disease pathogens will be put forward, and the argument for future research involving the application of many tools and strategies will be discussed. In the final section, we describe, amenably, the basic criteria to select pathogen drug targets, and the PINs of neglected-disease pathogens will be described in such a manner that the chapter will work as a source of key literature references for students and researchers. Papers will be reviewed to describe these basic principles, using key publications containing data and quantitative analyses (models, figures, tables) for PINs of some neglected-disease pathogens. We will describe novel lines of research; pros and cons of the use of PINs for prioritizing and identifying drug targets of neglected-disease pathogens.

2. Systems and network biology: Basic concepts

Systems biology is a holistic approach that involves the study of the inter-relationships of all the different elements in a biological system in order to understand non-deterministic behaviors that emerge from interaction between the cellular components and their environment and not by studying them in an isolated manner, one at a time (Hood and Perlmutter 2004, Weston and Hood 2004, Kohl and Noble 2009). Thus, the cell's behavior can be understood as a consequence of the complex interactions between its numerous constituents such as DNA, RNA, proteins, and metabolites. These interactions are also responsible for performing processes critical to cellular survival. For example, during transcription process the regulatory proteins can activate or inhibit the expression of genes or regulate each other as part of gene regulatory networks. Likewise, the cellular metabolism can be integrated into a metabolic network whose fluxes are regulated by enzymes. Similarly, the PINs represent how the proteins work together through interactions that lead to the modification of protein functions or new roles in protein complexes.

The biological systems consisting of interacting cellular components have led to the use of graph theory and mathematical tools based on graphs where the individual components are represented by nodes and the interactions by links (Fig. 1). Albert and Barabási (2002) have shown the general properties found among several networks ranging from the Internet to social and biological networks (Albert and Barabási 2002). The analysis of topology of those networks showed that they deviate substantially from randomly built networks as studied by Erdös and Rényi (Fig. 1a) (Erdös and Rényi 1960). Also, these networks did not show a well-shaped frequency distribution of the number of links per node as expected from randomly formed networks; instead, they showed a power-law distribution, which is characteristic of scale-free networks (Fig. 1b and 1c) (Amaral *et al.*, 2000, Albert 2005).

In scale-free network, the majority of nodes have only a few links, whereas very few nodes have a large number of links. Those nodes are called hubs and they represent the most vulnerable points of a network (Barabasi and Albert 1999, Albert *et al.*, 2000, Jeong *et al.*, 2001, Yu *et al.*, 2004a, Tew *et al.*, 2007). The topological features of networks can be quantified by measuring topological parameters whose information content provides a description from local (e.g., single nodes or links) to network-wide level (e.g., connections and relationships between nodes). For example, the nodes of a graph can be characterized by means of the number of links they have (the number of other nodes to which they are connected). This parameter is called "node degree". In directed networks, it is possible to distinguish the number of directed links that points toward the node (in-degree), and the number of directed edges that points outward the node (out-degree). The node degree characterizes individual nodes; however, in order to relate this parameter to whole network, a network degree distribution can be defined. The degree distribution P(k) represents the fraction of nodes that have degree k and it is obtained by counting the number of nodes N(k) that have k = 1, 2… links and dividing it by the total number of nodes *N*. The degree distributions of numerous networks such as the Internet, social, and biological networks, follow a power law (Fig. 1b and 1c) which is defined by the functional equation $P(k) \sim k^{\gamma}$, where γ represents the degree exponent, taking usually values in the range between $2<\gamma<3$ (Barabasi and Oltvai 2004). This function is intimately linked to the growth of the network in which new nodes are preferentially attached to already established nodes, a property that is also thought to characterize the evolution of biological systems (Jeong *et al.*, 2000).

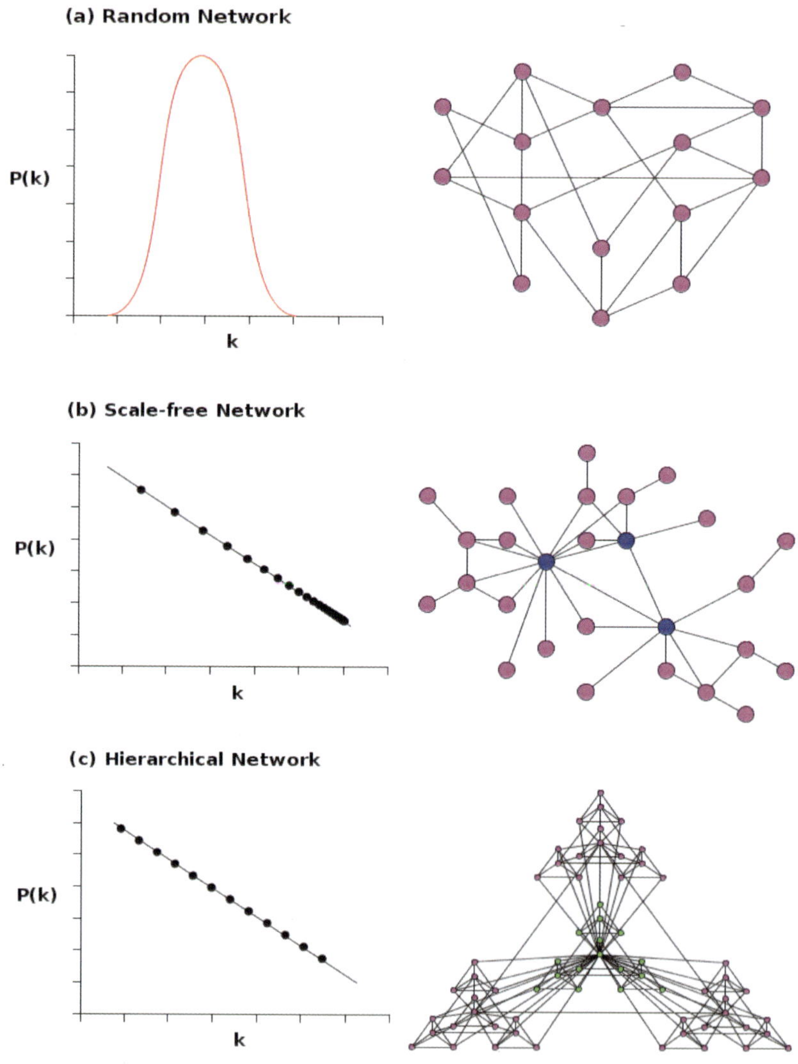

Fig. 1. Three types of network models and their associated distributions: (a) random network, (b) scale-free network, and (c) hierarchical network.

The distance between any two nodes in a network could be defined by the path length. In other words, it represents how many links we need to pass between two nodes. Nevertheless, it could have many alternative paths between two nodes in a network. The path with the smallest number of links between the selected nodes (shortest path) is of special interest. A common characteristic of several biological networks, including metabolic networks (Jeong *et al.*, 2000, Wagner and Fell 2001) and PINs (Giot *et al.*, 2003, Yook *et al.*, 2004) is that any two nodes can be connected with a path of a few links only. The main biological implications of this characteristic are related to: i) how the biological networks are capable of rapid responses to perturbations; ii) its capacity to employ alternative roads for the same input and output; and iii) the ability to efficiently compensate the perturbations in essential pathways.

Another important issue derived from network analysis is the concept of modularity, which can be used to describe how a group of physically or functionally linked nodes work together to achieve a particular function. The topological parameter used to quantify the modularity in a network is the clustering coefficient *Ci*, which represents the ratio between the number of links connecting nodes adjacent to node *i* and the total possible number of links among them (Watts and Strogatz 1998). It is worth noting that in first instance, the modularity concept might be in contradiction of the scale-free nature of the networks because the presence of modules implies that there are clusters of nodes that are relatively isolated from the rest of the network. However, it has been demonstrated that modularity and scale-free properties naturally co-occur in biological networks indicating that modules are not independent, instead, they are combined to form a hierarchical network (Fig. 1c) (Ravasz *et al.*, 2002).

Biological networks, including PINs and metabolic networks are good examples of network modularity because they exhibit high average *Ci*, which are associated to a high level of network robustness (Alon *et al.*, 1999, Ravasz *et al.*, 2002, Barabasi and Oltvai 2004). The most common representation of a module or cluster in a network is as a highly interconnected group of nodes. The biological implication of the modularity concept is that the nodes that integrate a module tend to participate in related biological processes and pathways; for example, protein and nucleic-acid synthesis, protein degradation, signal transduction, and metabolic pathways (Ma'ayan *et al.*, 2005). The analysis of experimental PINs have shown to have a remarkably modularity character (Giot *et al.*, 2003, Yook *et al.*, 2004). These findings in experimental PIN maps have been used to improve the understanding of the pleiotropic effects, and how perturbations on genes or proteins can propagate through the network and produce, in appearance, unrelated or extensive effects.

In addition to the modules, within a network, small and recurring sub-graphs, known as interaction motifs, with well-defined topologies can be identified (Fig. 2). The frequency analysis of these interaction motifs in networks revealed that they are over-represented when compared to a randomized version of the same network, suggesting that not all sub-graphs are equally significant in networks and that interaction motifs form functionally separable building blocks of cellular networks (Mangan and Alon 2003, Wuchty *et al.*, 2003, Alon 2007). For example, triangle motifs, also called feed-forward loops in directed networks, appear in both transcription-regulatory and neural networks. Likewise, there is evidence suggesting that specific motif type aggregates to form large motif clusters and that also appear to be commonly involved with certain functional roles (Milo *et al.*, 2002, Shen-

Orr *et al.,* 2002, Wuchty *et al.,* 2003). For example, in the *E. coli* transcription regulatory network, most motifs overlap, in which the specific motifs are no longer clearly separable (Shen-Orr *et al.,* 2002).

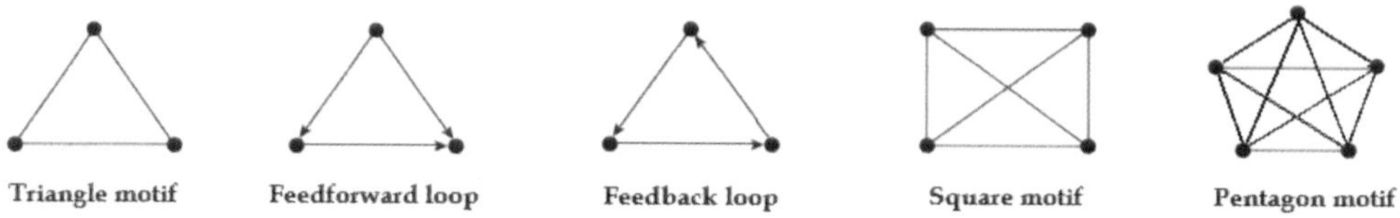

Fig. 2. Some types of interaction motifs found in biological networks.

The relevance of any node in mediating the communications flow among other nodes in the network is quantified by its betweenness centrality, which is defined as the total number of non-redundant shortest paths going through a certain node or edge (Freeman 1977). Girvan and Newman (2002), have proposed that the edges with high betweenness are the ones that are "between" network clusters; therefore, the information flow within a network could be altered by removing these edges (Girvan and Newman 2002). Dunn *et al.,* (2005) using an edge betweenness based-method have shown that clusters in PINs tend to share similar functions (Dunn *et al.,* 2005). Moreover, Yu *et al.,* (2007) have reconsidered the classical meaning of betweenness as a measure of the centrality of the nodes in a PIN. They have defined those nodes as "bottlenecks" with the highest betweenness centrality and find that bottlenecks nodes have a higher probability to be essential (Yu *et al.,* 2007).

It is worth noting that the topological parameters might be combined between them or with additional information of functional annotations regarding the network nodes (genes or proteins). Thus, a network provides testable predictions ranging from single interactions to essential genes and functional modules (del Rio *et al.,* 2009). Likewise, the functions of un-annotated genes or proteins can be also predicted on the basis of the annotation of their interacting partners. This approach to predict the protein/gene function is known as "guilty by association". Additionally, the integration of information related to diseases or specific phenotypes with network approaches also enhances the understanding of human diseases, pharmacology response, and phenotype prediction (Ideker and Sharan 2008, Lee *et al.,* 2008a, Lee *et al.,* 2010, Wang and Marcotte 2010, Lee *et al.,* 2011).

3. Methods to identify protein interactions networks (PINs)

3.1 Experimental methods

In the postgenomic era, the accumulation of protein-protein interaction data has enabled the biology systems studies at PINs levels (von Mering *et al.,* 2002). However, PIN analysis requires methods amenable to high throughput (HT) screening, such as large-scale versions of techniques like yeast two hybrid (Y2H) and tandem affinity purification coupled to mass spectrometry (TAP-MS) for performing systematic screens (Ito *et al.,* 2001a, Cusick *et al.,* 2005). In addition, there are a wide variety of methods to detect, analyze, and quantify protein interactions, including surface plasmon resonance spectroscopy, nuclear magnetic resonance (NMR), x-ray crystallography, and fluorescence-based technologies. These techniques provide detailed information on physical properties of protein interactions.

These methods are of paramount usefulness; however, herein, the techniques that can be applied to determine protein-protein interactions, at large-scale level, will be highlighted. In particular, the outcomes of Y2H system and TAP-MS are used further to perform *in silico* global network analysis. Both techniques were intensively applied to map the PIN of yeast, the first model organism with available PINs (Uetz *et al.*, 2000, Ito *et al.*, 2001b, Gavin *et al.*, 2002, Ho *et al.*, 2002, Ito *et al.*, 2002, Tong *et al.*, 2004, Yu *et al.*, 2008). Afterwards, large-scale efforts have been made to determine PINs for other model minor eukaryotic organisms: *D. melanogaster* (Giot *et al.*, 2003), and *C. elegans* (Li *et al.*, 2004); pathogenic microorganisms: *Helicobacter pylori, Campylobacter jejuni, Treponema pallidum, M. tuberculosis* (Wang et al., 2010), herpes simplex virus 1 (Lee *et al.*, 2008b), and Kaposi's sarcoma-associated herpesvirus (Uetz *et al.*, 2006, Rozen *et al.*, 2008), and major eukaryotic organisms: *Arabidopsis thaliana* (de Folter *et al.*, 2005) and humans (Rual *et al.*, 2005, Stelzl *et al.*, 2005, Gandhi *et al.*, 2006). Even though the PINs are not completed, the available PINs provide insight into how particular properties of proteins are integrated at systems level, and also, as a useful resource to predict the functional role of genes or proteins.

3.1.2 Yeast two-hybrid (Y2H) system

The Y2H system has considerably accelerated the *in vivo* large-scale screening of protein interactions enabling the detection of physically interacting proteins by using the modular organization of eukaryotic transcriptional activators. The eukaryotic transcription activators are formed by at least two distinct domains, one responsible of binding to a DNA region (BD) promoter and the other of activating the transcriptional processes (AD). It is well-known that splitting BD and AD domains will inactivate the transcriptional processes, but the transcription can be restored if a BD domain is re-associated with an AD domain (Fields and Song 1989). Thus, the standard Y2H system includes a DB domain fused to the "bait" protein-coding region and an AD domain fused to the "prey" protein-coding region. When DB-bait and AD-prey domains are co-expressed in the nucleus of yeast cells, "bait"-"prey" domain interaction reconstitutes a functional transcription factor that activates the transcription of one reporter gene (Fig. 3). The most used Y2H system is based on GAL4/LexA, where the GAL4 protein controls the expression of the LacZ gene encoding beta-galactosidase.

The main advantages of Y2H system are: i) the DNA (not the protein) is manipulated to study both bait and prey proteins (Walhout and Vidal 2001a); ii) it allows to identify protein interactions *in vivo*; iii) to identify transitory protein interactions, and iv) it is amenable to high-throughput screening methods (Buckholz *et al.*, 1999, Uetz and Hughes 2000, Walhout and Vidal 2001b, Ito *et al.*, 2002, Rual *et al.*, 2005).

The drawbacks include: i) a high proportion of false-positives and negatives (Vidal and Legrain 1999, Ito *et al.*, 2002); ii) it forces sub-cellular localization of bait and prey in the yeast nucleus which might preclude certain interactions from taking place (Cusick *et al.*, 2005). For example, membrane protein interactions cannot be identified by standard Y2H system because the AD-prey fusion will be retained at the membrane, thus, avoiding the reconstitution of a functional transcription factor (Xia *et al.*, 2006); iii) the over-expression of tested proteins, thus modifying the relative concentrations of potential interaction partners in comparison to the *in vivo* state; iv) the presence of auto-activators, i.e. proteins initiating transcription by themselves (Cusick *et al.*, 2005), and v) the differences in post-translational modifications and protein folding processes between yeasts and other organisms (Shoemaker and Panchenko 2007). Given these cons, several modifications have been made to improve the quality of the Y2H system results, including the development of membrane Y2H, the inclusion of different promoters of reporter genes, the use of low copy vectors, and the reduction of auto-activators. Once that these drawbacks are reduced, the quality of the Y2H system is significantly improved (Lehner *et al.*, 2004, Li *et al.*, 2004, Rual *et al.*, 2005, Yu *et al.*, 2008).

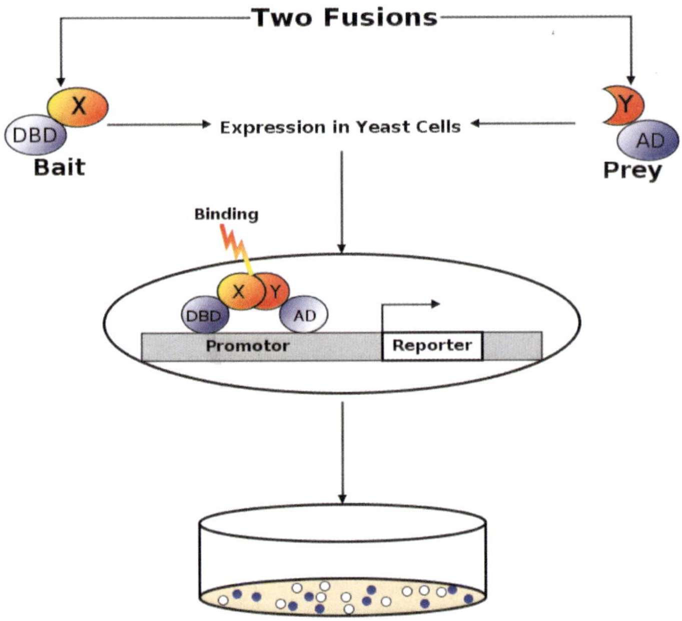

Fig. 3. The Y2H system. Y2H detects interactions between proteins X and Y, where X is linked to BD domain which binds to DNA region promoter.

3.1.3 Tandem affinity purification-tag coupled to mass spectrometry (TAP-MS)

TAP-MS method is a powerful approach to determine the composition of relevant protein complexes. In this method, a target protein-coding region is fused with a DNA sequence encoding an affinity tag which will be expressed with other cellular proteins, followed by two-step affinity purification (AP) and elucidation of the complex components by mass spectrometry (MS). A typical TAP tag is formed by an immunoglobulin interacting domain of protein A (protA) and a calmodulin-binding peptide (CBP) (Fig. 4). The protA/CBP binding domains are separated by a short recognition sequence for the site-specific tobacco-etch virus protease (TEV protease). The TEV site allows proteolytic elution of the protein complex from IgG-sepharose after the first affinity-purification step, which is based on the protA/IgG-sepharose interaction. The eluted protein complex is further purified by binding to a calmodulin affinity resin, eluted with EGTA and processed for identification with MS analyses.

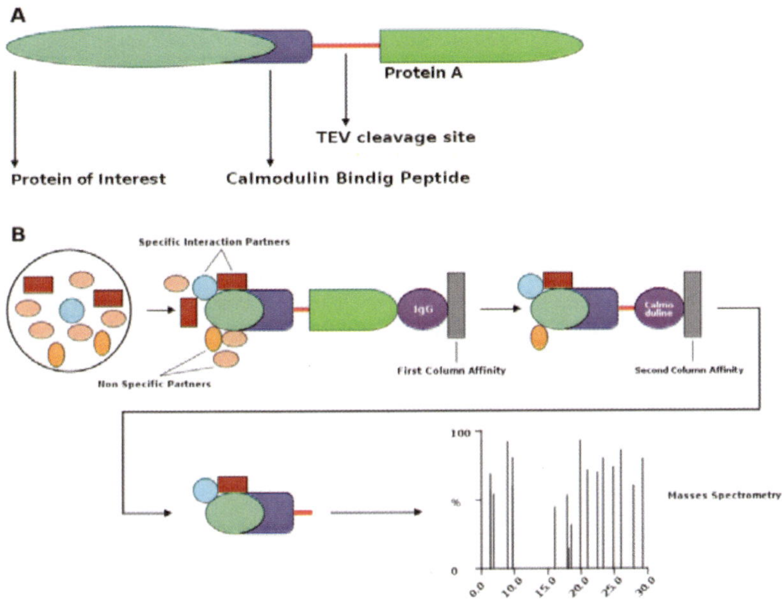

Fig. 4. TAP-MS method. TAP purifies protein complexes and removes the molecules of contaminants and MS identifies the complex components.

Similar to Y2H system results, TAP–MS method shows a high rate of false-positives and negatives, missing many transient interactions. In contrast to the Y2H system, the TAP–MS method can elucidate higher-order interactions beyond binary interactions and, therefore, provides direct information on protein complexes. Several large-scale studies of protein complexes have been performed using the TAP–MS method (Gavin *et al.*, 2002, Ho *et al.*, 2002, Gavin *et al.*, 2006). For example, Gavin *et al.*, (2006) used 5,500 ORFs fused to DNA sequences encoding an affinity tag to analyze PIN of *S. cerevisiae*. They found 491 complexes, of which 257 are novel, showing that PIN in *S. cerevisiae* has a modular organization (Gavin *et al.*, 2006). In addition, Stingl *et al.*, (2008), have elucidated the urease interactome of *H. pylori*. They combined the tandem affinity purification protocol with *in vivo* cross-link in order to capture transient interactions, which represent an improvement to TAP–MS method (Stingl *et al.*, 2008).

The use of experimental orthogonal approaches has demonstrated that Y2H and TAP-MS interaction data sets contain mostly highly reliable interactions. It has been suggested that the integration of data from the two approaches can also serve to increase confidence in either data set, and has provided support to derivate predictions from these approaches (Cusick *et al.*, 2005). Moreover, Venkatesan *et al.*, (2009) have developed a framework to estimate various quality parameters associated with currently used methods to identify PINs. The combination of these quality parameters (screening completeness, assay sensitivity, sampling sensitivity, and precision), has shown an estimate of the size of human binary interactome and a path toward the completion of its mapping (Venkatesan *et al.*, 2009).

Despite the technical or biological limitations (Cusick et al., 2005) of the aforementioned methods, that does not preclude a reduction on their impact in PINs studies, instead they are marking a paradigm change from one-gene/one-function reductionist approach to a more systemic approach that can capture all potential interactions encoded in a genome or proteome.

3.1.4 Protein interaction databases

The huge amounts of protein interaction data produced by high-throughput experimental methods as Y2H and TAP-MS and analyzed by bioinformatics have led to the conformation of several research groups aimed at conducting important efforts in designing and setting up databases that include carefully analyzed information to provide useful scientific knowledge about protein-protein interactions. Table 1 shows a summary of most significant public databases of protein-protein interactions published to date. These databases contain interactions obtained by direct submission from experimentalists, text-mining and other data sources. Also, there are other online resources integrating information from several of the databases that are listed in Table 1, or tools to browse and visualize such data; for example resources like APID (Prieto and De Las Rivas 2006, Hernandez-Toro *et al.*, 2007) and PINA (Wu *et al.*, 2009). The information deposited in these databases is verified using automated algorithms or manual curation like in the DIP database (Deane *et al.*, 2002). Altogether, protein interaction databases are an invaluable resource to develop projects that aims to analyze PINs of organisms ranging from viruses to humans.

Database	Type of data	Number of interactions	Website
DIP	E,C,S	71,589	http://dip.doe-mbi.ucla.edu
MINT	E,C	235,635	http://mint.bio.uniroma2.it
IntAct	E,C	275,144	http://www.ebi.ac.uk/intact/
BioGRID	E,C	282,005	http://thebiogrid.org/
HPRD	E,C	39,194	http://www.hprd.org/
APID	I	322,579	http://bioinfow.dep.usal.es/apid/apid2net.html
PINA	I	221,702	http://cbg.garvan.unsw.edu.au/pina

Table 1. Most representative databases of protein-protein interactions. (E) high-throughput experimental data; (S) structural data; (C) manual curation, and (I) integrative resource. The number of interactions was updated on September 29, 2011.

3.2 Computational methods to predict protein interactions networks (PINs)

Parallel to the experimental methods, several computational methods have been designed to predict protein-protein interactions. Initially, these methods were strictly limited to proteins whose three-dimensional structures had been determined (structure-based methods). The completion of genome sequences has provided large amounts of genomic information enabling the analysis from a genomic context of a given gene. Thus, a number of computational methods and resources have been developed for the prediction of protein interactions resulting from genomic information (genomic context-based methods), even in those cases where the three-dimensional structures are unknown yet (Galperin and Koonin 2000, Huynen *et al.*, 2000, Huynen and Snel 2000).

Hereinafter, we will describe computational methods and resources available for protein interaction prediction that exploit the genomic and biological contexts of proteins for complete genomes.

3.2.1 Genomic context-based methods

3.2.1.1 Gene neighborhood

The gene neighborhood method exploits the notion that genes which physically interact or are functionally associated to the same process or functional pathway will be adjacent to each other in the genome (Fig. 5a) (Tamames *et al.*, 1997, Overbeek *et al.*, 1999, Bowers *et al.*, 2004). For example, Dandekar et al. (2005), have shown that the neighborhood relationship could be used as fingerprint, suggesting that the proteins encoded by these genes may physically interact (Dandekar *et al.*, 1998). The most representative example of this phenomenon can be found in bacterial operons, where genes that work together are generally transcribed as a unit. Furthermore, operons which encode for co-regulated genes

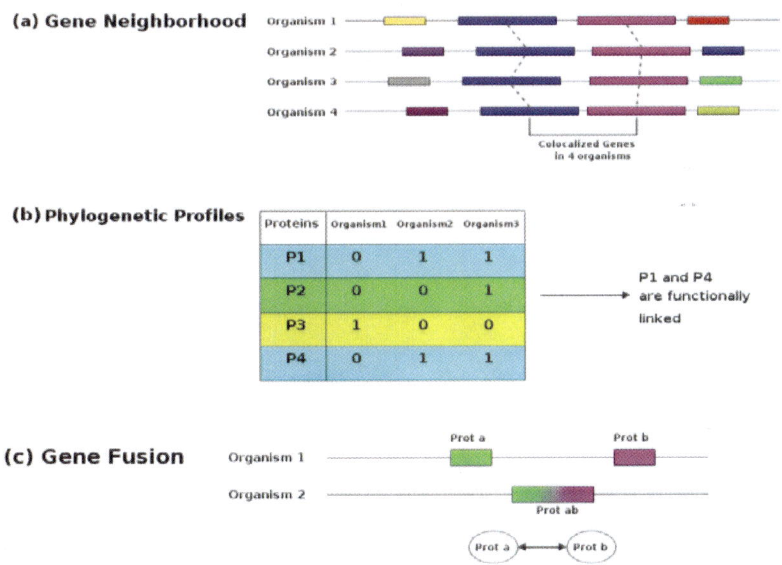

Fig. 5. Genomic context-based methods. (a) Gene neighborhood plots for four organisms, showing a pair of genes (blue and magenta) which are in close proximity in all four organisms. (b) Example phylogenetic profiles of four proteins from the three organisms. The proteins 1 and 4 have the same patterns of co-occurrence in all three organisms, and may physically interact based on this evidence. (c) A gene fusion event between two proteins (green and magenta) in two organisms is shown. Thus, the proteins a y b from organism 1 is predict to interact because they form part of a single protein in organism 2.

are usually conserved. The neighborhood relationship tends to be more relevant when it is conserved across different species (Tamames *et al.*, 1997). Hence, the gene neighborhood method, like many of the comparative genomics approaches, increases its robustness when a larger numbers of genomes are used for the prediction. Since operons and genes neighborhood are uncommon in eukaryotic species (Zorio *et al.*, 1994, Blumenthal 1998, Liu and Han 2009, Fitzpatrick *et al.*, 2010), this method is principally applicable to bacteria where such genome properties are relevant.

3.2.1.2 Phylogenetic profiles

The phylogenetic profile method is based on the co-occurrence of pairs of genes across multiple genomes (Fig. 5b). Consequently, a pair of orthologous genes remains together across many distant species representing a concerted evolution mechanism and indicating that these genes need to be simultaneously present to participate in the same biological process, pathway or physically interacting. A phylogenetic profile is commonly represented as a vector for the presence or absence of a gene across multiple genomes (Fig.), where "0" or "1" denoted the presence/absence at each position of a profile (Ouzounis and Kyrpides 1996, Rivera *et al.*, 1998, Pellegrini *et al.*, 1999).

The main drawbacks of this method are: it can only be applied to complete genomes; the prediction robustness is dependent on the number and distribution of genomes used to build the profile, thus, a pair of genes with similar profiles across many bacterial, archaeal and eukaryotic genomes is much more likely to interact each other than those genes found to co-occur in a small number of closely related species; its high computational cost since it needs to compare many complete genomes; and, fails in homology detection between distant organisms.

Like others genomic context methods, with the increasing number of completely sequenced genomes, it is expected that the accuracy of these predictions will be improved over time.

3.2.1.3 Gene fusion

The gene fusion method is based on the fact that some interacting protein domains (termed the rosetta stones) have homologs in other genomes that are fused into one protein chain (Fig. 5c). Thus, gene fusion events have been proposed for the identification of potential protein-protein interactions, metabolic or regulatory networks (Sali 1999, Galperin and Koonin 2000). The information about gene fusion events can be combined with phylogenomic profiling and identification of conserved chromosomal localization, to test hypotheses leading to the characterization of proteins of unknown function (Marcotte *et al.*, 1999a, Marcotte 2000, Enright and Ouzounis 2001). Marcotte *et al.*, (1999) found 6,809 potentially interacting pairs of non-homologous proteins in *E. coli*, revealing that, for more than half of the pairs, both involved members were functionally associated. More approaches with similar results have been used, including in eukaryotic genomes (Enright and Ouzounis 2001).

The drawbacks of this method are related with the domain complexity of eukaryotic proteins, the presence of promiscuous domains, and large degrees of paralogy (Enright *et al.*, 2002).

Currently, there are excellent resources implementing the genomic context-based methods. The most notable are the Search Tool for the Retrieval of Interacting Genes/Proteins

(STRING) and ProLinks. The STRING (URL: http://string-db.org) and ProLinks (URL: http://prl.mbi.ucla.edu) resources provide a web interface giving comprehensive access to gene context information in 1,100 and 900 complete genomes, respectively (Szklarczyk *et al.*, 2011, Bowers *et al.*, 2004).

3.2.2 Interologs

The use of homology relationships is a key paradigm in molecular biology and genomics. This approach has been extensively exploited to predict protein structure (Abagyan and Batalov 1997, Brenner *et al.*, 1998, Rost 1999), to study sub-cellular localization (Nair and Rost 2002), enzymatic activity (Devos and Valencia 2001, Todd *et al.*, 2001), and for comparative genomics (Marcotte *et al.*, 1999b, Pellegrini *et al.*, 1999). Thus, interologs is defined as a conserved interaction between a pair of proteins of a given organism which have interacting homologs in another organism (Yu *et al.*, 2004b). For example, the experimental observation that two yeast proteins interact is extrapolated to predict that the two corresponding homologs in human also interact in a similar way. Walhout (Walhout and Vidal 2001b) and Vidal (2001) have used yeast experimental interaction data (Uetz *et al.*, 2000, Ito *et al.*, 2001b) to infer similar interactions in worm (Fig. 6). Mika and Rost (2006) suggested that the extrapolation of interactions between distant organisms has to be undertaken with some caution. They found that the homology transfers are only accurate at high levels of sequence identity, and it is more reliable for protein pairs from the same species than for two protein pairs from different organisms (Mika and Rost 2006). Likewise, Wiles *et al.*, (2010) have developed a scoring schema to assess the confidence of interologs prediction. They have predicted protein interactions across five species (human, mouse, fly, worm, and yeast) based on available experimental evidence and conservation across species (Wiles *et al.*, 2010). Also, they developed the Interolog Finder (URL: http://www.interologfinder.org) to provide access to these data.

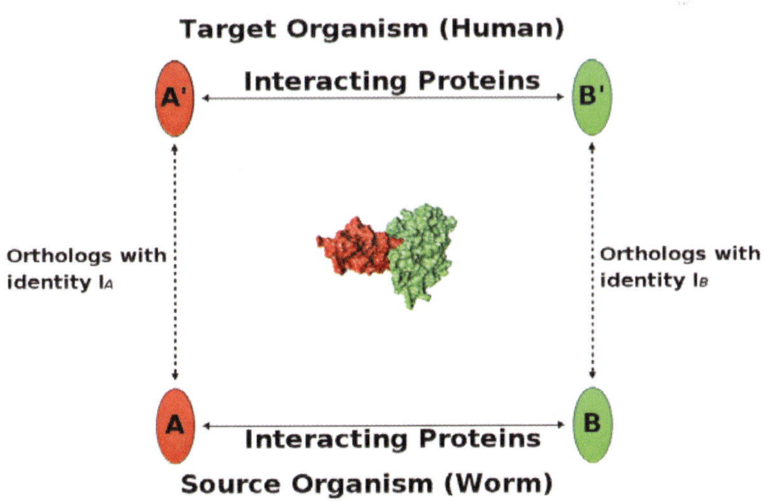

Fig. 6. The Interlog method. The A and B are interacting proteins in worm, and A′ and B′ are homologs in human of A and B proteins. Then A′ and B′ in human also interact in a similar way.

3.2.3 Integrative approaches

Currently, high-confidence PINs data sets are limited; however, they still provide a framework onto which other types of biological information can be integrated. Thus, new approaches that integrate other types of data, including protein-protein interactions, text mining, homology-based, and functional genomics approaches (Lee *et al.*, 2004, Chua *et al.*, 2007, Lee *et al.*, 2008a, Pena-Castillo *et al.*, 2008, Linghu *et al.*, 2009, Lee *et al.*, 2010, Wu *et al.*, 2010, Lee *et al.*, 2011, Szklarczyk *et al.*, 2011), have shown to be the most effective way to assign function to uncharacterized proteins that are components of the network (Fig. 7).

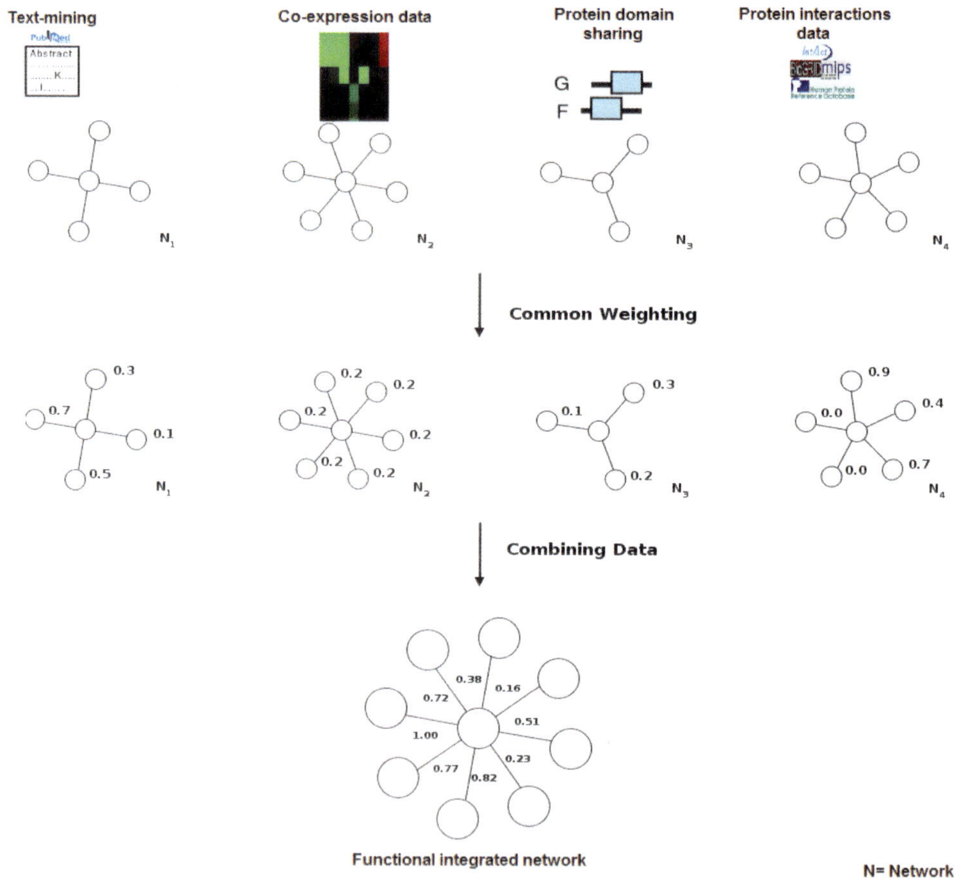

Fig. 7. General scheme for integrative approaches. N1, N2, N3 and N4 are networks representing four data sources. Each node is a protein, while each edge is a binary relationship. The edges are weighted into common weight that is consistent across different data sources. N1, N2, N3 and N4 are then combined and re-scored to form the final high confidence network N'.

The most representative example of these approaches is STRING which integrates experimental as well as predicted interaction information, mostly from the methods aforementioned. STRING provides ease of access to explore this integrated information (URL: http://string-db.org). Moreover, for each protein-protein interaction it provides a confidence score, and supplementary information such as protein domains and 3D structures, all within a stable and consistent identifier space. The version 9.0 of STRING includes the information of more than 1,100 completely sequenced organisms, ranging from bacteria and archaea to humans allowing to periodically execute interaction prediction algorithms and update such data depending on genome sequence information (Szklarczyk *et al.*, 2011).

Similarly, several groups have integrated multiple networks to predict protein functions, interactions and functional modules including data from multiple sources, ranging from co-expression patterns, sequence similarity to genomic context-based methods (Kemmeren *et al.*, 2002, Jansen *et al.*, 2003, Lee *et al.*, 2004, Lu *et al.*, 2005, Chua *et al.*, 2007, Lee *et al.*, 2008a, Pena-Castillo *et al.*, 2008, Linghu *et al.*, 2009, Lee *et al.*, 2010, Wu *et al.*, 2010, Lee *et al.*, 2011). For example, Marcotte´s group have shown the predictive power of an integrated functional network for *C. elegans* (Lee *et al.*, 2008a). Firstly, they computationally built an integrated functional network covering approximately 82% of *C. elegans* genes. Second, they used this network to predict the effects of perturbing individual genes on the organism's phenotype, identifying genes causing specific phenotypes ranging from cell cycle defects in single embryonic cells to life-span alterations, neuronal defects, and altered patterning of specific tissues. They select a set of candidate genes and their interactions associated to a phenotype and used RNAi to test whether targeting these candidate genes suppressed such phenotype. They found that 20% of such interactions suppressed the studied phenotype; instead, using only an RNAi, at large-scale screening, inactivation of 0.9% of genes produces such effect. Therefore, predictions arising from interactions of integrated network are 21-fold better than those expected by chance. They suggested a network-guided schema to accelerate research by using screening methods to identify genes and interactions for pathways of interest in human diseases.

The main limitation of integrative approaches is related with the availability of functional association data of genes/proteins. For example, these methods will not be able to make extensive predictions if no associations are available, as in the case of a novel genome with no known sequence or domain homology with known sequences, poorly studied genomes, and lack of functional genomics studies.

4. PINs as a tool to prioritize drug targets of neglected-disease pathogens

4.1 Drug targets prioritization

Despite the advent of the high-throughput techniques sparked by the genomics revolution, discovery and development of new drugs for neglected-disease pathogens has lagged in recent years due to the serious problems such as high cost, poor compliance, low efficacy, poor safety, evolution of antibiotic resistance, among others (Schmid 1998).

Target identification is the first step in the drug discovery process and such task can provide the foundation for years of dedicated research in the pharmaceutical industry (Read *et al.*, 2001). As compared with all the other steps in drug discovery, this stage is complicated by the fact that the identified drug target must satisfy a variety of criteria to permit progression to the next step. For example, the target must be selectively present in the pathogen, i.e.

target coding genes that are conserved across different pathogens and have no human homologs represent attractive target candidates for new broad-spectrum drugs (Schmid 2006); relevant for the pathogenesis process (Galperin and Koonin 1999, Sakharkar *et al.*, 2004); and, the essentiality of the target to the pathogen's growth and survival (Koonin *et al.*, 1998, Thanassi *et al.*, 2002, Galperin and Koonin 2004); suitability of the target for expression and assayability, and the availability of structures or models to initiate rational drug design (Aguero *et al.*, 2008). Hence, the integrated uses of above-mentioned strategies are considered as the basic schema in the drug target prioritization approaches. The criteria values of this basic schema can be found by querying publicly available bioinformatics resources and databases. For example, using metabolic pathway databases such as Kyoto Encyclopedia of Genes and Genomes (KEGG) (Ogata *et al.*, 1999, Kanehisa and Goto 2000), protein classification sets such as Clusters of Orthologous Groups (COGs), Gene Ontology (GO), and resources to evaluate the "druggability" of proteins (Hopkins and Groom 2002, Russ and Lampel 2005, Hambly *et al.*, 2006), like "Structure-based DrugEBIlity" online service at EBI (URL: https://www.ebi.ac.uk/chembl/drugebility/structure). For drug targets of neglected-disease pathogens, the TDR Targets Database (URL: http://tdrtargets.org) is an extensive resource for neglected tropical diseases (Aguero *et al.*, 2008). This database includes extensive genetic, biochemical, and pharmacological data related to tropical disease pathogens and computationally predicted druggability for potential targets. The database contains the data on the tuberculosis pathogen *M. tuberculosis*; the leprosy pathogen *M. leprae*; the malaria parasites *Plasmodium falciparum* and *P. vivax*, the toxoplasmosis parasite *Toxoplasma gondii*; the trematode *Schistosoma mansoni*; the filariasis helminth *Brugia malayi* and its intracellular symbiont bacterium *Wolbachia*; and the kinetoplastid parasites *Leishmania major, Trypanosoma brucei,* and *T. cruzi,* which are responsible for kala-azar and other forms of leishmaniasis, sleeping sickness, and Chagas disease, respectively.

4.2 PINs, drug targets, and neglected-disease pathogens

Networks analysis is a broadly applicable tool for the drug discovery and development process. Any type of association data linking one gene to another, a protein or a compound, can be modeled, visualized and analyzed as networks (Lee *et al.*, 2004, Chua *et al.*, 2007, Lee *et al.*, 2008a, Linghu *et al.*, 2009, Lee *et al.*, 2010, McGary *et al.*, 2010, Wu *et al.*, 2010, Lee *et al.*, 2011). Hence, data from pre-clinical and clinical trial studies can be included in network analyses (Nikolsky *et al.*, 2005). Thus, networks could represent the standard for data integration and analysis. Network analysis involving neglected-disease pathogens is a very young area of research. Moreover, despite the availability experimentally PINs of model organisms as *S. cerevisiae, C. elegans*, and *D. melanogaster*, and some bacterial pathogens like *H. pylori, C. jejuni, Treponema pallidum,* the number of experimentally neglected-disease pathogens PINs is limited. For example, LaCount *et al.*, (2005) identified protein-protein interactions of *P. falciparum* through a high throughput screening version of the yeast two-hybrid system (LaCount *et al.*, 2005). They found 2,846 unique interactions in more than 32,000 *P. falciparum* protein fragments. In order to determine clusters of interacting proteins they used computational methods such as analysis of network connectivity, gene co-expression, and enrichment of Gene Ontology terms. The results of the network analysis was the identification of two protein clusters, one of which related to the chromatin modification, transcription, messenger RNA stability, and ubiquitination and the other implicated in the invasion of host cells. They suggested that the information provided by this network may be relevant to understand the basic biology of the parasite and to discover new drug and vaccine targets. Wang *et al.*, (2010) built a PIN of the *M. tuberculosis* H37Rv strain based on a high-throughput bacterial two-hybrid method. They found more than 8,000 novel interactions and performed a cross-species PINs comparison, showing 94 conserved sub-networks between *M. tuberculosis* and several prokaryotic PINs (Wang *et al.*, 2010).

Additionally, even the lack of data, several computational studies aims to predict PINs of neglected-disease pathogens and prioritize drug targets have been performed. Florez *et al.*, (2010) built an *in silico* PIN of *L. major* by combining information of PSIMAP, PEIMAP, iPfam databases, and using the interologs method (Florez *et al.*, 2010). They predicted 33,861 interactions for 1,366 proteins, and also analyzed the PIN by calculating topology parameters such as connectivity and betweenness centrality detecting 142 potential and specific drug targets without human orthologs (Fig. 8). Pedamallu and Posfai (2010) have developed a simple open source package module (OpenPPI_predictor) to predict putative PIN for target genomes (Pedamallu and Posfai 2010). The package is based on interologs method and uses experimental data from a related organism. Thus, they assayed OpenPPI_predictor to infer a PIN for *B. malayi* using experimental PIN data from *C. elegans*. They identified 118 and 143 clusters in *B. malayi* and *C. elegans* interactomes,

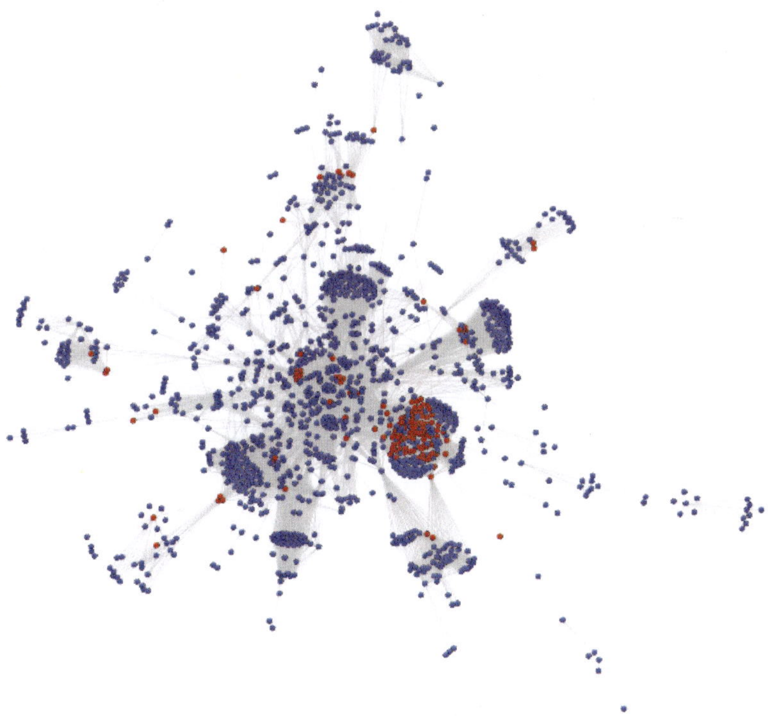

Fig. 8. Predicted PIN of *Leishmania major* by Florez *et al.*, (2010). The nodes in color red represent predicted essential proteins without human orthologs.

respectively, and found that highly connected region contains 363 and 340 proteins in *B. malayi* and *C. elegans* PINs. They suggests that core cellular functions of the two related organisms have similar complexity and that further analysis of these highly connected regions may provide clues about genes missing from a conserved pathway, or proteins missing from a complex.

Similarly, computational studies have been developed in order to model host-neglected-disease pathogens PINs. For example, Dyer *et al.*, (2007) integrated public intra-species PINs datasets with protein–domain profiles to predict a Human–*P. falciparum* PIN. They found 516 protein interactions between these two organisms, and showed that *Plasmodium* proteins interacting with human proteins are co-expressed in DNA microarray datasets, associated with developmental stages of the *Plasmodium* life cycle (Dyer *et al.*, 2007). Dyer *et al.*, (2008) have analyzed the landscape of human proteins interacting with pathogens. They integrated human–pathogen PINs for 190 pathogen strains from seven public databases and found that both viral and bacterial pathogens tend to interact with proteins with many interacting partners (hubs) and those that are central to many paths (bottlenecks) in the human PIN (Dyer *et al.*, 2008). Similar results were obtained by Navratil *et al.*, (2011). They used a high-quality dataset manually curated and validated of virus-host protein interactions to depict the "human infectome" (Navratil *et al.*, 2011). Additionally, they showed, by using functional genomic RNAi data, that the high centrality of targeted proteins was correlated to their essentiality for viruses' lifecycle. Also, they perform a simulation of cellular network perturbations and showed a stealth-attack of viruses on proteins bridging cellular functions, which is a property that could be essential in the molecular etiology of some human diseases (Fig. 9). Doolittle and Gomez (2011) have predicted interactions between dengue

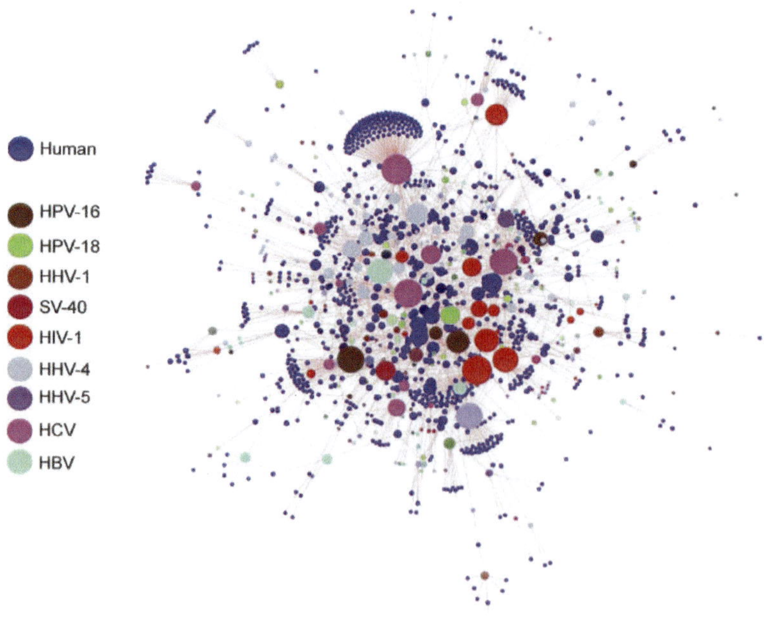

Fig. 9. The human infectome by Navratil *et al.*, (2011).

virus (DENV) and its hosts, both human and the insect vector *Aedes aegypti*. They implemented a protocol based on structural similarity between DENV and host proteins, and also they supported a subset of the predictions via mining from the literature. They predicted, after filtering and based on shared Gene Ontology cellular component, over 2,000 interactions between DENV and humans, as well as 18 interactions between DENV and the *A. aegypti* vector (Doolittle and Gomez 2011). They suggested those specific interactions between virus and host proteins are involved in interferon signaling, transcriptional regulation, stress, and the unfolded protein response.

The most relevant outcome of such computational studies is the identification of human and pathogen proteins to target experimentally for developing new drugs. It also provides different roadmaps and emerging approaches to develop projects to model and analyze PINs of neglected-disease pathogens. For example, novel therapies for human diseases employ multi-target drugs (Borisy *et al.,* 2003, Csermely *et al.,* 2005) and compounds targeted to inhibit protein-protein interactions (Emerson *et al.,* 2003, Klein and Vassilev 2004, Vassilev 2004, Vassilev *et al.,* 2004).

5. Conclusions

Because of the development of massive analysis technologies in genomics and computational biology, we can outline a trend to interplay and integrate the computational and experimental techniques. Thus, the methods and resources to identify protein interactions that combine both approaches will be used as a routine protocol in the future.

Even though the use of network biology approaches to drug discovery are in their initial stages, they already contributed to meaningful drug development decisions by accelerating hypothesis-driven biology, modeling specific physiologic problems in target validation or clinical physiology and, providing rapid characterization and interpretation of disease-relevant cell systems.

Despite the lack of experimental functional genomics and PINs data for neglected-disease pathogens, computational approaches represent a starting point and complementary approach to current high-throughput screening projects whose aim is to delineate the complete genomes of neglected-disease pathogens. Moreover, integrative computational approaches have shown to be a powerful tool as guide for large scale-studies improving and facilitating the rational identification of therapeutic targets.

It is clear that for those organisms whose genome has not been sequenced yet, it will be difficult to implement the aforementioned protocols. That is the case for some nematodes and trypanosomal parasites as *T. cruzi*, *S. mansoni*, *B. malayi*, and *O. volvulus*, and the soil-transmitted helminthes (e.g., species of *A. lumbricoides*, and *T. trichura)*. However, according to NCBI Entrez Genome (URL:, http://www.ncbi.nlm.nih.gov/genomes/leuks.cgi; Sep 29, 2011), the status of most of them is in "assembly"stage. Once the genome of the neglected-disease pathogen is available, we can use the information of experimental PINs of model organism as *C. elegans* to model and predict PINs of such pathogens enabling the discovery of those hubs and bottlenecks proteins that modulate the infectious process and prioritize them as drug targets.

While the computational approaches analyzed here are by nature probabilistic, i.e. it offers the likelihood of association of a given pair of proteins, nevertheless it clearly indicates the utility of inferring functionally relevant correlations from the available genomic databases for systematic drug target identification. The further improvement of computational approaches will help to increasing the availability of systematically collected biologic data and will provide an easy schema for the integration of different types of data within network analysis, thus enhancing the role of such approaches in drug discovery.

Finally, comprehensive repositories of functional genomic data for neglected-disease pathogens will be created. Hence, as soon as large molecular datasets are processed with the help of network analysis, a growing set of predicted pathways and PINs will emerge and will offer a new paradigm for re-thinking about how to revolutionize the drug discovery process.

6. Acknowledgments

The authors thank BioMed Central for allowing the reproduction of figures 8 and 9 (Florez *et al.*, 2010, Navratil *et al.*, 2011). Mario A. Rodríguez-Pérez and Xianwu Guo holds a scholarship from Comisión de Operación y Fomento de Actividades Académicas (COFAA)/IPN.

7. References

Abagyan, R. A., and S. Batalov. (1997). Do aligned sequences share the same fold? *J Mol Biol* 273: 355-368: Oct 17.

Aguero, F., B. Al-Lazikani, M. Aslett, M. Berriman, F. S. Buckner, R. K. Campbell, S. Carmona, I. M. Carruthers, A. W. Chan, F. Chen, G. J. Crowther, M. A. Doyle, C. Hertz-Fowler, A. L. Hopkins, G. McAllister, S. Nwaka, J. P. Overington, A. Pain, G. V. Paolini, U. Pieper, S. A. Ralph, A. Riechers, D. S. Roos, A. Sali, D. Shanmugam, T. Suzuki, W. C. Van Voorhis, and C. L. Verlinde. (2008). Genomic-scale prioritization of drug targets: the TDR Targets database. *Nat Rev Drug Discov* 7: 900-907: Nov.

Albert, R. (2005). Scale-free networks in cell biology. *J Cell Sci* 118: 4947-4957: Nov 1.

Albert, R., and A. L. Barabási. (2002). Statistical mechanics of complex networks. *Rev. Modern Phys* 1: 30.

Albert, R., H. Jeong, and A. L. Barabasi. (2000). Error and attack tolerance of complex networks. *Nature* 406: 378-382: Jul 27.

Alon, U. (2007). Network motifs: theory and experimental approaches. *Nat Rev Genet* 8: 450-461: Jun.

Alon, U., M. G. Surette, N. Barkai, and S. Leibler. (1999). Robustness in bacterial chemotaxis. *Nature* 397: 168-171: Jan 14.

Amaral, L. A., A. Scala, M. Barthelemy, and H. E. Stanley. (2000). Classes of small-world networks. *Proc Natl Acad Sci U S A* 97: 11149-11152: Oct 10.

Barabasi, A. L., and R. Albert. (1999). Emergence of scaling in random networks. *Science* 286: 509-512: Oct 15.

Barabasi, A. L., and Z. N. Oltvai. (2004). Network biology: understanding the cell's functional organization. *Nat Rev Genet* 5: 101-113: Feb.

Blumenthal, T. (1998). Gene clusters and polycistronic transcription in eukaryotes. *Bioessays* 20: 480-487: Jun.

Borisy, A. A., P. J. Elliott, N. W. Hurst, M. S. Lee, J. Lehar, E. R. Price, G. Serbedzija, G. R. Zimmermann, M. A. Foley, B. R. Stockwell, and C. T. Keith. (2003). Systematic discovery of multicomponent therapeutics. *Proc Natl Acad Sci U S A* 100: 7977-7982: Jun 24.

Bowers, P. M., M. Pellegrini, M. J. Thompson, J. Fierro, T. O. Yeates, and D. Eisenberg. (2004). Prolinks: a database of protein functional linkages derived from coevolution. *Genome Biol* 5: R35.

Brenner, S. E., C. Chothia, and T. J. Hubbard. (1998). Assessing sequence comparison methods with reliable structurally identified distant evolutionary relationships. *Proc Natl Acad Sci U S A* 95: 6073-6078: May 26.

Buckholz, R. G., C. A. Simmons, J. M. Stuart, and M. P. Weiner. (1999). Automation of yeast two-hybrid screening. *J Mol Microbiol Biotechnol* 1: 135-140: Aug.

Csermely, P., V. Agoston, and S. Pongor. (2005). The efficiency of multi-target drugs: the network approach might help drug design. *Trends Pharmacol Sci* 26: 178-182: Apr.

Cusick, M. E., N. Klitgord, M. Vidal, and D. E. Hill. (2005). Interactome: gateway into systems biology. *Hum Mol Genet* 14 Spec No. 2: R171-181: Oct 15.

Chua, H. N., W. K. Sung, and L. Wong. (2007). An efficient strategy for extensive integration of diverse biological data for protein function prediction. *Bioinformatics* 23: 3364-3373: Dec 15.

Dandekar, T., B. Snel, M. Huynen, and P. Bork. (1998). Conservation of gene order: a fingerprint of proteins that physically interact. *Trends Biochem Sci* 23: 324-328: Sep.

de Folter, S., R. G. Immink, M. Kieffer, L. Parenicova, S. R. Henz, D. Weigel, M. Busscher, M. Kooiker, L. Colombo, M. M. Kater, B. Davies, and G. C. Angenent. (2005). Comprehensive interaction map of the Arabidopsis MADS Box transcription factors. *Plant Cell* 17: 1424-1433: May.

Deane, C. M., L. Salwinski, I. Xenarios, and D. Eisenberg. (2002). Protein interactions: two methods for assessment of the reliability of high throughput observations. *Mol Cell Proteomics* 1: 349-356: May.

del Rio, G., D. Koschutzki, and G. Coello. (2009). How to identify essential genes from molecular networks? *BMC Syst Biol* 3: 102.

Devos, D., and A. Valencia. (2001). Intrinsic errors in genome annotation. *Trends Genet* 17: 429-431: Aug.

Doolittle, J. M., and S. M. Gomez. (2011). Mapping protein interactions between Dengue virus and its human and insect hosts. *PLoS Negl Trop Dis* 5: e954.

Dunn, R., F. Dudbridge, and C. M. Sanderson. (2005). The use of edge-betweenness clustering to investigate biological function in protein interaction networks. *BMC Bioinformatics* 6: 39.

Dyer, M. D., T. M. Murali, and B. W. Sobral. (2007). Computational prediction of host-pathogen protein-protein interactions. *Bioinformatics* 23: i159-166: Jul 1.

Dyer, M. D., T. M. Murali, and B. W. Sobral. (2008). The landscape of human proteins interacting with viruses and other pathogens. *PLoS Pathog* 4: e32: Feb 8.

Emerson, S. D., R. Palermo, C. M. Liu, J. W. Tilley, L. Chen, W. Danho, V. S. Madison, D. N. Greeley, G. Ju, and D. C. Fry. (2003). NMR characterization of interleukin-2 in complexes with the IL-2Ralpha receptor component, and with low molecular weight compounds that inhibit the IL-2/IL-Ralpha interaction. *Protein Sci* 12: 811-822: Apr.

Enright, A. J., and C. A. Ouzounis. (2001). Functional associations of proteins in entire genomes by means of exhaustive detection of gene fusions. *Genome Biol* 2: RESEARCH0034.

Enright, A. J., S. Van Dongen, and C. A. Ouzounis. (2002). An efficient algorithm for large-scale detection of protein families. *Nucleic Acids Res* 30: 1575-1584: Apr 1.

Erdös, P., and A. Rényi. (1960). On the evolution of random graphs. *Publ. Math. Inst. Hung. Acad. Sci*: 4.

Fields, S., and O. Song. (1989). A novel genetic system to detect protein-protein interactions. *Nature* 340: 245-246: Jul 20.

Fitzpatrick, D. A., P. O'Gaora, K. P. Byrne, and G. Butler. (2010). Analysis of gene evolution and metabolic pathways using the Candida Gene Order Browser. *BMC Genomics* 11: 290.

Florez, A. F., D. Park, J. Bhak, B. C. Kim, A. Kuchinsky, J. H. Morris, J. Espinosa, and C. Muskus. (2010). Protein network prediction and topological analysis in Leishmania major as a tool for drug target selection. *BMC Bioinformatics* 11: 484.

Freeman, L. C. (1977). Set of measures of centrality based on betweenness. *Sociometry* 40: 7.

Galperin, M. Y., and E. V. Koonin. (1999). Searching for drug targets in microbial genomes. *Curr Opin Biotechnol* 10: 571-578: Dec.

Galperin, M. Y., and E. V. Koonin. (2000). Who's your neighbor? New computational approaches for functional genomics. *Nat Biotechnol* 18: 609-613: Jun.

Galperin, M. Y., and E. V. Koonin. (2004). 'Conserved hypothetical' proteins: prioritization of targets for experimental study. *Nucleic Acids Res* 32: 5452-5463.

Gandhi, T. K., J. Zhong, S. Mathivanan, L. Karthick, K. N. Chandrika, S. S. Mohan, S. Sharma, S. Pinkert, S. Nagaraju, B. Periaswamy, G. Mishra, K. Nandakumar, B. Shen, N. Deshpande, R. Nayak, M. Sarker, J. D. Boeke, G. Parmigiani, J. Schultz, J. S. Bader, and A. Pandey. (2006). Analysis of the human protein interactome and comparison with yeast, worm and fly interaction datasets. *Nat Genet* 38: 285-293: Mar.

Gavin, A. C., P. Aloy, P. Grandi, R. Krause, M. Boesche, M. Marzioch, C. Rau, L. J. Jensen, S. Bastuck, B. Dumpelfeld, A. Edelmann, M. A. Heurtier, V. Hoffman, C. Hoefert, K. Klein, M. Hudak, A. M. Michon, M. Schelder, M. Schirle, M. Remor, T. Rudi, S. Hooper, A. Bauer, T. Bouwmeester, G. Casari, G. Drewes, G. Neubauer, J. M. Rick, B. Kuster, P. Bork, R. B. Russell, and G. Superti-Furga. (2006). Proteome survey reveals modularity of the yeast cell machinery. *Nature* 440: 631-636: Mar 30.

Gavin, A. C., M. Bosche, R. Krause, P. Grandi, M. Marzioch, A. Bauer, J. Schultz, J. M. Rick, A. M. Michon, C. M. Cruciat, M. Remor, C. Hofert, M. Schelder, M. Brajenovic, H. Ruffner, A. Merino, K. Klein, M. Hudak, D. Dickson, T. Rudi, V. Gnau, A. Bauch, S. Bastuck, B. Huhse, C. Leutwein, M. A. Heurtier, R. R. Copley, A. Edelmann, E. Querfurth, V. Rybin, G. Drewes, M. Raida, T. Bouwmeester, P. Bork, B. Seraphin, B. Kuster, G. Neubauer, and G. Superti-Furga. (2002). Functional organization of the yeast proteome by systematic analysis of protein complexes. *Nature* 415: 141-147: Jan 10.

Giot, L., J. S. Bader, C. Brouwer, A. Chaudhuri, B. Kuang, Y. Li, Y. L. Hao, C. E. Ooi, B. Godwin, E. Vitols, G. Vijayadamodar, P. Pochart, H. Machineni, M. Welsh, Y. Kong, B. Zerhusen, R. Malcolm, Z. Varrone, A. Collis, M. Minto, S. Burgess, L. McDaniel, E. Stimpson, F. Spriggs, J. Williams, K. Neurath, N. Ioime, M. Agee, E. Voss, K. Furtak, R. Renzulli, N. Aanensen, S. Carrolla, E. Bickelhaupt, Y. Lazovatsky, A. DaSilva, J. Zhong, C. A. Stanyon, R. L. Finley, Jr., K. P. White, M.

Braverman, T. Jarvie, S. Gold, M. Leach, J. Knight, R. A. Shimkets, M. P. McKenna, J. Chant, and J. M. Rothberg. (2003). A protein interaction map of Drosophila melanogaster. *Science* 302: 1727-1736: Dec 5.

Girvan, M., and M. E. Newman. (2002). Community structure in social and biological networks. *Proc Natl Acad Sci U S A* 99: 7821-7826: Jun 11.

Hambly, K., J. Danzer, S. Muskal, and D. A. Debe. (2006). Interrogating the druggable genome with structural informatics. *Mol Divers* 10: 273-281: Aug.

Hernandez-Toro, J., C. Prieto, and J. De las Rivas. (2007). APID2NET: unified interactome graphic analyzer. *Bioinformatics* 23: 2495-2497: Sep 15.

Ho, Y., A. Gruhler, A. Heilbut, G. D. Bader, L. Moore, S. L. Adams, A. Millar, P. Taylor, K. Bennett, K. Boutilier, L. Yang, C. Wolting, I. Donaldson, S. Schandorff, J. Shewnarane, M. Vo, J. Taggart, M. Goudreault, B. Muskat, C. Alfarano, D. Dewar, Z. Lin, K. Michalickova, A. R. Willems, H. Sassi, P. A. Nielsen, K. J. Rasmussen, J. R. Andersen, L. E. Johansen, L. H. Hansen, H. Jespersen, A. Podtelejnikov, E. Nielsen, J. Crawford, V. Poulsen, B. D. Sorensen, J. Matthiesen, R. C. Hendrickson, F. Gleeson, T. Pawson, M. F. Moran, D. Durocher, M. Mann, C. W. Hogue, D. Figeys, and M. Tyers. (2002). Systematic identification of protein complexes in Saccharomyces cerevisiae by mass spectrometry. *Nature* 415: 180-183: Jan 10.

Hood, L., and R. M. Perlmutter. (2004). The impact of systems approaches on biological problems in drug discovery. *Nat Biotechnol* 22: 1215-1217: Oct.

Hopkins, A. L., and C. R. Groom. (2002). The druggable genome. *Nat Rev Drug Discov* 1: 727-730: Sep.

Huynen, M., B. Snel, W. Lathe, 3rd, and P. Bork. (2000). Predicting protein function by genomic context: quantitative evaluation and qualitative inferences. *Genome Res* 10: 1204-1210: Aug.

Huynen, M. A., and B. Snel. (2000). Gene and context: integrative approaches to genome analysis. *Adv Protein Chem* 54: 345-379.

Ideker, T., and R. Sharan. (2008). Protein networks in disease. *Genome Res* 18: 644-652: Apr.

Ito, T., T. Chiba, and M. Yoshida. (2001a). Exploring the protein interactome using comprehensive two-hybrid projects. *Trends Biotechnol* 19: S23-27: Oct.

Ito, T., T. Chiba, R. Ozawa, M. Yoshida, M. Hattori, and Y. Sakaki. (2001b). A comprehensive two-hybrid analysis to explore the yeast protein interactome. *Proc Natl Acad Sci U S A* 98: 4569-4574: Apr 10.

Ito, T., K. Ota, H. Kubota, Y. Yamaguchi, T. Chiba, K. Sakuraba, and M. Yoshida. (2002). Roles for the two-hybrid system in exploration of the yeast protein interactome. *Mol Cell Proteomics* 1: 561-566: Aug.

Jansen, R., H. Yu, D. Greenbaum, Y. Kluger, N. J. Krogan, S. Chung, A. Emili, M. Snyder, J. F. Greenblatt, and M. Gerstein. (2003). A Bayesian networks approach for predicting protein-protein interactions from genomic data. *Science* 302: 449-453: Oct 17.

Jeong, H., S. P. Mason, A. L. Barabasi, and Z. N. Oltvai. (2001). Lethality and centrality in protein networks. *Nature* 411: 41-42: May 3.

Jeong, H., B. Tombor, R. Albert, Z. N. Oltvai, and A. L. Barabasi. (2000). The large-scale organization of metabolic networks. *Nature* 407: 651-654: Oct 5.

Kanehisa, M., and S. Goto. (2000). KEGG: kyoto encyclopedia of genes and genomes. *Nucleic Acids Res* 28: 27-30: Jan 1.

Kemmeren, P., N. L. van Berkum, J. Vilo, T. Bijma, R. Donders, A. Brazma, and F. C. Holstege. (2002). Protein interaction verification and functional annotation by integrated analysis of genome-scale data. *Mol Cell* 9: 1133-1143: May.

Klein, C., and L. T. Vassilev. (2004). Targeting the p53-MDM2 interaction to treat cancer. *Br J Cancer* 91: 1415-1419: Oct 18.

Kohl, P., and D. Noble. (2009). Systems biology and the virtual physiological human. *Mol Syst Biol* 5: 292.

Koonin, E. V., R. L. Tatusov, and M. Y. Galperin. (1998). Beyond complete genomes: from sequence to structure and function. *Curr Opin Struct Biol* 8: 355-363: Jun.

LaCount, D. J., M. Vignali, R. Chettier, A. Phansalkar, R. Bell, J. R. Hesselberth, L. W. Schoenfeld, I. Ota, S. Sahasrabudhe, C. Kurschner, S. Fields, and R. E. Hughes. (2005). A protein interaction network of the malaria parasite Plasmodium falciparum. *Nature* 438: 103-107: Nov 3.

Lee, I., S. V. Date, A. T. Adai, and E. M. Marcotte. (2004). A probabilistic functional network of yeast genes. *Science* 306: 1555-1558: Nov 26.

Lee, I., U. M. Blom, P. I. Wang, J. E. Shim, and E. M. Marcotte. (2011). Prioritizing candidate disease genes by network-based boosting of genome-wide association data. *Genome Res* 21: 1109-1121: Jul.

Lee, I., B. Lehner, C. Crombie, W. Wong, A. G. Fraser, and E. M. Marcotte. (2008a). A single gene network accurately predicts phenotypic effects of gene perturbation in Caenorhabditis elegans. *Nat Genet* 40: 181-188: Feb.

Lee, I., B. Lehner, T. Vavouri, J. Shin, A. G. Fraser, and E. M. Marcotte. (2010). Predicting genetic modifier loci using functional gene networks. *Genome Res* 20: 1143-1153: Aug.

Lee, J. H., V. Vittone, E. Diefenbach, A. L. Cunningham, and R. J. Diefenbach. (2008b). Identification of structural protein-protein interactions of herpes simplex virus type 1. *Virology* 378: 347-354: Sep 1.

Lehner, B., J. I. Semple, S. E. Brown, D. Counsell, R. D. Campbell, and C. M. Sanderson. (2004). Analysis of a high-throughput yeast two-hybrid system and its use to predict the function of intracellular proteins encoded within the human MHC class III region. *Genomics* 83: 153-167: Jan.

Li, S., C. M. Armstrong, N. Bertin, H. Ge, S. Milstein, M. Boxem, P. O. Vidalain, J. D. Han, A. Chesneau, T. Hao, D. S. Goldberg, N. Li, M. Martinez, J. F. Rual, P. Lamesch, L. Xu, M. Tewari, S. L. Wong, L. V. Zhang, G. F. Berriz, L. Jacotot, P. Vaglio, J. Reboul, T. Hirozane-Kishikawa, Q. Li, H. W. Gabel, A. Elewa, B. Baumgartner, D. J. Rose, H. Yu, S. Bosak, R. Sequerra, A. Fraser, S. E. Mango, W. M. Saxton, S. Strome, S. Van Den Heuvel, F. Piano, J. Vandenhaute, C. Sardet, M. Gerstein, L. Doucette-Stamm, K. C. Gunsalus, J. W. Harper, M. E. Cusick, F. P. Roth, D. E. Hill, and M. Vidal. (2004). A map of the interactome network of the metazoan C. elegans. *Science* 303: 540-543: Jan 23.

Linghu, B., E. S. Snitkin, Z. Hu, Y. Xia, and C. Delisi. (2009). Genome-wide prioritization of disease genes and identification of disease-disease associations from an integrated human functional linkage network. *Genome Biol* 10: R91.

Liu, X., and B. Han. (2009). Evolutionary conservation of neighbouring gene pairs in plants. *Gene* 437: 71-79: May 15.

Lu, L. J., Y. Xia, A. Paccanaro, H. Yu, and M. Gerstein. (2005). Assessing the limits of genomic data integration for predicting protein networks. *Genome Res* 15: 945-953: Jul.

Ma'ayan, A., S. L. Jenkins, S. Neves, A. Hasseldine, E. Grace, B. Dubin-Thaler, N. J. Eungdamrong, G. Weng, P. T. Ram, J. J. Rice, A. Kershenbaum, G. A. Stolovitzky, R. D. Blitzer, and R. Iyengar. (2005). Formation of regulatory patterns during signal propagation in a Mammalian cellular network. *Science* 309: 1078-1083: Aug 12.

Mangan, S., and U. Alon. (2003). Structure and function of the feed-forward loop network motif. *Proc Natl Acad Sci U S A* 100: 11980-11985: Oct 14.

Marcotte, E. M. (2000). Computational genetics: finding protein function by nonhomology methods. *Curr Opin Struct Biol* 10: 359-365: Jun.

Marcotte, E. M., M. Pellegrini, M. J. Thompson, T. O. Yeates, and D. Eisenberg. (1999a). A combined algorithm for genome-wide prediction of protein function. *Nature* 402: 83-86: Nov 4.

Marcotte, E. M., M. Pellegrini, H. L. Ng, D. W. Rice, T. O. Yeates, and D. Eisenberg. (1999b). Detecting protein function and protein-protein interactions from genome sequences. *Science* 285: 751-753: Jul 30.

McGary, K. L., T. J. Park, J. O. Woods, H. J. Cha, J. B. Wallingford, and E. M. Marcotte. (2010). Systematic discovery of nonobvious human disease models through orthologous phenotypes. *Proc Natl Acad Sci U S A* 107: 6544-6549: Apr 6.

Mika, S., and B. Rost. (2006). Protein-protein interactions more conserved within species than across species. *PLoS Comput Biol* 2: e79: Jul 21.

Milo, R., S. Shen-Orr, S. Itzkovitz, N. Kashtan, D. Chklovskii, and U. Alon. (2002). Network motifs: simple building blocks of complex networks. *Science* 298: 824-827: Oct 25.

Nair, R., and B. Rost. (2002). Sequence conserved for subcellular localization. *Protein Sci* 11: 2836-2847: Dec.

Navratil, V., B. de Chassey, C. R. Combe, and V. Lotteau. (2011). When the human viral infectome and diseasome networks collide: towards a systems biology platform for the aetiology of human diseases. *BMC Syst Biol* 5: 13.

Nikolsky, Y., T. Nikolskaya, and A. Bugrim. (2005). Biological networks and analysis of experimental data in drug discovery. *Drug Discov Today* 10: 653-662: May 1.

Ogata, H., S. Goto, K. Sato, W. Fujibuchi, H. Bono, and M. Kanehisa. (1999). KEGG: Kyoto Encyclopedia of Genes and Genomes. *Nucleic Acids Res* 27: 29-34: Jan 1.

Ouzounis, C., and N. Kyrpides. (1996). The emergence of major cellular processes in evolution. *FEBS Lett* 390: 119-123: Jul 22.

Overbeek, R., M. Fonstein, M. D'Souza, G. D. Pusch, and N. Maltsev. (1999). The use of gene clusters to infer functional coupling. *Proc Natl Acad Sci U S A* 96: 2896-2901: Mar 16.

Pedamallu, C. S., and J. Posfai. (2010). Open source tool for prediction of genome wide protein-protein interaction network based on ortholog information. *Source Code Biol Med* 5: 8.

Pellegrini, M., E. M. Marcotte, M. J. Thompson, D. Eisenberg, and T. O. Yeates. (1999). Assigning protein functions by comparative genome analysis: protein phylogenetic profiles. *Proc Natl Acad Sci U S A* 96: 4285-4288: Apr 13.

Pena-Castillo, L., M. Tasan, C. L. Myers, H. Lee, T. Joshi, C. Zhang, Y. Guan, M. Leone, A. Pagnani, W. K. Kim, C. Krumpelman, W. Tian, G. Obozinski, Y. Qi, S. Mostafavi, G. N. Lin, G. F. Berriz, F. D. Gibbons, G. Lanckriet, J. Qiu, C. Grant, Z. Barutcuoglu, D. P. Hill, D. Warde-Farley, C. Grouios, D. Ray, J. A. Blake, M. Deng, M. I. Jordan, W. S. Noble, Q. Morris, J. Klein-Seetharaman, Z. Bar-Joseph, T. Chen, F. Sun, O. G. Troyanskaya, E. M. Marcotte, D. Xu, T. R. Hughes, and F. P. Roth. (2008). A critical assessment of Mus musculus gene function prediction using integrated genomic evidence. *Genome Biol* 9 Suppl 1: S2.

Prieto, C., and J. De Las Rivas. (2006). APID: Agile Protein Interaction DataAnalyzer. *Nucleic Acids Res* 34: W298-302: Jul 1.

Ravasz, E., A. L. Somera, D. A. Mongru, Z. N. Oltvai, and A. L. Barabasi. (2002). Hierarchical organization of modularity in metabolic networks. *Science* 297: 1551-1555: Aug 30.

Read, T. D., S. R. Gill, H. Tettelin, and B. A. Dougherty. (2001). Finding drug targets in microbial genomes. *Drug Discov Today* 6: 887-892: Sep 1.

Rivera, M. C., R. Jain, J. E. Moore, and J. A. Lake. (1998). Genomic evidence for two functionally distinct gene classes. *Proc Natl Acad Sci U S A* 95: 6239-6244: May 26.

Rost, B. (1999). Twilight zone of protein sequence alignments. *Protein Eng* 12: 85-94: Feb.

Rozen, R., N. Sathish, Y. Li, and Y. Yuan. (2008). Virion-wide protein interactions of Kaposi's sarcoma-associated herpesvirus. *J Virol* 82: 4742-4750: May.

Rual, J. F., K. Venkatesan, T. Hao, T. Hirozane-Kishikawa, A. Dricot, N. Li, G. F. Berriz, F. D. Gibbons, M. Dreze, N. Ayivi-Guedehoussou, N. Klitgord, C. Simon, M. Boxem, S. Milstein, J. Rosenberg, D. S. Goldberg, L. V. Zhang, S. L. Wong, G. Franklin, S. Li, J. S. Albala, J. Lim, C. Fraughton, E. Llamosas, S. Cevik, C. Bex, P. Lamesch, R. S. Sikorski, J. Vandenhaute, H. Y. Zoghbi, A. Smolyar, S. Bosak, R. Sequerra, L. Doucette-Stamm, M. E. Cusick, D. E. Hill, F. P. Roth, and M. Vidal. (2005). Towards a proteome-scale map of the human protein-protein interaction network. *Nature* 437: 1173-1178: Oct 20.

Russ, A. P., and S. Lampel. (2005). The druggable genome: an update. *Drug Discov Today* 10: 1607-1610: Dec.

Sakharkar, K. R., M. K. Sakharkar, and V. T. Chow. (2004). A novel genomics approach for the identification of drug targets in pathogens, with special reference to Pseudomonas aeruginosa. *In Silico Biol* 4: 355-360.

Sali, A. (1999). Functional links between proteins. *Nature* 402: 23, 25-26: Nov 4.

Schmid, M. B. (1998). Novel approaches to the discovery of antimicrobial agents. *Curr Opin Chem Biol* 2: 529-534: Aug.

Schmid, M. B. (2006). Crystallizing new approaches for antimicrobial drug discovery. *Biochem Pharmacol* 71: 1048-1056: Mar 30.

Shen-Orr, S. S., R. Milo, S. Mangan, and U. Alon. (2002). Network motifs in the transcriptional regulation network of Escherichia coli. *Nat Genet* 31: 64-68: May.

Shoemaker, B. A., and A. R. Panchenko. (2007). Deciphering protein-protein interactions. Part I. Experimental techniques and databases. *PLoS Comput Biol* 3: e42: Mar 30.

Stelzl, U., U. Worm, M. Lalowski, C. Haenig, F. H. Brembeck, H. Goehler, M. Stroedicke, M. Zenkner, A. Schoenherr, S. Koeppen, J. Timm, S. Mintzlaff, C. Abraham, N. Bock, S. Kietzmann, A. Goedde, E. Toksoz, A. Droege, S. Krobitsch, B. Korn, W. Birchmeier, H. Lehrach, and E. E. Wanker. (2005). A human protein-protein interaction network: a resource for annotating the proteome. *Cell* 122: 957-968: Sep 23.

Stingl, K., K. Schauer, C. Ecobichon, A. Labigne, P. Lenormand, J. C. Rousselle, A. Namane, and H. de Reuse. (2008). In vivo interactome of Helicobacter pylori urease revealed by tandem affinity purification. *Mol Cell Proteomics* 7: 2429-2441: Dec.

Szklarczyk, D., A. Franceschini, M. Kuhn, M. Simonovic, A. Roth, P. Minguez, T. Doerks, M. Stark, J. Muller, P. Bork, L. J. Jensen, and C. von Mering. (2011). The STRING database in 2011: functional interaction networks of proteins, globally integrated and scored. *Nucleic Acids Res* 39: D561-568: Jan.

Tamames, J., G. Casari, C. Ouzounis, and A. Valencia. (1997). Conserved clusters of functionally related genes in two bacterial genomes. *J Mol Evol* 44: 66-73: Jan.

Tew, K. L., X. L. Li, and S. H. Tan. (2007). Functional centrality: detecting lethality of proteins in protein interaction networks. *Genome Inform* 19: 166-177.

Thanassi, J. A., S. L. Hartman-Neumann, T. J. Dougherty, B. A. Dougherty, and M. J. Pucci. (2002). Identification of 113 conserved essential genes using a high-throughput gene disruption system in Streptococcus pneumoniae. *Nucleic Acids Res* 30: 3152-3162: Jul 15.

Todd, A. E., C. A. Orengo, and J. M. Thornton. (2001). Evolution of function in protein superfamilies, from a structural perspective. *J Mol Biol* 307: 1113-1143: Apr 6.

Tong, A. H., G. Lesage, G. D. Bader, H. Ding, H. Xu, X. Xin, J. Young, G. F. Berriz, R. L. Brost, M. Chang, Y. Chen, X. Cheng, G. Chua, H. Friesen, D. S. Goldberg, J. Haynes, C. Humphries, G. He, S. Hussein, L. Ke, N. Krogan, Z. Li, J. N. Levinson, H. Lu, P. Menard, C. Munyana, A. B. Parsons, O. Ryan, R. Tonikian, T. Roberts, A. M. Sdicu, J. Shapiro, B. Sheikh, B. Suter, S. L. Wong, L. V. Zhang, H. Zhu, C. G. Burd, S. Munro, C. Sander, J. Rine, J. Greenblatt, M. Peter, A. Bretscher, G. Bell, F. P. Roth, G. W. Brown, B. Andrews, H. Bussey, and C. Boone. (2004). Global mapping of the yeast genetic interaction network. *Science* 303: 808-813: Feb 6.

Uetz, P., and R. E. Hughes. (2000). Systematic and large-scale two-hybrid screens. *Curr Opin Microbiol* 3: 303-308: Jun.

Uetz, P., Y. A. Dong, C. Zeretzke, C. Atzler, A. Baiker, B. Berger, S. V. Rajagopala, M. Roupelieva, D. Rose, E. Fossum, and J. Haas. (2006). Herpesviral protein networks and their interaction with the human proteome. *Science* 311: 239-242: Jan 13.

Uetz, P., L. Giot, G. Cagney, T. A. Mansfield, R. S. Judson, J. R. Knight, D. Lockshon, V. Narayan, M. Srinivasan, P. Pochart, A. Qureshi-Emili, Y. Li, B. Godwin, D. Conover, T. Kalbfleisch, G. Vijayadamodar, M. Yang, M. Johnston, S. Fields, and J. M. Rothberg. (2000). A comprehensive analysis of protein-protein interactions in Saccharomyces cerevisiae. *Nature* 403: 623-627: Feb 10.

Vassilev, L. T. (2004). Small-molecule antagonists of p53-MDM2 binding: research tools and potential therapeutics. *Cell Cycle* 3: 419-421: Apr.

Vassilev, L. T., B. T. Vu, B. Graves, D. Carvajal, F. Podlaski, Z. Filipovic, N. Kong, U. Kammlott, C. Lukacs, C. Klein, N. Fotouhi, and E. A. Liu. (2004). In vivo activation of the p53 pathway by small-molecule antagonists of MDM2. *Science* 303: 844-848: Feb 6.

Venkatesan, K., J. F. Rual, A. Vazquez, U. Stelzl, I. Lemmens, T. Hirozane-Kishikawa, T. Hao, M. Zenkner, X. Xin, K. I. Goh, M. A. Yildirim, N. Simonis, K. Heinzmann, F. Gebreab, J. M. Sahalie, S. Cevik, C. Simon, A. S. de Smet, E. Dann, A. Smolyar, A. Vinayagam, H. Yu, D. Szeto, H. Borick, A. Dricot, N. Klitgord, R. R. Murray, C. Lin, M. Lalowski, J. Timm, K. Rau, C. Boone, P. Braun, M. E. Cusick, F. P. Roth, D. E. Hill, J. Tavernier, E. E. Wanker, A. L. Barabasi, and M. Vidal. (2009). An empirical framework for binary interactome mapping. *Nat Methods* 6: 83-90: Jan.

Vidal, M., and P. Legrain. (1999). Yeast forward and reverse 'n'-hybrid systems. *Nucleic Acids Res* 27: 919-929: Feb 15.

von Mering, C., R. Krause, B. Snel, M. Cornell, S. G. Oliver, S. Fields, and P. Bork. (2002). Comparative assessment of large-scale data sets of protein-protein interactions. *Nature* 417: 399-403: May 23.

Wagner, A., and D. A. Fell. (2001). The small world inside large metabolic networks. *Proc Biol Sci* 268: 1803-1810: Sep 7.

Walhout, A. J., and M. Vidal. (2001a). High-throughput yeast two-hybrid assays for large-scale protein interaction mapping. *Methods* 24: 297-306: Jul.

Walhout, A. J., and M. Vidal. (2001b). Protein interaction maps for model organisms. *Nat Rev Mol Cell Biol* 2: 55-62: Jan.

Wang, P. I., and E. M. Marcotte. (2010). It's the machine that matters: Predicting gene function and phenotype from protein networks. *J Proteomics* 73: 2277-2289: Oct 10.

Wang, Y., T. Cui, C. Zhang, M. Yang, Y. Huang, W. Li, L. Zhang, C. Gao, Y. He, Y. Li, F. Huang, J. Zeng, C. Huang, Q. Yang, Y. Tian, C. Zhao, H. Chen, H. Zhang, and Z. G. He. (2010). Global protein-protein interaction network in the human pathogen Mycobacterium tuberculosis H37Rv. *J Proteome Res* 9: 6665-6677: Dec 3.

Watts, D. J., and S. H. Strogatz. (1998). Collective dynamics of 'small-world' networks. *Nature* 393: 440-442: Jun 4.

Weston, A. D., and L. Hood. (2004). Systems biology, proteomics, and the future of health care: toward predictive, preventative, and personalized medicine. *J Proteome Res* 3: 179-196: Mar-Apr.

Wiles, A. M., M. Doderer, J. Ruan, T. T. Gu, D. Ravi, B. Blackman, and A. J. Bishop. (2010). Building and analyzing protein interactome networks by cross-species comparisons. *BMC Syst Biol* 4: 36.

Wu, J., T. Vallenius, K. Ovaska, J. Westermarck, T. P. Makela, and S. Hautaniemi. (2009). Integrated network analysis platform for protein-protein interactions. *Nat Methods* 6: 75-77: Jan.

Wu, M., X. Li, H. N. Chua, C. K. Kwoh, and S. K. Ng. (2010). Integrating diverse biological and computational sources for reliable protein-protein interactions. *BMC Bioinformatics* 11 Suppl 7: S8.

Wuchty, S., Z. N. Oltvai, and A. L. Barabasi. (2003). Evolutionary conservation of motif constituents in the yeast protein interaction network. *Nat Genet* 35: 176-179: Oct.

Xia, Y., L. J. Lu, and M. Gerstein. (2006). Integrated prediction of the helical membrane protein interactome in yeast. *J Mol Biol* 357: 339-349: Mar 17.

Yook, S. H., Z. N. Oltvai, and A. L. Barabasi. (2004). Functional and topological characterization of protein interaction networks. *Proteomics* 4: 928-942: Apr.

Yu, H., D. Greenbaum, H. Xin Lu, X. Zhu, and M. Gerstein. (2004a). Genomic analysis of essentiality within protein networks. *Trends Genet* 20: 227-231: Jun.

Yu, H., P. M. Kim, E. Sprecher, V. Trifonov, and M. Gerstein. (2007). The importance of bottlenecks in protein networks: correlation with gene essentiality and expression dynamics. *PLoS Comput Biol* 3: e59: Apr 20.

Yu, H., N. M. Luscombe, H. X. Lu, X. Zhu, Y. Xia, J. D. Han, N. Bertin, S. Chung, M. Vidal, and M. Gerstein. (2004b). Annotation transfer between genomes: protein-protein interologs and protein-DNA regulogs. *Genome Res* 14: 1107-1118: Jun.

Yu, H., P. Braun, M. A. Yildirim, I. Lemmens, K. Venkatesan, J. Sahalie, T. Hirozane-Kishikawa, F. Gebreab, N. Li, N. Simonis, T. Hao, J. F. Rual, A. Dricot, A. Vazquez, R. R. Murray, C. Simon, L. Tardivo, S. Tam, N. Svrzikapa, C. Fan, A. S. de Smet, A. Motyl, M. E. Hudson, J. Park, X. Xin, M. E. Cusick, T. Moore, C. Boone, M. Snyder, F. P. Roth, A. L. Barabasi, J. Tavernier, D. E. Hill, and M. Vidal. (2008). High-quality binary protein interaction map of the yeast interactome network. *Science* 322: 104-110: Oct 3.

Zorio, D. A., N. N. Cheng, T. Blumenthal, and J. Spieth. (1994). Operons as a common form of chromosomal organization in C. elegans. *Nature* 372: 270-272: Nov 17.

2

Kojic Acid Derivatives

Mutlu D. Aytemir* and G. Karakaya
Hacettepe University, Faculty of Pharmacy
Department of Pharmaceutical Chemistry, Ankara
Turkey

1. Introduction

Melanin is one of the most important pigments which exist ubiquitously from microorganisms to plants and animals. It is secreted by melanocyte cells and determines the color of skin and hair in mammalians. It protects the skin from photocarcinogenesis by absorbing UV sunlight and removing reactive oxygen species (ROS) (Gupta, 2006; Kim, 2005; Sapkota, 2011). It is formed by enzymatically catalyzed chemical reactions (Chang, 2009). The modifications in melanin biosynthesis occur in many disease states. The excessive level of melanin pigmentation causes various dermatological disorders including hyperpigmentations such as senile lentigo, melasma, postinflammatory melanoderma, freckles, ephelide, age spots and sites of actinic damage which can give rise to esthetic problems (Briganti, 2003; Curto, 1999). Hyperpigmentation usually becomes a big problem as people age because darker spots will start to be seen on the face, arms and body. Also, hormonal changes such as pregnancy and drugs manipulating hormone levels may cause hyperpigmentation.

Inhibitors of the enzyme tyrosinase (EC 1.14.18.1, syn.polyphenol oxidase, PPO; monophenol; dihydroxy-L-phenylalanin; oxidoreductase) can be used to prevent or treat melanin hyperpigmentation disorders. Therefore, they have become increasingly important in cosmetic and medical products. Besides being used in the treatment of some dermatological disorders associated with melanin hyperpigmentation, tyrosinase inhibitors are found to have an important role in cosmetic industry for their skin lightening effect and depigmentation after sunburn (Briganti, 2003; Chang, 2009; Khan, 2007; Parvez, 2007; Seo, 2003). Tyrosinase is a common multifunctional copper-containing enzyme from the oxidase superfamily found in plants, animals and fungi. It is responsible for melanin biosynthesis, which determines the color of skin, hair and fur. It is at the moment a well-characterized enzyme. As an enzyme that produces pigment, tyrosinase catalyzes two key reactions in the melanin biosynthesis pathway: the addition of a hydroxyl group (-OH) to the amino acid tyrosine, which then becomes 3,4-dihydroxypheylalanine (L-DOPA). The tyrosinase enzyme then converts L-DOPA into *o*-dopaquinone by an oxidation reaction. Following these two main steps, melanin is then generated after further enzymatic steps (Scheme 1) (Gupta, 2006; Parvez, 2007). Melanin formation is considered to be deleterious to the color quality and flavor, and loss of nutritional and market values of foods. So, it causes the enzymatic

* Corresponding Author

browning in fruits and vegetables. In the food industry, tyrosinase is important in controlling the quality and economics of fruits and vegetables. Hence, tyrosinase inhibitors from natural sources have great potential in the food industry, as they are considered to be safe and largely free from adverse effects. Also in insects, tyrosinase is involved in melanogenesis wound healing, parasite encapsulation and sclerotisation (Seo, 2003). Therefore, tyrosinase inhibitors used as insecticides and insect control agents. Moreover, the tyrosinase is responsible from melanization in animals and is the key enzyme for the regulation of melanogenesis in mammals. Melanogenesis is the process by which melanin is produced and subsequently distributed by melanocytes within the skin and hair follicles. This process results in the synthesis of melanin pigments, which play a protective role against skin photocarcinogenesis (Khan, 2007; Kim, 2005).

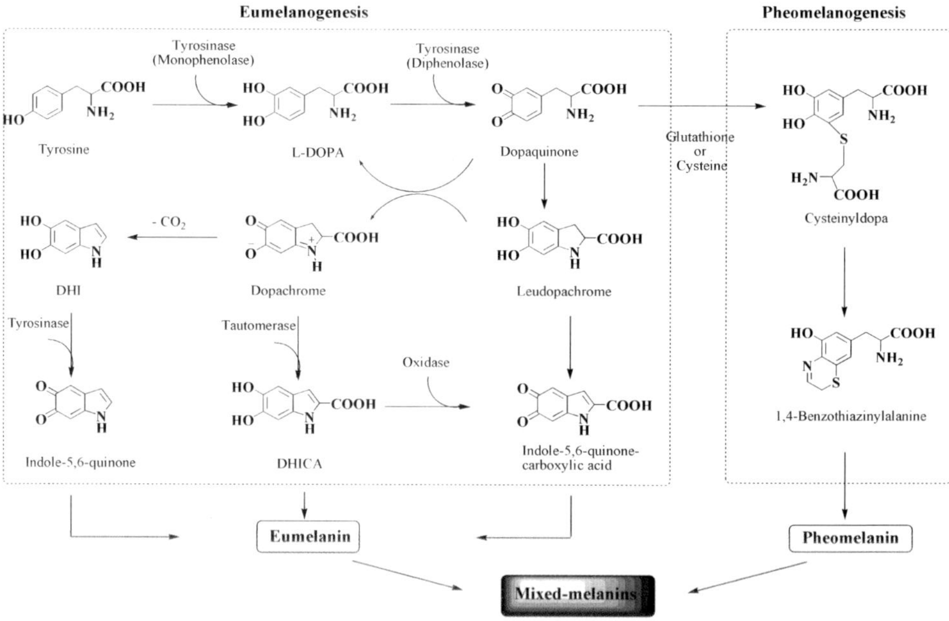

Scheme 1. Biosynthetic pathway of melanin (Chang, 2009; Kim, 2005; Seo, 2003). DOPA, 3,4-dihydroxyphenylalanine; DHI, 5,6-dihydroxyindole; DHICA, 5,6-dihydroxyindole-2-carboxylic acid.

Safety is a primary consideration for tyrosinase inhibitors, especially when utilized in unregulated quantities on a regular basis. On the other hand, the use of the inhibitors is primary in the cosmetic industry due to their skin-whitening effects. Since a huge number of tyrosinase inhibitors have been developed, assessing the validation of these inhibitors in skin-whitening efficiency has become more important. Most inhibitors have rarely been incorporated in topically applied cosmetics, often due to a lack of parallel human clinical trials (Chang, 2009; Khan, 2007; Kim, 2005).

Compounds called inhibitors are being synthesized to hinder or completely stop the enzyme's function. Natural products have already been discovered, experimented upon and proved to be safe and viable. However, due to depleting resources, synthetic derivatives based on naturally occurring compounds have opened up this research to a broad range of possible tyrosinase inhibitors (Diaz, 2009). There are several inhibition mechanisms of tyrosinase but only two types' inhibitors are regarded as "true inhibitors". These are specific tyrosinase inactivators and specific tyrosinase inhibitors. Specific tyrosinase inactivators such as mechanism-based inhibitors are also called suicide substrates. These inhibitors can be catalyzed by tyrosinase and form covalent bond with the enzyme, thus irreversibly inactivating the enzyme during catalytic reaction. They inhibit tyrosinase activity by inducing the enzyme catalyzing "suicide reaction." Specific tyrosinase inhibitors reversibly bind to tyrosinase and reduce its catalytic capacity (Chang, 2009). Therefore, the inhibition of tyrosinase is very essential in controlling the economy of foods and agriculture. Development of high-performance tyrosinase inhibitors is currently needed for these fields (Parvez, 2007).

Mushroom tyrosinase is popular among researchers as it is commercially available and inexpensive. It plays a critical role in tyrosinase inhibitor studies for its use in cosmetics as well as in food industries, and many researches have been conducted with this enzyme, which is well studied and easily purified from the mushroom *Agaricus bisporus*. No matter in terms of inhibitory strength, inhibitory mechanism, chemical structures, or the sources of the inhibitors, the search for new inhibitors based on mushroom tyrosinase has been so successful that various different types of inhibitors have been found in the past 20 years (Chang, 2009; Parvez, 2007; Seo, 2003).

In cosmetic products, tyrosinase inhibitors are used for skin-whitening effect, preventing formation of freckles and skin depigmentation after sunburn. Use of them is becoming increasingly important in the cosmetic and medicinal industries due to their preventive effect on pigmentation disorders. A number of tyrosinase inhibitors have been reported from both natural and synthetic sources, but only a few of them are used as skin-whitening agents, primarily due to various safety concerns, e.g. high toxicity toward cells, and low stability toward oxygen and water, resulting with their limited application (Chang, 2009; Kim, 2005).

Inhibitors of tyrosinase enzyme have a huge impact on industry and economy. Therefore, researchers around the world are studying on the discovery of several classes of these inhibitors. Although a large number of tyrosinase inhibitors have been reported from both natural resources or semi- and full synthetic pathways, only a few of them are used as skin lightening agents, primarily due to various safety concerns. For example, kojic acid and catechol derivatives, well-known hypopigmenting agents, inhibit enzyme activity but also exhibit harmful side effects (Fig. 1) (Seo, 2003).

Kojic acid (5-hydroxy-2-hydroxymethyl-4*H*-pyran-4-one) (Fig. 1, 4) and arbutin (4-hydroxyphenyl-β-D-glucopyranoside), extracted from leaves of common bearberry, are often used in skin care products as a lightening agent (Fig. 1). It has been shown to be safe and effective for topical use (Burdock, 2001). Recently, bibenzyl analogues are reported to have potent anti-tyrosinase activity with almost 20-fold stronger than kojic acid. However, the inhibitory activity of kojic acid is not sufficiently potent or unstable for storage for use in cosmetics. Kojic acid, a well-known tyrosinase inhibitor, alone or together with tropolone and L-mimosine are often used as the positive control in the literature for comparing the inhibitory strength of the newly inhibitors (Briganti, 2003; Chang, 2009; Khan, 2007; Parvez, 2007). L-mimosine, kojic acid and tropolone, having structural similarity to phenolic subsrates and showing competitive inhibition with respect to these substrates, are known as slow binding inhibitors (Seo, 2003). In addition, most tyrosinase inhibitors listed below are not currently commercially available, especially those from natural sources, and this limits their further evaluation in an *in vivo* study, where usually a large amount is needed for a tested inhibitor (Chang, 2009).

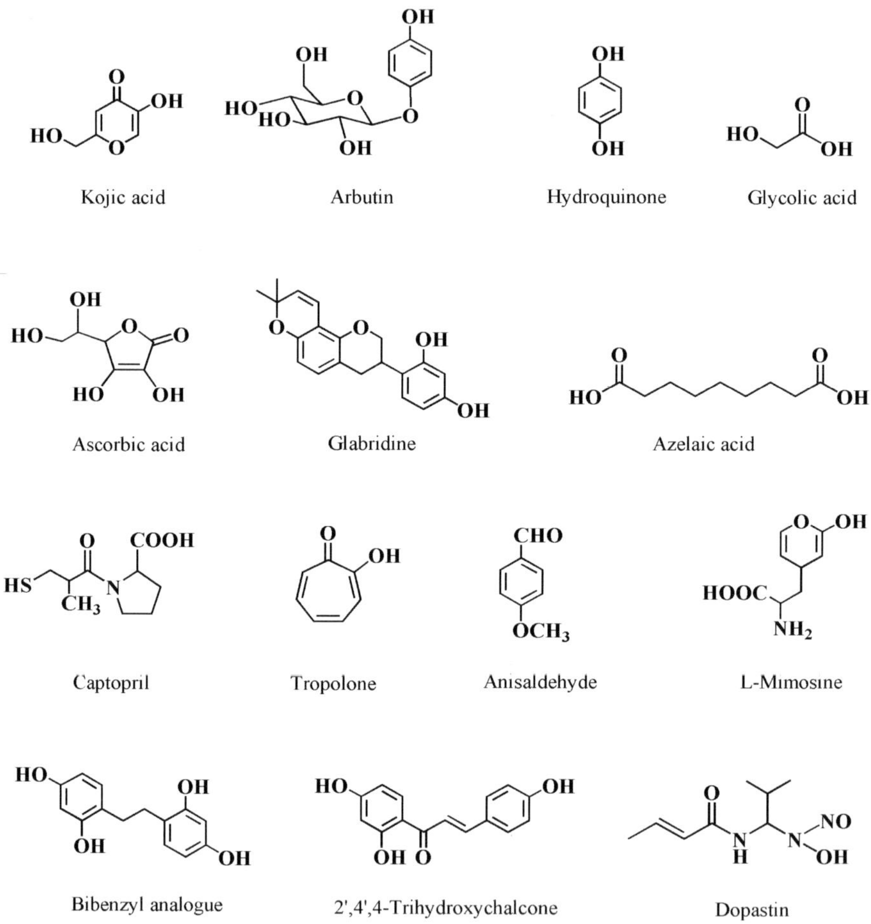

Fig. 1. Some tyrosinase inhibitors.

To treat hyperpigmentation through chemical treatments or bleaching creams are used. Most of the inhibitors are phenol or catechol derivatives, structurally similar to tyrosine or DOPA (Briganti, 2003). Hydroquinone (Fig. 1), a widely used skin lightening agent, is probably the most used bleaching cream on the market but it has a laundry list of warnings, including risk of hepatotoxicity. However, it is the most widely used bleaching cream in the world, despite the potential health side effects. It is also a reliable treatment for melasma. Kojic acid is used as an antioxidant and alternative to hydroquinone for skin lightening by the cosmetic industry (Gupta, 2006).

Although the huge number of reversible inhibitors has been identified, rarely irreversible inhibitors of tyrosinase have been found until now. Captopril, used as an antihypertensive drug, is able to prevent melanin formation as a good example of irreversible inhibitors (Khan, 2007). Another example for tyrosinase inhibitor azelaic acid, has anti-inflammatory, antibacterial, and antikeratinizing effects, which make it useful in a variety of dermatologic conditions (Briganti, 2003; Gupta, 2006). Besides, 4,4'-biphenyl derivative exhibited strong tyrosinase inhibitory activity and also assessed for the melanin biosynthesis in B16 melanoma cells (Kim, 2005).

2. Kojic acid

Kojic acid, the most intensively studied inhibitor of tyrosinase, was discovered by K. Saito in 1907. Since the early twentieth century, it has been known as an additive to prevent browning of food materials such as crab, shrimp, and fresh vegetables in food industry (*e.g.*, as an antioxidant or antibrowning agent) in order to preserve their freshness and to inhibit discoloration. It shows a competitive inhibitory effect on monophenolase activity and a mixed inhibitory effect on the diphenolase activity of mushroom tyrosinase. The ability of kojic acid to chelate copper at the active site of the enzyme may well explain the observed competitive inhibitory effect. In addition, it is reported to be a slow-binding inhibitor of the diphenolase activity of tyrosinase (Cabanes, 1994). It is a biologically important natural antibiotic produced by various fungal or bacterial strains such as *Aspergillus oryzae*, *Penicillium* or *Acetobacter spp.* in an aerobic process from a wide range of carbon sources (Bentley, 2006; Brtko, 2004; Burdock, 2001). It plays an important role in iron-overload diseases such as β-thalassemia or anemia, since it possesses iron chelating activity (Brtko, 2004; Moggia, 2006; Stenson, 2007; Sudhir, 2005; Zborowski, 2003). Also, it forms stable complexes of metal kojates via reaction of kojic acid with metal acetate salts such as tin, beryllium, zinc, copper, nickel, cobalt, iron, manganese, chromium, gold, palladium, indium, gallium, vanadium, and aluminium (Fig. 2) (Barret, 2001; Cecconi, 2002; Emami, 2007; Finnegan, 1987; Hryniewicz, 2009; Masoud, 1989; Moggia, 2006; Naik, 1979; Sudhir, 2005; Yang, 2008; Zaremba, 2007; Zborowski, 2005). They were used as new drugs in the therapy of some diseases such as diabetes, anemia, fungal infections and neoplasia (Brtko, 2004; Song, 2002; Wolf, 1950). Tris(kojic acid) aluminium(III) and -gallium(III) complexes have lipid solubility; therefore, they can cross the blood-brain barrier with considerable facility (Finnegan, 1987).

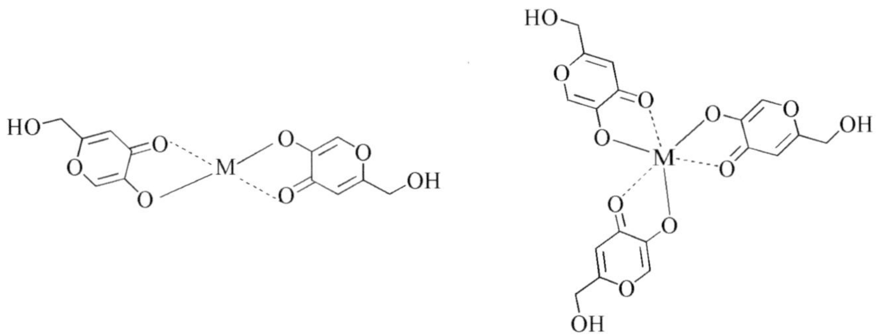

Fig. 2. M(Kojic acid)n (n=2,3) metal complexes.

Kojic acid has weaker activity than ethylmaltol (2-ethyl-3-hydroxy-4*H*-pyran-4-one) against the convulsions induced by pentetrazole and strychnine. It is generally accepted that the lipid solubility of a drug is an important factor in connection with its transfer into the central spinal fluid and brain. The increase of inhibitory effect of 2-alkyl-3-hydroxy-4*H*-pyran-4-ones on the pentetrazole-induced convulsion with increasing carbon number of the alkyl group might be due to the enhancement of lipid solubility (Aoyagi, 1974; Kimura, 1980).

In acute, chronic, reproductive and genotoxicity studies, kojic acid was not found as a toxicant. Due to slow absorption into the circulation from human skin, it would not reach the threshold at tumor promotion and weak carcinogenicity effects were seen. The Cosmetic Ingredient Review (CIR) Expert Panel concluded that it is safe for use in cosmetic products up to a concentration level of 1%. The available human sensitization data support the safety of kojic acid at a concentration of 2% in leave-on cosmetics, suggesting that a limit of 2% might be appropriate. In an industrial survey of current use concentrations, it is used at concentrations ranging from 0.1% to 2%. The European Commission's Scientific Committee on Consumer Products (SCCP) determined that, based on a margin of safety calculation, the use of kojic acid at a maximum concentration of 1.0% in skin care formulations poses a risk to human health due to potential systemic effects (thyroid side effects). The SCCP also found it to be a potential skin sensitizer (Burnett, 2011).

2.1 Kojic acid as a tyrosinase inhibitor

It is well recognized that kojic acid, of high purity (99%) made by a certain pharmaceutical manufacture, began to be used extensively as a cosmetic skin-whitening product (quasi-drug) especially in Japan, for topical application. Because of its slow and effective reversible competitive inhibition of human melanocyte tyrosinase, kojic acid prevents melanin formation. So, it can play an important role at the formation of cellular melanins (Cabanes, 1994; Jun, 2007; Kahn, 1997; Kang, 2009; Kim, 2003; Lin, 2007; Noh, 2007; Raku, 2003; Saruno, 1979). Noncosmetic uses reported for kojic acid include therapeutic uses for melasma, antioxidant and preservative in foods, antibiotic, chemical intermediate, metal chelate, pesticide, and antimicrobial agents. Because of its well-documented ability to inhibit tyrosinase activity, kojic acid has been used in numerous studies as a positive control. It was showed that kojic acid have inhibitory effect on mushroom, plant (potato and apple), and crustacean (white shrimp, grass prawn, and Florida spiny lobster) tyrosinase. The inhibition mushroom, potato, apple, white shrimp and spiny lobster tyrosinase was found to be related with the kojic acid inhibited melanosis by interfering with the uptake of O_2 required for enzymatic browning (Chen, 1991). It was well-known that tyrosinase containing two copper ions in the active center and a lipophilic long-narrow gorge near to the active center. It has been reported that kojic acid inhibits the activity of tyrosinase by forming a chelate with the copper ion in the tyrosinase through the 5-hydroxyl and 4-carbonyl groups. There are several types of assays determining tyrosinase inhibition. Cabanes *et al.* stated that kojic acid is a slow-binding inhibitor of catecholase activity of frog tyrosinase in a nonclassical manner (Cabanes, 1994). In a study of several mammalian melanocyte tyrosinase inhibitors, kojic acid was considered a potent free enzyme inhibitor (Curto, 1999). Kojic acid was a positive control in a study of the inhibitory effects of oxyresveratrol and hydroxystilbene compounds on mushroom and murine melanoma B-16 tyrosinase (Kim, 2002). Melanoma-specific anticarcinogenic activity is also known to be linked with tyrosinase activity (Kim, 2005). Malignant melanoma continues to be a serious clinical problem with a high mortality rate among the human beings (Seo, 2003). Therefore, the potential therapies targeting tyrosinase activity have a paramount importance.

The beauty industry agrees with the statement regarding kojic acid is one of the best natural based lotions as far as skin lightening agents go. The definition of beauty for some cultures consists of fair, even toned skin, so many women resort to using skin lightening products, such as kojic acid, to achieve a lighter skin tone. It has been used for years in the Far East as an alternative to hydroquinone for its bleaching effects but many women are using it to treat hyperpigmentation as well as sun spots, freckles, liver spots and a number of other pigment problems related to beauty. The majority of lightening lotions contains a healthy dose of kojic acid in it beside vitamin C (ascorbic acid), bearberry extract, licorice or mulberry; in some cases, kojic acid is the main active ingredient. Most skin lightening lotions that use kojic acid as one of their ingredients also use small amounts of hydroquinone as well as glycolic acid (Fig. 1).

In addition, kojic acid is found to prevent photodamage and subsequent wrinkling of the skin in the hairless mouse. It is a good chelator of transition metal ions and a good scavenger of free radicals therefore it is an effective agent for photoprotection (Mitani, 2001). Also, it is used as bleaching agent in cosmetics (Burdock, 2001; Lin, 2007). Current evidence suggests that it induces skin depigmentation through suppression of free tyrosinase, mainly due to chelation of its copper at the active site of the enzyme (Chen, 1991; Jun, 2007; Lee, 2006). It has been demonstrated to be responsible for therapy and prevention of pigmentation, both *in vitro* and *in vivo* and being used for topical application. Melasma is often affecting women, especially those living in areas of intense UV radiation. In treatment of melasma which continues to be a difficult problem, the addition of kojic acid in a gel containing glycolic acid and hydroquinone improved melasma. Kojic acid is found as effective as hydroquinone in reducing the pigment. The combination of both agents augments this inhibition further (Gupta, 2006).

Previous antimicrobial activity studies showed that kojic acid was more active against gram negative bacteria than against gram positive ones (Bentley, 2006). However, some of its derivatives have shown adverse effects different from kojic acid's antibacterial activity results (Aytemir, 2003a, 2003b; Fassihi, 2008; Kotani, 1978; Masoud, 1989; Petrola, 1985; Veverka, 1992). Also, its derivatives especially have significant antifungal activity against *C. albicans* and *C. krusei* (Aytemir, 2003b, 2004; Brtko, 2004; Fassihi, 2008; Kayahara, 1990; Mitani, 2001; Veverka, 1992). According to its antibacterial and fungicidal properties, kojic acid is used as a food additive (Burdock, 2001). There are several forms of kojic acid containing products including soap, cream, lotion and gel. Kojic acid also has antifungal and antibacterial properties in it, making it a perfect ingredient to be used in soap. Women who choose a kojic acid lotion tend to use it to treat smaller areas of the skin that have been affected by hyperpigmentation, age spots or hormone related skin conditions brought on by pregnancy or birth control pills. Some women favor this lotion because it absorbs directly into the skin much better than creams or soaps. One of the greatest benefits to using kojic acid is reduction of getting wrinkles when you use the lotion before exposure to the sun. So it makes this also a perfect anti-aging lotion. Based on such tyrosinase-inhibiting activity of kojic acid, there have been proposed a lot of cosmetic compositions containing kojic acid as an active ingredient. There are a variety of kojic acid creams available for purchase online and in certain specialty stores. Each one has its own unique blend of ingredients which set them apart from one another. Some creams combine various vitamins like A and E which give them different effects. The reason many people mix these vitamins within the kojic acid creams is to help them alleviate the skin irritation that has been said to occur with kojic acid products. Another cream combines retinol, vitamin C, with kojic acid, and glycolic acid. These ingredients are added to this base to help counteract the sensitivity that is associated with prolonged use of kojic acid when it is used by itself. According to FDA kojic acid is used in a total of 16 products. Some of the trade names of kojic acid having skin-whitening usage are AEC Kojic acid, Kojic acid SL, Melanobleach-K, Oristar KA, Rita KA and Tonelite Kojic acid. Besides these there are trade name mixtures in markets Botacenta SLC 175, Dermawhite HS, Melarrest A, Melarrest L and Vegewhite (Burnett, 2011; FDA, 2009).

The development of tyrosinase inhibitors is of great concern in the medical, agricultural, and cosmetic fields. Among the many kinds of tyrosinase inhibitors, kojic acid has been intensively studied. It acts as a good chelator of transition metal ions such as Cu^{2+} and Fe^{3+} and a scavenger of free radicals. This fungal metabolite is currently applied as a cosmetic skin-lightening agent and food additive to prevent enzymatic browning. Kojic acid shows a competitive inhibitory effect on the monophenolase activity and a mixed inhibitory effect on the diphenolase activity of mushroom tyrosinase. However, its use in cosmetics has been limited, because of the skin irritation caused by its cytotoxicity and its instability during storage. Accordingly, many semi-synthetic kojic acid derivatives have been synthesized to improve its properties by converting the alcoholic hydroxyl group into an ester, hydroxyphenyl ether, glycoside, amino acid derivatives, or tripeptide derivatives (Kang, 2009; Lee, 2006).

2.2 Some studies on synthetic kojic acid derivatives

Recently, it was found that kojic acid-tripeptide amides showed similar tyrosinase inhibitory activities to those of kojic acid-tripeptide free acids but exhibited superior storage stability than those of kojic acid and kojic acid tripeptide free acids (Noh, 2007). To find further kojic acid derivatives with higher tyrosinase inhibitory activity, stability, and synthetic efficiency, a library of kojic acid-amino acid amides (KA-AA-NH_2) prepared and screened for their tyrosinase inhibitory activities. It was also confirmed that the kojic acid-phenylalanine amides reduced the amount of dopachrome production during the melanin formation. It was suggested that a tyrosinase inhibition mechanism of KA-AA-NH_2 based on the possible hydrophobic interactions between the side chain of KA-AA-NH_2 and tyrosinase active site by a docking program (Noh, 2009; Kim, 2004).

Kojic acid is a potential inhibitor of NF-κB(transcription factor) activation in human keratinocytes, and suggests the hypothesis that NF-κB activation may be involved in kojic acid induced anti-melanogenic effect. It was reported that the inhibitory effect of kojic acid on the activation of NF-κB in two human keratinocytes and suggest the hypothesis that the modulation of NF-κB in keratinocytes may be involved in anti-melanogenic effect induced by kojic acid (Moon, 2001).

The metal complexes of kojic acid-phenylalanine-amide exhibited potent tyrosinase inhibitory activity both *in vitro* enzyme test and in cell-based assay system. These results demonstrated that metal complex formation could be applied as a delivery system for hydrophilic molecules which have low cell permeability into cells. In addition, these new materials can be used as an effective whitening agent in the cosmetic industry or applied on irregular hyperpigmentation (Kwak, 2010). Furthermore, kojic acid was shown to inhibit different enzymes relevant to the undesirable melanosis of agricultural products, which is related to its coordination ability to, e.g., copper, in the active site of tyrosinase (Naik, 1979; Stenson, 2007; Synytsya, 2008). The kojic acid scaffold was modified by a Mannich reaction with piperidine derivatives with the aim to link it to Ru(II)–arene fragments and to obtain compounds with anticancer activity (Kasser, 2010).

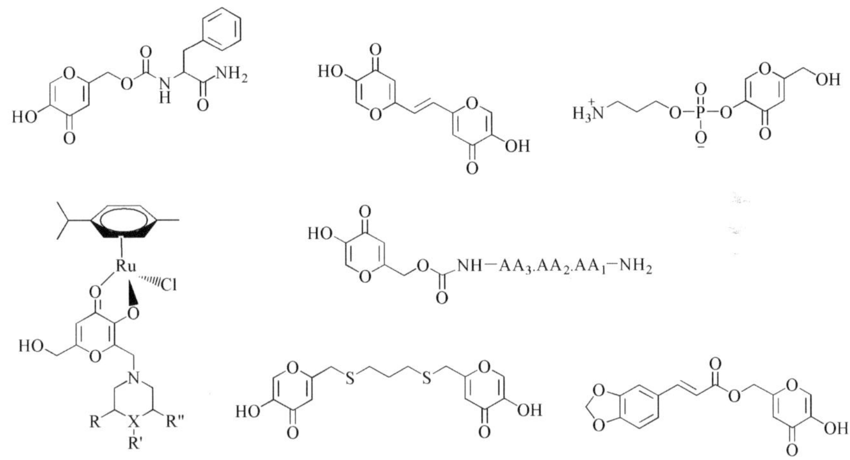

Fig. 3. Chemical structure of some synthetic kojic acid derivatives as tyrosinase inhibitors.

It was reported that compound, joining to two pyrone rings of kojic acid through an ethylene linkage, exhibited 8 times more potent mushroom tyrosinase inhibitory activity than that of kojic acid and also showed superior melanin synthesis inhibitory activity using B16F10 melanoma cell (Lee, 2006). A series of kojic acid derivatives containing thioether, sulfoxide and sulfone linkages were synthesized. Sulfoxide and sulfone derivatives decreased and kojyl thioether derivatives containing appropriate lipophilic various alkyl chains increased tyrosinase inhibitory activity (Rho, 2010). Kojic acid derivatives, containing ester linkages such as hydrophobic benzoate or cinnamate groups, increased the inhibitory activity of kojic acid. When the enolic hydroxyl group of ester derivatives was protected by a methyl group the activity was lost completely. These results indicated that the kojic acid moiety may have blocked the copper active site of tyrosinase (Rho, 2011). 5-[(3-aminopropyl)phosphinooxyl]-2-(hydroxymethyl-4*H*-pyran-4-one (Kojyl-APPA) was showed tyrosinase inhibition effect *in situ*, but not *in vitro*. It means that Kojyl-APPA was converted to kojic acid and 3-aminopropane phosphoric acid enzymatically in cells. Kojyl-APPA was showed the inhibitory activity to same extent as kojic acid on melanin synthesis in mouse melanoma and normal human melanocytes (Kim, 2003).

In a recent study, the correlations of the inhibition of cell-free mushroom tyrosinase activity with that of cellular tyrosinase activity and melanin formation in A2058 melanoma cell line using kojic acid were evaluated. Kojic acid (10 µM) exhibited the best inhibitory effects with % inhibition values 33.3, 52.7 and 52.5 respectively against mushroom tyrosinase activity, cellular tyrosinase activity and cellular melanin formation. Also, ultraviolet A irradiation of melanoma cells A2058 markedly improved the correlation between the inhibition of cellular tyrosinase and of melanin formation (Song, 2009).

Kojic acid contains a polyfunctional heterocyclic, oxygen containing ring with several important centers enabling additional reactions like as oxidation and reduction, alkylation and acylation, substitution nucleophilic reactions, substitution electrophilic reactions, a ring opening of the molecule, and chelation (Aytemir, 1999; Brtko, 2004; Dehkordi, 2008; O'Brien, 1960; Pace, 2004). Since kojic acid is freely soluble in water, ethanol, acetone, and sparingly soluble in ether, ethylacetate, and chloroform, its various derivatives were advantageously prepared (Brtko, 2004; Burdock, 2001; Krivankova, 1992).

Kojic acid provides a promising skeleton for development of new more potent derivatives such as chlorokojic acid (2-chloromethyl-5-hydroxy-4*H*-pyran-4-one), allomaltol (5-hydroxy-2-methyl-4*H*-pyran-4-one) and pyromeconic acid (3-hydroxy-4*H*-pyran-4-one) (Fig. 4). Allomaltol was synthesized from commercially available kojic acid in a two-step reaction according to the literature (Aytemir, 2004; 2010a; 2010b). Chlorination of the 2-hydroxymethyl moiety of kojic acid using thionyl chloride at room temperature afforded chlorokojic acid, with the ring hydroxyl being unaffected. Reduction of chlorokojic acid with zinc dust in concentrated hydrochloric acid resulted in the production of allomaltol (Scheme 2) (Aytemir, 2004; 2010a; 2010b; Ellis 1996).

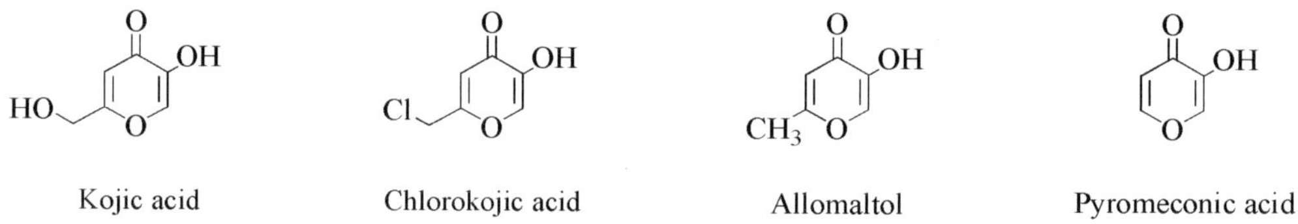

Fig. 4. Hydroxypyranone derivatives.

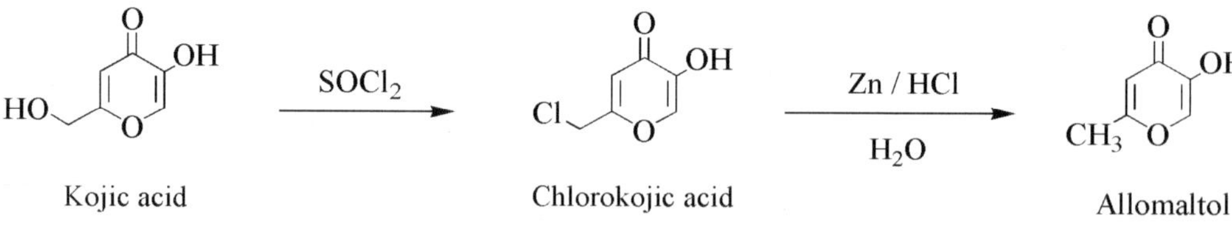

Scheme 2. Synthesis of some hydroxypyrone derivatives from kojic acid.

Wolf and Westveer showed that chlorokojic acid contains catechol group-inhibited *Aeromonas aerogenes, Micrococcus pyogenes* var. *aureus, Salmonella typhosa, Penicilium digitalum, Russula nigricans* and *Saccharomyces cerevisiae* (Wolf, 1950). Also, chlorokojic acid and other halogen derivatives have significant antifungal activity. Moreover, their copper(II) salts' complex derivatives were prepared and found to be more active than chlorokojic acid (Brtko, 2004). Chlorokojic acid was found to be more potent inhibitor of tyrosinase than kojic acid. Moreover, allomaltol has been described as a treatment for pigmentation disorders, sunburn prevention and as an antioxidant for oils and fats (Wempe, 2009). Ester derivatives of allomaltol were described as new tyrosinase inhibitors.

It is well known that hydroxypyranones can exist in cationic and anionic forms due to the protonation or deprotonation reactions, respectively. The hydroxyl group that is directly bound to the pyranone ring was probable more deprotonated than the hydroxymethyl group. The results of quantum mechanical investigations on tautomeric equilibria of kojic acid were determined. Because of two intramolecular hydrogen bonds, the enolic structure of neutral kojic acid is expected to be the most stable one. One of these two bonds is located between keto and hydroxyl group and the other hydrogen bond can be formed weakly between hydroxymethyl moiety and intra-ring oxygen (Beelik, 1955).

On the other hand, kojic acid and other hydroxypyranones having catechol groups are also known as effective metal chelation agents which form complexes with various metal ions that are potentially useful in medicinal therapy. These complexes have reasonable hydrolytic stability, neutral charge, and significant lipophilicity (Masoud, 1989; Thompson, 2001). Additionally, kojic acid and its derivatives have shown to possess various pharmacological activities such as herbicidal (Veverka, 1990; 1990), anti-speck (Uchino, 1988), pesticide and insecticide (Higa, 2007; Kahn, 1997; Uher, 1994), antitumor (Uher, 1994; Yamato, 1987), anti-diabetes (Xiong, 2008), slight anti-inflammatory effects (Brtko, 2004), antiproliferative properties (Fickova, 2008) antiepileptic (Aytemir, 2004, 2006, 2007, 2010a, 2010b) and antiviral (Aytemir, 2010c, 2011) activity.

3. Mannich derivatives with biological activities

Multicomponent reactions are the major parts of the synthetic organic chemistry with advantages ranging from lower reaction times and temperatures to higher yields. Mannich-type reactions are a three component condensation reaction involving carbonyl compounds, which exist as keto-enol tautomeric forms, formaline and a primary or secondary amine. Due to phenol-like properties of kojic acid readily undergoes aminomethylation in the Mannich reaction *ortho* to enolic hydroxyl group at room temperature. It was reported that di-Mannich derivatives which were formed at 3- and 6-positions, were obtained in an acidic medium by the reaction of kojic acid, formaline and aromatic amine derivatives. Woods has reported di-Mannich derivatives were obtained in an acidic medium from kojic acid, formaline and aromatic amine (Woods, 1946). However, O'Brien *et al.* showed that derivatives of Mannich bases occurred at only 6-position of kojic acid, which were synthesized using dimethylamine, diethylamine, pyrrolidine, morpholine, piperidine or 4-methylpiperazine, and chlorokojic acid. Additionally, 6-morpholino or piperidinomethyl chlorokojic acid were prepared via Mannich reaction (O'Brien, 1960). At the latter study, Mannich bases of kojic acid and pyromeconic acid were synthesized in either acidic and basic medium using aliphatic or heterocyclic secondary amines such as dimethylamine, diethylamine or morpholine, respectively (Ichimoto, 1965).

Using the methodology shown in Scheme 3, having 6-chloromethyl/hydroxymethyl/methyl-3-hydroxy-2-substituted 4*H*-pyran-4-one structure, 130 derivatives were synthesized as Mannich bases. The basic substituent was introduced in the 6-position of allomaltol/chlorokojic acid/kojic acid via a Mannich-type reaction, using formaline and an appropriate substituted piperidine, piperazine and morpholine derivatives in methanol at room temperature (Scheme 3). The reaction proceeded very rapidly (Aytemir, 2004, 2006, 2007, 2010a, 2010b, 2010c, 2011 and unpublished data).

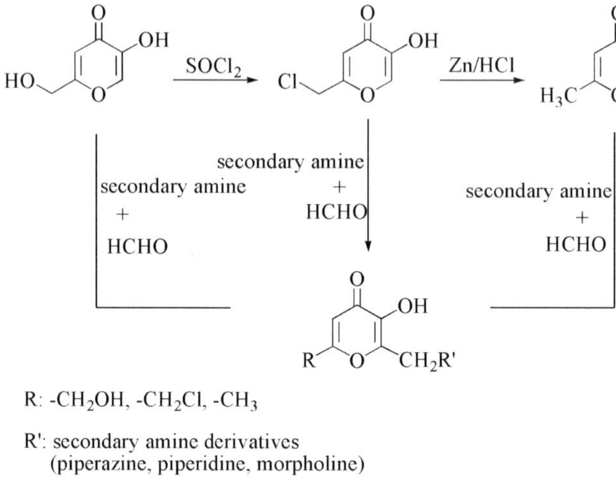

Scheme 3. Synthesis of Mannich bases of kojic acid/chlorokojic acid/allomaltol.

Structure of some Mannich bases was determined by X-Ray analysis. The conformation of the molecule is determined by intra- and intermolecular hydrogen bonds. Some weak intramolecular interactions helped to stabilize the structure. The piperazine ring displayed an almost perfect chair conformation (İskeleli, 2005; Köysal, 2004; Ocak, 2004).

3.1 Anticonvulsant activity

In our previous studies, we reported that Mannich bases of 3-hydroxy-6-hydroxymethyl/methyl-2-substituted *4H*-pyran-4-one derivatives anticonvulsant activity (Aytemir, 2004, 2006, 2007, 2010a, 2010b). Anticonvulsant activity was examined by maximal electroshock (MES) and subcutaneous Pentylenetetrazol (scPTZ)-induced seizure tests. Substitution of different lipophilic phenyl derivatives at 4th position of piperazine ring enables penetration of the blood-brain barrier. The effects of mono substitution of an electron donating or electron-withdrawing groups at the ortho, meta and para position of the phenyl group were examined. According to the results, these compounds, especially 4-chlorophenyl and 3-trifluoromethylphenylpiperazine derivatives, had valuable anticonvulsant activity against scPTZ and MES induced seizure tests (Aytemir, 2004). When substituted piperidine derivatives and morpholine ring at 2nd positions of allomaltol (Fig. 1) were used instead of piperazine ring, anticonvulsant activity of these Mannich bases derivatives was decreased (Aytemir, 2007, 2010a). Both kojic acid and allomaltol derivatives including 4-chloro and 3-trifluoromethylphenylpiperazine were determined to be protective against all seizures. When the effect of different piperazine ring upon activity examined, kojic acid derivatives were found to be more active than allomaltol derivatives. The difference between these two starting materials is just methyl or hydroxymethyl groups at 6th positions at pyranone ring. On the other hand, when the results of the studies are compared to each other, replacement of hydroxymethyl with methyl group at 6th position at pyranone ring increases the protective effect against both tests, because of two hydrogen bonds of kojic acid, which are located between keto and hydroxyl group and/or hydroxymethyl moiety and intra-ring oxygen (Aytemir, 2010b).

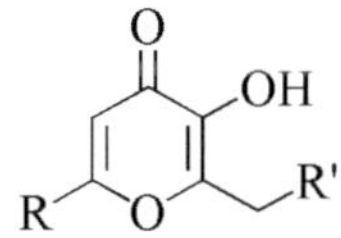

R	R′	MES		scPTZ	
		0.5 h (mg/kg)	4 h (mg/kg)	0.5 h (mg/kg)	4 h (mg/kg)
-CH$_3$	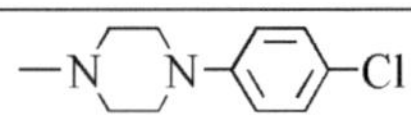	30	300	-	300
-CH$_3$	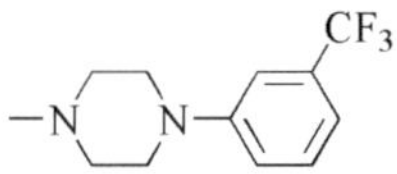	-	300	300	30
-CH$_3$	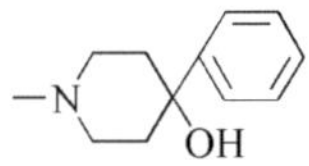	300	30	30	-
-CH$_3$	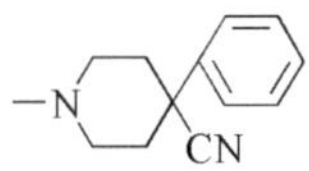	100	300	30	-
-CH$_3$	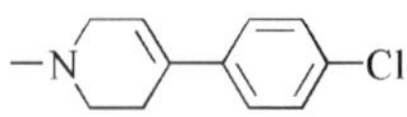	100	30	-	30
-CH$_2$OH	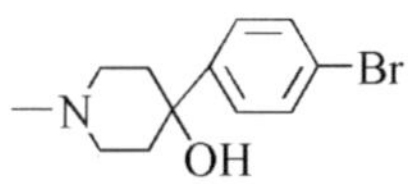	300	-	30	30
-CH$_2$OH	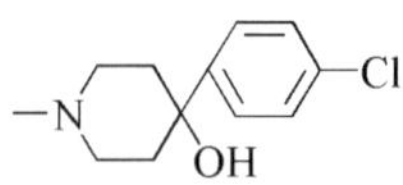	300	-	-	30
-CH$_2$OH	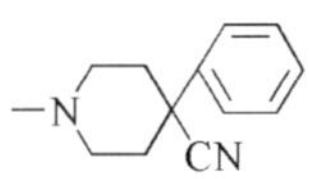	-	-	-	30
-CH$_2$OH	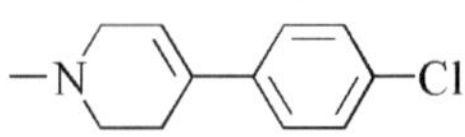	-	30	100	300
-CH$_2$OH	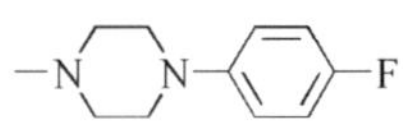	-	300	30	100
-CH$_2$OH	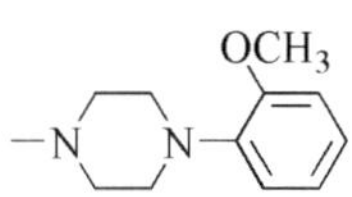	-	-	30	30
-CH$_2$OH	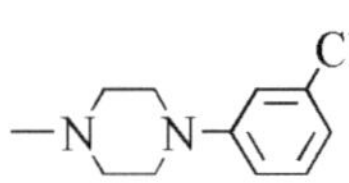	300	-	300	30
-CH$_2$OH	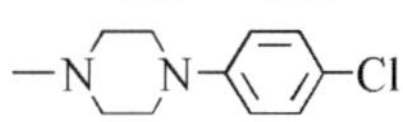	30	30	100	300
-CH$_2$OH	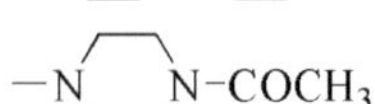	30	300	-	-

Table 1. Anticonvulsant activities of the synthesized compounds.

3.2 Antiviral activity

All compounds were assayed against both *herpes simplex* virus-1 (*HSV*-1) and human *parainfluenza* virus type 3 (*PI*-3) by using Madin Darby Bovine Kidney and Vero cell lines with the aim to capture structure relationship in each of the compounds. Acyclovir and oseltamivir were used as control agents. Correlation between toxicity on uninfected cells (Vero, MDBK) and antiviral activity of the synthesis compounds were determined in the same microtiter plate. The results of the antiviral study are presented in Table 2.

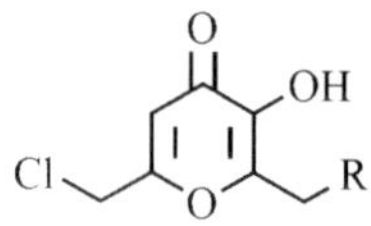

		MDBK Cells			Vero Cells		
	R	MNTCs [a] (µg/mL)	CPE [b] Inhibitory Concentration *HSV*-1 [c]		MNTCs [a] (µg/mL)	CPE [b] Inhibitory Concentration *PI*-3 [d]	
			Max.	Min.		Max.	Min.
1	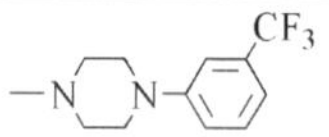	0.8	0.8	0.05	0.8	0.4	0.025
2	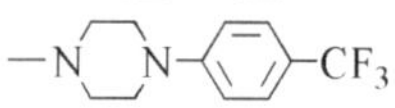	0.8	0.8	0.05	0.4	0.4	0.025
3	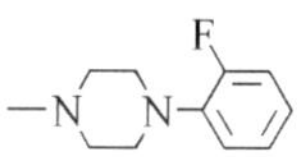	0.8	0.8	0.05	0.8	0.2	0.025
4	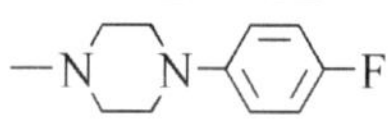	0.8	0.8	0.05	1.6	0.2	0.025
5	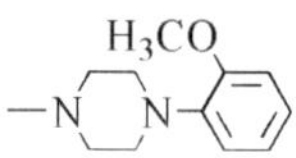	0.8	0.8	0.2	1.6	0.2	0.05
6	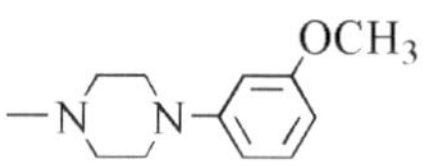	0.8	0.8	0.2	1.6	0.4	0.1
7	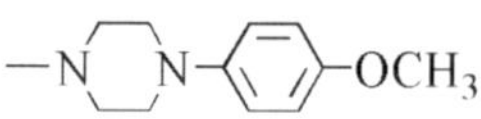	1.6	1.6	0.1	1.6	0.8	0.05
8	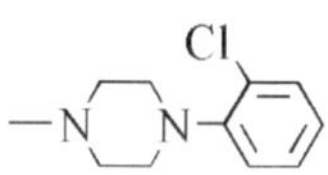	1.6	0.4	0.1	0.4	0.4	0.2
9	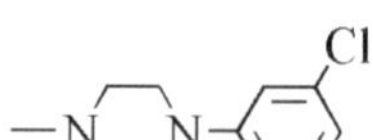	1.6	0.8	0.1	0.8	0.8	0.025
10	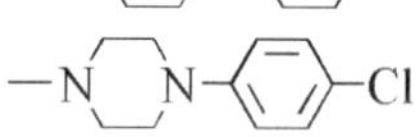	1.6	0.4	0.1	0.4	0.4	0.025
11	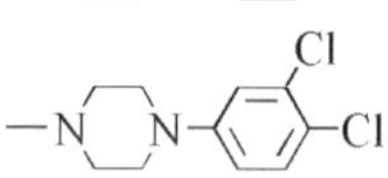	1.6	0.4	0.1	0.4	0.4	0.05

	R	MDBK Cells: MNTCs a) (µg/mL)	MDBK Cells: CPE b) Inhibitory Concentration *HSV*-1 c) Max.	MDBK Cells: CPE b) Inhibitory Concentration *HSV*-1 c) Min.	Vero Cells: MNTCs a) (µg/mL)	Vero Cells: CPE b) Inhibitory Concentration *PI-3* d) Max.	Vero Cells: CPE b) Inhibitory Concentration *PI-3* d) Min.
12	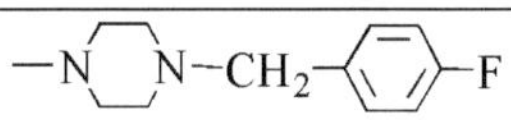	1.6	0.4	0.1	0.4	0.4	0.05
13	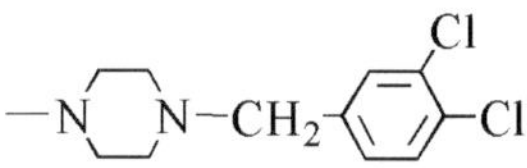	0.4	-	-	0.8	0.8	0.05
14	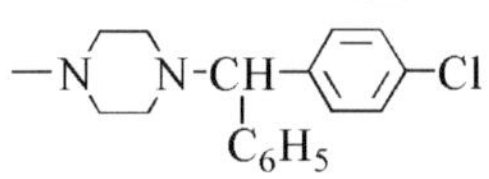	0.4	-	-	0.4	0.2	0.1
15	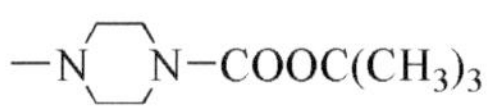	0.8	0.8	0.4	0.4	0.4	0.2
16	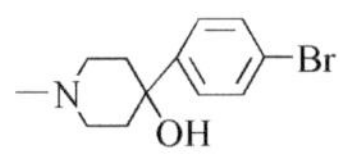	0.4	-	-	0.8	0.2	0.05
17	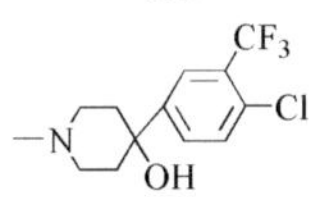	0.8	0.8	0.2	0.4	0.2	0.05
18	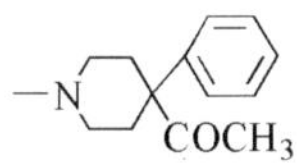	0.4	-	-	0.4	0.4	0.05
	Acyclovir	1.6	1.6	<0.012			
	Oseltamivir	-	-	-	1.6	1.6	<0.012

a) MNTCs: Maximum non-toxic concentrations
b) CPE: Cytopathogenic effect
c) *HSV*-1: *Herpes simplex* virus Type-1
d) *PI-3: Parainfluenza*-3 virus Max: Maximum
Min: Minimum - : Not done; activity observed

Table 2. Cytotoxicity on MDBK and Vero Cells as well as antiviral activity against HSV-1 and PI-3 results of the compounds **1-18**.

As given in CPE inhibitory concentration ranging, compound **7** bearing 4-methoxyphenylpiperazine substituent showed significant activity against *HSV*-1 as potent as the reference compound acyclovir, but limited activity at maximum and minimum concentration ranges of 1.6-<0.1 µg/mL with the maximum non-toxic concentration (MNTCs) value of 1.6 µg/mL. Additionally, compound **9** (0.8-0.1 µg/mL) was shown anti-*Herpes simplex* activity but less potent. On the other hand, compounds **1-4** were shown as same activity as compound **7** but on higher non-toxic concentrations (MNTC: 0.8 µg/mL). Among the tested Mannich bases derivatives, compounds **5**, **6**, **8**, **10**, and **11** were less active against DNA virus. Take into account CPE inhibitory concentration ranging against the

RNA viruses *PI*-3, compound **9** (0.8-0.025 μg/mL) and compound **13** (0.8-0.05 μg/mL) had remarkable antiviral activity in Mannich base derivatives. Furthermore, compounds **1, 7, 12** and **18** were less active than compounds **9** and **13**. While the activities of compounds **2** and **10** (0.4-0.025 μg/mL) against *PI*-3 were in similar CPE inhibitory concentration range, compounds **3, 4** and **11** had lower activity than those had. Also, compounds **5** and **6** were negligible values as seen in Table 2. Compounds **12** and **17** showed anti-*Herpes simplex* activity with less potency. While the activities of compounds **12** and **18** (0.4-0.05 μg/mL) against *PI*-3 were in similar CPE inhibitory concentration range, compounds **5** and **6** had lower activity than those that had (Aytemir, 2010c, 2011).

3.3 Antimicrobial activity

The antibacterial and antifungal activity profiles of the newly synthesized compounds were assessed for antimicrobial activity against both standard and the isolated strains of bacteria. For antibacterial activity assessment, standard strains (*Escherichia coli, Pseudomonas aeruginosa, Proteus mirabilis, Klebsiella pneumoniae, Acinetobacter baumannii, Staphylococcus aureus, Enterococcus faecalis* and *Bacillus subtilis*) and their drug-resistant isolates were tested; and for antifungal activity *Candida albicans* and *C. parapsilosis* were used. Ampicillin, vancomycin, gentamicin, ofloxacin, levofloxacin, ketoconazole, and fluconazole were also tested under identical conditions for comparison in antibacterial and antifungal assays, respectively. Tables 3 and 4 describe the *in vitro* antimicrobial activity with MIC values of compounds **1-18**.

According to our data (Table 3 and 4), the synthesized compounds showed a broad spectrum of activity against gram positive and gram negative standard strains with MIC values between 1 and 64 μg/mL. In the meantime, the synthesized compounds showed activity against drug-resistant isolated both gram positive and negative strains with MIC values of 2 to ≥128 μg/mL.

As given in Table 3, the antibacterial activity against gram negative bacteria of the synthesized compounds **14, 16**, and **17** bearing (4-chlorophenyl)benzylpiperazine, 4-bromophenyl-4-hydroxypiperidine and 4-chloro-3-(trifluoromethyl) phenyl-4-hydroxypiperidine moiety respectively at the 2-position of pyran-4-one ring, was found to have significantly high antibacterial potential against standard strains of *E. coli, P. aeruginosa, K. pneumoniae, A. baumannii* with a bacterial inhibition between 2 and 4 μg/mL. Also, these compounds showed more activity (MIC: 2 μg/mL) against *E. coli* and *P. aeruginosa* than the other gram negative bacteria compared with control drugs ampicillin (MIC: 2 μg/mL), ofloxacin (1 μg/mL) and levofloxacin (1 μg/mL). As for compounds **13** and **15**, it was found that they had the same effect against all gram negative bacteria. The MIC values of both compounds were 4 μg/mL against *P. aeruginosa*; 8 μg/mL against *E. coli, K. pneumoniae*, and *A. baumannii*; and 16 μg/mL against *P. mirabilis*. Furthermore, in comparison, compound **18** had similar antibacterial activity with MIC values between 4 and 16 μg/mL as these (compounds **13** and **15**). In the entire series, compounds **1-7, 9, 12** was less effective (MIC: 16-32 μg/mL) and compound **18** with MIC values between 4 and 16 μg/mL towards standard strains of all gram negative bacteria. Especially, compound **13** which has 3,4-dichlorobenzylpiperazine moiety showed remarkable activity against ESβL(+)

strains of *E. coli* and *K. pneumoniae* with MIC values of 4 μg/mL, compared with the reference drugs, ampicillin (MIC: ≥128 μg/mL), ofloxacin (MIC: 0.5 μg/mL) and levofloxacin, (MIC: 0.5-1 μg/mL) respectively. As for structure-activity relationship (SAR), fluoro substitution in *para* position of the benzyl ring (compound **12**) has the worst activity with MIC values between 16 and 32 μg/mL in this series, whereas the 3,4-dichloro substitution (compound **13**) of benzyl ring increases antibacterial activity with four-folds (MIC: 4-8 μg/mL) towards isolated strains of *A. baumannii* and *P. aeruginosa* and two-folds (MIC: 8 μg/mL) against *E. coli* and *K. pneumoniae.* Moreover, antibacterial activity of the compounds **12** and **13** against *P. mirabilis* was determined to be the same. Furthermore, compounds **13** and **15** showed same activity against all bacteria except from *P. aeruginosa.* In the Mannich base derivatives bearing piperazine ring, compound **14** was the most remarkable and active one (MIC: 2-8 μg/mL). There were diphenyl rings in the structure of in which one of them was a p-chlorophenyl ring and the other a nonsubstituted phenyl ring. When compounds **13** and **15** were compared, the addition of phenyl ring on the structure of compound **14** increased the activity two-folds against all gram negative bacteria and *S. aureus.* When antibacterial activities of compounds **16-18** possessing piperidine ring were investigated, it was observed that compounds **16** and **17** were found to have the same activity and higher effect than compound **18** without halogen substitution at its structure. Hence, when hydroxy substitution at the 4-position of piperidine ring was changed with acetyl, antibacterial activity was decreased. In addition, there was no difference in the antimicrobial activity with the location and type of the halogen substituted on phenyl ring. Also, these compounds (**16** and **17**) had exactly the same activity as compound **18** possessing piperazine ring against all gram negative bacteria.

Among gram positive bacteria, *S. aureus* has been recognized for so long as one of the major resistant pathogens that can cause diseases in humans. Likewise, multi-drug resistant Enterococci have become a serious threat for public health. High level resistance for penicillin and aminoglycosides are being reported of this bacterium. According to the obtained data (Table 4), antibacterial activity results of compounds **13-18** (MIC: 1-2 μg/mL) and 8-11 (MIC: 8 μg/mL) against standard gram positive bacteria were encouraging, although compound **1-7** and **12** were found to manifest moderate (MIC: 16-64 μg/mL) activity against standard strains of *S. aureus.* Compounds **13-18** were found to be highly active against *B. subtilis* showing a bacterial inhibition value at 1 μg/mL. The antibacterial potential against *E. faecalis* was exhibited by compounds **2**, **8-11**, and **15** at concentration 8 μg/mL among the synthesized compounds. *Candida* species are the most widespread and threatening fungal pathogens today, and are responsible for many of the invasive and non-invasive fungal infections. Among all *Candida* species, *Candida albicans* is the most frequent pathogen. The results obtained clearly indicate that the series of Mannich bases discussed here are active towards growth inhibition of pathogenic fungi. In general, **1-7** (MIC: 8 μg/mL) and **13-18** (MIC: 4 μg/mL) exhibited excellent antifungal activity against *C. albicans* and at MIC values at 8 μg/mL against *C. parapsilosis* when compared to the reference drugs, ketoconazole (MIC: 1 μg/mL) and fluconazole (MIC: 2-4 μg/mL). The compounds **1-7** and **13-18** may be promoted as fungicides. In general, the compounds showed an improved antibacterial activity when compared to their antifungal activity (Aytemir, 2010c, 2011).

	Gram-negative Standard and Clinic Isolated Strains									
	E. coli	*P. aeruginosa*		*P. mirabilis*		*K. pneumoniae*		*A. baumannii*		
	ATCC 35218	Isolated strain ESβL+	ATCC 10145	Isolated strain	ATCC 7002	Isolated Strain ESβL+	RSKK 574	Isolated Strain ESβL+	RSKK 02026	Isolated strain
1	16	64	16	64	16	64	16	64	32	64
2	16	64	16	64	16	64	32	64	16	64
3	16	64	32	64	32	64	16	64	32	64
4	16	64	32	64	16	64	16	64	32	64
5	32	64	32	64	32	64	32	64	32	64
6	32	64	32	64	32	64	32	64	32	64
7	32	64	16	64	32	64	16	32	16	32
8	64	>128	64	>128	64	>128	64	>128	64	>128
9	32	64	32	64	32	64	32	64	32	64
10	64	>128	64	>128	64	>128	64	>128	64	>128
11	64	64	16	64	32	64	32	64	64	32
12	16	64	16	64	16	64	16	64	32	64
13	8	4	4	16	16	64	8	4	8	16
14	4	64	2	16	8	64	4	64	4	16
15	8	64	4	16	16	64	8	64	8	16
16	4	64	2	16	8	64	4	64	4	16
17	4	64	2	16	8	64	4	64	4	16
18	8	64	4	16	16	64	8	64	4	16
AMP [a)]	2	>128	-	-	2	>128	2	>128	2	>128
OFX [b)]	0.12	-	0.5	2	-	-	-	-	-	-
LVX [c)]	<0.12	0.5	1	64	<0.12	1	<0.12	0.5	0.12	64

[a)] AMP: ampicillin,
[b)] OFX: ofloxacin,
[c)] LVX: levofloxacin
-: No activity observed, *E. coli* isolates; (resist to trimethoprim-sulfamethoxazole, cefepime, tazobactam), *P. aeruginosa* isolates (resist to Trimethoprim-Sulfamethoxazole, tazobactam), *P.mirabilis* isolates (resist to trimethoprim-sulfamethoxazole, cefepime, tazobactam), *K. pneumoniae* isolates (resist to trimethoprim-sulfamethoxazole, amoxicillin clavulonate, ceftriaxone, cefepime, aztreonam) *A. baumannii* isolates (resist to trimethoprim-sulfamethoxazole, cefepime).

Table 3. Antibacterial activity of the synthesized compounds **1-18** and the control drugs (MIC in μg/mL).

Comp.	Gram-positive standard and Clinic Isolated Strain Bacteria						Fungi	
	S. aureus		*E. faecalis*		*B. subtilis*		*C. albicans*	*C. parapsilosis*
	ATCC 25923	Isolated Strain MRSA	ATCC 29212	Isolated Strain	ATCC 6633	Isolated Strain	ATCC 10231	ATCC 22019
1	32	64	16	32	32	64	8	8
2	16	64	8	32	8	64	8	8
3	16	64	16	32	8	16	8	8
4	16	64	16	32	16	32	8	8
5	64	128	64	128	16	32	8	8
6	64	128	64	128	16	32	8	8
7	32	64	32	64	32	64	8	8
8	8	>128	8	>128	16	>128	16	16
9	8	128	8	128	16	32	16	16
10	8	>128	8	>128	16	>128	16	16
11	8	64	8	64	16	64	16	16
12	32	64	16	32	32	64	16	16
13	2	128	16	128	1	2	4	8
14	1	64	16	32	1	2	4	8
15	2	128	8	128	1	2	4	8
16	1	64	16	32	1	2	4	8
17	1	64	16	32	1	2	4	8
18	2	128	64	128	1	2	4	8
AMP[a)]	<0.12	>128	0.5	>128	0.12	0.5	-	-
VAN[b)]	0.12	2	-	-	-	-	-	-
OFX[c)]	0.25	64	1	32	-	-	-	-
LVX[d)]	0.25	128	0.5	32	-	-	-	-
KET[e)]	-	-	-	-	-	-	1	1
FLU[f)]	-	-	-	-	-	-	2	4

[a)] AMP: ampicillin,
[b)] VAN: vancomycin,
[c)] OFX: ofloxacin,
[d)] LVX: levofloxacin,
[e)] KET; ketoconazole,
[f)] FLU: fluconazole
-: No activity observed, *S. aureus* isolates (resist to oxacillin, gentamicin, aztreonam, trimethoprim-sulfamethoxazole), *E. faecalis* isolates (resist to cephalosporins & beta-lactam), *B. subtilis* isolates (resist to ceftriaxone).

Table 4. Antibacterial and antifungal activities of the synthesized compounds **1-18** and the control drugs (MIC in μg/mL).

4. Conclusions

A number of research groups around the world are engaged and are expending much effort in the discovery of tyrosinase inhibitors. Various limitations are associated with many of these inhibitors, such as high cytotoxicity, poor skin penetration and low stability in formulations. Therefore, it is very important to discover novel and potent inhibitors with potent activity and lower side effect.

Kojic acid is currently used as tyrosinase inhibitors which are commercially available. Unfortunately, unstability during storage limits its use and new tyrosinase inhibitors of novel kojic acid derivatives are needed in cosmetics industry. More expended studies on this subject will be helpful in designing more suitable tyrosinase inhibitors for human use.

In our continuing search, a huge number of Mannich bases are being examined as inhibiting mushroom tyrosinase activity at the moment, and few of them will have confirmed in melanogenesis inhibiting activity in cell or skin models. Mannich bases compounds are more hydrophobic than kojic acid. Therefore, disadvantages of kojic acid might be decreased by increasing skin penetration and stability in formulation. In the light of these findings we will undertake further synthetic and biological studies on the new compounds in the future.

5. Acknowledgement

The authors thank to TUBITAK (Project no: TBAG 2021) and Hacettepe Univ. Research Center Office (Project no: 03 02 301 001, 09D01301002) and L'Oréal Türkiye Fellowships for Young Women in Science supported by The Turkish Academy of Sciences for financial support.

6. References

Alverson, J. (2003) Effects of mycotoxins, kojic acid and oxalic acid, on biological fitness of *Lygus hesperus* (Heteroptera: Miridae) *J. Inverteb. Pathol.*, Vol.83, pp.60-62.

Aoyagi N.; Kimura R.; Murata T. (1974)Studies on *Passiflora incarnata* Dry Extract. I. Isolation of Maltol and Pharmacological Action of Maltol and Ethyl Maltol, *Chem. Pharm. Bull.*, Vol.22(5), pp.1008-1013.

Aytemir, M.D.; Uzbay, T.; Erol, D.D. (1999) New 4(1H)-pyridinone Derivatives as Analgesic Agents. *Arzneim.-Forsch./Drug Res.* Vol.49(1), pp.250-254.

Aytemir, M.D.; Hider, R.C.; Erol, D.D.; Özalp, M.; Ekizoğlu, M. (2003a) Synthesis of New Antimicrobial Agents; Amide Derivatives of Pyranones and Pyridinones, *Turk J. Chem.*, Vol.27(4), pp.445-52.

Aytemir, M.D.; Erol, D.D.; Hider, R.C.; Özalp, M. (2003b) Synthesis and Evaluation of Antimicrobial Activity of New 3-Hydroxy-6-methyl-4-oxo-4*H*-pyran-2-carboxamide Derivatives, *Turk J. Chem.*, Vol.27(6), pp.757-64.

Aytemir, M.D.; Çalış, Ü.; Özalp, M. (2004) Synthesis and Evaluation of Anticonvulsant and Antimicrobial Activities of 3-Hydroxy-6-methyl-2-substituted 4*H*-Pyran-4-one Derivatives. *Arch. Pharm. Pharm. Med. Chem.* Vol.337, pp.281-288.

Aytemir, M.D.; Çalış, Ü. (2006) Synthesis of Some New Hydroxypyranone Derivatives and Evaluation of Their Anticonvulsant Activities. *FABAD J. Pharm. Sci.* Vol.31, pp.23-29.

Aytemir, M. D.; Çalış, Ü. (2007) Synthesis of some novel mannich bases derived from allomaltol and evaluation of their anticonvulsant activities. *H U J Fac Pharm,* Vol.27(1), pp.1-10.

Aytemir, M.D., Septioğlu, E., Çalış, Ü. (2010a). Synthesis and anticonvulsant activity of new kojic acid derivatives. *Arzneim. Forsch. Drug Res.,* Vol.60(1), pp.22-29.

Aytemir, M.D.; Çalış, Ü. (2010b) Anticonvulsant and Neurotoxicity Evaluation of Some Novel Kojic Acids and Allomaltol Derivatives. *Archiv Pharm. Med. Chem. Life Sci.* Vol.343(3), pp.173-181.

Aytemir, M.D.; Özçelik, B. (2010c) A study of cytotoxicity of novel chlorokojic acid derivatives with their antimicrobial and antiviral activities. *Eur. J. Med. Chem.* Vol.45, pp.4089-4095.

Aytemir, M.D.; Özçelik, B. (2011) Synthesis and biological activities of new Mannich bases of chlorokojic acid derivatives. *Med. Chem. Res.* Vol.20, pp.443-452.

Barret, M.C.; Mahon, M.F.; Molloy, K.C.; Steed, J.W.; Wright, P. (2001) Synthesis and structural characterisation of Tin(II) and Zinc(II) derivatives of cyclic α-Hydroxyketones, including the structures of $Sn(maltol)_2$, $Sn(tropolone)_2$, $Zn(tropolone)_2$ and $Zn(hinokitiol)_2$. *Inorg. Chem.,* Vol.40, pp.4384-4388.

Beelik, A.; Purves, C. B. (1955) Some new reactions and derivatives of kojic acid. *Can. J. Chem. Soc.,* Vol.33, pp.1361.

Bentley, R. (2006). From *miso, saké* and *shoyu* to cosmetics: a century of science for kojic acid. *Nat. Prod. Rep.* Vol.23 pp.1046-1062.

Brtko, J.; Rondahl, L.; Fickova, M.; Hudecova, D.; Eybl, V.; Uher, M. (2004). Kojic acid and its derivatives: History and present state of art. *Cent. Eur. J. Publ. Health,* Vol.12, pp.16-18.

Briganti, S.; Camera, E.; Picardo, M. (2003) Chemical and Instrumental Approaches to Treat Hyperpigmentation. Pigment Cell Res. Vol.16, pp.101-110.

Burdock, G. A.; Soni, M.; Carabin, I. G. (2001) Evaluation of health aspects of kojic acid in food. *Regul. Toxic. Pharm.* Vol.33, pp.80-101.

Burnett, C.L.; Bergfeld, W.F.; Belsito, D.V.;. Hill, R.A.; Klaassen, C.D.; Liebler, D.C.; Marks, J.G.; Shank, R.C.; Slaga, T.J.; Snyder, P.W.; Andersen, F.A. (2010) Final Report of the Safety Assessment of Kojic Acid as Used in Cosmetics. *Int. J. Toxic.* Vol.29(4), pp.244-273.

Cabanes, J.; Chazarra, S.; Carmona, F.G. (1994). Kojic Acid, a cosmetic skin whitening agent, is a slow-binding inhibitor of catecholase activity of tyrosinase. *J. Pharm. Pharmacol.* Vol.46, pp.982-985.

Cecconi, F.; Ghilardi, C.A.; Ienco, A.; Mariani, P.; Mealli, C.; Midollini, S.; Orlandini, A.; Vacca, A. (2002) Different complexation properties of some hydroxy keto heterocycles toward Beryllium(II) in aqueous solutions: Experimental and Theoretical Studies. *Inorg. Chem.,* Vol.42, pp.4006-4017.

Chang, T. S. (2009) An Updated Review of Tyrosinase Inhibitors. *Int. J. Mol. Sci.* Vol.10, 2440-2475.

Chen, J.S.; Wei, C.; Marshall, M.R. (1991) Inhibition Mechanism of Kojic Acid on Polyphenol Oxidase. *J. Agric. Food Chem.* Vol.39(11), pp.1899-1901.

Curto, E.V.; Kwong, C.; Hermersdörfer, H.; Glatt, H.; Santis, C.; Virador, V.; Hearing, V.J. ; Dooley, T.P. (1999) Inhibitors of Mammalian Melanocyte Tyrosinase: *In Vitro* Comparisons of Alkyl Esters of Gentisic Acid with Other Putative Inhibitors. *Biochem. Pharmacol.*, Vol.57, pp.663–672.

Dehkordi, L.S., Liu, Z.D., Hider, R.C. (2008) Basic 3-hydroxypyridine-4-ones: Potential antimalarial agents. *Eur. J. Med. Chem.*, Vol.43, pp.1035-1047.

Ellis, B.L.; Duhme, A.K.; Hider, R.C.; Hossain, M.B.; Rizvi, S.; van der Helm, D. (1996) Synthesis, physicochemical properties, and biological evaluation of hydroxypyranone and hydroxypyridinones: novel bidentate ligands for cell-labeling. *J. Med. Chem.*, Vol.39, pp.3659-3670.

Emami, S.; Hosseinimehr, S.J.; Taghdisi, S.M.; Akhlaghpoor, S. (2007) Kojic acid and its manganase and zinc complexes as potential radioprotective agents. *Bioorg. Med. Chem. Lett.*, Vol.17, pp.45-48.

Fassihi, A.; Abedi, D.; Saghaie, L.; Sabet, R.; Fazeli, H.; Bostaki, G.; Deilami, O.; Sadinpour, H. (2008) Synthesis, antimicrobial evaluation and QSAR study of some 3-hydroxypyridine-4-one and 3-hydroxypyran-4-one. *Eur. J. Med. Chem.* Vol.44, pp.2145-2157.

Food and Drug Administration (FDA), (2009) Frequency of use of Kojic Acid in cosmetic ingredients, FDA database.

Fickova, M.; Pravdova, E.; Rondhai, L.; Uher, M.; Brtko, J. (2008) In vitro antiproliferative and cytotoxic activities of novel kojic acid derivatives: 5-benzyloxy-2-selenocyanotomethyl- and 5-methoxy-2- selenocyanotomethyl-4-pyranone. *J. App. Toxicol.*, Vol.28, pp.554-559.

Finnegan, M.M.; Lutz, T.G.; Nelson, W.O.; Smith, A.; Orvig, C. (1987) Neutral water-soluble post-transition-metal chelate complexes of medical interest: aluminium and gallium tris(3-hydroxy-4-pyronates), *Inorg. Chem.*, Vol.26, pp.2171-2176.

Futamura, T.; Okabe, M.; Tamura, T.; Toda, K.; Matsunobu, T.; Park, Y.S. (2001) Improvement of production of Kojic acid by a mutant strain Aspergillus oryzae, MK107-39. *J. Biosci. Bioeng.*, Vol.91(3), pp.272-276.

Gomes, A.J.; Lunardi, C.N.; Gonzales, S.; Tedesco, A.C. (2001) The antioxidant action of Polypodium leucotomos extract and kojic acid: reactions with reactive oxygen species. *Braz. J. Med. Biol. Res.* Vol.34, pp.1487–1494.

Gupta, A.K.; Gover, M.D.; Nouri, K.; Taylor, S. (2006) The treatment of melasma: A review of clinical trials. *J. Am. Acad. Dermatol.* Vol.55(6), pp.1048-1065.

Higa, Y.; Kawawbe, M.; Nabae, K.; Toda, Y.; Kitamoto, S.; Hara, T.; Tanaka, N.; Kariya, K.; Takahashi, M. (2007) Kojic acid-absence of tumor-initiating activity in rat liver, and of carcinogenic and phoo-genotoxic potential in mouse skin. *J. Toxicol. Sci.*, Vol.32(2), pp.143-159.

Hryniewicz, K.; Stadnicka, K.; Pattek-Janczyk, A. (2009) Crystal structure and vibrational spectra of 2-chloromethyl-5-hydroxy-4*H*-pyran-4-one as potential ligands for Fe (III) complexes. *J. Mol. Struct.* Vol.919, pp.255-270.

Ichimoto, I.; Ueda, H.; Tatsumi C. (1965) Studies on kojic acid and its related γ-Pyrone compounds. Part VII. The alkylation of Kojic Acid and Pyromeconic Acid through their Mannich Base. *Agric. Biol. Chem.*, Vol.1(2), pp.94-98.

İskeleli, N.; Işık, Ş.; Aytemir, M.D. (2005) 3-Hydroxy-2-[4-(2-hydroxyethyl)piperazine-1-yl-methyl]-6-methyl-pyran-4-one. *Acta Cryst. Section* E61, pp.o1947-o1949.

İyidoğan, N.F.; Bayındırlı, A. (2004) Effect of L-cysteine, kojic acid and 4-hexylrezorcinol combination on inhibition of enzymatic browning in Amasya apple juice. *J. Food Eng.* Vol.62, pp.299-304.

Jun, N.; Hong, G.; Jun, K. (2007) Synthesis and evaluation of 20,40,60-trihydroxychalcones as a new class of tyrosinase inhibitors. *Bioorg. Med. Chem.* Vol.15, pp.2396-2402.

Kahn, V.; Ben-Shalom, N.; Zakin, V. (1997) Effect of kojic acid on the oxidation of N-acetyl-dopamine (NADA) by mushroom tyrosinase. *J. Agric. Food Chem.* Vol.45, pp.4460-4465.

Kang, S.S.; Kim, H.J.; Jin, C.; Lee, S.L. (2009) Synthesis of tyrosinase inhibitory (4-oxo-4*H*-pyran-2-yl)acrylic acid ester derivatives. *Bioorg. & Med. Chem. Lett.* Vol.19, pp.188-191.

Kasser, J. H.; Kandioller, W.; Hartinger, C. G.; Nazarov, A. A.; Arion, V. B.; Dyson, P. J.; Keppler, B. K. (2010) Mannich products of kojic acid and N-heterocycles and their Ru(II)–arene complexes: Synthesis, characterization and stability. *J. Organomet. Chem.* Vol.695, pp.875–881.

Kayahara, H.; Shibata, N.; Tadasa, K.; Maeda, H.; Kotani, T.; Ichimoto, I. (1990) Amino acid and Peptide Derivatives of Kojic Acid and Their Antifungal Properties, *Agr. Biol. Chem.*, Vol.54(9), pp.2441-42.

Khan, M.T.H. (2007). Molecular design of tyrosinase inhibitors: A critical review of promising novel inhibitors from synthetic origins. *Pure Appl.Chem.* Vol.29(12), pp.2277-2295.

Kim, D.H.; Hwang, J.S.; Baek, H.S.; Kim, K.J.; Lee, B.G.; Chang, I.; Kang, H.H.; Lee, O.S. (2003) Development of 5-[(3-Aminopropyl)phosphinooxy]-2-(hydroxymethyl)-4H-pyran-4-one as a Novel Whitening Agent. *Chem. Pharm. Bull.* Vol.51(2) pp.113-116.

Kim, H.; Choi, J.; Cho, J.K.; Kim, S.Y.; Lee, Y.S. (2004) Solid phase synthesis of kojic acid-tripeptides and their tyrosinase inhibitory activity, storage stability, and toxicity. *Bioorg. Med. Chem. Lett.* Vol.14, pp.2843-2846.

Kim, Y.J.; Uyama, H. (2005) Tyrosinase inhibitors from natural and synthetic sources: structure, inhibition mechanism and perspective for the future. *Cell. Mol. Life Sci.* Vol.62, pp.1707–1723.

Kimura, R.; Matsui, S.; Ito, S.; Aimoto, T.; Murata, T.; (1980) Central Depressant Effects of Maltol Analogs in Mice, *Chem. Pharm. Bull.*, Vol.28, pp.2570-2579.

Kotani, T.; Ichimoto, I.; Tatsumi, C.; Fujita, T. (1975) Structure-activity Study of Bacteriostatic Kojic Acid Analogs, *Agr. Biol. Chem.*, Vol.39(6), pp.1311-1317.

Köysal, Y., Işık, Ş., Aytemir, M. D. (2004). 3-Hydroxy-6-methyl-2-[4-(3-trifluoro-methylphenyl)piperazine-1-ylmethyl]-4*H*-pyran-4-one. *Acta Cryst. Section* E60, pp.o112-o114.

Krivankova, I.; Marcisinova, M.; Söhnel, O. (1992) Solubility of Itaconic and Kojic Acids. *J. Chem. Eng. Data*, Vol.37, pp.24-28.

Kwak, S.Y.; Noh, J.M.; Park, J.S.H.; Byun, W.; Choi, H.R.; Park, K.C. ; Lee, Y.S. (2010) Enhanced cell permeability of kojic acid–phenylalanine amide with metal complex. *Bioorg. Med. Chem. Lett.* Vol.20, pp.738–741.

Lee, Y.S.; Park, J.H.; Kim, M.H.; Seo, S.H.; Kim, H.J. (2006) Synthesis of Tyrosinase Inhibitory Kojic acid Derivative. *Arch. Pharm. Chem. Life Sci.*, Vol.339, pp.111-114.

Lim, J. (1999) Treatment of Melasma Using Kojic Acid in a Gel Containing Hydroquinone and Glycolic Acid. *Dermatol. Surg.* Vol.25, pp.282-284.

Lin, C.H.; Wu, H.L.; Huang, Y.L. (2007) Combining high-performance liquid chromatography with on-line microdialysis sampling for the simultaneous determination of ascorbyl glucoside, kojic acid, and niacinamide in bleaching cosmetics. *Anal. Chim. Acta*, Vol.581, pp.102-107.

Lin, H.Y., Yang, Y.H., Wu, S.M. (2007) Experimental design and capillary electrophoresis for simultaneous analysis of arbutin, kojic acid and hydroquinone in cosmetics. *J. Pharm. Biomed. Anal.* Vol.44, pp.279-282.

Masoud, M.S.; El-Tahana, S.A.; El-Enein, A. (1989) Palladium(II)-kojic Acid Interaction, *Transition Met. Chem.*, Vol.14, pp.155-156.

Mitani, H.; Koshiishi, I.; Sumita, T.; Imanari, T. (2001) Prevention of photodamage in the hairless mouse dorsal skin by kojic acid as an iron chelator. *Eur. J. Pharm.*, Vol.411, pp.169-174.

Moggia, F.; Brisset, H.; Fages, F.; Chaix, C.; Mandrand, B., Dias, M.; Levillain, E. (2006) Design, Synthesis and Redox Properties of Two Ferrocene-Containing Iron Chelators, *Tetrahedr. Lett.*, Vol.47, pp.3371-74.

Moon, K.Y.; Ahn, K.S.; Lee, J.; Kim, Y.S. (2001) Kojic Acid, a Potential Inhibitor of NF-KB Activation in Transfectant Human HaCaT and SCC-13 Cells. *Arch. Pharm. Res.*, Vol.24(4), pp.307-311.

Naik, D.V. (1979) Interaction of Kojic Acid with Gold(III) Ions. *Analytic. Chim. Acta*, Vol.106, pp.147-50.

Noh, J.M.; Kwak, S.Y.; Kim, D.H.; Lee, Y.S. (2007) Kojic Acid–Tripeptide Amide as a New Tyrosinase Inhibitor. *Biopolymers (Peptide Science)* Vol.88(2), pp.300-307.

Noh, J. M.; Kwak, S. Y.; Seo, H. S.; Kim, B. G.; Lee, Y. S. (2009) *Bioorg. Med. Chem. Lett* Vol.19, pp.5586–5589.

O'Brien, G.J.; Patterson, M.; Meadow, J.R. (1960) Amino derivatives of Kojic acid, *J. Org. Chem.*, Vol.25, pp.86-89.

Ocak, N.; Işık, Ş.; Aytemir, M.D. (2004) Ethyl [4-(3-Hydroxy-6-methyl-4-oxo-4*H*-pyran-2-ylmethyl)piperazine]-1-carboxylate. *Acta Cryst. Section* E60, pp.o561-o563.

Pace, P.; Nizi, E.; Pacini, B.; Pesci, S.; Matassa, V.; Francesco, R.D.; Altamura, S.; Summa, V. (2004) The monoethyl ester of meconic acid is an active site inhibitor of HCV NS5B RNA-dependent RNA polymerase. *Bioorg. Med. Chem. Lett.*, Vol.14, pp.3257-3261.

Parejo, I.; Viladomat, F.; Bastida, J.; Codina, C. (2001) A Single Extraction Step in the Quantitative Analysis of Arbutin in Bearberry (Arctostaphylos uva-ursi) Leaves by High- Performance Liquid Chromatography. *Phytochem. Anal.* Vol.12, pp.336-339.

Parvez, S.; Kang, M.; Chung, H.S.; Bae, H. (2007) Naturally occuring tyrosinase inhibitors: Mechanism and applications in skin health, cosmetics and agriculture industries. *Phytother. Res.*, Vol.21, pp.805-816.

Petrola, R.; Repetti, L.; (1985) The complex formation between Ni^{2+} and substituted 3-hydroxy-4H-pyran-4-ones in aqueous solution. *Finn. Chem. Lett.*, Vol.5, pp.213.

Raku, T.; Tokiwa, Y. (2003) Regioselective synthesis of kojic acid esters by Bacillus subtilis protease. *Biotech. Lett.* Vol.25, pp.969-974.

Rho, H.S.; Ahn, S.M.; Yoo, D.S.; Kim, M.K.; Cho, D.H.; Cho, J.Y. (2010) Kojyl thioether derivatives having both tyrosinase inhibitory and anti-inflammatory properties. *Bioorg. Med. Chem. Lett.* Vol.20, pp.6569–6571.

Rho, H.S.; Goh, M.; Lee, J.; Ahn, S.M.; Yeon, J.; Yoo, D.S.; Kim, D.H.; Kim, H.G.; Cho, J.Y. (2011) Ester Derivatives of Kojic Acid and Polyphenols Containing Adamantane

Moiety with Tyrosinase Inhibitory and Anti-inflammatory Properties. *Bull. Korean Chem. Soc.* Vol. 32(4), pp.1411-1414.

Sapkota, K.; Roh, E.; Lee, E.; Ha, E.; Yang, J.; Lee, E.S.; Kwon, Y.; Kim, Y.; Na, Y. (2011) Synthesis and anti-melanogenic activity of hydroxyphenyl benzyl ether analogues. *Bioorg. Med. Chem.* Vol.19, pp.2168-2175.

Saruno, R.; Kato, F.; Ikeno, T. (1979) Kojic acid, a tyrosinase inhibitor from *Aspergillus albus. Agric. Biol. Chem.* Vol.43(6), pp.1337-1338.

Seo, S.Y.; Sharma, V.K.; Sharma, N. (2003) Mushroom tyrosinase: Recent Prospects. *J. Agric. Food Chem.* Vol.51, pp.2837-2853.

Son, S.M.; Moon, K.D.; Lee, C.Y. (2001) Inhibitory effects of various antibrowning agent on apple slices. *Food Chem.* Vol.73, pp.23-30.

Song, B.; Saatchi, K.; Rawji, G.H.; Orvig, C. (2002) Synthesis and solution studies of the complexes of pyrone analogue ligands with vanadium(IV) and vanadium(V). *Inorg. Chim. Acta*, Vol.339, pp.393-399.

Stenson, A.C.; Cioffi, E.A. (2007) Speciation of M^{+3}-hydroxypyrone chelation complexes by electrospray ionization ion trap and Fourier transform ion cyclotron resonance mass spectrometry. *Rapid. Commun. Mass Spectrom.*, Vol.21, pp.2594-2600.

Sudhir, P.R.; Wu, H.F.; Zhou, Zi.C. (2005) Probing the interaction of kojic acid antibiotics with iron(III) chloride by using electrospray tandem mass spectrometry, *Rapid Commun. Mass Spectrom*, Vol.19, pp.209-212.

Synytsya, A.; Blafková, P.; Synytsya, A.; Čopíková, J.; Spěváček, J.; Uher, M. (2008) Conjugation of kojic acid with chitosan. *Carbohydrate Polymers*, Vol.72, pp.21-31.

Thompson, K.H.; Orvig, C. (2001) Coordination chemistry of vanadium in metallopharmaceutical candidate compounds. *Coord. Chem. Reviews*, Vol.219-221, pp.1033-1053.

Uchino, K.; Nagawa, M.; Tanasaki, Y.; Oda, M.; Fukuchi, A. (1988). Kojic acid as an anti-speck agent. *Agric. Biol. Chem.*, Vol.52, pp.2609-2610.

Uher, M.; Konecny, V.; Rajniakova, O. (1994). Synthesis of 5-Hydoxy-2-hydroxymethyl-4H-pyran-4-one Derivatives with Pesticide Activity. *Chem. Pap-Chem. Zvesti*, Vol.48(4), pp.282-284.

Veverka M.; Kralovicova E. (1990) Synthesis of Some Biologically Active Derivatives of 2-Hydroxymethyl-5-hydroxy-4H-pyran-4-one, *Collect. Czech. Chem. Commun.*, Vol.55, pp.833-40.

Veverka, M. (1992) Synthesis of Some Biologically Active Derivatives of 2-Hydroxymethyl-5-hydroxy-4H-pyran-4-one. II. Synthesis and Biological Properties of S-Substituted 2-Thiomethyl-5-O-acyl Derivatives, *Chem. Papers*, Vol.46(3), pp.206-210.

Wan, H.M.; Chen, C.C., Giridhar, R.; Chang, T.S.; Wu, W.T. (2005) Repeated-batch production of kojic acid in a cell-retention fermenter using Aspergillus oryae. M3B9 *J. Ind. Microbiol. Biotechnol.* Vol.32, pp.227-233.

Wempe, M.; Fitzpatrick, M. (2009) 5-Hydroxy-2-methyl-4H-pyran-4-one-esters as novel tyrosinase inhibitors, WO 2009/108271 A1.

Wolf, P.A.; Westveer, W.M. (1950) The antimicrobial activity of several substituted pyrones. *Arch. Biochem.* Vol.28, pp.201-206.

Woods, L.L. (1946) Mannich Bases from Kojic acid and aryl amines. *J. Am. Chem. Soc.*, Vol.68, pp.2744–2745.

Xiong, X.; Pirrung, M.C. (2008) Modular synthesis of candidate ındole-based insulin mimics by Claisen rearrangement. *Org. Lett.*, Vol.10(6), pp.1151-1154.

Yamato, M.; Hashigaki, K.; Yasumoto, Y.; Sakai, J.; Luduena, R.F.; Banerjee, A.; Tsukagoshi, S.; Tashiro, T.; Tsuruo, T. (1987) Synthesis and antitumor activity of tropolone derivatives. 6. Structure-activity relationships of antitumor-active tropolone and 8-hyroxyquinolone derivatives. *J. Med. Chem.*, Vol.30, pp.1897-1900.

Yang, C.T.; Sreerama, S.G.; Hsieh, W.Y.; Liu, S. (2008) Synthesis and Characterisation of a Novel Macrocyclic Chelator with 3-Hydroxy-4-Pyrone Chelating Arms and Its Complexes with Medicinally Important Metals. *Inorg. Chem.*, Vol.47, pp.2719-2727.

Zaremba, K.; Lasocha, W.; Adamski, A.; Stanek, J.; Pattek-Janczyk. A. (2007) Crystal structure and magnetic properties of tris(2-hydroxymethyl-4-oxo-4H-pyran-5-olato-κ^2O^5,O^4)iron(III), *J. Coord. Chem.*, Vol.60(14), pp.1537-1546.

Zborowski, K.; Grybos, R.; Proniewicz, L.M. (2003) Determination of the most stable structures of selected hydroxypyrones and their cations and anions. *J. Mol. Struct. (Theochem)*, Vol.639, pp.87-100.

Zborowski, K.; Grybos, R,; Proniewicz, L.M. (2005)Molecular structure of oxovanadium (IV) complexes with maltol and kojic acid: aquantum mechanical study, *Inorg. Chem. Commun.*, Vol.8, pp.76-78.

3

Recent Applications of Quantitative Structure-Activity Relationships in Drug Design

Omar Deeb
Al-Quds University, Faculty of Pharmacy, Jerusalem
Palestine

1. Introduction

One of the most important challenges that face medicinal chemists today is the design of new drugs with improved properties and diminished side-effects for treating human disease such as AIDS and others. Medicinal chemists began the process by taking a lead structure and then finding analogs exhibiting the preferred biological activities. Next, they used their experience and chemical insight to eventually choose a nominee analog for further development. This process is difficult, expensive and took a long time. The conventional methods of drug discovery are now being supplemented by shortest approaches made possible by the accepting of the molecular processes involved in the original disease. In this view, the preliminary point in drug design is the molecular target which is receptor or enzyme in the body as an option of the existence of known lead structure.

The lock-and-key concepts at present are considered in drug design. Samples of protein targets were isolated and X-ray crystallography discovered their molecular structural design. Molecules are conceived either on the basis of similarities with recognized reference structures or on the basis of their complementarily with the three dimensional (3D) structure of well-known active sites.

The techniques currently on hand provide widespread insight into exact molecular features that are in charge for the regulation of biological processes: molecular geometries, electronic features and others. All these structural characteristics are of crucial importance in the understanding of structure-activity relationships and in rational drug design.

Rational drug design is based on the belief that the biological properties of drugs are related to their actual structural features. What has changed along the years is the way molecules are perceived and defined. In the past, medicinal chemists considered molecules as simple two-dimensional (2D) entities with related chemical and physicochemical properties. Quantitative structure-activity relationships (QSAR) concepts began to be considered and became very accepted.

However, most of these properties have not been well represented by the basic numerical parameters considered to characterize these features: the interactions between a ligand and a protein require much more information than the ones included in substituent indexes characterizing the molecular properties. Now, it has shown that consideration of the full detailed properties in 3D is necessary in allowing the understated stereochemical features to be respected.

The effective design of chemical structures with the desirable therapeutic properties is directed towards computer aided-drug design (CADD) a well established area of computer aided molecular design (CAMD). These techniques cover new methodologies, such as molecular modeling and quantitative structure-activity relationships (QSAR). Molecular modeling can be simply considered as a range of automated techniques based on theoretical chemistry methods and experimental data that can be used to predict molecular and biological properties.

The main applications of CAMD are the clarification of the basic requirements for a compound to obtain a determined activity, the simulation of the binding between a ligand and the receptor, the discovery of new active compounds and the prediction of activities for non-synthesised analogues. These applications convert CAMD to be used in drug design.

Computer aided molecular design (CAMD) is predictable to contribute to the discovery of "bright" molecules conceived on the basis of exact three-dimensional details. Two major modeling strategies right now used in the designing of new drugs. In the first strategy, the three-dimensional features of a known receptor site are directly considered whereas in the second strategy, the design is based on the comparative analysis of the structural features of known active and inactive molecules that are interpreted in terms of their complementarily with a supposed receptor site model.

The improvements in computer speed and capacity increased the number of lead compounds available for further research. But not only the number of feasible drug candidates increased, but also the costs and time devoted in various drug discovery processes was reduced, improving the effectiveness of the drug development.

One of the initial approaches to decrease these costs were attempted by correlating the biological function of a compound with its chemical structure, expressed in terms of molecular structural descriptors, by means of QSAR techniques. This discipline was promoted by Hansch and his group (Fujita, 1990). It was based on the determination of mathematical equations expressing the biological activities as a function of molecular parameters.

QSAR believe that the biological activity of a compound is a result of its chemical structure. Within the QSAR approach, the descriptor variable are not physically measured but computed, therefore, they are easy and cheap to generate even for large molecular sets.

2. Quantitative structure activity relationships (QSAR)

QSAR is a way of finding a simple equation that can be used to calculate some property from the molecular structure of a compound. QSAR attempt to correlate structural molecular features (descriptors) with physicochemical properties such as biological activities for a set of compounds, by means of statistical methods. As a result, a simple mathematical relationship is established.

Applications of QSAR can be extended to any molecular design purpose, including prediction of different kinds of biological activities, lead compound optimization and prediction of novel structural leads in drug discovery. The process of building a QSAR model is similar, apart from what type of property is being predicted. It consists of several steps which hopefully lead to the design of new compounds with the desired activity profile.

The first step in building a QSAR model is to select a training set of compounds with their experimental activities. Ideally, each of these activities should cover the range of possible values for that activity. The next step is to compute descriptors that contain sufficient relevant information about the biological phenomenon. However, it is difficult to predict in advance which descriptor variables will be valuable. Once descriptors have been calculated, it is necessary to pick which should be included in the QSAR model. A correlation coefficient gives a quantitative measure of how well each descriptor describes the activity. Thus, the descriptor with the highest correlation coefficient can be picked. Next step, a data analysis is needed to calculate the best mathematical expression linking together the descriptors and biological activities, in which information relating the essential features of the chemical and biological data structure is obtained. In the final step, validation and predictions for non-tested compounds will take place. However, the predictive capability of the model first is verified experimentally. This is talented by biological testing of some additional compounds (test set) in the same way as the training set and then comparing the experimental finding with the values predicted by the QSAR model. If the QSAR predicts within acceptable restrictions, it may be used for a more extensive prediction of more compounds. An interpretation of results should be done for the proposal and design of new compounds with the desired activity outline.

2.1 History of QSAR

Crum-Brown and Fraser expressed the suggestion that the physiological action of a substance was a function of its chemical composition. Later, in 1893, Richet showed that the cytotoxicities of a dissimilar set of uncomplicated organic compounds were inversely related to their corresponding water solubility. After that, Meyer and Overton independently recommended that the narcotic action of a group of organic molecules correlated with their olive oil/water partition coefficients. The extensive work of Albert, and Bell and Roblin established the importance of ionization of bases and weak acids in bacteriostatic activity. In the physical organic border, great progress was being made in the clarification of substituent effects on organic reactions, led by the influential job of Hammett. Taft invented a way for separating polar, steric, and resonance effects and introducing the first steric parameter, *ES*.

The contributions of Hammett and Taft together laid the mechanistic source for the progress of the QSAR model by Hansch and Fujita. In 1962 Hansch et al. (Hansch et al., 1962) published their bright study on the structure-activity relationships of plant growth regulators and their dependency on Hammett constants and hydrophobicity. A Linear Free Energy Relationships (LFER) related model published by Fujita et al. and Hansch et al., (Fujita et. al., 1964, Hansch et. al., 1964) considered to be the official beginning for QSAR. Their fragment and additive group contribution idea added two things: the use of calculated properties to correlate with biological activities and the detection that multiple properties may influence the biological activity. For this purpose, they implemented the use of the computer to fit QSAR equations.

The so-called Hansch equation (Hansch, 1969) was developed to correlate physicochemical properties (descriptors) with biological activities is given in a general form by:

$$\log 1/C = a (\log P)^2 + b\log P + c\sigma + \ldots k \quad (1)$$

where C is the molar concentration that produces the biological effect; P is the octanol/water partition coefficient and σ is the electronic Hammett constant.

Besides the Hansch approach, other methodologies were also developed to deal with structure- activity questions. The Free-Wilson approach (Free and Wilson, 1964) addresses structure-activity studies in a congeneric series in which the contribution of each structural feature was a parameter of interest. These parameters, also called indicator variables, codify the presence or absence of particular structural feature. They are assigned the binary values of 1 and 0, accordingly.

2.2 Descriptors

A common question in QSAR is how to describe molecules and their physicochemical properties (descriptors). The nature of the descriptors used and the extent to which they instruct the structural properties related to the biological activity is a critical part of a QSAR study (Downs, 2004). It has been estimated that thousands of molecular descriptors are now existing (Devillers and Balaban 1999; Karelson, 2000; Todeschini et. al., 2002). Most of them can be calculated by using commercial software packages such as CODESSA (Katritzky et. al., 2002), DRAGON (Todeschini et. al., 2002) and others. The various descriptors in use can be largely categorized as being constitutional, topological, electrostatic, geometrical, or quantum chemical.

Constitutional descriptors give a simple description of what is in the molecule. For example, the number of heteroatoms, the number of rings, the number of double bonds, etc. Constitutional descriptors often appear in a QSAR equation when the property being predicted varies with the size of the molecule.

Topological descriptors are numbers that give information about the bonding collection in a molecule. They are derived from graph representation of chemical structures; they attempt to encode the size, shape, or branching in the compound by handling of graph-theoretical aspects of the structures (Silipo and Vittoria, 1990). Some examples are Randic indices, Kier and Hall indices, Weiner index (sum of the chemical bonds existing between all pairs of heavy atoms in the molecule), the connectivity index and others.

Electrostatic descriptors are single values that give information about the molecular charge division. Some examples are polarity indices and polarizability. One of the most commonly used electrostatic descriptors is the topological polar surface area (TPSA), which gives an indication of the portion of the molecular surface composed of polar groups against nonpolar groups. Another deeply used descriptor is the octanol–water partition coefficient, which is designated by a specific prediction scheme such as ClogP or MlogP.

Geometrical descriptors are single values that describe the molecule's size and shape as well as the degree of complementarity of a ligand and the receptor. They are developed from three-dimensional models of molecules, and derived from molecular surface area calculations. Some examples are moments of inertia, molecular volume molecular surface area, and other parameters that describe length, height, and width.

Quantum chemical descriptors give information about the electronic structure of the molecule. They are obtained by molecular orbital calculations and they mainly describe electronic interaction. These includes, the energy of the highest occupied molecular orbital, E_{HOMO}, which is a quantitative measure for the chemical reactivity of the compound-ionization potential of a molecule, the energy of the lowest unoccupied molecular orbital, E_{LUMO}, which accounts for the electron affinity, refractivity, and total energy. The E_{HOMO}–E_{LUMO} gap or ionization potential can be important descriptors for predicting how molecules will react.

New nodal angle quantum descriptors - the Frontier Orbital Phase Angles - suggested by Clare (Clare, 1998) which considered as novel QSAR descriptors for benzene derivatives will be discussed in the application part.

2.3 Statistical methods

Statistical methods are the mathematical basis for the development of QSAR models. Chemometric methods (Eriksson et al., 2001) are used to extract information from QSAR data using tools of statistics and mathematics. The applications of these methods are combined with the important goal of explanation and prediction of non-synthesised test compounds. Many different statistical methods are available in the literature and the selection of the appropriate method is critical (Xu and Zhang, 2001).

Multiple Linear Regression (MLR) (Montgomery and Peck, 1992) can be considered as an easy interpretable regression-based method. Regression analysis correlates independent X variables or descriptors (physicochemical parameters) with dependent Y variables (biological data). The regression model assumes a linear relationship between *m* molecular descriptors and the response (biological activity) variable. This relationship can be expressed with the single multiple-term linear equation:

$$Y = b_0 + b_1X_1 + b_2X_2 + \dots + b_mX_m + e \quad (2)$$

The MLR analysis calculates the regression coefficients, b_i, by minimizing the residuals, **e**, which quantify the deviations between the data (Y) and the model (Y'), as in the case of simple linear regression.

Partial Least Squares (PLS) (World et al., 1993) which in turn decrease the information content of data matrices. It projects multivariate data into a space of lower size, and certainly providing insight to see and model huge sets of data. The Partial Least Squares (PLS) regression method carries out regression using latent variables from the independent and dependent data that are along their axes of most variation and are highly correlated. It is applied when the numbers of independent variables are more than the number of observations. Under these circumstances, it gives a more strong QSAR equation than multiple linear regressions. Thus, PLS is able to examine complex structure-activity problems and to examine data in a more realistic way. PLS gives a condensed statistically strong solution and, in fact, it contains MLR as a special case when a MLR be present.

Another way to reduce the dimensionality of the data set descriptors X is the so called **Principal Component Analysis** (PCA) technique (Jolliffe, 1986). It seeks to find out a new set of variables named Principal Components (PC) showing the data in order of decreasing variance with the aim to state the main information in the variables by the principal components of X. The primary Principal Component (PC1) describes the maximum deviation in the whole data set. The subsequent principal component (PC2) describes the maximum remaining variance, and so forth, with each axis linearly independent, to the preceding axis. Some of the last components may be discarded to decrease the size of the model and stay away from over-fitting.

The **Principal Components Regression (PCR)** method uses linear regression to generate a model by means of the principal components as independent descriptors. PCR applies the scores from PCA as regressors in the QSAR model. Therefore, a multiple-term linear equation is generated and derived from a principal components analysis transformation of the independent variables.

Artificial Neural Networks (ANN) method (Tetko, 1996; Novi et al., 1997; Duprat et al., 1998) is non-linear technique inspired in the human brain, composed of many simple processing units called neurons. This method is also recognized as learning algorithms. The aim is to simulate the various shells of the neurones, where each neuron is connected to a number of neighbouring neurones with variable coefficients of connectivity that signify the strength of these associations. The learning process consists of adjusting the coefficient so that the network provided as an output the suitable results. In neural networks, a training set is used to train the network, and then the network is used to predict the property (biological activity) that it was trained to predict. This technique can be associated with principal components analysis in which it is referred as **PC-ANN.**

Support Vector Machine (SVM) can be applied to regression by the introduction of an alternative loss function. In support vector regression (SVR) (Gunn, 1997), the basic idea is to map the data X into a higher-dimensional feature space via a nonlinear mapping and then to do linear regression in this space. Therefore, regression approximation addresses the problem of estimating a function based on a given data set.

2.4 Validation of QSAR models

After the model equation is obtained, moreover the stability and the goodness of fit of the model, it is also significant to estimate the power and the validity of the model before using it to predict the biological activity. Validity is to establish the reliability and significance of the method for a particular use. Therefore, validation of a QSAR model must be done. There are two validation methods used for a QSAR model: internal and external validation techniques to establish the confidence and strength of the model.

2.4.1 Internal validation

Internal validation uses the dataset from which the model is built and checks for internal stability. **Cross-Validation (CV) technique** is widely employed as an internal validation method of statistical models (Allen, 1974; World, 1978, 1991). Usually, one compound of the set is extracted each time, and then the model is recalculated using as training set the *n-1* (where n is number of compounds) remaining compounds, so that the biological activity value for the extracted compound is predicted once for all compounds. This process is repeated *n* times for all the compounds of the initial set, thus obtaining a prediction for each object. This process referred as leave-**one-out (LOO)** method. Also an alternative method can be defined when leaving out more than a compound of the data set at each time. This method is called **leave n-out** or **Leave-many-Out (LMO) CV method or sometimes it is referred as leave-group-out (LGO)**. Calculation of the correlation coefficient of the cross-validation procedure, that is, the **coefficient of prediction** q^2 must be done and it is by definition smaller or equal than the overall r^2 (correlation coefficient) for a QSAR equation. It is used as an investigative tool to estimate the predictive power of an equation obtained by using a regression method. Another procedure to test the validity of the model is the **randomization test.** Even with a huge number of compounds and a small number of descriptors, an equation can still have very poor predictive power. One way to test for this is by **randomization** of the compounds. The set of biological activity values is re-assigned arbitrarily to different compounds, and a new regression is done. This process is repeated many times. If the random models' biological activity prediction is analogous to the original equation within a given estimated self-confidence level, this means that the original model was obtained by chance. The random test analyses the ability of the model to derive actual structure-activity relationships.

2.4.2 External validation

A QSAR model with excellent goodness of fit and acceptable predictions may be deficient in real relationship between structural descriptors and biological activity. The perfect validity of the model is examined by **external validation**, which evaluates how well the model generalizes. If a sufficiently huge series of compounds with known activity is obtainable, the original data set can be divided into two subgroups, the **training set** and the **test set.** The training or calibration set is used to derive a calibration model that will be used later to predict the activities of the test or validation set compounds. On the other hand, an external test set that has not been included in any stage of the building of the model can be used as **test set.**

The obtained predictions of the new generated model for the test set determine the validity of the model. The parameters quantifying the superiority of prediction of the external test set may be the same used for the internal validation. The Sum of Squares Prediction Errors (SSPE) is extensively used to account for the inconsistency.

3. Recent applications of QSAR in drug design

3.1 Nodal angle quantum descriptors and flip regression

When implementing QSAR on flat, symmetrical, usually aromatic molecules, symmetry considerations often affirm that alternative orientations should be inspected. For phenethylamines, for example, there are five substitution sites on the benzene nucleus. If substituents with property P_i were introduced to site i (i = 2-6), an equation may be formulated:

$$log\ A = \sum_i C_i P_i + C_0 \quad (3)$$

where A is activity and C_i are constants to be determined by regression techniques (Clare and Supuran, 2005a). Hence, both 2-methoxyphenethylamine and 6-methoxyphenethylamine may be predicted to have the same activity for both molecules. Apparently, it may appear that C_2 must equal C_6 and C_3 must equal C_5, but it can be shown that this is not the case when considering 2,3,4-trimethoxyamphetamine and 2,4,5-trimethoxyamphetamine. Equating the C values would predict the same activity for both substances, but experimentally one of these is a potent hallucinogen and the other is inactive (Shulgin et al., 1991).

At the molecular level, the flat aromatic molecule may lay in two ways on the receptor, corresponding to the 5- or 6-membered rings swapping positions, or flipping. All combinations of each drug flipped and unflipped must be considered. In the absence of structural data the only way in which we can proceed is to carry out regressions with every combination of each drug in both orientations and find which regression fits best. For the case of N drugs, 2^N regressions must be considered. A full treatment is possible only to the smallest groups of compounds, so the approach used is to employ simulated annealing as a method of combinatorial optimization. This problem was first addressed by Kishida and Manabe (Kishida and Manabe, 1980), in perspective of QSAR of substituted benzenedisulfonamides. In a study by Clare (Clare, 1998), a descriptor for QSAR calculations on benzene derivatives was proposed, and shown to be highly effective in correlating activities in humans of a large class of phenylalkylamine hallucinogens.

Moreover, in a number of studies (Clare, 1998; Clare, 2000; Clare, 2001; Clare, 2002; Clare and Supuran, 2004), it has been shown that a small number of descriptors can account for the activity of diverse aromatic drugs, and a method for dealing with the symmetry nature in some groups of planar aromatic molecules has also been outlined. Particularly, it has been verified that in most cases the orientations of nodes in π -like orbitals of aromatic molecules are a significantly important feature in understanding their activity. This was first established in phenylalkylamine hallucinogens (Clare, 1998), and then also in benzenoid and heteroaromatic carbonic anhydrase, trypsin, thrombin and bacterial collagenase inhibitors (Clare and Supuran, 2004), as well as in tryptamine hallucinogens (Clare, 2004).

The descriptors are based on the similarity of the frontier orbitals of the molecule in question to those of benzene and involves an analytical least squares fitting of the molecules frontier orbitals, calculated by any semiempirical or ab initio method to those carefully calculated for unsubstituted benzene. Both the highest occupied molecular orbital (HOMO) and lowest unoccupied molecular orbital (LUMO) of benzene are degenerate, and each consists of two components that may be mixed in any proportion with normalization to form an infinity of equally acceptable frontier orbitals. In benzene itself, each of these mixtures is equivalent. When the benzene is substituted, the degeneracy is lifted, and each of the resulting separate orbitals may be considered as being approximately derived from one particular linear combination of the original two components.

The significance of orbital symmetry in the interactions of atoms to form molecules has been known for a long time. It appears that this is directly transferable to the association of molecules in pharmacology, at least insofar as π orbitals are involved. Many QSAR studies on aromatic molecules have involved the HOMO and LUMO energies or their sum or difference as descriptors. Consideration of the nodal angles, especially if the aromatic moiety is benzene could profit any of these studies. The π-like orbitals involved are standing waves of probability of finding an electron in a given location in the field of the atomic nuclei, and have no classical counterpart. Therefore, the dependence of activity on these variables (Clare, 2000; Clare, 2001) is perhaps the best indication yet of the essential quantum mechanical nature of drug-receptor interactions. Conventional 3D-QSAR programs, which employ classical interactions, such as coulombic charge-charge forces and empirical van der Waals interactions, may benefit from the incorporation of π orbital wave mechanical interactions such as those discussed in (Clare, 2000; Clare, 2001).

The calculation of nodal orientation is performed with the program NODANGLE (Clare and Supuran, 2005b). NODANGLE calculates the angle between the nodes in π -like orbitals and a reference point on the aromatic ring. NODANGLE works by comparing the coefficients of the p_z atomic orbitals on a 5- or 6-membered ring with those of the cyclopentadienide anion (for a 5-membered ring) or the benzene molecule (for a 6-membered ring), of known nodal orientation.

3.1.1 QSAR of protein tyrosine kinase inhibitory activity of flavonoid analogues

Flavonoids are a group of low molecular weight plant (Wang and Wang, 2002; Cronin et al, 1998) products, based on the parent compound, flavone (2-phenylchromone) and have shown potential for application in a variety of pharmacological targets. A large number of natural and synthetic flavonoids are being tested as specific inhibitors of protein tyrosine kinase (PTK). The flavonoid-inhibitory activity is expressed as log 1 / IC_{50}, which is the molar concentration of the flavonoid necessary to give half-maximal inhibition compared to the control assay carried out in the absence of inhibitor, but in the presence of dimethyl sulphoxide carrier. Clare and Deeb in (Deeb and Clare, 2007) have investigated the flavonoid-inhibitory activity of 54 analogues using the nodal angle descriptors (Clare, 2000; Clare and Supuran, 2005b) and flipstep regression analysis (Clare, 2000; Clare, 2001) mentioned above.

For the flavonoid, calculating the angles in the three rings can be accomplished by entering the atom as numbered in Figure 1. The three rings are 6-membered rings numbered 1–6, 5–10 and 11-16 for rings 1, 2 and 3 respectively. The angles calculated by NODANGLE (Clare and Supuran, 2005b) are then Θ_1, Θ_2 and Θ_3 in the figure, measured at atoms 1, 5 and 11 respectively. A problem arises from the symmetry of the parent molecule; therefore, the

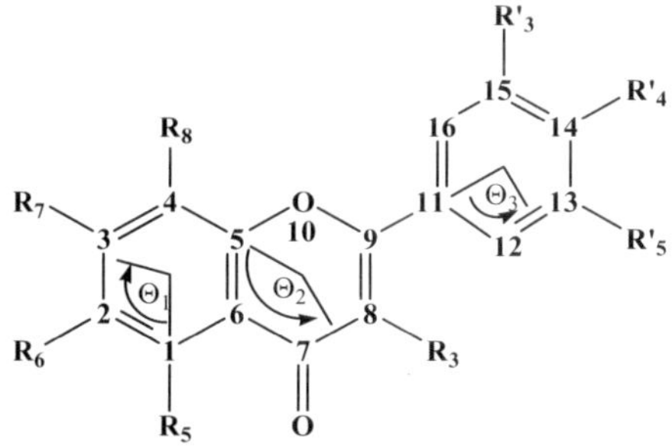

Fig. 1. Numbering of flavonoids skeleton used in MOPAC and NODANGLE calculations and angles used in the interpretations. The angle subscript indicates the ring number.

program FLIPSTEP, a component of the MARTHA statistical package (Clare and Supuran, 2005a) was used. This set of flavonoids separates into two parts (symmetry wise): the chromone moiety and the phenyl ring. The chromone ring system has no vertical mirror planes or axes. Hence, ring 1 cannot be flipped into ring 2. Thus for this part of the molecule flip regression is not applied. The phenyl ring has C_{2v} symmetry, so flip regression is applicable to this. Thus only ring 3 should be flipped.

In the study carried out by Deeb and Clare (Deeb and Clare, 2007), it was demonstrated that the charge on O_{10} proved to be the most important factor. Low charge on O_{10} was found to be favourable to high activity. Furthermore, it was found that the charge on C_7 and the mean of absolute charge are significant variables. Moreover, it was shown that the orientation of the nodes on ring 3 are significant factors which indicate the importance of the electrostatic and quantum chemical descriptors for the interaction of flavonoids with the specific enzymatic active site plays an important role. Exactly which rings are involved becomes clear from the identity of the descriptors included in the regression equation:

$$\log 1/IC_{50} = 7.4417\ (\pm 2.0652) - 0.65265\ (\pm 0.1569) \times HOP1 + 0.81601\ (\pm 0.1348) \times SHOP1$$
$$+ 0.35316\ (\pm 0.1422) \times HOP3 - 0.32482\ (\pm 0.0974) \times S2\Theta 1H - 0.21638\ (\pm 0.0778) \times C2\Theta 1H$$
$$- 0.00235\ (\pm 0.0008) \times Vol - 14.69500\ (\pm 6.1426) \times QC_7 - 27.77900\ (\pm 5.1297) \times QO_{10}$$
$$+ 14.14800\ (\pm 3.0611) \times Q_{mean} + 0.46973\ (\pm 0.1042) \times C2\Theta 3H + 1.57150\ (\pm 0.1779) \times S2\Theta 3H$$
$$- 0.26624\ (\pm 0.0889) \times C4\Theta 3L - 12.75700\ (\pm 1.6295) \times S4\Theta 3L \quad (4)$$
$$N = 54,\ R^2 = 0.8240,\ F = 14.403,\ S = 0.30537,\ Q^2 = 0.6612$$

where HOP1 is the highest occupied π orbital on ring 1, SHOP1 is the second highest occupied π orbital on ring 1, HOP3 is the highest occupied π orbital on ring 3, S2Θ1H is sin(2× the nodal angle in the highest occupied π orbital in ring 1), C2Θ1H is cos(2× the nodal angle in the highest occupied π orbital in ring 1), Vol is molecule volume, QC_7 is charge on C_7, QO_{10} is charge on O_{10}, Q_{mean} is the mean absolute Mulliken charge, C2Θ3H is cos(2× the nodal angle in the highest occupied π orbital in ring 3), S2Θ3H is sin(2× the nodal angle in the highest occupied π orbital in ring 3), C4Θ3L is cos(4× the nodal angle in the lowest unoccupied π orbital in ring 3), S4Θ3L is sin (4× the nodal angle in the lowest unoccupied π orbital in ring 3), N is number of compounds, R^2 is the coefficient of determination, F is Fisher variance ratio, S is standard deviation and Q^2 is the square of the multiple correlation coefficients based on the leave-one-out residuals.The numbers in parentheses are the standard errors.

The work of Deeb and Clare (Deeb and Clare, 2007) demonstrated that the nodal orientation terms have a powerful explanatory importance in that they account for more of the variance in activity than is possible using the classical descriptors alone. However, a combination of the classical descriptors and the nodal orientation term gives even better explanatory of activity of the flavone analogues. The chromone moiety of the flavonoid structure is envisaged to be a mixed region for hydrophobic and electronic interactions, while the phenyl ring moiety, especially the substituents at the 3' and 4' position, are involved in electronic interactions with the enzyme. S4Θ3L, that is cos (4 × the nodal angle in the lowest unoccupied π orbital in ring 3), was identified to be an important descriptor.

3.1.2 QSAR of EGFR inhibitory activity of quinazoline analogues

Epidermal growth factor receptor (EGFR) that has been identified as a kind of PTK and has been demonstrated to be related to many human cancers such as breast and liver cancers, leading many to believe that EGFR is an attractive target for anti-tumor drug discovery (Yang et al., 2001).

Deeb and Clare in (Deeb and Clare, 2008a) have applied the flip regression procedure applied on classical and quantum nodal oreinetation angles descriptors to investigate the quinazoline-inhibitory activity of 63 analogues expressed as log IC_{50}. IC_{50} is the effective concentration of the compound required to inhibit by 50% the phosphorylation of a 14-residue fragment of phosphorylase $C_{\gamma\text{-}1}$ (prepared from A431 human epidermoid carcinoma cells through immunoaffinity chromatography) by EGFR. For the quinazoline, calculating the angles in the three rings can be accomplished by entering the atom as numbered in Figure 2(a). The three rings are 6-membered rings numbered 1–6, 5–10 for ring 1 and 2, respectively. Ring 3 is also a 6-membered ring numbered 12–17. The angles calculated by NODANGLE are then Θ_1, Θ_2 and Θ_3 in that figure, measured at atoms 1, 5 and 12 respectively.

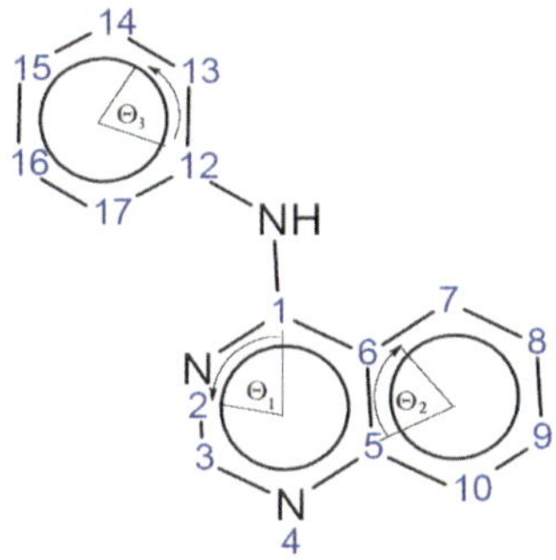

Fig. 2. (a) Numbering of quinazolines skeleton and angles used in the interpretations. The angle subscription indicates the ring number

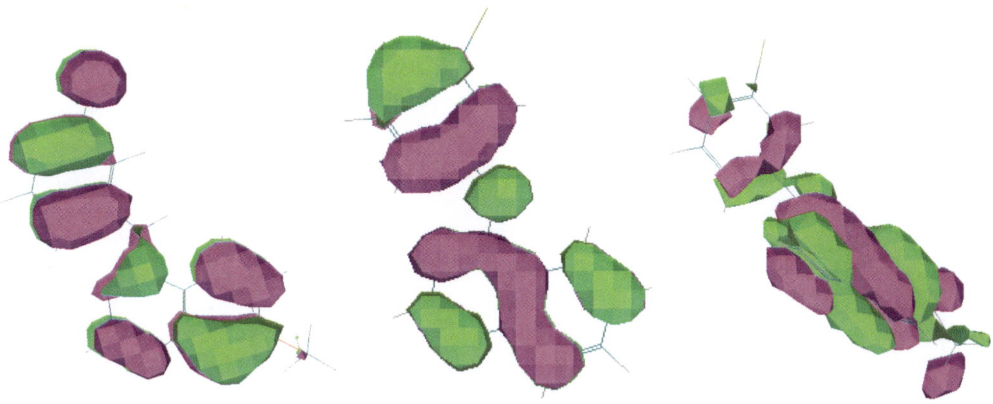

Fig. 2. (b) HOMO orbitals for quinazolines.

In this study (Deeb and Clare, 2008a) it is shown that the benzene rings of the quinazolines are interacting with aromatic systems on the receptor and that alignment occurs between the π orbital nodes on the pair. Exactly which rings are involved becomes clear from the identity of the descriptors included in the regression equation:

$$\begin{aligned} \log 1/IC_{50} = &- 8.7912\ (2.80) - 0.30044\ (3.36)\ SHOP2 \\ &+ 1.1489\ (7.10)\ LUP3 \\ &- 1.2589\ (8.19)\ SLUP3 \\ &- 0.47012\ (6.30)\ C2\Theta1H - 0.84000\ (7.73)\ C4\Theta1L \\ &- 0.27740\ (3.07)\ S2\Theta2H + 0.77819\ (7.80)\ P_{xx} \\ &- 0.55845\ (6.55)\ P_{zz} \\ &- 0.17269\ (3.34)\ C2\Theta3H + 0.03004\ (0.57)\ S2\Theta3H \\ &- 0.03340\ (0.51)\ C4\Theta3L + 0.5871\ (11.27)\ S4\Theta3L \end{aligned} \quad (5)$$

$$N = 63,\ S = 0.49766,\ F = 38.21,\ R^2 = 0.9017,\ Q^2 = 0.8550$$

where SHOP2 is the second highest occupied π orbital on ring 2 (see Figure 2(b)), LUP3 is the lowest unoccupied π orbial in ring 3, SLUP3 is the second lowest unoccupied occupied π orbital on ring 3, C4Θ1L is cos(4× the nodal angle in the lowest unoccupied π orbital in ring 1), P_{xx} is diagonal components of polarizability in x-direction, P_{zz} is diagonal components of polarizability in z-direction and S2Θ2H is sin(2× the nodal angle in the highest occupied π orbital in ring 2). The numbers in parentheses are student's *t* values.

Equation (5) shows that the second lowest unoccupied π orbital on ring 3 was identified to be an important descriptor. The only classical variables found to be significant were the polarizability components. High polarizability in the highest inertia direction was found to be favorable to high activity, while high polarizability in the lowest inertia direction was detrimental.

3.1.3 QSAR of phenylisopropylamines MAO-inhibition: Comparison of AM1 and B3LYP-DFT

Monoamine oxidase plays a critical role in the regulation of monoamine neurotransmitters such as serotonin, noradrenaline, and dopamine. MAO isoenzymes are classified on the basis of their substrate preference, sensitivity toward specific inhibitors, and tissue distribution into MAO-A and MAO-B. Selective MAO-A inhibitors have been used clinically in the treatment of depression and anxiety, while MAO-B inhibitors have been used in the treatment of Parkinson's and Alzheimer's diseases. Many plant-derived and synthetic compounds such as isoquinolines and xanthones have been identified as MAO inhibitors. In (Deeb and clare, 2008b) the monoamine oxidase (MAO)-inhibitory activity of 46 phenylisopropylamines expressed as pIC50 is modeled with the orientations of nodes in π-like orbitals of the phenyl ring and some other descriptors using flip regression analysis. The authors aim to provide an initial clue regarding the scope and limitations of some state-of-the-art methods in computational chemistry, including semiempirical (AM1) and density functional theory (B3LYP), in the flip regression procedure applied to the inhibition of phenylisopropylamines.

Calculating the angles for the aromatic ring in the each phenylisopropylamines can be accomplished by entering the atoms as numbered in Figure 3. The ring is six-membered and is numbered 1 to 6. The angle calculated by NODANGLE is then Θ measured at atom 1. The flip regression is applicable to the phenyl ring of C_{2v} symmetry.

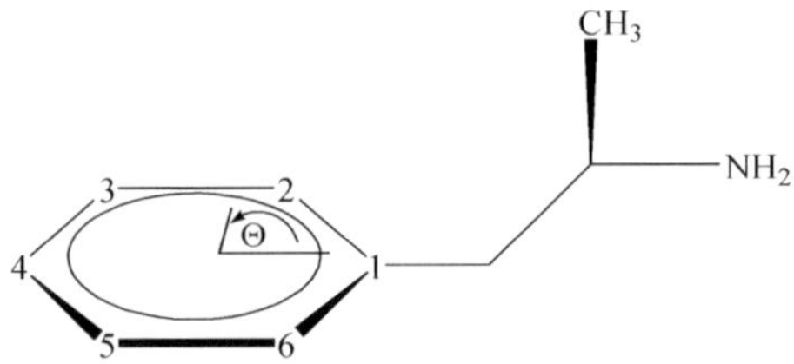

Fig. 3. Ring substitution pattern of the phenylisopropylamines.

Again, it was found that a combination of the classical descriptors and the nodal orientation terms gives better explanatory of activity of the phenylisopropylamines as it can be seen in the following regression equation:

$$\begin{aligned} pIC_{50} = {} & 14.961\ (\pm 2.2558) + 1.2957\ (\pm 0.28952)\ SHOP \\ & - 3.957\ (\pm 0.34587)\ LUP - 7.4769\ (\pm 2.52)\ LDI \\ & - 1.8473\ (\pm 0.22595)\ C2\Theta H \\ & - 1.8104\ (\pm 0.18915)\ S2\Theta H \\ & + 0.75002\ (\pm 0.10146)\ C4\Theta L \\ & + 1.1693\ (\pm 0.13404)\ S4\Theta L \end{aligned} \qquad (6)$$

$$N = 32,\ R^2 = 0.9309,\ F = 46.222,\ S = 0.28690,\ Q^2 = 0.8587$$

where SHOP is the second highest occupied π orbital, LUP is the lowest unoccupied π orbital, LDI is the local dipole index, C2ΘH is cos(2* the nodal angle in the highest occupied π orbital), S2ΘH is sin(2* the nodal angle in the highest occupied π orbital) and S4ΘL is sin(4* the nodal angle in the lowest unoccupied π orbital).The numbers in parentheses are the standard errors.

From equation (6), it can be predicted that the phenyl moiety of phenylisopropylamines is involved in electronic interactions with the enzyme. Lowest unoccupied π energy was identified to be an important descriptor. Adding classical variables, improves the correlation. The classical variables found to be significant are LUP and LDI which were found to be favorable to high activity. This is based on the concept that the stability of stacked aromatic systems is highly orientation-dependent, and is also dependent on the energies of those orbitals in the two aromatic systems that resemble the degenerate HOMO and LUMO of benzene. Furthermore, the results show that the models established based on DFT-B3LYP method are better than those based on AM1 method. The B3LYP model gives more reasonable interpretation of phenylisopropylamines MAO inhibition activity.

3.2 Applications of QSAR using PC-ANN

3.2.1 Correlation ranking and stepwise regression procedures in principal components artificial neural networks modeling with application to predict toxic activity and human serum albumin binding affinity

A successful drug should be able to reach its target without generating toxic effects in addition to possessing intrinsic activity. Considering the substantial failure rate of drug candidates in late stage development and the expensive and time-consuming process of measuring toxic effects, predictive tools that eliminate inappropriate compounds become necessary. Prediction of toxicity from the structure of compounds can help in designing the new beneficial compounds and hence, screening of large number of chemicals for toxic effects as well as interpreting the mechanisms of toxicity. Development of QSARs relating toxicity potency and structural properties can be an alternative that has the advantage of high speed and low costs in comparison with experiments. Because most toxicology predictions engage a diverse set of compounds belonging to different classes and multiple toxic mechanisms, some nonlinear relations between the properties of compounds and their toxicity parameters are expected and linear regression approaches may not be accurate and can lead to imprecision.

Human serum albumin (HSA) is the most abundant protein in plasma. It is characterized by its surprising capacity to bind a large variety of drugs. Extensive biochemical studies resulted in the proposition of two main drug-binding sites in HSA, denoted as I and II. Site I was shown to prefer large heterocyclic and negatively charged compounds, while site II was the one for small aromatic carboxylic acids. When the crystal structures of HSA with ligands were available, these sites were localized at subdomains IIA and IIIA. Analytical techniques have been employed to measure drug-binding affinities to HSA. These techniques have low throughput and they require relatively large quantities of both drug and protein. The recent development of high-performance affinity chromatography (HPAC) columns with immobilized HSA has allowed the medium-throughput determination of drug binding to this protein in a way that requires small amounts of both drug and HSA. Developing a model for predicting the drug-binding affinity based on molecular structure is very important goal for medicinal chemist. Several studies aim to generate models that predict drug-binding affinities to HSA such as QSAR and molecular modeling.

Two data sets were used in this study (Deeb, 2010). The first was an extensive toxicity data set that contains 278 substituted benzenes (Feng et al., 2003). The logarithm of half maximal inhibitory concentration (log IC_{50}) toxicity to T. pyriformis is used as the toxicity end point. Another data set of 95 HSA drug and drug-like compounds and their binding affinities were reported by Colmenarejo (Colmenarejo, 2003). The 3D molecular structures of the compounds were optimized by Hyperchem software using the semiempirical AM1 level of theory. In this study, a total of 1233 and 698 molecular descriptors were calculated for each molecule of the substituted benzenes and HSA drug and drug-like compounds, respectively. These descriptors are belonging to 17 different types of theoretical descriptors (Table 1).

Dragon software was used to calculate 1217 and 684 descriptors gathered into 16 groups for the toxic compounds and HSA drug and drug-like compounds, respectively. A group of 16 and 14 quantum descriptors for the toxic and HSA drug and drug-like compounds, respectively, describing the electronic properties of molecules were calculated by Hyperchem software. SPSS Software was used for the simple principal component regression (PCR) analysis. PCA and ANN regressions were performed in the MATLAB environment.

J *	Descriptors	No. of descriptors calculated for toxicity of substituted benzenes	No. of descriptors calculated for HSA binding affinity
1	Quantum descriptors	16	14
2	Constitutional descriptors	34	31
3	Topological descriptors	228	89
4	Molecular walk counts	15	7
5	Burden eigenvalue (BCUT) descriptors	64	18
6	Galvz topological charge indices 21	21	21
7	2D autocorrelations	96	68
8	Charge descriptors	14	8
9	Aromaticity indices	4	0
10	Randic molecular profiles	41	5
11	Geometrical descriptors	38	29
12	RDF descriptors	142	51
13	3D-MoRSE descriptors	160	95
14	WHIM descriptors	99	30
15	GETAWAY descriptors	197	131
16	Functional group counts	27	40
17	Atom-centred fragments	37	61

* J is the index of the group of descriptors.

Table 1. Types of descriptors used in this study.

Aiming to test the final model performances, the data set was divided into training (60%), validation (20%) and prediction (20%) sets based on descriptor spaces. For this purpose, the data matrix containing the total descriptors was subjected to PCA and the first two PCs were plotted against each other. PCA was run twice, once by grouping of descriptors and analysis of each group separately. This approach is referred to as the individual PCA approach, PCA(I). And once, by analysis of the entire set of calculated descriptors simultaneously. This approach is referred as the combined PCA approach, PCA(C). In PCA(I) procedure, each group of descriptors was subjected to PCA separately and the subset of PCs that explained 95% of the variances in the original descriptors data matrix were extracted from each set. The PCs extracted from this approach are named in the form "PCi-j" where "i" indicates the descriptors group and "j" indicates the PC number in the ith group which is related to its ranked eigenvalue. In a similar manner, in PCA(C) procedure all calculated PCs were collected in a single data matrix and the PCs were extracted. A feed-forward neural network with back-propagation of an error algorithm was constructed to model the structure–activity relationship. Our network has one input layer, one hidden layer, and one output layer. The input vectors were the set of PCs, selected according to PCA(I) and PCA(C) in combination with stepwise regression (SR) and correlation ranking (CR) procedures. The number of nodes in the input layer is dependent on the number of PCs introduced in the network. The number of nodes in the hidden layer is optimized through a learning procedure. Fgure 4 illustrates the four ANN analyses carried out in this study.

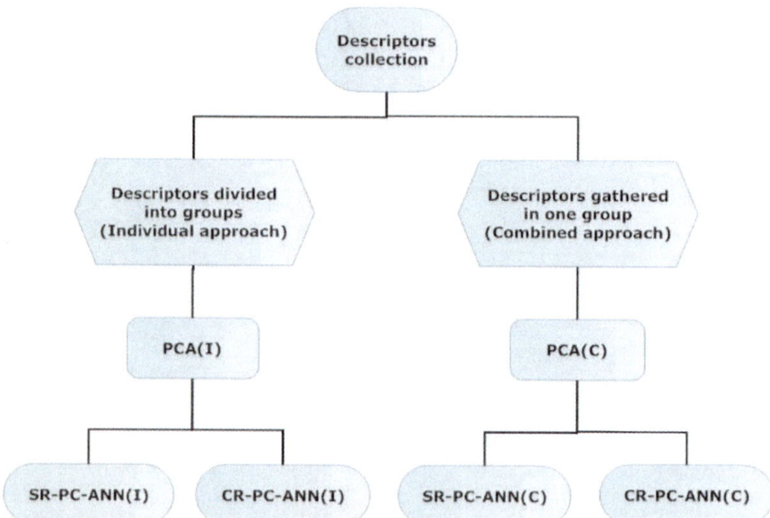

Fig. 4. PC-ANN approaches used in this study.

The results of modeling the toxicity data indicates that the residual plots for the training, validation and test sets are not scattered and they do not warranty the stability of the models. There is a strong relationship between the residual and actual values which reflects that the obtained models have systematic error, therefore a correction scheme is done to correct this issue. The cross-validation parameters for the chosen models before and after correction are shown in Table 2. This table shows that the correction term improves the cross-validation parameters by lowering the RMSE and increasing the R^2CV values. Considering the number of variables entered to the regression model for the SR-PC-ANN approach, PCA(I) based-model which has lower number of variables (3 variables) is superior over the PCR(C) based-model which has 13 variables due to chance correlation possibilities. It also shows that, after applying the correction scheme, model 3 obtained from the SR-PC-ANN(I) explains 58.5% of the data variances and has a 0.471 RMSE of prediction. This model has regression coefficients of 0.811 and 0.858 for the training and test sets, respectively. The RMSE of prediction for the CR-PC-ANN(I) model is less than that of the CR-PC-ANN(C) optimal model (0.571 and 0.590, respectively). The optimal model obtained using the CR-PC-ANN (I) procedure has correlation coefficients of 0.817 and 0.866 for the training and test sets, respectively and explains 53.4% of the data variances while the optimal model obtained from the CR-PC-ANN(C) procedure explains 51.1% of the data variances.

Approach used	PCs entered in the model	$RMSE^c$	$R^2_{CV}{}^c$	$RMSE^p$
SR-PC-ANN(I)	PC2-1 + PC17-3 + PC13-2	0.657	0.496	0.668
		0.498	0.585	0.471
SR-PC-ANN(C)	PC2 + PC5 + PC6 + PC30 + PC29 + PC8 + PC3 + PC48 + PC1 + PC24 + PC11 + PC10 + PC18	0.618	0.558	0.619
		0.404	0.734	0.451
CR-PC-ANN(I)	PC2-1, PC17-3, PC16-2	0.691	0.443	0.691
		0.525	0.534	0.571
CR-PC-ANN(C)	PC2, PC1, PC3, PC12, PC4, PC5, PC45, PC34, PC24, PC26, PC48, PC43, PC27	0.682	0.452	0.643
		0.551	0.511	0.590

Table 2. Cross validation parameters for the original models (grey background) and the corrected ones (white background) for the optimal ANN models of the different approaches used for modeling the toxicity data.

A randomization test was performed and the results obtained for five trails shows that the probability of obtaining chance models (with high correlation coefficients) from the PCA(C) approach is more than that for the PCA(I) approach. Furthermore, it is noticed that the chance correlation coefficients obtained for the CR-PCANN(I) approach are lower than those obtained for the SR-PC-ANN(I) approach. This indicates that model obtained from the CR-PC-ANN(I) approach is more accurate than the other models.

Following the same procedure used for modeling the toxicity of substituted benzenes, the SR-PC-ANN and CR-PC-ANN approaches were compared for modeling the HSA binding affinity with the PCs extracted according to PCA(I) and PCA(C) approaches. The results of this analysis are summarized in table 3.

Approach used	PCs entered in the model	$RMSE^{c}$	$R^2_{CV}{}^{c}$	$RMSE^{P}$
SR-PC-ANN(I)	PC16-1 + PC15-1 + PC6-1 + PC5-1 + PC4-1 + PC14-1 + PC1-1 + PC8-1 + PC2-2 + PC11-1	0.361	0.441	0.245
		0.258	0.509	0.077
SR-PC-ANN(C)	PC4 + PC8 + PC1 + PC33 + PC9 + PC3 + PC22 + PC12 + PC17 + PC31 + PC28 + PC7 + PC34 + PC10 + PC46 + PC20 + PC26	0.282	0.642	0.419
		0.270	0.747	0.388
CR-PC-ANN(I)	PC17-1, PC2-3, PC2-2, PC7-1, PC4-1, PC15-1, PC8-1, PC5-1, PC16-1, PC6-1, PC13-1, PC11-1, PC1-1, PC14-1	0.339	0.414	0.545
		0.419	0.583	0.586
CR-PC-ANN(C)	PC4 , PC8 , PC1 , PC33 , PC9 , PC3 , PC22 , PC12 , PC17 , PC31 , PC28 , PC7 , PC34 , PC10 , PC46 , PC20 , PC26 , PC27 , PC6 , PC25	0.284	0.633	0.454
		0.258	0.764	0.321

Table 3. Cross validation parameters for the original models (grey background) and the corrected ones (white background) for the optimal ANN models of the different approaches used for modeling the HSA binding affinity.

It shows that the correction terms improve the cross-validation parameters by increasing the R^2CV and decreasing the RMSE values. This table shows also that the RMSE of prediction of the model obtained from the SR-PC ANN(I) approach is smaller than those for of the models obtained from the other approaches. The corrected model explains 50.9% of the data variances and has a RMSE of prediction of 0.077, regression coefficients of 0.714 and 0.670 for the training and test sets, respectively. On the other hand, the corrected model obtained from the CR-PC-ANN(I) approach explains 53.7% of the data variances and has a RMSE of prediction of 0.586, regression coefficients of 0.733 and 0.675 for the training and test sets, respectively.

In summary, the performance of the two novel QSAR algorithms, principal component-artificial neural network modeling method, named SR-PC- ANN and CR-PC-ANN, combined with two factor selection procedures, named PCA(I) and PCA(C), is compared. These methods are applied to predict the toxic activity of a large set of compounds (278 substituted benzenes) as well as HSA binding affinity (94 compounds). The optimal model for the toxicity data set has a prediction RMSE of 0.471 while the optimal model for the HSA binding affinity has a prediction RMSE of 0.077. Comparison of the models shows that the results obtained by the CR-PC-ANN procedure are more accurate than those obtained from the SR-PC-ANN procedure. Generally, the models obtained from the PCA(I) approach are better than those obtained from the PCA(C) approach regardless which approach was used to perform the ANN analysis. Both the external and cross-validation methods are used to validate the performances of the resulting models.

Randomization test is employed to check the suitability of the models and to investigate the possibility of obtaining chance models.

3.2.2 Exploring QSARs of some analgesic compounds

Analgesics are a class of drugs used to reduce pain. The pain relief induced by analgesics occurs either by blocking pain signals going to the brain or by interfering with the brain's interpretation of the signals, without loss of awareness. There are essentially two kinds of analgesics: non-narcotics and narcotics. Because of the potential to relieve pain, they play an important role in medical therapy. The dose required to produce analgesia frequently does not change the functions of central nervous system. Analgesia is believed to engage activation of μ-receptors largely at supraspinal sites and k-receptors mainly within the spinal cord. It has been demonstrated that log IC, where IC refers to the half maximal (50%) inhibitory concentration of a drug, can be successfully used to predict analgesic activity. The aim of this study is to apply PC-ANN with different molecular descriptors in the development of new statistically validated QSAR models. This model will predict the analgesic activity of the heterogeneous data set of different types of analgesics (narcotic, opioid, and non-opioid) as a whole without splitting them into categorizes. The strength and the predictive performance of the proposed models were verified using both internal (cross-validation and randomization) and external statistical validations.

In this study (Deeb and Drabh, 2010), a data set of 95 analgesic compounds and their analgesic activity (log IC) obtained from reference (Mathur, 2003) were used in this study. HyperChem software was used to optimize the structure of the different compounds on AM1 semi-empirical level. The optimization was preceded by the Polak-Rebiere algorithm to reach 0.01 root mean square gradient. In this study, a pool of molecular descriptors including constitutional, topological, chemical, quantum, and functional descriptors were calculated using Hyperchem and Dragon software. A condensed set of 150 descriptors were obtained by removal of highly intercorrelated ($r > 0.95$) descriptors in addition to descriptors having constant values. Descriptors that have zero for almost all the cases were also removed together with those descriptors that include outliers' values to enclose a set of 132 descriptors. This set was then declined to 24 descriptors by stepwise regression.

In the MLR analysis, different regression models were suggested in which the number of descriptors in these models varied between 1 and 20. The best correlation coefficient obtained is 0.760 for a regression model with 20 descriptors. The linear relationships according to MLR analysis provide models with poor cross-validation parameters. Therefore, ANNs algorithm was used to investigate non-linear relationships for the best MLR models according to the cross-validation coefficient of determination (R^2CV).

In PC-ANN, the inputs of the ANN were the subset of the descriptors used in different MLR models. From the correlation data matrix for these descriptors, some of them represent considerable degree of collinearity. Therefore, the PCA was performed first to classify the molecules into training, validation, and prediction (test) sets. Performing PCA on the whole data of 95 compounds, 132 descriptors and plotting the first and second principals (Figure 5), shows that 11 compounds behave differently (outliers) from other compounds with respect to both molecular structure (descriptors) and analgesic activity. Therefore, these compounds are not used in the future analysis (Figure 6).

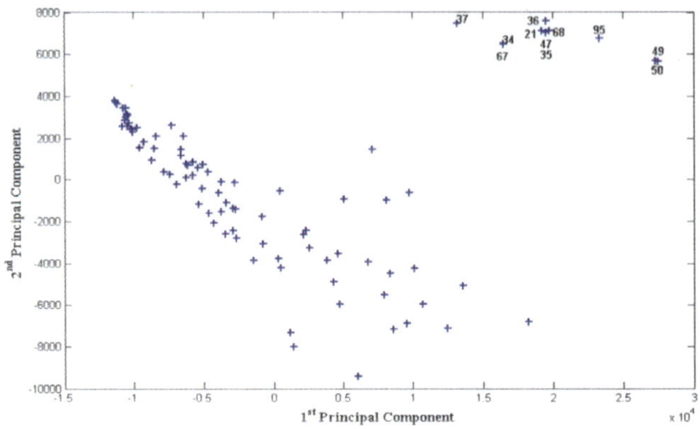

Fig. 5. First and second principal components for the factor spaces of the descriptors and analgesic activity data.

Checking the structure of the outlier compounds shown in Figure 6 reveals that they all morphine derivatives and belong to the same family of opiates analgesic.

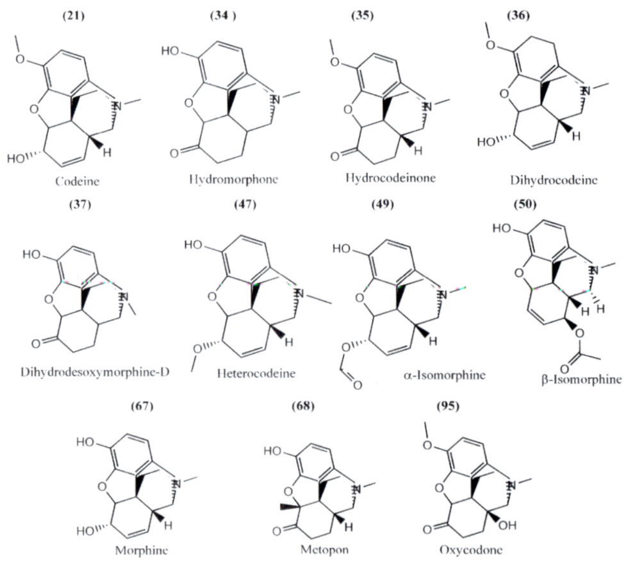

Fig. 6. Structure of outliers suggested from principal component analysis.

According to the pattern of the distribution of the data in factor spaces (Figure 5), the training, validation, and prediction compounds were selected homogenously, so that compounds in different zones of Figure 5 belong to all three subsets. After removing the outliers, the classified data were used as an input for the ANN. In this study, a three-layered feed-forward ANN model with back-propagation learning algorithm was employed. At first, non-linear relationship between the subset of descriptors selected by stepwise selection-based MLR and analgesic activity was preceded by PC-ANN models with similar structure. The number of hidden layer's nodes was set to 8 for all models, and the number of nodes in the input layer was the number of PCs extracted for each subset of descriptors. After that, for the best models, optimization of the number of hidden nodes was done.

Cross-validation parameters show that the prediction ability is improved for model the best model which has a relative standard error of prediction of 5.396% and the correlation coefficient of 0.834 ands 0.846 for the training and test sets, respectively. The cross-validation coefficient of determination is 0.656 which means that the six PCs selected by eigenvalue ranking procedure can explain at least 63.6% variances in log IC for the calibration. Consequently, the optimal performance occurs for the best model when using nine hidden nodes. A randomization test was performed to investigate the probability of chance correlation for the optimal model. The results of randomization test indicate that the correlation coefficients obtained by chance are low in general, while the predicted error values are high. This indicates that the model obtained from PCA-ANN is better than those obtained by chance.

In summary, the results obtained by principal component-artificial neural network give advanced regression models with good prediction ability using a relatively low number of principal components. A 0.834 correlation coefficient was obtained using principal component- artificial neural network with six extracted principal components.

3.2.3 QSAR Model of drug-binding to human serum albumin

In this study (Deeb and Hemmateenejad, 2007), a data set of 94 HSA drug and drug-like compounds and their binding affinities reported by Colmenarejo (Colmenarejo, 2003) are used in this study. HYPERCHEM software was used to optimize the structure of the different compounds on AM1 semi-empirical level. The optimization was preceded by the Polak-Rebiere algorithm to reach 0.01 root mean square gradient (298 K, gas phase). Esbelen (compound number 8) was dropped from this set because Se is not parameterized for AM1 semiempirical method. In this study, a set of 60 molecular descriptors including constitutional, topological, chemical, and quantum descriptors were calculated using Hyperchem and Dragon software.

Multiple linear regression analysis with stepwise selection and elimination of variables was employed to model the binding affinity (log K'hsa) relationships with different set of descriptors. The number of descriptors in the suggested MLR models is varied between 1 and 25. The best correlation coefficient obtained is 0.912 for a regression model with 25 descriptors. The number of descriptors is large according to the rule of the thumb, whereas the statistical parameters are not so high. Therefore, ANNs algorithm was used seeking for better regression model.

In PC-ANN, the inputs of the ANN were the subset of the descriptors used in different MLR models. The correlation data matrix for these descriptors indicated that some descriptors represent high degree of collinearity. Principal component analysis groups together descriptors that are collinear to form a composite indicator capable of capturing as much of common information of those descriptors as possible. Application of PCA on a descriptor data matrix results in a loading matrix containing factors or PCs, which are orthogonal. These factors used as the inputs of ANN instead of the original descriptors.

The procedure used in this study is similar to that used in the QSAR study of some analgesics compounds. Performing PCA on the whole data of 94 compounds and 60 descriptors and plotting the first and second principal, shows that compounds 62 and 91 are outliers. According to the pattern of the distribution of the data in factor spaces the training, validation, and prediction molecules were selected homogenously. After removing the outliers the classified data was used as an input for the ANN. A three-layered feed-forward ANN model with backpropagation learning algorithm was employed. At the first, the nonlinear relationship between the subset of descriptors selected by stepwise selection-based MLR and drug HSA binding constant was proceeded by PC-ANN models with similar structure. The number of hidden layer's nodes was set 3 for all models and the number of nodes in the input layer was the number of PCs extracted for each subset of descriptors. The results of PC-ANN modeling for MLR model numbers 15–25 shows that the best model which has almost the highest correlation coefficient for the external test set (0.8065) which indicates a high predictive power. This model has also a relatively low PRESS/SST ratio (0.4485) compared with other models which make it the most reasonable model among all. The R^2 values for the cross-validation and prediction for this model are 0.5515 and 0.5100, respectively, which means that the six PCs selected by eigenvalue ranking procedure can explain at least 55.2% and 51% variances in log K'hsa for the calibration and prediction, respectively. In order to optimize the performance of the ANN model , we trained the ANN using different number of hidden nodes starting from 1 hidden node to 20 hidden nodes. The results for the optimization indicate that an ANN with eight hidden nodes resulted in the optimum network model. Using eight hidden nodes, we obtained almost the highest correlation coefficient for both the training set (0.9218) and the prediction set (0.8302). This model gives the lowest PRESS/SST ratio (0.2757) which makes it the most reasonable. The results of the randomization test shows that the correlation coefficients obtained by chance are low in general while PRESS and PRESS/SST ratio are high. This indicates that the model obtained from PCA-ANN is better than those obtained by chance.

3.3 Exploring QSARs for inhibitory activity of non-peptide HIV-1 protease inhibitors by GA-PLS and GA-SVM

Human immunodeficiency virus (HIV), the causative agent of AIDS infects millions of people worldwide. Although a treatment has not been found yet for this serious disease, rapid advances in molecular biology along with the 3-D elucidation of HIV proteins have led to new drug-targeting approaches for designing antiviral agents that specifically bind to key regulatory proteins that are essential for HIV replication. Thus, by developing new inhibitors of HIV-1 protease activity, the treatment of AIDS can be advanced. Several peptidic inhibitors are currently under clinical trials and significant efforts to improve their pharmacology continues. In this study, we picked out small non-peptide HIV protease inhibitors with potentially better pharmacological characteristics based on the structural features of peptidic inhibitors bound to the enzyme, and performed QSAR study.

In this study (Deeb and Goodarzi, 2010), a data set of 46 non-peptide HIV-1 protease inhibitors and their inhibitory activity reported by Tummino et al. (Tummino et al. 1996) are used in this study. Molecular chemical structure was built using Hyperchem. AM1 method was applied to optimize the molecular structure of the compounds. All calculations were carried out at the restricted Hartree-Fock level with no configuration interaction. The molecular structures were optimized using the Polak–Ribiere algorithm until the root mean square gradient was 0.01 Kcal/mol.

One thousand four hundred eighty one descriptors belonging to eighteen different theoretical descriptors were calculated for each molecule. The calculated descriptors were first analyzed for the existence of constant or near constant variables. The detected ones were then removed. Correlation among descriptors with the activity of the molecules was examined and collinear descriptors (i.e. $r > 0.9$) were detected. Descriptors that contain a high percentage (> 90%) of identical values were discarded to decrease the redundancy existing in the descriptor data matrix. Among the collinear descriptors, the one presenting the highest correlation with the activity was retained and others were removed from the data matrix. The dataset was splitted into two sets based on activity range; training set (85%) with activity ranges from 3.921 to 8.444 and test set (15%) with activity ranges from 4.538 to 8.208. In this work, genetic algorithm (GA) variable subset selection method (Leardi et al., 1992) was used for the selection of the most relevant descriptors from the pool of remaining descriptors. These descriptors would be used as inputs for PLS and SVM in the construction of QSAR models.

In GA-PLS, model validation was achieved through leave-one-out cross-validation (LOO CV) to find the best number of latent variables (Lv) to be used in calibration and prediction. External validation (for a test set), and the predictive ability was statistically evaluated through the root mean square errors of calibration (RMSEC) and validation (RMSECV). The results indicate that four latent variables are the best number to make a model. The following equation represents the best model achieved by GA-PLS:

$$
\begin{aligned}
pIC_{50} = {} & -3.405737\ (\pm 1.447) + 0.525607\ (\pm 0.052)\ TE2 \\
& + 0.911090\ (\pm 0.236) Ui \\
& + 2.586873\ (\pm 0.369)\ GATS5e \\
& - 47.069316\ (\pm 8.558) Mor13e \\
& - 0.207581\ (\pm 0.027)\ ATS7m \\
& + 13.338116\ (\pm 3.599)\ Ss \\
& - 0.001142\ (\pm 0.000)\ Mor27e \\
& + 49.494231\ (\pm 7.841)\ RDF035e
\end{aligned}
\tag{7}
$$

The best model shown above reveals that the most significant contribution comes from the RDF035e. Table 4 gives brief description of these descriptors.

In GA-SVM, the quality of SVM for regression depends on several parameters namely, kernel type k, which determines the sample distribution in the mapping space, and its corresponding parameter σ, capacity parameter C, and ε-insensitive loss function. The three parameters were optimized in a systematic grid search-way and the final optimal model was determined. Six general statistical parameters were selected to evaluate the prediction ability of the constructed model. These parameters are: root mean square error of prediction

(RMSEP), relative standard error of prediction (RSEP), mean absolute error (MAE), square of correlation coefficient (R2), F-statistical and t test. Table 5 shows the results of GA-PLS and GA-SVM and the calculated statistical parameters. This table shows that the results of the GA-SVM are better than GA-PLS.

No	Symbol	Class	Meaning
1	TE2	Charge descriptors	Topographic electronic descriptor(bond resctricted)
2	Ui	Empirical descriptors	Unsaturation index
3	GATS5e	2D autocorrelations	Geary autocorrelation-lag5/weighted by atomic Sanderson electronegativities
4	Mor13m	3D-MoRSE descriptors	3D MoRSE-signal13/weighted by atomic masses
5	ATS7m	2D autocorrelations	Broto-Moreau autocorrelation of a topological structure- lag7/ weighted by atomic masses
6	Ss	Constitutional descriptors	Sum of Kier-Hall electrotopological States
7	Mor27e	3D-MoRSE descriptors	3D MoRSE-signal27/weighted by atomic Sanderson electronegativities
8	RDF035e	RDF descriptors	Radial Distribution function-3.5/weighted by atomic Sanderson electronegativities

Table 4. Description of the selected descriptors in this study.

Parameters		GA-SVM	GA-PLS
NOC[a]			4
Q^2 LOO[b]		0.9672	0.8259
σ		0.5	
ε		0.06	
C		8	
RMSEP	Training set	0.2027	0.3934
	Test set	0.2751	0.3962
RSEP(%)	Training set	3.1520	6.1156
	Test set	4.0216	5.7928
MAE(%)	Training set	6.5080	8.9351
	Test set	18.093	21.745
R^2	Training set	0.9800	0.8935
	Test set	0.9355	0.8603
F statistical	Training set	1815.2	310.26
	Test set	72.481	30.792
T test	Training set	42.606	17.614
	Test set	8.5136	5.5491

[a] Number of components

[b] Q^2 Leave-one-out Cross-validation

Table 5. Results and statistical parameters of GA-PLS and GA-SVM.

Figure 7A shows calculated pIC_{50} against experimental values, while Figure 7B shows their residual values against the experimental pIC_{50} using GA-SVM.

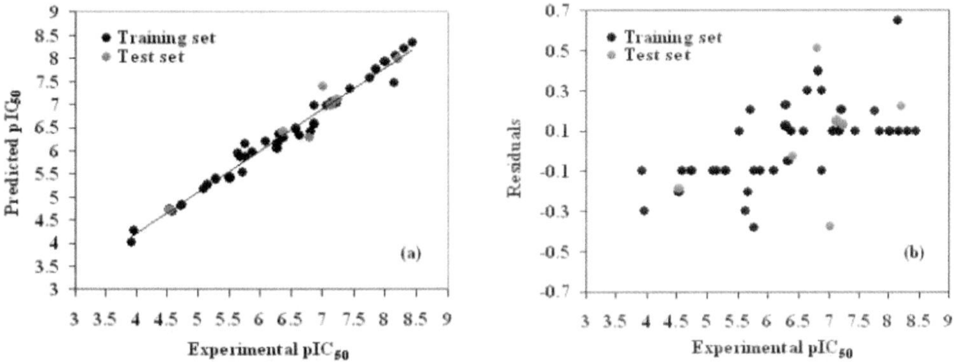

Fig. 7. A) Calculated pIC_{50} against the experimental values using GA-SVM. B) Residual values against experimental pIC_{50} using GA-SVM.

In summary, the support vector machine (SVM) and partial least square (PLS) methods were used to develop quantitative structure activity relationship (QSAR) models to predict the inhibitory activity of nonpeptide HIV-1 protease inhibitors. Genetic algorithm (GA) was employed to select variables that lead to the best-fitted models. A comparison between the obtained results using SVM with those of PLS revealed that the SVM model is much better than that of PLS. The root mean square errors of the training set and the test set for SVM model were calculated to be 0.2027, 0.2751, and the coefficients of determination (R^2) are 0.9800, 0.9355 respectively. Furthermore, the obtained statistical parameter of leave-one-out cross-validation test (Q^2) on SVM model was 0.9672, which proves the reliability of this model. Omar Deeb is thankful for Al-Quds University for financial support.

4. Acknowledgment

Omar Deeb is thankful for Al-Quds university for financial support.

5. References

Allen, D.M. (1974) The relationship between variable selection and data augmentation and a method for prediction. *Technometrics, 16*, 125-127.

Clare, B.W. (1998). The Frontier Orbital Phase Angles: Novel QSAR Descriptors for Benzene Derivatives, Applied to Phenylalkylamine Hallucinogens. *J. Med. Chem.* 41, 3845 – 3856.

Clare, B.W. (2000). The frontier orbital phase angles: a theoretical interpretation. *Theochem*, 507, 157-164.

Clare, B.W. (2001). Erratum to "The frontier orbital phase angles: a theoretical interpretation". *J. Mol. Struct. (Theochem)* 507 (2000) 157-167]. *Theochem*, 535 , 301-301.

Clare, B.W. (2002). QSAR of benzene derivatives: comparison of classical descriptors, quantum theoretic parameters and flip regression, exemplified by phenylalkylamine hallucinogens. *J. Comput.-Aided Mol. Des.* 16, 611-633.

Clare, B.W. (2004). A novel quantum theoretic QSAR for hallucinogenic tryptamines: a major factor is the orientation of π orbital nodes. *Theochem*, 712, 143-148.

Clare, B.W. and Supuran, C.T. (2004). Quantum Theoretic QSAR of Benzene Derivatives: Some Enzyme Inhibitors. *J. Enz. Inhib. Med. Chem.* 19, 237-248.

Clare, B.W. and Supuran, C.T. (2005a). Predictive Flip Regression: A Technique for QSAR of Derivatives of Symmetric Molecules, *J. Chem. Inf. Model.* 45, 1385-1391.

Clare, B.W. and Supuran, C.T (2005b). A physically interpretable quantum-theoretic QSAR for some carbonic anhydrase inhibitors with diverse aromatic rings, obtained by a new QSAR procedure. *Bioorg. Med. Chem.*, 13, 2197–2211.

Colmenarejo G. (2003). In silico prediction of drug-binding strengths to human serum albumin. *Med Res Rev*, 23, 275–301.

Cronin M.T.D., Gregory B.W. and Schultz T.W. (1998) Quantitative structure-activity analyses of nitrobenzene toxicity to Tetrahymena pyriformis. *Chem. Res. Toxicol.*, 11, 902–908.

Deeb O. and Hemmateenejad B., (2007). ANN-QSAR Model of Drug-binding to Human Serum Albumin, *Chem. Biol. Drug Des.* 70, 19-29.

Deeb O., (2010). Correlation ranking and stepwise regression procedures in principal components artificial neural networks modeling with application to predict toxic activity and human serum albumin binding affinity, *Chemometrics and Intelligent Laboratory Systems* 104, 181–194.

Deeb O. and Drabh M.,(2010). Exploring QSARs of some analgesic compounds by PC-ANN, *Chem Biol, Drug Des.* 76, 255-262.

Deeb O. and Goodarzi M., (2010), Exploring QSARs for Inhibitory Activity of Non-peptide HIV-1 Protease Inhibitors by GA-PLS and GA-SVM, *Chem. Biol. Drug Des.* 75, 506-514.

Deeb, O. and Clare, B.W., (2007). QSAR of Aromatic Substances: Protein Tyrosine Kinase Inhibitory Activity of Flavonoid Analogues. *Chem. Biol. Drug. Des.*, 70, 437–449.

Deeb, O. and Clare, B.W. (2008a) QSAR of aromatic substances: EGFR inhibitory activity of quinazoline Analogues. *J Enz. Inhib. Med. Chem.* 23, 763–775.

Deeb, O. and Clare, B.W.; (2008b) Comparison of AM1 and B3LYP-DFT for Inhibition of MAO-A by Phenylisopropylamines: A QSAR Study. *Chem. Biol. Drug. Des.*, 71, 352–362.

Devillers, J. and Balaban, A.T. (1999) *Topological Indices and Related Descriptors in QSAR and QSPR.* Gordon Breach Scientific Publishers: Amsterdam, 811.

Downs, G.M. (2004). Molecular Descriptors. In *Computational Medicinal Chemistry for Drug Discovery.* Bultinck, P.; De Winter, H.; Langenaeker, W.; Tollenaere, J. P. (Eds.). Marcel Dekker; New York, 515-538.

Duprat, A.F., Huynh, T. and Dreyfus, G.(1998). Toward a principled methodology for neural network design and performance evaluation in QSAR. Application to the prediction of log P. *J. Chem. Inf. Comput. Sci.*, *38*, 586-594.

Eriksson, L., Johansson, E., Kettaneh-Wold, N. and Wold S.(2001). *Multi- and Megavariate Data Analysis. Principles and Applications.* Umetrics: Umea.

Feng J., Lurati L., Ouyang H, Robinson T., Wang Y, Yuan Y. and Young S. (2003) Predictive toxicology: benchmarking molecular descriptors and statistical methods, *J. Chem. Inf. Comput. Sci.* 43, 1463–1470.

Free S. M. and Wilson J. W. , (1964). A Mathematical Contribution to Structure-Activity Studies. *J. Med. Chem.*, 7, 395-399.

Fujita, T., Iwasa, J. and Hansch, C. (1964). A new substituent constant,π, derived from partition coefficients. *J. Am. Chem. Soc.*, *86*, 5175-5180.

Fujita, T. (1990). The extrathermodynamic approach to drug design. In "*Comprehensive Medicinal Chemistry*" (C. Hansch, P. G. Sammes, and J. B. Taylor, eds.), Vol. 4, Pergamon, Elmsford, NY. pp. 497-560.

Gunn S.R. (1997) Support Vector Machines for Classification and Regression. UK: University of Southampton.

Hansch C., Maloney P. P., T. Fujita and Muir R. M. , (1962), Correlation of Biological Activity of Phenoxyacetic Acids with Hammett Substituent Constants and Partition Coefficients. *Nature*, 194, 178.

Hansch, C. and Fujita, T. (1964). ρ-σ-π analysis. A method for the correlation of biological activity and chemical structure. *J. Am. Chem. Soc.*, *86*, 1616-1626.

Hansch, C. (1969). A quantitative approach to biochemical structure-activity relationships. *Acct. Chem.Res.*, *2*, 232-239.

Jolliffe, I.T. (1986) *Principal Component Analysis*. Springer-Verlag: New York

Karelson, M. *(2000). Molecular Descriptors in QSAR/QSPR*. Wiley-InterScience; New York.

Katritzky, A.R., Lobanov, V.S. and Karelson, M.(1994) CODESSA, Reference Manual. Gainesville, FL University of Florida. Available: http://www.semichem.com/codessarefs.html

Kishida, K. and Manabe, R. (1980). The role of the hydrophobicity of the substituted groups of dichlorphenamide in the development of carbonic anhydrase inhibition. *Med. J. Osaka Univ.* 30, 95-100.

Leardi R., Boggia R. and Terrile M. (1992) Genetic algorithms as a strategy for feature selection. *J Chemom.* 6, 267–281.

Mathur K.C., Gupta S. and Khadikar P.V. (2003) Topological modeling of analgesia. *Bioorg Med Chem*, 11, 1915–1928.

Montgomery, D.C. and Peck, E.A.(1992) *Introduction to linear regression analysis*. Wiley: New York

Novi , M.; Nikolovska-Coleska, Z. and Solmajer, T.(1997) Quantitative structure-activity relationship of flavonoid p56 protein tyrosine kinase inhibitors. A neural network approach. *J. Chem. Inf. Comput. Sci.*, *37*, 990-998.

Shulgin, A., Shulgin A. and Pihkal A. (1991). A Chemical Love Story; Transform Press: Box 13675, Berkeley, CA, pp 864-869.

Silipo, C. and Vittoria, A. (1990) Three-Dimensional Structure of Drugs. In *Comprehensive Medicinal Chemistry. Vol 4. Quantitive Drug Design*. Hansch, C. Sammes, P.G.; Taylor, J.B.; eds. Pergamon Press, New York, 154-204.

Todeschini, R.; Consonni, V. and Pavan, M. (2001). DRAGON-Software for the Calculation of Molecular Descriptors. Release 1.12 for Windows. Available: http://www.disat.unimib/chm

Tetko, I.V.; Alessandro, E.; Villa, P. and Livingstone, D.J. (1996) Neural network studies. 2. Variable selection. *J. Chem. Inf. Comput. Sci.*, *36*, 794-803.

Tummino P.J., Prasad J.V.N.V., Ferguson D., Nouhan C., Graham N., Domagala J.M., Ellsworth E. et al. (1996) Discovery and optimization of nonpeptide HIV-1 protease inhibitors. *Bioorg Med Chem.*, 4, 1401–1410.

Wang X., Yin C. and Wang L. (2002) Structure–activity relationships and response–surface analysis of nitroaromatics toxicity to the yeast (Saccharomyces cerevisiae). *Chemosphere*, 46, 1045–1051.

Wold, S. (1978) Cross-validatory estimation of the number of components in factor and principal component models. *Technometrics, 20,* 397-405.

Wold, S. (1991) Validation of QSARs. *Quant. Struct.-Act. Relat., 10,* 191-193.

Wold, S., Johansson, E. and Cocchi, M.(1993) PLS—partial least squares projections to latent structures. In *3D-QSAR in Drug Design, Theory, Methods, and Applications*. Kubinyi, H. (Ed). ESCOM Science Publishers: Leiden, 523–550

Xu, L. and Zhang, W.J.(2001) Comparison of different methods for variable selection. *Anal. Chim. Acta, 446,* 477–483.

Yang E.B., Guo Y.J., Zhang K., Chen Y.Z. and Mack P. (2001) Inhibition of epidermal growth factor receptor tyrosine kinase by chalcone derivatives. *Biochim. Biophys. Acta.,* 1550, 144-152.

4

Inhibitors of Serine Proteinase – Application in Agriculture and Medicine

Rinat Islamov, Tatyana Kustova and Alexander Ilin
Scientific Centre for Anti-Infectious Drugs
Kazakhstan

1. Introduction

Inhibitors are important elements of regulation of enzyme activity. They can be named ubiquitous components in living organisms (Fan & Wu, 2005). There is a number of inhibitors, such as protein and nonprotein. Among all inhibitors, the most significant are inhibitors of hydrolytic enzymes. Hydrolases are enzymes that catalyze the hydrolysis of chemical bonds. For example, proteolytic enzymes (peptidases or proteinases) hydrolyse the peptide bond, glycosidic glycosidases, esterases hydrolytically cleave the ester bond (The Enzyme List, 2010). The inhibitors of hydrolases was found in bacteria, plants, fungi and animals (Rawlings et al., 2004).

In the homeostatic state the ratio of proteinases and their inhibitors in the tissues of animals and humans is balanced, but at various pathological conditions, this equilibrium is disturbed. For example, at carcinogenesis, seeking to destroy the tissue barrier, synthesized mainly protease (Duffy et al., 2002).

Changes in the ratio of activity of proteases and their inhibitors are observed in the fungal and bacterial skin lesions, traumatic lesions of the eye, burns, apoptosis and other pathological processes (Garcia-Carreno, 1996; Bohm et al., 1998; Thorburn et al., 2003; Wouters et al., 2008). Thus, some inhibitors are actively affected both the cellular environment and on the cell proteome, changing its composition (Vincent & Zivy, 2007).

Most of them are used for medical purposes. For example, inhibitors of thrombin, a key factor in blood clotting. Thrombin (clotting factor II) is the trypsin-like proteases, which circulate in the blood in an inactive zymogen form. The search for new thrombin inhibitors began long before receiving the full 3D structure of thrombin. Initially, were synthesized short peptides containing the amino acid arginine, for example, H-Gly-Pro-Arg-H or H-DPhe-Pro-Arg-H. Then were obtained effective non-specific serine protease inhibitors – ketone-derivatives of 4-amidinophenylpyruvic acid and 4-aminopyridine (Smith & Simons, 2004).

One of the key enzymes of hepatitis C virus replication is a trypsin-like serine protease NS3. Obtained multiple protease inhibitors NS3, including macrocyclic and peptidomimetics (Harper et al., 2009).

Inhibitors of hydrolytic enzymes also play an important role in plant protection. They are widely used use in protecting plants from fungal and bacterial diseases as well as in insect control. Harvest losses associated with damage to plants by various pathogens, can reach 100%, leading to economic disaster (Mehrabadi et al., 2010). The Republic of Kazakhstan is also concerned about the problem of protecting crops from pests because it is one of durum wheat exporter. At this reason Kazakhstan is paying attention to the study of inhibitors contained in wheat, barley and rice. Besides studies in agriculture sector, studies in medicine sector are conducted, for example in the Scientific Centre for Anti-Infectious Drugs were developed iodine-polymer complexes as inhibitors of HIV integrase (Yuldasheva et al., 2011).

2. Serine proteinase inhibitors

Serine proteinase inhibitors long time were classified according to their characteristics, for example, inhibits the enzyme (trypsin inhibitors, subtilisin, etc.) or source selection - the chicken or ovomucoid pancreatic trypsin inhibitor or by the location of the amino acid residue of lysine or arginine in the reactive centre (Laskowski Jr. & Kato, 1980). This nomenclature is often confusing. One of the challenges ranges of inhibitors is the presence of several homologous domains in a single polypeptide chain (Fan & Wu, 2005; Hejgaard et al., 2005; Dunwiddie et al., 1989).

Typically, the inhibitors are divided by at least 10 families or types of proteinase inhibitors (Laskowski Jr. & Kato, 1980). Among the most studied can be noted soybeans Kunitz inhibitor. To the family of Kunitz inhibitors are proteins with a long polypeptide chain of about 170 - 200 amino acids that contain one or two disulfide bonds and a rather conservative N-site, and generally inhibit the activity of trypsin or chymotrypsin. One well-studied is the soybean Kunitz inhibitor, which is a protein type globulin with a molecular weight of about 21.5 kDa, contains carbohydrate residues, is stable over a wide pH range 1,0-12,0, at a temperature below 40°C. Inhibitor molecule consists of 198 amino acids at the N-terminal aspartic acid is located on the C-terminal leucine. Reactive centre includes the residue arginine-64 (Valueva & Mosolov, 2002). By the way, due to the high content of inhibitor in soybeans, raw soybeans, and raw foods are warming, causing the digestive system in mammals (Duranti M., et al. 2003).

Inhibitors of Bowman-Birk types are widely distributed in plants and significantly different from the Kunitz inhibitor in their amino acid composition and are able to interact not only with trypsin, but with chymotrypsin (Valueva & Mosolov, 2002; Rawlings et al., 2004). Inhibitors of Bowman-Birk type characterized by the presence of two reactive centers on a single polypeptide chain rich in cysteine (7 or more residues in one polypeptide), and the lack of amino acid residues tryptophan and tyrosine. The molecular weight of such inhibitors can vary from 8 to 16 kDa. Sometimes there are inhibitors that contain two domains on one polypeptide chain and active only in relation to one type of enzyme (Valueva & Mosolov, 2002; Yan et al., 2009; Mosolov & Valueva, 2008).

Kazal family inhibitors - the type of trypsin inhibitor-like proteinase, commonly found in animals, including invertebrates. Molecules consist of one or more domains, and three disulfide bridges. The sequence of many often conservative, but the site of binding to the enzyme can be variable (Li et al., 2009; Rimphanitchayakit & Tassanakajon, 2010) Kazal inhibitors are involved in various pathologies of the pancreas. In particular inhibitor Kazal SPINK1 is expressed not only in normal cells of the pancreas, but also transformed. It is assumed that SPINK1 is able to stimulate proliferation of pancreatic cancer through epidermal growth factor receptor / proteinkinase cascade. Inhibitor SPINK1 is also expressed in other organs and tissues. Apparently, this indicates that the value of SPINK1 is not only in preventing proteolysis non-secretory of proteinases in the gut, but he also has some regulatory function (Ozaki et al., 2009).

Seprpins (serin proteinase inhibitors) group of proteins, which have inhibitory activity, but it is not an inhibitor in the strict sense of the body and performs a different function. Among the most studied serpin antithrombin may be noted, ovalbumin, cortisol binding globulin, precursors of peptide hormones, etc. (Valueva & Mosolov, 2002; Rawlings et al., 2004). Serpins widespread in the proteome, and despite the name, serpins inhibit also other proteases, such as cysteine, aspartate etc.

The examples of classification and nomenclature of inhibitors, really confusing and complicated. Therefore, the team (Rawlings et al., 2004) developed a classification system of inhibitors based on sequence relationship and the relationship of protein fold on the inhibitory domain. An inhibitor domain is defined as the segment of the amino acid sequence containing a single reactive site after removal of any parts that are not directly involved in the inhibitor activity. Their searches of the amino acid sequence databases led to the retrieval of 2500 sequences homologous to those of known peptidase inhibitors. On the basis of sequence homologies of their inhibitor domain proteinase inhibitors been classified into 48 families. As expected, the greatest numbers of inhibitors with a similar sequence were in the family serpin, I4, with over 500 sequences. In turn, families are divided into clans. The study of inhibitors of proliferation of living organisms found, only three families are known so far from Archaea, two of which (I4 (serpins) and I42 (chagasin)) are present in all three superkingdoms. I4 is the most widespread of all, being found even in viruses (Rawlings et al., 2004).

3. The use of protease inhibitors in medicine

The discovery, development, and registration of a pharmaceutical are an immensely expensive operation and represent a rather unique challenge. For every 9000 to 10,000 compounds specifically synthesized or isolated as potential therapeutics, one (on average) will actually reach the market. Each successive stage in the process is more expensive, making it of great interest to identify as early as possible those agents that are likely not to go the entire distance, allowing a concentration of effort on the compounds that have the highest probability of reaching the market (Das & Suresh, 2008).

Throughout most of history, humanity has used as medicines from natural sources, such as medicinal plants, by-products of animals and insects, etc. After isolation of these active substances and determine their molecular structure, drug manufacturing has become more ambitious. This is confirmed by the fact that all 250 of the main structures of existing drugs, as well as their prototypes, 60% were derived from natural sources or has a common molecular structure (Spainhour, 2005; Molinari, 2009). Only a small number have been developed and synthesized "from scratch" (Spainhour, 2005).

So, natural products have been the single most productive source of leads for the development of drugs. Over a 100 new products are in clinical development, particularly as anti-cancer agents and anti-infection (Harvey, 2008).

Mainly drugs are protein-based categories namely, recombinant proteins and enzymes, monoclonal antibodies and their derivatives, and synthetic peptides (Das & Suresh, 2008). Although there are studies that propose to use protein inhibitors as drugs. One of the problems of using proteins as drugs of instability in the gastrointestinal tract (GIT), and intravenous administration response from the immune system (Das & Suresh, 2008).

To protect the protein drugs from cleavage by enzymes in the GIT using of encapsulation or complexation with inhibitors. Some researchers propose to encapsulation with an inhibitor aprotinin (Larionova et al., 1999a). Aprotinin - basic pancreatic trypsin inhibitor, which inhibits trypsin and related proteolytic enzymes. By inhibiting kallikrein, aprotinin indirectly inhibits the formation of activated factor XII, a biochemical reaction normally amplified by inhibition of the contact system and of fibrinolysis by aprotinin. Aprotinin inhibits the initiation of both coagulation and fibrinolysis induced by the contact of blood with a foreign surface (Mannucci, 1998). Further studies have shown the effectivity aprotinin for suppressing viral replication rhinotracheitis and adenovirus in vitro (Larionova et al., 2000b).

Russian researchers (Valuev et al., 2001) have proposed as a protection from destruction of proteins in the digestive tract ovomucoid inhibitor included in the hydrogel. In the hydrogel also included insulin. As a result, the mechanism of action, this involves the inhibition of proteolysis of insulin due to neutralizing proteolytic enzymes and increasing the rate of diffusion of insulin from the particles through the small intestine. Rapid diffusion provided by interaction of the carbohydrate bonds of the hydrogel and of the ovomucoid with of lectins intestinal mucosa.

Inhibitors of serine proteinase can be used in the therapy of diseases associated with bowels surgery. Under intestinal resection, as well as ulcerative colitis, a high activity of proteolytic enzymes in the faeces are observed, which is highly undesirable (Bohe, 1987). Studies have shown that inhibitors of serine proteinases from potato significantly reduce the depression of the skin in the anogenital region in patients with intestinal resection, as well as healthy children, in which the activity of proteinases in the feces is physiologically increased (Ruseler-van Embden et al., 2004).

Proteinase inhibitors (aprotinin, ilomastat) can be used in the treatment of acute and chronic damage to lung tissue (Anderson et al., 2009; Weinberger et al., 2011). Chronic lung disease due to interstitial fibrosis can be a consequence of acute lung injury and inflammation. The inflammatory response is mediated through the migration of inflammatory cells (neutrophil granulocyte et al), actions of proinflammatory cytokines, and the secretion of matrix-degrading proteinases. The activation of circulating granulocytes was characterized by increased production of serine proteinases and reactive oxygen metabolites. After the initial inflammatory insult, successful healing of the lung may occur, or alternatively, dysregulated tissue repair can result in scarring and fibrosis. On the basis of recent insights into the mechanisms underlying acute lung injury and its long-term consequences, data suggest that proteinases may not only be involved in the breakdown and remodelling that occurs during the injury but may also cause the release of growth factors and cytokines known to influence growth and differentiation of target cells within the lung (Neumann et al., 1999; Winkler & Fowlkes, 2001).

The effectiveness of proteinase inhibitors as anti-oxidants has been investigated on a model venom-induced tissue damage in rats by Scorpion venom toxins (Fatani et al., 2006).As an antioxidant was used inhibitor aprotinin. Aprotinin alone significantly reduces the venom-elicited increase in glucose-6-phosphate dehydrogenase and lactate dehydrogenase activities and the decrease in glutathione peroxidase levels. But the best results were obtained when the joint application of extract of *Gingko biloba* leaves and aprotinin (Fatani et al., 2006).

As we see the role of proteinase inhibitors in the pathogenesis of disease is significant. In our view, it is important to note the significance of inhibitors in tumours processes. Various types of proteinases are implicated in the malignant progression of tumours and increase oxidative stress (Koblinski et al., 2000; Aoshiba al., 2001). To be fair, it is not always proteases have been associated with cancer progression (Lypez-Otin & Matrisian, 2007).

Nevertheless, proteinase inhibitors may therefore be useful as therapeutic agents in anti-invasive and anti-metastatic treatment. Studies have shown that potato cysteine proteinase inhibitor PCPI 8.7 inhibited invasion B16 mouse melanoma cell by 21% and serine proteinase inhibitor reduced invasiveness by up to 24 % (Sever et al., 2005). Overexpression of cathepsin B excessively associated with adenocarcinoma of the esophagus and other cancers (Kos & Lah, 1998).

Trypsin inhibitor from soybean BBI 3 can suppress the growth of cancer cells (Armstrong et al., 2000). Because of its inhibitory properties BBI3 can be used inside in the form of capsules and tablets, dispersible in the gut, not worrying about what will be split by proteases of the gastrointestinal tract.

A very interesting example may be the use of Bowman-Birk Inhibitor (BBI) from soybeans in the treatment of multiple sclerosis. Proteases generated during inflammation are involved in the induction of tissue damage during inflammatory demyelination in the central nervous system. Both in vitro and ex vivo, BBI inhibited myelin basic protein-specific proliferation of lymph node cells. BBI reduced the activity of matrix metalloproteinase-2 and -9 in spleen cell supernatants and was detected in the central nervous system of treated rats. BBI suppresses experimental autoimmune encephalomyelitis, it can be administered orally, and it is safe and relatively inexpensive. It may have a therapeutic role in patients with MS (Gran et al., 2006).

Bifunctional inhibitor of xylanase and aspartic proteases from extremophilic microorganism Bacillus sp. aspartic proteinase inhibits HIV-1 (Dash et al., 2001).

The Bowman-Birk trypsin-chymotrypsin inhibitor (BBI) from soybean has been proposed as anticarcinogenic drugs. The BBI inhibited the growth of human colorectal adenocarcinoma HT29 cells in vitro (Clemente et al., 2005).

The trypsin inhibitor from *Peltophorum dubium* seeds (PDTI), as well as soybean trypsin inhibitor (SBTI), both belonging to the Kunitz family, have lectin-like properties and trigger rat lymphoma cell apoptosis. It was shown that PDTI and SBTI induce human leukemia Jurkat cell death. Induction of apoptosis was confirmed by flow cytometry (Troncoso et al., 2009).

In our research studies the cytotoxicity of trypsin inhibitor extract (Islamov & Fursov, 2007) from wheat seeds was evaluated by counting the cells at the time of harvest, with a haemocytometr. Cytotoxicity in treated cultures was assessed by Relative increase in cell counts (Fellows & O'Donovan, 2007; Lorge et al., 2008). This study was made on L5178Y TK +/- clone 3.7.2c mouse lymphoma cells which were obtained from American Type Culture Collection. Cells were cultured in RPMI 1640 medium supplemented with 10% heat-inactivated horse serum, 200 U/ml penicillin, 50 μg/ml streptomycin, 2.5 μg/ml amphotericin B, 200 μg/ml L-glutamine, 200 μg/ml sodium pyruvate and 500 μg/ml pluronic acid. Cell cultures were grown in a humidified atmosphere with 5% CO2 in air at 37°C. Cells tested negative for mycoplasma contamination and were routinely passaged to maintain exponential growth. Three concentration of trypsin inhibitor substance was tested 1/1000, 1/100, 1/10 (v/v). The exposure was 24-h and 0-h recovery. Utilizing exponentially proliferating cells, 96 V-bottomed wells were seeded at a concentration of 6×10^4 cells per well. Each concentration was performed in triplicate. At the end of treatment time 20 μl of cells from each concentration was mix with trypan blue 1:1 (v/v). An aliquot of the cell suspension was then transferred to a hemacytometer for cell counts. The cell counts were used to determine Relative increase in cell counts. Representative results for trypsin inhibitor extract are shown in Table 1.

Concentration of trypsin inhibitors (μg/ml)	% Toxicity RICC*
Negative control	0
500	100%
50	91%
5	14%

*Relative increase in cell counts

Table 1. Cytotoxicity trypsin inhibitors from grain wheat

Our studies have shown the cytotoxic effect of trypsin inhibitors. Similar results were obtained in cell culture H28 of malignant mesothelioma. When adding Bowman-Birk protease inhibitor from soybeans at concentrations of 200-400 μg/ml Inhibition of cell growth (Kashiwagi et al., 2011). Currently, research is continuing to explore mechanisms of toxicity. Apparently, this may be related to the processes of apoptosis (Troncoso et al., 2009).

A completely different example of the serpin CrmA (cytokine response modifier A), which expresses Cowpox virus. The targets of CrmA are members of the caspase family of proteases that either initiate the extrinsic pathway of apoptosis (caspases 8 and 10) or trigger activation of the pro-inflammatory cytokines interleukin-1β and interleukin-18 (caspase 1). CrmA has the typical fold of a cleaved serpin, even though it lacks the N-terminal half of the A helix, the entire D helix, and a portion of the E helix that are present in all other known serpins. Thus, the inhibitory proteins can be not only drugs. They may also viral countermeasures to host defenses against infection may contribute significantly to the pathology associated with poxvirus infections (Renatus et al., 2000).

Such examples are very much (Polya, 2003). All this points to the crucial regulate the activity inhibitors of proteinase activity. In addition, the study of mechanisms of interaction enzyme with inhibitor can tell researchers how to develop new drugs - semi synthetic (including modified) and synthetic (non-protein). So, after some modification of the reactive site serpin, they acquire the ability to block angiogenesis and induce tumor regression (Carrell, 1999). Successfully completed Phase 2 clinical trials engineered protein inhibitor of human neutrophil elastase (Dyax Corp. & Debiopharm). Human neutrophil elastase, an enzyme produced as part of the inflammatory response, is implicated in the loss of lung function in patients with cystic fibrosis and other clinical conditions. (Dyax Corp. & Debiopharm). The inhibitor of human neutrophil elastase is derived from the Kunitz-type domain of inter-α-inhibitor which is a natural inhibitor of human neutrophil elastase normally present in plasma (Grimbert et al., 2003).

There is enough work, in which information about the protease inhibitors and their application (Wenzel & Tschesche, 1995; Polya, 2003).

4. Inhibitors in agriculture

Considering the basic properties of inhibitors - inhibition of enzyme activity, they have successfully used to control pests. It is known that plants are often damaged by many different pathogens - fungi, bacteria and viruses (Selitrennikoff, 2001; Franco et al., 2002). Also, insects and parasitic worms of plants are cause illness and death of plants frequently, causing great agricultural economic losses. However, during infection of plants by infectious agents, not all plants of one population or species ill. This is due to phytoimmunity - the ability to resist pathogens (Valueva & Mosolov, 2002; Mosolov & Valueva, 2008). Protective mechanisms were elaborated in the long process of co-existence of host and parasite. The major components of the existing protection mechanisms are substances of protein nature. These include enzymes - glucanase, chitinase and protease inhibitors and α-amylase. For example, damage to tomato leaves (*Licopersicon esculentum* Mill.) by insects or microorganisms induce the synthesis of more than twenty different proteins, including inhibitors of serine, cysteine proteinases and aspartilnyh and α-amylase (Valueva & Mosolov, 2002).

Inhibitors of trypsin and chymotrypsin from soybeans, beans and potato to suppress proteinase from phytopathogenic fungus (*Fusarium solani*). Moreover, the inhibitors belonging to the family of Bowman-Birk inhibit the growth of hyphae and conidia germination of fungi *Fusarium solani, F. culmorum* and *Botrytis cinerea,* etc. (Loreti et al., 2002). Along with trypsin and chymotrypsin inhibitors in plants and detected proteins that inhibit proteases of microorganisms.

Quite interesting are bifunctional inhibitors. Bifunctional inhibitors - proteins that contain two active sites, interacting as one of the enzymes, eg trypsin/trypsin, and various enzymes - trypsin/chymotrypsin or proteinase/amylase (Sreerama et al., 1997; Valueva & Mosolov, 2002; Mosolov & Valueva, 2008).

Bifunctional (double-headed) inhibitors of proteases, traditionally, belong to the family Bowman-Birk inhibitors. Bifunctional inhibitors are assumed to have arisen by duplication of an ancestral single headed inhibitor gene and subsequently diverged into different classes and with a network of highly conserved disulfide bridges (Odani et al., 1983; Qi et al., 2005). However, interest bifunctional inhibitors active against both proteases and amylases (Table 2).

The first three bifunctional inhibitor (BASI, WASI and RASI) show significant similarities in the structure and properties (Ohtsubo & Richardson, 1992; Franco et al., 2002; Nielsen et al., 2004).

Inhibitors	Family or subfamily	Source	Molecular weight, kDa	Isoelectric points	Residue numbers	Reference
α-amylase/subtilisin (BASI)	I3A (Kunitz (plant)	*Hordeum vulgare* L	19,879	7,2	181	(Nielsen et al., 2004)
α-amylase/subtilisin (WASI)	I3A (Kunitz (plant)	*Triticum aestivum* L	20,5	7,2	187	(Mundy et al., 1984)
α-amylase/subtilisin (RASI)	I3A (Kunitz (plant)	*Orysa sativa* L.	21	9,05	189	(Yamasaki et al., 2006)
α-amylase/proteinase K (PKI3)	-	*Triticum aestivum* L	19,6	> 7	180	(Zemke et al., 1991)
α-amylase/trypsin (BIAT)	I6 (cereal)	*Triticum aestivum* L	14,0	10	-	(Islamov & Fursov, 2007)
α-amylase/trypsin (RBI)	I6 (cereal)	*Eleusine coracana* Gaertneri	13,3	10	122	(Maskos et al., 1996)

Table 2. Bifunctional inhibitors of amylase/protease of cereals

Thanks to the "dual" activity, the bifunctional inhibitor of amylase/proteinase appears to provide synergetic effect in protecting against pathogens. Bifunctional inhibitors of the subject of many articles and studies (Konarev et al., 1999; Franco et al., 2002; Birk, 2003; Salcedo et al., 2004; Pouvreau, 2004; Habib & Fazil, 2007).

The essential role of inhibitors in plant protection from insects and other pests inspired the creation of transgenic plants. Transgenic plants with enhanced resistance to insects, containing the genes of proteinase inhibitors. Trypsin inhibitor gene (SrTI) of cowpea (*Vigna unguiculata* L.) was transferred into tobacco plants (*Nicotiana tabacum* L.). Plants content SrTI reached 1% of total soluble protein, the defeat of the tobacco cutworm larvae plants decreased by 50% (Valueva & Mosolov, 2002). Along with transgenic plants containing genes of serine protease inhibitors were obtained plants expressing genes of inhibitors of cysteine proteinases. Extracts of potato containing the gene of LS-1, effectively inhibited the activity of proteinases from the digestive tract Colorado potato beetle (*Leptinotarsa decemlineata* Say) (Mosolov & Valueva, 2008).

Differential expression of the CaMV proteinase inhibitor obtained the transfer of the corresponding gene using Agrobacterium transformation into the genome of tobacco culture (*Solanum nigrum*) and alfalfa (*Medicago sativa*). Expression was studied by measuring mRNA levels in leaves of CaMV. It was also shown the accumulation of inhibitors in the vacuoles of Solanum nigrum to 125 mg per 1 g of tissue, tobacco, 75 mcg / g, alfalfa 20mkg / g (Valueva & Mosolov, 2002). In a similar way shape transgenic peas (*Pisum sativum*), which is introduced into a plant α-amylase cDNA inhibitor I bean (*Phaseolus vulgaris*) and "substituted" under a strong promoter of phytohemagglutinin. As a result, the inhibitor content increased to 3% of soluble protein, compared with the control (1%). Although I inhibitor inhibits α-amylase man, his concentration was not sufficient to disrupt the digestive proces (Schroeder et al., 1995).

Inhibitors of proteolytic enzymes may play an important role in plant protection not only from harmful insects, but also other pests: nematodes, the nematodes. Many nematodes are parasitic on plants and cause significant damage to agricultural production. In the gut of nematodes contains active cysteine and serine proteases, including chymotrypsin and kallikrein is similar. It is interesting that when infected with worms, among transcripts of tomato were found proteins related to the family of Kunitz inhibitor (SBTI) (Valueva & Mosolov, 2002; Schroeder et al., 1995).

Expression of proteinase inhibitor chimera-II-CAT in tissues of potato tobacco prevailed 50 times under the influence of 1% sugar (maltose, glucose and fructose) in the farmed environment. Adding mannitol to the nutrient medium in place of these sugars does not affect the synthesis inhibitor-II-CAT (Valueva &Mosolov, 2002). The resulting transgenic plants from cell cultures of tobacco leaves revealed sensitivity to a 3% sucrose, which results in increased synthesis inhibitor-II-CAT 3-fold (Mundy et al., 1986). In addition, a mechanical failure of one of the leaves of the plant stimulates the transcription of genes encoding proteinase inhibitors are not only damaged but also in intact tissues. Systemic induction of gene expression was also observed with wounds or infected tomatoes (Valueva & Mosolov, 2002). Similar results, mostly on potatoes are presented in studies and reviews (Rolland et al., 2002).

In the process of co-existence of plants and their vermins, every organism has developed a protection system, and ways to overcome this protection. Plants synthesize a large number of different inhibitors, which makes them not edible. In response, many vermin have developed a system of protection against these inhibitors. Especially, began to secrete enzymes are not susceptible to inhibition by inhibitors of the existing (Maarten & Jules, 2011). For example, instead of trypsin, which is actively suppressed by inhibitors of trypsin and which are enriched with plants, insects began to synthesized chymotrypsin-like enzymes (Valueva & Mosolo, 2002). So, in future research the question of the co-evolution of insect proteases and plant inhibitors should be better approached from a systems level.

Apart from the use of inhibitors in the creation of transgenic plants resistant to certain pathogens, they are also of interest as genetic markers to study diversity, evolution and plant breeding. In many Compositae plants shows monogenic control, while interline crosses, loci coding for many protein inhibitors, have demonstrated linked inheritance. For example, the cyclic inhibitor, with a mass of 1.5 kDa and trypsin inhibitor, three groups of sunflowers, which, according to the results of mating, gave the values of the recombination frequencies for different pairs of loci from 0.23 to 0.40 in F2. Small molecule inhibitors of the information on the TI better match the taxonomy of Asteridae, based on data for molecular markers than the classical (Lawrence & Koundal, 2002).

A number of cereal caryopsis contains two clearly divided groups of inhibitors with a mass of 12 and 24 kDa. A comparative study of intraspecific polymorphism of these proteins and their components of different species showed that the evolution of the spectrum there is a complication of inhibitors and most complete range of typical soft hexaploid wheat (Schroeder et al., 1995).

In the works of A. Konarev (Konarev et al. 1999; Konarev et al., 2004) shows in detail the variability of inhibitors of trypsin-like proteinases in cereals due to resistance to various grain pests. So in wheat trypsin inhibitors are represented by several genetically independent systems of proteins controlled by the genome and B chromosomes 1D (endosperm), 3Dβ (aleurone layer), 1DS and 3Aβ (leaf). Trypsin inhibitors of rye are controlled chromosome 3R and barley 3H. The most complex structure of inhibitors was wheat leaves, with the genomic formula AABBDD. In general, it is the sum of the spectra of trypsin inhibitors from several tetraploid (T. turgidum) (AABB) and (Aegilops tauschii Coss.) (DD) (Konarev, 1986; Konarev et al., 2004).

In addition to the trypsin inhibitors are very interesting inhibitors of chymotrypsin and subtilisin, which are the most heterogeneous structure and variability of all species of wheat and corn and barley, which are controlled by fifth chromosome, while the wheat and rye - I homoeologous group of chromosomes of different genomes. In diploid wheat, a number of species (*T. timopheevii*) identified the protein components capable of inhibiting both subtilisin and chymotrypsin, which are characterized by low variability (Konarev et al., 2004).

Investigation of the stability of different wheat varieties to pest insect (*Rhyzopertha dominica* F) showed some dependence on composition of trypsin inhibitors and chymotrypsin. Grades Kirghiz 16, Saratov 41 had low levels of trypsin inhibitors and demonstrated the instability to the pest insect. Whereas grade Kalayan Sona, Saba, Diamond, Aurora 44, Zernogardskaya 39 were resistant to grain pest insect. This is also confirmed by the fact that part of the digestive enzymes *R. dominica* F. are trypsin-like proteases. In addition, a variety Zernogardskaya 39 contained a number of specific inhibitors of α-amylase insects (Konarev, 1986; Konarev et al., 1999; Konarev, 2006).

As we see the potential use of inhibitors in agriculture and in particular, to protect plants from pests wide. Such an approach to crop protection against loss of environmentally safer and economically more advantageous. Since there is no need to conduct expensive toxicological studies of new insecticides. The products of these plants are safe for humans and animals. And the use of transgenic technology will accelerate the development of new, resistant to insect pests, plant varieties.

5. Conclusion

Presented data from studies of protein inhibitors of serine proteases confirm their crucial role in the regulation of proteolytic enzymes. Examples of their use as drugs, crop protection agents, antioxidants, etc. are given in this chapter. No less interesting is the diversity of the whole family of inhibitory proteins - Serpin. Nevertheless, there are several obstacles to widespread use of inhibitors:

1. Several inhibitors of serine proteases can cause allergies.
2. Intravenous application of inhibitors is extremely difficult because of their antigenic properties.
3. Increased production of one of the inhibitor in the plant is inefficient, since most vermins are able to quickly adapt to it.

At the same time, there are positive aspects for the development of research inhibitors. It should also be noted.

1. Studying the mechanisms of interaction of natural protein inhibitors of enzymes provides an opportunity to develop approaches to the preparation of synthetic, small molecule inhibitors.
2. The prevalence of proteinase inhibitors in all kingdom, from viruses to eukaryotes, and indicates their important role in the regulation of proteolysis.
3. The use of two or more inhibitors at the same time to protect plants from pests, reducing the ability of pathogens to adapt.

So, enzyme - inhibitor interactions are very important process into living organisms. To date, a variety of genetic and biochemical methods exist for studying enzyme - inhibitor interactions and identifying of such interactions.

As mentioned earlier, of methods of the quantum chemistry, not only managed to learn in detail about HIV integrase, but also to develop an algorithm for obtaining drugs based on organic complexes of iodine. The next step is to study the inhibition of organic complexes of iodine with HIV proteinase.

Quite promising direction is also in search of new plants, small inhibitors. Examples of the serpin showed that any protein can potentially be an inhibitor that expands the range of functional significance of the proteome.

6. References

Anderson, D.R., Taylor, S.L., Fetterer, D.P., Holmes, W.W. (2009). Evaluation of protease inhibitors and an antioxidant for treatment of sulfur mustard-induced toxic lung injury. *Toxicology,* Vol. 263, No. 1, (Sep. 2009), pp. 41-46, ISSN 0300-483X

Aoshiba, K., Yasuda, K., Yasui, Sh., Tamaoki, J., Nagai, A. (2001). Serine proteases increase oxidative stress in lung cells. *Am. J. Physiol. Lung Cell Mol. Physiol.,* Vol. 281, L. 556–L564, ISSN 1522-1504

Armstrong, W.B., Kennedy, A.R., Wan, X.S. (2000). Single-dose administration of Bowman-Birk inhibitor concentrate in patients with oral leukoplakia. *Cancer Epidemiol. Biomarkers Prev.,* Vol. 9, pp. 43-47, ISSN 1538-7755

Birk, Y. (2003). *Plant protease inhibitors: significance in nutrition, plant protection, cancer prevention, and genetic engineering,* Springer, ISBN 3540001182, Germany

Bohe, M. (1987). Pancreatic and granulocytic endoproteases in faecal extracts from patients with active ulcerative colitis. *Scand. J. Gastroenterol.,* Vol. 22, No. 1, pp. 59-64, ISSN 1502-7708

Bohm, S.K., McConalogue, K., Kong, W., Bunnett, N.W. (1998). Proteinase-activated receptors: new functions for old enzymes. *News in Physiological Sciences,* Vol. 13, No. 5, pp. 231-240, ISSN 1522-161X

Carrell, R.W. (1999). How serpins are shaping up. *Science.* Vol. 285, No. 35, pp. 1861-1863, ISSN 1095-9203

Clemente, A., Gee, J.M., Johnson, I.T., Mackenzie, D.A., Domoney, C. (2005). Pea (Pisum sativum L.) protease inhibitors from the Bowman-Birk class influence the growth of human colorectal adenocarcinoma HT29 cells in vitro. *J. Agric. Food Chem.,* Vol. 16, No. 23, pp. 8979-8986, ISSN 0021-8561

Das, D., Suresh, M.R. (2008). Preclinical Development of Protein Pharmaceuticals: An Overview. In: *Preclinical development handbook,* Ed. Sh.C. Gad, pp. 713-740, John Wiley & Sons, ISBN 978-0-470-24846-1, USA

Dash, Ch., Rao, R. (2001). Interactions of a novel inhibitor from an extremophilic Bacillus sp. with HIV-1 protease. *J. Biol. Chem.,* Vol. 276, No. 4, pp. 2487-2493, ISSN 0021-9258

Duffy, M.J., Maguire, T.M., Hill, A., McDermott, E., O'Higgins, H. (2000). Metalloproteinases: role in breast carcinogenesis, invasion and metastasis. *Breast Cancer Research,* Vol. 2, No. 4, pp. 252-257, ISSN 1465- 5411

Dunwiddie, Ch., Thornberry, N.A., Bull, H.G., Sardana, M., Friedman, P.A., Jacobs, J.W., Simpson, E. (1989). Antistasin, a leech-derived inhibitor of factor Xa. *J. Biol. Chem.,* Vol. 264, No. 28, pp. 16694-16699, ISSN 0021-9258

Duranti, M., Barbiroli, A., Scarafoni, A., Tedeschi, G., Morazzoni, P. (2003). One-step purification of Kunitz soybean trypsin inhibitor. *Protein Expr. Purif.,* Vol. 30, pp.167-170, ISSN 1096-0279

Fan, S., Wu, G. (2005). Characteristics of plant proteinase inhibitors and their applications in combating phytophagous insects. *Bot. Bull. Acad. Sin.,* Vol. 46, pp. 273-292, ISSN 1817-406X

Fatani, A.J., Al-Zuhair, H.A., Yaquob, H.I., Abdel-Fattah, A.A., El-Sayed, M.I., El-Sayed, F.A. (2006). Protective effects of the antioxidant *Ginkgo biloba* extract and the protease inhibitor aprotinin against *Leiurus quinquestriatus* venom-induced tissue damage in rats. *J. Venom. Anim. Toxins. Incl. Trop. Dis.,* Vol. 12, No. 2, pp. 255-275, ISSN 1678-9199

Dyax Corp. and Debiopharm S.A. Report positive results from phase IIa clinical trial with DX-890 (EPI-hNE4) in children with cystic fibrosis, < www.debiopharm.com/images/files/doc3fddb49b39b70.pdf>

Franco, O.L., Rigden, D.J., Melo, F.R., Grossi-de-Sa, M.F. (2002). Plant alpha-amylse inhibitors and their interaction with insect alpha-amylases. *European Journal Biochemistry,* Vol. 269, pp. 397-412 ISSN 1432-1033

Fellows, M.D., O'Donovan, M.R. (2007). Cytotoxicity in cultured mammalian cells is a function of the method used to estimate it. *Mutagenesis,* Vol. 22, No. 4, pp. 275–280, ISSN 1464-3804

Garcia-Carreno, F.L. (1996). Proteinase inhibitors. *Trend in food science & Technology,* Vol. 7, pp. 197-204, ISSN 0924-2244

Gran, B., Tabibzadeh, N., Martin, A., Ventura, E.S., Ware, J.H., Zhang, G-X., Parr, J.L., Kennedy, A.R., Rostami, A.M. (2006). The protease inhibitor, Bowman-Birk inhibitor, suppresses experimental autoimmune encephalomyelitis: a potential oral therapy for multiple sclerosis. *Mult. Scler. J.,* Vol. 12, No. 6, pp. 688-697, ISSN 1477-0970

Grimbert, D., Vecellio, L., Delepine, P., Attucci, S., Boissinot, E., Poncin, A., Gauthier, F., Valat, C., Saudubray, F., Antonioz, P., Diot, P. (2003). Characteristics of EPI-hNE4 aerosol: a new elastase inhibitor for treatment of cystic fibrosis. *J. Aerosol. Med.,* Vol. 16, pp. 121–129, ISSN 0894-2684

Habib, H., Fazil, K.M. (2007). Plant protease inhibitors: a defense strategy in plants. *Biotechnology and Molecular Biology Review,* Vol. 2, No. 3, pp. 068-085, ISSN 1538-2273

Harper, S., Ferrara, M., Crescenzi, B. (2009). Inhibitors of the hepatitis C virus NS3 protease with basic amine functionality at the P3-amino acid N-terminus: Discovery and optimization of a new series of P2-P4 macrocycles. *J. Med. Chem.,* Vol. 52, No. 15, pp. 4820-4837, ISSN 1520-4804

Harvey, A.L. (2008). Natural products in drug discovery. *Drug Discov. Today,* Vol. 13, No. 19-20, pp. 894-901 ISSN 1359-6446

Hejgaard, J., Laing, W.A., Marttila, S., Gleave, A.P., Roberts, T.H. (2005). Serpins in fruit and vegetative tissues of apple (Malus domestica): expression of four serpins with distinct reactive centres and characterisation of a major inhibitory seed form, MdZ1b. *Functional Plant Biology,* Vol. 32, No. 6, pp. 517-527, ISSN 1445-4408

Islamov, R.A., Fursov, O.V. (2007). Bifunctional inhibitor of alpha-amylase/trypsin from wheat grain. *Applied Biochemistry and Microbiology,* Vol. 43, No. 4, pp. 379-382, ISSN 0003-6838

Kashiwagi, K., Virgona, N., Yamada, J., Sato, A., Ota, M., Yazawa, T., Yano, T. (2011). Bowman-Birk protease inhibitor from soybeans enhances cisplatin-induced cytotoxicity in human mesothelioma cells. Experimental and Therapeutic Medicine, Vol. 2, No. 4, pp. 719-724, ISSN 1792-1015

Koblinski, J.E., Ahram, M., Sloane, B.F. (2000). Unraveling the role of proteases in cancer. *Clinica Chimica Acta,* Vol. 291, pp. 113–135 ISSN 0009-8981

Konarev, Al.V. (1986). Analysis of proteinase inhibitors from wheat grain by gelatin replicas. *Biochemistry,* Vol. 51, No. 2, pp. 195-200, ISSN 1608-3040

Konarev, Al.V., Anisimova, I.N., Konechnaya, G,Y., Shewry P.R. (2004). Polymorphism of inhibitors of serine proteinases of animals and microorganisms in the Compositae and other Asteridie, *Proceedings of International Conference "Genetics and plant breeding"*, Moscow, 2004

Konarev, Al.V., Anisimova, I.N., Gavrilova, V.A., Shewry, P.R. (1999). Polymorphism of inhibitors of hydrolytic enzymes present in cereal and sunflower seeds, In: *Genetics and breeding for crop quality and resistance: proceedings of the XV EUCARPIA Congress, Viterbo, Italy, September 20-25,* Eds G.T. Scarascia Mugnozza, E. Porceddu, M.A. Pagnotta, Springer, pp.135-144, ISBN 0792358449, Netherlands

Konarev, Al.V., (2006). Use of molecular markers in solving the problems of plant genetic resources and breeding. *Agrarnaya Rossiya,* No. 6, pp. 4-23, ISSN 1999-5636

Kos, J., Lah, T.T. (1998). Cysteine proteinases and their endogenous inhibitors: target proteins for prognosis, diagnosis and therapy in cancer (review). *Oncol Rep.,* Vol. 5, No. 6, pp. 1349-1361, ISSN 1791-2431

Larionova, N.V., Kazanskaya, N.F., Larionova, N.I., Ponchel, G., Duchene, D. (1999). Preparation and characterization of microencapsulated proteinase inhibitor aprotinin. *Biochemistry (Moscow),* Vol. 64, No. 8, 1999, pp. 857-862.

Larionova, N.V., Dushen, D., Belousova, R.V. (2000). Effect of native and microencapsulated protease inhibitor - aprotinin on the reproduction of respiratory and intestinal viruses in cattle. *Vestinik Moscow University, Seria Khim.,* Vol. 41, No. 6, pp. 417-419, ISSN 1728-2101

Laskowski, Jr. M., Kato, I. Protein inhibitors of proteinases. *Annual Review of Biochemistry*, Vol. 49, pp. 593-626, ISSN 0066-4154

Lawrence, P.K., Koundal, K.R. (2002). Plant protease inhibitors in control of phytophagous insects. *Journal of Biotechnology*, Vol. 5, No. 1, pp. 93-109, ISSN 0168-1656

Li, Y., Qian, Y-Q., Ma, W-M., Yang, W-J. (2009). Inhibition mechanism and the effects of structure on activity of male reproduction-related peptidase inhibitor Kazal-type (MRPINK) of Macrobrachium rosenbergii. *J. Mar. Biotechnol.*, Vol. 11, pp.252–259, ISSN 1432-1408

Loreti, E., Bellicampi, D., Millet, C. (2002). Elicitors of defense responses repress a GA signaling pathway in barley embryos. *Plant Physiology*, Vol. 159, pp. 1383-1386, ISSN 1532-2548

Lorge, E., Hayashi, M., Albertini, S., Kirkland, D. (2008). Comparison of different methods for an accurate assessment of cytotoxicity in the in vitro micronucleus test I. Theoretical aspects. *Mutation Research*, Vol. 655, pp. 1–3, ISSN 0027-5107

Lypez-Otin, C., Matrisian, L.M. (2007). Emerging roles of proteases in tumour suppression. *Nature Reviews Cancer*, Vol. 7, pp. 800-808, ISSN 1474-1768

Maarten, A.J., Jules, B. (2011) Co-evolution of insect proteases and plant protease inhibitors. *Current Protein and Peptide Science*, Vol. 12, No. 5, pp. 437-447, ISSN 1389-203

Mannucci, P.M. (1998). Hemostatic drugs. *N. Engl. J. Med.*, Vol. 339, No. 4, pp. 245–253 ISSN 0028-4793

Maskos, K., Huber-Wunderlich, M., Glockshuber, R. (1996). RBI, a one-domain alpha-amylase/trypsin inhibitor with completely independent binding sites. *FEBS*, Vol. 397, pp. 11-16, ISSN 1742-4658

Mehrabadi, M., Bandani, A.R., Saadati, F. (2010). Inhibition of Sunn pest, Eurygaster integriceps, alpha-amylases by alpha-amylase inhibitors (T-alpha-AI) from Triticale. *Journal of Insect Science*, Vol. 10, pp. 179-185, ISSN 1536-2442

Molinari, G. (2009). Natural products in drug discovery: present status and perspectives. *Adv Exp Med Biol.*, Vol. 655, pp. 13-27 ISSN 0065-2598

Mosolov, V.V., Valueva, T.A (2008). Proteinase inhibitors in plant biotechnology: A review. *Applied Biochemistry and Microbiology*, Vol. 44, No. 3, pp. 233-241, ISSN 0003-6838

Mundy, J., Hejgaard, J., Svendsen, I. (1984). Characterization of a bifunctional wheat inhibitor of endogenous alpha-amylase and subtilisin. *FEBS*, Vol. 167, pp. 210-214, ISSN 1742-4658

Neumann, B., Zantl, N., Veihelmann, A., Emmanuilidis, K., Pfeffer, K., Heidecke, C-D., Holzmann, B. (1999). Mechanisms of acute inflammatory lung injury induced by abdominal sepsis. *Int. Immunol.*, Vol. 11, No. 2, pp. 217-227, ISSN 1460-2377

Nielsen, P.K., Bønsager, B.C., Fukuda, K., Svensson, B. (2004). Barley α-amylase/subtilisin inhibitor: structure, biophysics and protein engineering. *Biochimica et Biophysica Acta - Proteins & Proteomics*, Vol. 1696, No. 2, (February 2004), pp. 157-164 ISSN 1570-9639

Odani, S., Koide, T., Ono, T. (1983). The complete amino acid sequence of barley trypsin inhibitor. *J. of Biological Chemistry*, Vol. 258, No. 13, pp. 7998-8003, ISSN 0021-9258

Ohtsubo, K., Richardson, V. (1992). The amino acid sequence of a 20 kDa bifunctional subtilisin alpha-amylase inhibitor from brain of rice (Oryza sativa L.) seeds. *FEBS*, Vol. 309, pp. 68-72, ISSN 1742-4658

Ozaki, N., Ohmuraya, M., Hirota, M. (2009). Serine protease inhibitor Kazal type 1 promotes proliferation of pancreatic cancer cells through the epidermal growth factor receptor. *Mol. Cancer. Res.*, Vol. 7, pp. 1572-1581, ISSN 1557-3125

Polya, G.M. (2003). Protein and non-protein proteinase inhibitors from plants, In: *Bioactive natural products*, Ed. by Atta-ur- Rahman, Vol. 29, Part 1, pp. 567-641, Elsevier, ISBN 978-0-444-53181-0, Netherlands

Pouvreau, P. (2004). Occurrence and physico-chemical properties of protease inhibitors from potato tuber (Solanum tuberosum), In: Ph.D. thesis Wageningen University, < http://library.wur.nl/wda/dissertations/dis 3602.pdf>

Qi, R-F., Song, Z-W., Chi, Ch-W. (2005). Structural features and molecular evolution of Bowman-Birk protease inhibitors and their potential application. *Acta Biochimica et Biophysica Sinica*, Vol. 37, No. 5, pp. 283–292 ISSN 1745-7270

Rawlings, N.D., Tolle, D.P., Barrett, A.J. (2004). Evolutionary families of peptidase inhibitors. *Biochem J.*, Vol. 15, No. 378, pp. 705–716, ISSN 1470-8728

Renatus, M., Zhou, Q., Stennicke, H.R, Snipas, S.J., Turk, D., Bankston, L.A., Liddington, R.C., Salvesen, S. (2000). Crystal structure of the apoptotic suppressor CrmA in its cleaved form. *Structure.*, Vol. 8, pp. 789–797, ISSN 0969-2126

Rimphanitchayakit, V., Tassanakajon, A. (2010). Structure and function of invertebrate Kazal-type serine proteinase inhibitors. *Dev. Comp. Immunol.*, Vol. 34, No. 4, pp. 377-386. ISSN 0145-305X

Rolland, F., Moore, B., Sheen, J. (2002). Sugar sensing and signaling in plants. *The Plant Cell*, Vol. 15, pp. 185-205, ISSN 1532-298X

Ruseler-van Embden, J.G., van Lieshout, L.M., Smits, S.A., van Kessel, I., Laman, J.D. (2004). Potato tuber proteins efficiently inhibit human faecal proteolytic activity: implications for treatment of peri-anal dermatitis. *Eur. J. Clin. Invest.*, Vol. 34, No. 4, pp. 303-311, ISSN 1365-2362

Salcedo, G., Sanchez-Monge, R., Garsia-Casado, G., Armentina, A., Gomez, L., Barber, D. (2004). The cereal amylase/trypsin inhibitor family associated with Bakers` asthma and food allergy, In: *Plant food allergens*, Eds E. N. Clare Mills, Peter R. Shewry pp. 70-86, Wiley-Blackwell, ISBN 0–632–05982–6, Great Britain

Schroeder, H.E., Gollasch, S., Moore, A. (1995). Been alpha-amylase inhibitor confers resistance to the pea weevil (Bruchus pisorum) in transgenic peas (Pisum sativum L.). *Plant Physiology*, Vol. 107. No. 4, pp. 1233-1239, ISSN 1532-2548

Selitrennikoff, C.P. (2001). Antifungal proteins. *Applied and Environmental Microbiology*, Vol. 67, No. 7, (July 2001), pp. 2883-2894, ISSN 1098-5336

Sever, N., Filipic, M., Brzin, J., Lah, T.T. (2002) Effect of cysteine proteinase inhibitors on murine B16 melanoma cell invasion in vitro. *Biol. Chem.*, Vol. 383, No. 5, pp. 839-842, ISSN 1431-6730

Smith, J.H., Simons, C. (2004). Development of Enzyme Inhibitors as Drugs, In: *Enzymes and their inhibitors drug development*, Eds. H.J. Smith and C. Simons, pp. 190-328, CRC Press, ISBN 978-0-203-41458-3

Sreerama, Y.N., Das, J.R., Rao, D.R., Gowda, L.R. (1997). Double-headed trypsin/chymotrypsin inhibitors from horse gram (Dolichos biflorus): purification, molecular and kinetic properties. *J. of Food Biochemistry*, Vol. 21, No. 1, pp. 461–477, ISSN 1745-4514

Spainhour, Ch.B. (2005). Natural products, In: *Drug discovery handbook*, Ed. Sh. Gad, pp. 12-63, John Wiley & Son, ISBN 13 978-0-471-21384-0, USA

The Enzyme List. Class 3 – Hydrolases. In: *(NC-IUBMB) Generated from the ExplorEnz database*, 2010, < http://www.enzyme-database.org/downloads/ec3.pdf>

Competitiveness and Private Sector Development. Kazakhstan sector competitiveness strategy. <www.oecd.org/daf/psd/eurasia>

Thorburn, J., Bender, L.M., Morgan, M.J., Thorburn, A. (2003). Caspase- and serine protease-dependent apoptosis by the death domain of FADD in normal epithelial cells. *Mol Biol Cell.*, Vol. 14, No. 1, pp. 67-77, ISSN 1939-4586

Troncoso, M.F., Biron, V.A., Longhi, S.A., Retegui, L.A., Wolfenstein-Todel, C. (2007). Peltophorum dubium and soybean Kunitz-type trypsin inhibitors induce human Jurkat cell apoptosis. *Int. Immunopharmacol.*, Vol. 7, No. 5, pp. 625-636, ISSN 1567-5769

Valuev, I.L., Sytov, G.A., Valuev, L.I., Valueva, T.A., Ul'yanova, M.V., Plate, N.A. (2001). Inhibitors of proteolytic enzymes in the therapy of diabetes. *Russian Journal Voprosy Meditsinskoi Khimii,* Vol. 47, No. 1, pp. 132-135, ISSN 0042-8809

Valueva, T.A., Mosolov, V.V. (2002). The role of inhibitors of proteolytic enzymes in plant protection. *Uspekhi Biologicheskoi Khimmii,* Vol. 42, pp. 193-216, ISSN 0006-2979

Vincent, D., Zivy, M. (2007). Plant proteome responses to abiotic stress. In: *Plant Proteomics,* Eds. J. Šamaj and J.J. Thelen, pp. 346-364, Springer, ISBN 13 978-3-540-72616-6, Germany

Weinberger, B., Laskin, J.D., Sunil, V.R., Sinko, P.J., Heck, D.E., Laskin, D.L. (2011). Sulfur mustard-induced pulmonary injury: therapeutic approaches to mitigating toxicity. *Pulm Pharmacol Ther.*, Vol. 24, No. 1, (Feb. 2011), pp. 92-99 ISSN 1094-5539

Wenzel, H.R. and Tschesche, H. (1995). Reversible inhibitors of serine proteinases. In: *Peptides: Synthesis, Structures, and Applications,* Ed. B. Gutte, pp. 321-362, Academic Press, ISBN 0123109205, USA

Winkler, M.K., Fowlkes, J.L.(2002). Metalloproteinase and growth factor interactions: do they play a role in pulmonary fibrosis? *AJP - Lung Physiol.,* Vol. 283, No. 1, (July 2002), L.1-11, ISSN 1522-1504

Wouters, D., Wagenaar-Bos, I., van Ham, M., Zeerleder, S. (2008). C1 inhibitor: just a serine protease inhibitor? New and old considerations on therapeutic applications of C1 inhibitor. Expert. Opin. Biol. Ther., Vol. 8, No. 8, pp. 1225-1240, ISSN 1744-7682

Yamasaki, T., Deguchi, M., Fujimoto, T., Masumura, T., Uno, T., Kanamaru, K., Yamagata, H. (2006). Rice bifunctional alpha-amylase/subtilisin inhibitor: cloning and characterization of the recombinant inhibitor expressed in Escherichia coli. *Biosci Biotechnol Biochem.,* Vol. 70, No. 5, pp. 1200-1209, ISSN 1347-6947

Yan, K-M., Chang, T., Soon, S-A., Huang, F-Y. (2009). Purification and characterization of Bowman-Birk protease inhibitor from rice coleoptiles. *J. of the Chinese Chemical Society,* Vol. 56, pp. 949-960, ISSN 2192-6549

Yuldasheva, G.A., Zhidomirov, G.M., Ilin, A.I. (2011). A quantum-chemical model of the inhibition mechanism of viral DNA HIV-1 replication by Iodine complex compounds. *Natural Science,* Vol. 3, No. 7, pp. 573-579, ISSN 2150-4091

Zemke, K.J., Muller-Fahrnow, A., Jany, K. (1991). The three-dimensional structure of the bifunctional proteinase K/alpha-amylase inhibitor from wheat (PKI3) at 2.5 A resolution. *FEBS,* Vol. 397, pp.240-242, ISSN 1742-4658

5

Atherosclerosis and Antihyperlipidemic Agents

Laila Mahmoud Mohamed Gad*
Faculty of Pharmacy, King Abdulaziz University KAU, Jeddah
Kingdom of Saudi Arabia

1. Introduction

1.1 Atherosclerosis & cholesterol

The link between cardiovascular disease (CVD) and lipids has been appreciated for a long time, but the individual role of specific lipids in predisposition to disease is constantly under question. Cardiovascular disease, including myocardial infarction (MI), heart failure, and stroke, represents the leading cause of mortality worldwide, accounting for half of the total number of deaths in the developed world (World Health Organization, 2002). CVD will result in 20.5 million deaths annually by 2020 (World Health Organization, 2002, Fig. 1), (Revkin et al. 2007).

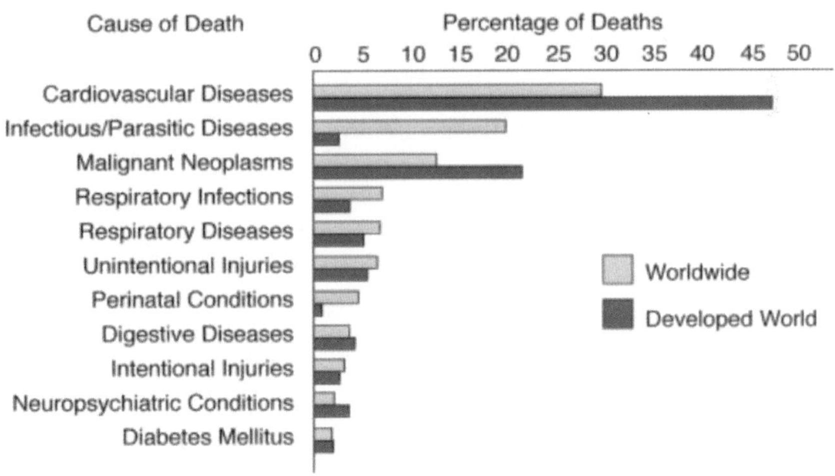

Fig. 1. Cardiovascular disease accounts for one third of deaths worldwide and half of deaths in the developed world. Data from World Health Organization (2002).

Atherosclerosis, or "athero" as we call it, is a condition underlying most cardiovascular diseases (Berliner et al. 1995) and results from an imbalance between uptake and efflux of

* *Associate prof. Pharmaceutical Organic Chemistry, Faculty of Pharmacy, Mansoura University, Egypt*

cholesterol by macrophages in the wall of blood vessels. It is the progressive buildup of plaque in the arteries over time causing narrowing of the vessels and severely limiting blood flow in advanced cases. Rupture of the plaque and thrombosis may result in complete occlusion of the vessel and, ultimately, myocardial infarction or stroke (Berliner and Glass). For many of us, this plaque starts building up in our arteries in early adulthood and gets worse over time (Fig.2, for illustrative purposes).

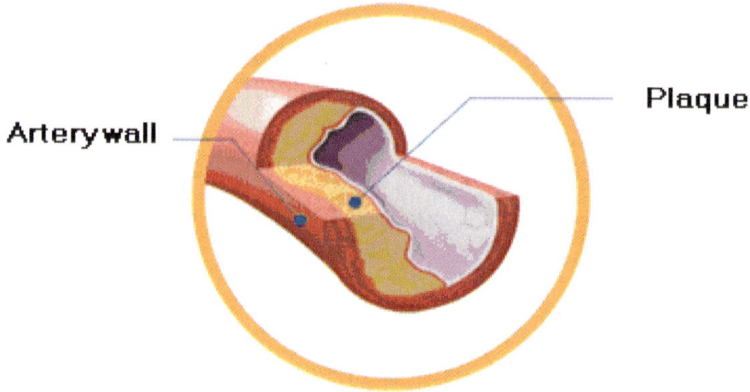

Fig. 2. Atherosclerosis; the progressive build up of plaque in arteries over time.

Cholesterol

Is a fatty substance, also called a lipid, which is produced by the liver. It is also found in foods high in saturated fat, like fatty meats, egg yolks, shellfish, and whole-milk dairy products. Since lipids are insoluble in blood, they are carried in association with proteins as lipoproteins, which allows their transport around the body. Lipoprotein complexes present in the serum have been the focus of much study in the etiology of cardiovascular disease (Goldstein, 1990).

There are five types of lipoproteins, and this classification is based on their densities. Those of lowest density, the chylomicrons, contain more lipids and less protein than those at the other extreme, high-density lipoproteins (HDLs). Between these classes are the very low-density lipoproteins (VLDLs), low-density lipoproteins (LDLs), and intermediate-density lipoproteins (IDLs). Plasma cholesterol is carried from the intestine and the liver to peripheral tissues largely in the form of LDLs. Most clinical studies concentrate on the relative abundance of HDLs and LDLs in the serum. LDL cholesterol is considered "bad" because too much of it in the blood stream can contribute to the progression of atherosclerosis, the buildup of plaque in the arteries. HDL cholesterol, on the other hand, is considered "good", it appears to be protective against cardiovascular disease (Miller, 2000), and this is generally considered to be due to the efficiency by which HDL returns cholesterol to the liver for metabolism and excretion, resulting in reduced serum cholesterol availability (Barter & Rye, 1994).

The elevated levels of the lipoprotein (LDL) and (VLDL) are usually associated with atheroma formation. Therefore, defects in cholesterol metabolism are a major cause of cardiovascular disease, this is apparent in patients with familial hypercholesterolemia, characterized by grossly elevated levels of serum cholesterol, in particular LDL. Reduction of plasma LDL-cholesterol (in patients with elevated levels) is associated with a decreased incidence of coronary heart disease (CHD) (Anderson; Boden; Farnier; Fruchart and Gordon). Also, there is an increasing evidence that serum triglycerides (TGs) are strong risk factors in cardiovascular disease in many patients with normal circulating LDL-cholesterol, but with high levels of plasma TGs and concomitantly low levels of HDL-cholesterol (Cullen; Krauss and Rubins).

LDL-cholesterol has been well established as an independent risk factor since reporting of the 1948 Framingham study (Gordon et al. 1977). HDL-cholesterol is recognized as being a negative risk factor for CHD (Fruchart et al. 1998). While LDL cholesterol is a major health factor, here are a few other factors that can contribute to the progression of athero.

- Family history of early heart disease
- Diabetes
- High blood pressure
- Cigarette smoking
- Overweight/obesity

In a prospective follow-up study of 56 individuals with known CVD, a relationship between progression of atherosclerosis in the left main coronary artery and coronary risk factors was demonstrated (von Birgelen et al. 2004) (Fig. 3). In this study, the investigators applied three different, commonly used cardiovascular risk scores to subjects (Anderson et al. 1991 & Assmann et al. 2002, and Conroy et al. 2003) and demonstrated a positive linear relationships between the calculated risk of CVD and plaque progression (Revkin et al. 2007).

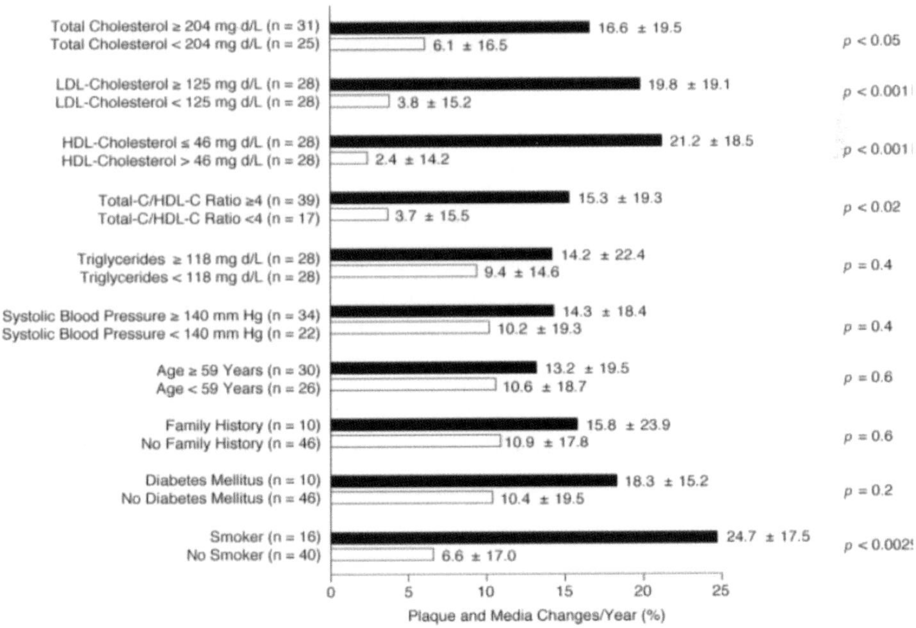

Fig. 3. Relationships between cardiovascular risk factors and atherosclerosis progression in the left main coronary artery. Data from von Birgelen et al. (2004). Reprinted from *Circulation* 110:1579–1585.

2. Biomarkers of atherosclerosis

Atherosclerosis as a disease characterized by low-level vascular inflammation is gaining much attention recently. Some lipid parameters i.e. total serum cholesterol TC, LDL cholesterol, HDL cholesterol and triglyceride contents and also, serum markers of inflammation are considered as predictive biomarker for the prevalence of atherosclerotic disease.

Biomarkers: A biomarker is defined as a characteristic that is objectively measured and evaluated as an indicator of normal biologic or pathogenic processes or as physiologic response to a therapeutic intervention. In clinical medicine, biomarkers are routinely used in disease diagnosis, prognostication, ongoing clinical decision-making, and follow-up to assess effects of therapy.

- Commonly used biomarkers: e.g. electrocardiogram, isotopic and ultrasound imaging studies applied in multiple areas of disease management, bone densitometry in the assessment of osteoporotic fracture risk.
- Commonly used soluble biomarkers include low- and high-density lipoprotein cholesterol (LDL-C and HDL-C), triglycerides (TG), serum creatinine, and hepatocellular enzymes, as well as a host of other routine clinical laboratory measurements.
- Surrogate endpoints are biomarkers that are predictors of clinical outcomes.. Typical surrogate endpoints used to assess the clinical efficacy of cardiovascular drugs include levels of LDL-C and blood pressure.

The need for more rapid drug development highlights the role that surrogate markers may play in establishing the efficacy of drugs for managing CVD, and more specifically, atherosclerosis (Revkin et al. 2007).

a. **Lipid markers of atherosclerosis**:

Plasma levels of lipids and lipoproteins have been well established as strong predictors of CHD. There is, also, a stronger positive correlation of **apolipoproteins** (apo) with atherosclerosis and coronary events than that of the plasma lipoproteins, either cholesterol carried by lipoprotein particles or their actual concentration expressed as **apo B** and **apo A-I**.

Lipoproteins are spherical molecules that transport different amounts of cholesterol and triglycerides in the blood stream. LDL and HDL particles are rich in cholesterol, while VLDL and chylomicron particles predominantly transport triglycerides The apo B is present on the surface of LDL, VLDL and chylomicrons (one molecule at each particle), while apo A-I resides on HDL particles (Fig.4). **Lipoprotein (a)** consist of two main components: low-density lipoprotein (LDL) and apolipoprotein (apo) (a) linked by a single disulphide bond between the C terminal of apo B100 and apo(a) kringle (K) IV type 9.The LDL particles may differ among individuals in the cholesteryl ester content of the lipid core that is surrounded by a monolayer of phospholipids, unesterified cholesterol, and apo B100. Apo (a) is made of 10 different type IV kringles (1-10) followed by kringleV and a catalytically inactive protease domain (P), (Angelo M. et al. 2008).

Conventional **lipid tests** determine the amount of cholesterol and triglycerides transported by all particles within the lipoprotein classes or in total plasma. Thus, cholesterol and triglycerides may be regarded as surrogate markers for their carrier-lipoprotein particles.

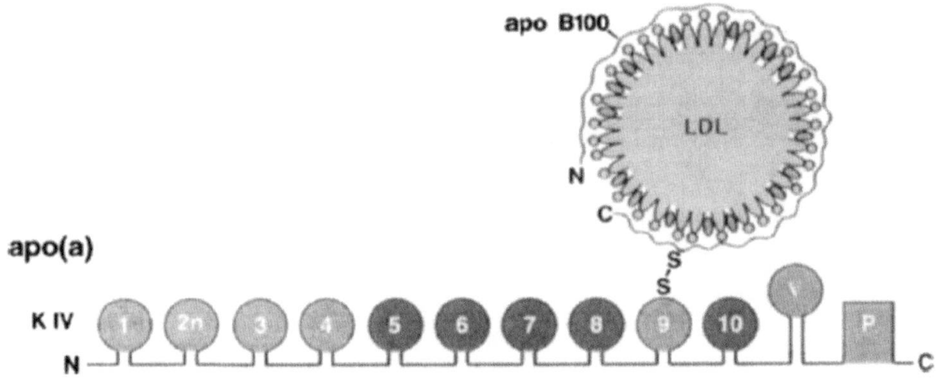

Fig. 4. Schematic representation of lipoprotein (a).

The **level of apoB-containing lipoprotein particles** is measured directly, mostly by immunonephelometric analysis of the plasma, on empty stomach or postprandially, whereas LDL cholesterol is mostly calculated indirectly as the difference of total cholesterol minus HDL-cholesterol and VLDL-cholesterol. In that respect, apo B can be considered a superior indicator of the global atherogenic risk over the sole quantification of LDL cholesterol and triglyceride levels, particularly in conditions of hypertriglyceridaemia characterized by high VLDL and low LDL levels. (JMB 2008, 27:148 –153).

Non-HDL cholesterol: Another approach to the measurement of atherogenic lipoproteins is the use Non-HDL cholesterol which is easily calculated by deducting the HDL cholesterol from the total cholesterol value, with no need for previous fasting of the patient. This is the cholesterol contained in VLDL and LDL particles, atherogenic triglyceride-rich lipoproteins, cholesteryl ester-enriched remnants of triglyceride-rich lipoproteins, and lipoprotein(a). Consequently, the non-HDL cholesterol is essentially the cholesterol analogue to an apo B level. The non-HDL cholesterol content is easily available within the primary screening of the lipid profile, and according to the recommendations of NCEP ATP III it is identified as a secondary therapeutic target after achieving the target levels of LDL cholesterol. (JMB, 2008, 27:148 –153).

b. **Circulating markers of inflammation and atherosclerosis**:

Epidemiologic and prospective studies evaluating the predictive value of the variety of circulating markers of vascular inflammation such as C-reactive protein (CRP), fibrinogen, serum amyloid A (SAA), leukocyte count in peripheral blood, immunoglobulin, adhesion molecules, cytokines and chemokines has been well established. Population studies demonstrated a moderate elevation of serum fibrinogen and leukocyte count in peripheral blood in individuals subsequently developed atherosclerotic disease. Increased fibrinogen levels were identified as strong predictors of stroke (JMB, 2008, 27:148 –153).

3. Metabolic syndrome

The metabolic syndrome has emerged in recent years as a major public health concern. By 2002 it was estimated that as many as 24% of American adults suffer from the metabolic syndrome as defined by the ATPIII criteria*).Individuals suffer from the metabolic syndrome have been demonstrated to be at increased risk of the development of hypertension, atherosclerosis, type II diabetes and cardiovascular disease. The term 'metabolic syndrome' refers to a cluster of metabolic abnormalities associated primarily with obesity including elevated plasma triglycerides (TG), low-density lipoprotein (LDL-cholesterol), and very low-density lipoprotein (VLDL-cholesterol), reduced high-density lipoprotein (HDL-cholesterol), and elevations in blood pressure and fasting glucose.

4. Dyslipidemia

Dyslipidemia is a disruption in the amount of lipids in the blood either by increase or decrease. Most dyslipidemias are hyperlipidemias; that is, an elevation of lipids in the blood, often due to diet and lifestyle. The increased type of dyslipidemia could be differentiated as:

- Hyperlipidemia: increase in lipids; either increase in cholesterol (Hypercholesterolemia), in glycerides (Hyperglyceridemia) or in triglycerides (Hypertriglyceridemia).
- Hyperlipoproteinemia: increase in lipoproteins (usually LDL).
- Combined hyperlipidemia: that is an increase in both LDL and triglycerides.

*Executive Summary of the Third Report of the National Cholesterol Education Program (NCEP) Expert Panel on Detection, Evaluation, and Treatment of High Blood Cholesterol In Adults (Adult Treatment Panel III; ATPIII) 2001, JAMA 285: 2486–97

5. Managing cholesterol

The elevated levels of the lipoprotein (high cholesterol level) may depend on the lifestyle of the patient. Eating a lot of fats and not getting enough exercise can cause cholesterol levels to rise. It's also, in part, a result of the genetic makeup. Some people inherit genes associated with elevated levels of cholesterol. One type is called familial hypercholesterolemia. People with this genetic makeup can eat a healthy diet and exercise, and still have high cholesterol. Managing high cholesterol may be different for one patient to another depending on the medical history and the health of the patient. Therefore, cholesterol test, also known as a **fasting lipid profile**, and, along with complete medical background can work together to manage cholesterol.

6. Cholesterol guidelines

National Cholesterol Education Program (NCEP) guidelines recommend that all adults over age 20 have their cholesterol checked at least once every 5 years. The guidelines below give a better idea of where the cholesterol numbers of any person should be.

Total cholesterol level

- Less than 200 mg/dL — Desirable
- 200-239 mg/dL — Borderline high
- 240 mg/dL or higher — High

Total cholesterol is based on your LDL cholesterol (LDL-C) and HDL cholesterol (HDL-C) counts. Generally, a lower number is better.

Triglycerides

• Less than 150 mg/dL	Normal
• 150-199 mg/dL	Borderline high
• 200-499 mg/dL	High
• 500 mg/dL or higher	Very high

Triglycerides, like cholesterol, are another substance that can be dangerous to your health. Like LDL-C, you want to keep your triglycerides low.

LDL-C

• Less than 100 mg/dL	Optimal
• 100-129 mg/dL	Near optimal /above optimal
• 130-159 mg/dL	Borderline high
• 160-189 mg/dL	High
• 190 mg/dL or higher	Very high

LDL-C is considered the "bad" cholesterol because if you have too much LDL-C in your bloodstream, it can lead to the buildup of plaque in your arteries known as atherosclerosis. Generally, lower is better.

HDL-C

• 60 mg/dL or higher	High
• Less than 40 mg/dL	Low

HDL-C is considered the "good" cholesterol because it helps return cholesterol to the liver, where it can be eliminated from the body. Generally, higher is better.

Source: National Cholesterol Education Program (NCEP), Webmed October 27, 2008

7. Peroxisome proliferator-activated receptor agonists

Peroxisome proliferator-activated receptors (PPARs) are a group of nuclear hormone receptors which function as transcription factors in the regulation of genes involved in glucose and lipid fatty acid metabolism and vessel wall function. Three PPAR subtypes have been identified: PPAR α, γ and δ.

PPARα is predominantly expressed in catabolically active tissues such as liver, heart, kidney, and muscle. It is involved in the uptake and oxidation of fatty acids as well as in lipoprotein metabolism. PPARγ is mainly expressed in adipose tissue and regulates insulin sensitivity, glucose and fatty acid utilization as well as adipocyte differentiation (Hao Zhang et al. 2009). Recent studies have found that PPARδ is also a regulator of serum lipids

There are many clinically useful drugs that produce their effects by acting on these receptors. The clinically used PPARα agonists are the fibrate class of drugs (including Fenofibrate and Gemfibrozil), which elevate HDL cholesterol levels and lower triglyceride and LDL cholesterol levels. Fibrate drugs are ligands for the fatty acid receptor PPARα (Fruchart et al. 1999).

The clinically used PPARγ agonists comprise the thiazolidinedione (TZD); class of anti-diabetic drugs. The thiazolidinediones (TZDs) drugs are PPARγ ligands and these have beneficial effects on serum lipids in diabetic patients. The fibrate class of drugs is agonists of the PPARα isoform, and the thiazolidinediones (TZDs) that activate PPARγ isoform. This is an area of great pharmaceutical interest concernining the dual α/γ agonists, which have the potential to combine the benefits of the fibrates and the TZDs, are under development (Helen V. et al. 2002).

It has been hypothesized that the combination of PPARγ and PPARα agonist activities in a single compound would result in synergistic improvements in insulin sensitivity and normalization of glucose metabolism as well as amelioration of the dyslipidemia associated with type 2 diabetes.

Currently marketed drugs targeting PPARγ like rosiglitazone used for the treatment of type 2 diabetes. We have recently reported the design and synthesis of Muraglitazar a dual PPARα/γ agonist which has shown excellent efficacy in animal models of type 2 diabetes and the associated dyslipidemia as well as in human clinical trial (Fig. 5), (Xiang-Yang Ye et al. 2008).

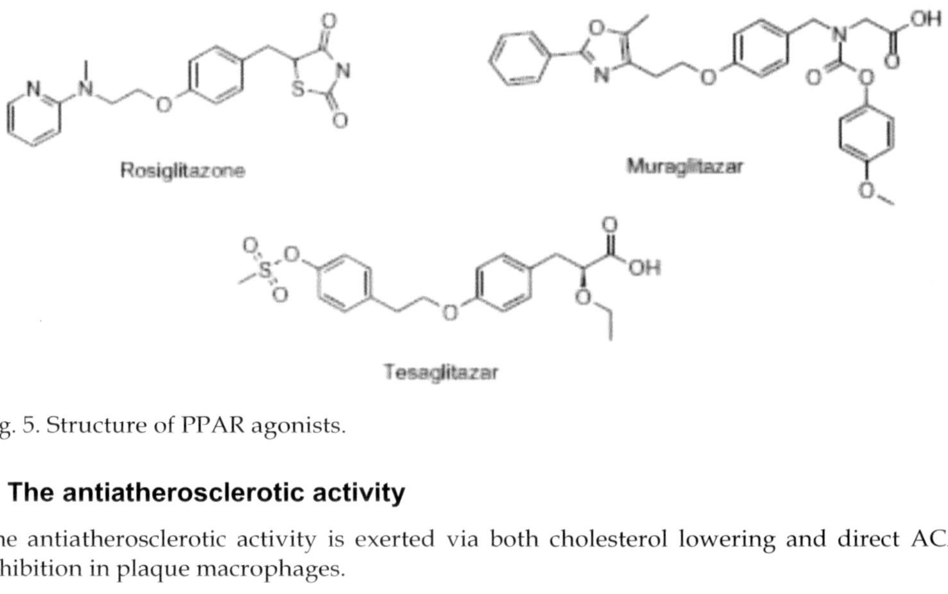

Fig. 5. Structure of PPAR agonists.

8. The antiatherosclerotic activity

The antiatherosclerotic activity is exerted via both cholesterol lowering and direct ACAT inhibition in plaque macrophages.

Acyl-CoA: cholesterol acyl transferase (ACAT) catalyzes the intracellular formation of cholesteryl esters (CE) in all mammalian cells. It has been implicated as a key enzyme involved in cholesterol absorption, very low density lipoprotein secretion, and the formation of lipid-laden macrophages. The accumulation of CE in macrophage-derived foam cells is characteristic of the early step in the development of atherosclerosis. ACAT inhibitors reduced TC levels without affecting HDL-C. This can be attributed to decreased intestinal cholesterol absorption based on binding to bile acid (Turley SD. and Herndon MW. 1994)

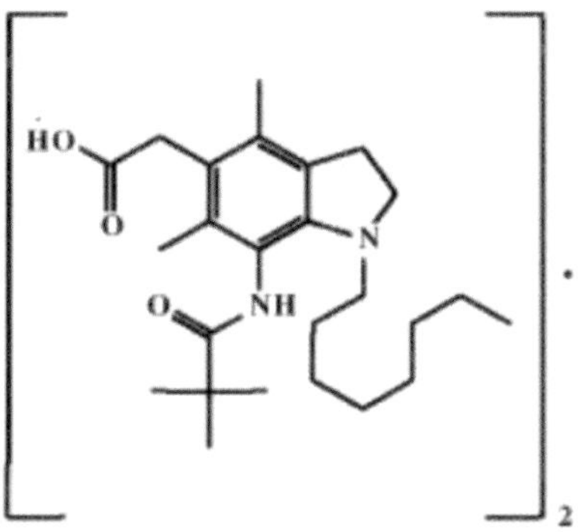

CS-505 (pactimibe sulfate)

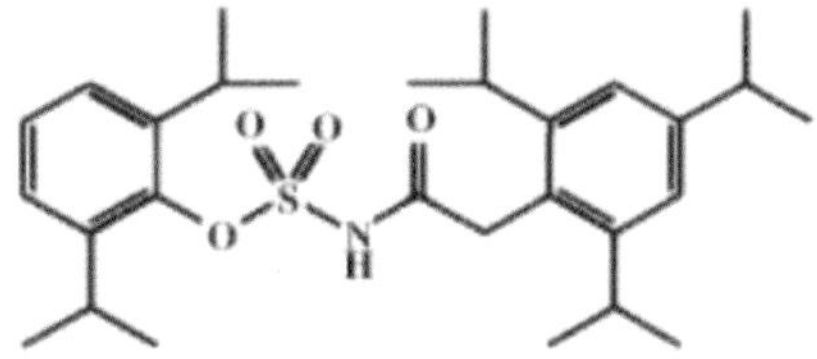

CI-1011 (avasimibe)

Fig. 6. Chemical structure of ACAT inhibitor CS-505 (pactimibe sulfate) & CI-1011(avasimibe).

Cholesterol esters (CE) are the main lipid components responsible for the development of atherosclerosis; hence they are present in the foam cells and extracellular plaque matrix, and susceptible to oxidation that could increase their atherogenic potential.

The treatment using novel ACAT inhibitor pactimibe sulfate (CS-505), avasimibe (CI-1011) (Fig.6), and a potent bile acid binding resin cholestyramine directly affects macrophages in atherosclerotic lesions. They would limit the increase in intracellular free cholesterol by its TC-lowering effect. This would allow free cholesterol to excrete into HDL, restoring the cholesterol influx/efflux balance, thus preventing foam cell formation. (Terasak N. et al. 2007).

Lipid lowering drugs (LLD)

Lipid-lowering drugs (LLD) or agents are a diverse group of pharmaceuticals that are used in the treatment of hyperlipidemia; some may lower "*bad cholesterol*" (LDL) more so than others, while others may prudentially increase (HDL), "*the good cholesterol*". Other studies showed that elevating the high-density lipoprotein (HDL), as well as, lowering the low-density lipoprotein (LDL) and triglyceride levels (TGs) in the serum are accepted measures in treating hyperlipidemia and atherosclerosis.

1. Clinical trials

The lipid lowering in hyperlipidemia is achieved clinically using **statins** and **fibrate** drugs. Since 1966, there have been 16 major trials investigating the efficacy of statin and fibrate therapy, both as a single drug treatment and as part of a multi-drug regimen (Napoli C. et al. 1997). These trials have involved the participation of some 30,000 patients, and have considered both primary and secondary prevention of coronary heart disease (CHD), myocardial infarction, stroke, and peripheral artery disease (Tylor, Faergeman, Boden). Studies by Nagao et al. (1998), involved the use of fibrate gemfibrozil to reduce cholesterol levels in hypercholesterolemia rats fed a cholesterol rich diet.

Other studies have confirmed these results (Bruckert and Rustemeijer), while some trials involving gemfibrozil, bezafibrate, and fenofibrate indicated that fibrates can reduce LDL-cholesterol to a degree comparable with that observed with statins (Feussner; Guay and Haffner). Most of the studies are of the general conclusion that statins are the drug of choice where the major dyslipidaemia is high-baseline LDL-cholesterol and that fibrates are particularly effective in the case of hypertriglyceridaemia (Farnier M. 1998). Other studies have confirmed these results while some trials involving bezafibrate, gemfibrozil, and fenofibrate indicated that fibrates can reduce LDL-cholesterol to a degree comparable with that observed with statins (Guay DR. 1999).

2. **The well-established lipid lowering drugs**
1. **Statins**: Current ATPIII guidelines for the treatment of patients with the metabolic syndrome encourage therapies that lower LDL-cholesterol and TG, and raise HDL-cholesterol. Primary intervention often involves treatment with statins to improve the lipid profiles of these patients. Statins act by competitively inhibiting 3-hydroxy-3-methylglutaryl-coenzyme A, (HMG-CoA) reductase, the rate-limiting enzyme in the cholesterol biosynthesis pathway in the liver (Fig.7), thus stimulates the LDL-receptors resulting in an increased clearance of LDL from the blood stream and a decrease in blood cholesterol levels. The first result can be seen after one week of use and the effect is maximal after four to six weeks. Statins are particularly well suited for lowering **LDL** in people at risk for cardiovascular diseases because of hypercholesterolemia .

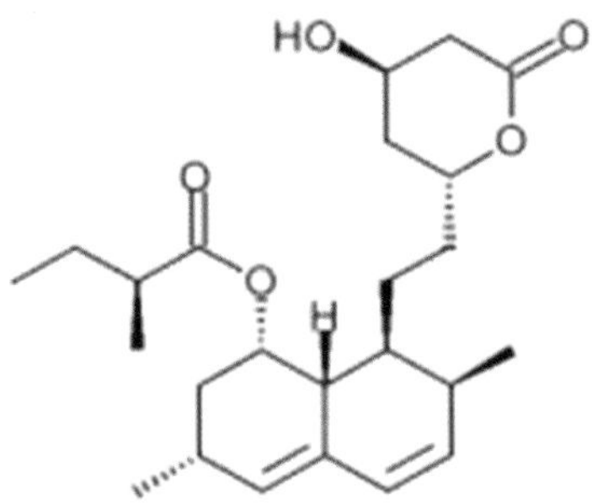

(1)

Lovastatin, the first statin to be marked

Statins are **Lovastatin (1), Mevastatin** -naturally-occurring compound found in red yeast rice**, and Pravstatin.** Statins exhibit action beyond lipid-lowering activity in the prevention of atherosclerosis; **i)** Improving endothelial function **ii)** Modulate inflammatory responses **,** **iii)** Maintain plaque stability, and **iv)** Prevent thrombus formation.

Rosuvastatin is a new member of the statin family with higher efficacy in reducing LDL cholesterol than other statins at comparable doses . Rosuvastatin has been shown to have an increased number of binding interactions with HMG-CoA reductase, compared to other statins. rosuvastatin also possesses a relatively long half-life and a high degree of selectivity for liver cells (the main site of cholesterol synthesis) compared with non-hepatic cells. Rosuvastatin (10 mg) has been shown to improve dyslipidemia in patients with the metabolic syndrome (Naples M. et al. 2008).

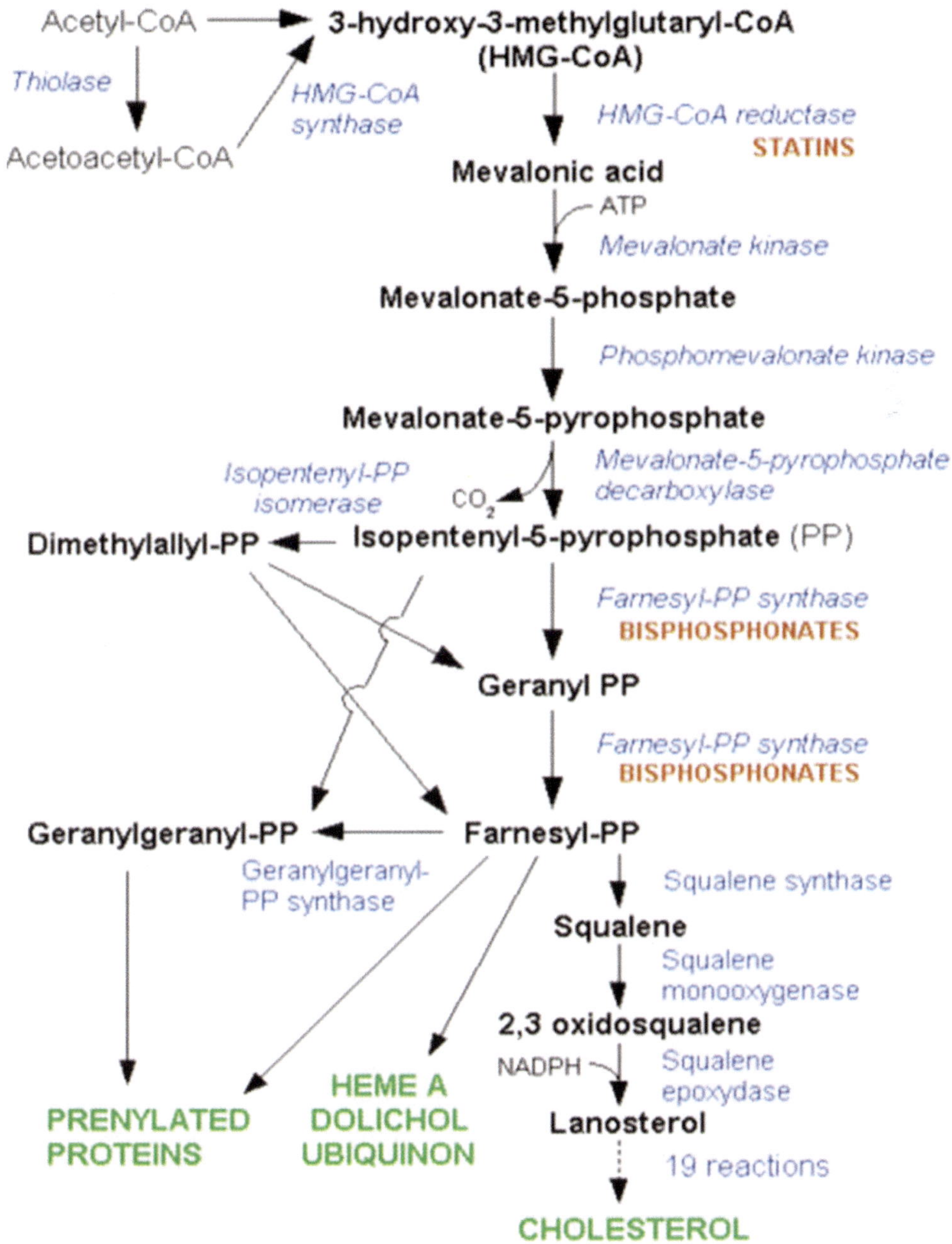

Fig. 7. Synthesis of Cholesterol through HMG-CoA reductase pathway.

2. **Fibrates**: Although fibrates (e,g. clofibrate 2) are used clinically since the early 1970s, the mechanism of action of fibrates remained unelucidated until, in the 1990s, it was discovered that fibrates activate PPAR (peroxisome proliferator-activated receptors), especially PPARα. The PPARs are a class of intracellular receptors that modulate carbohydrate, fat metabolism and adipose tissue differentiation (Staels B. 1998) ; (Fruchart JC. et al. 1999). They typically lower triglyceride by 20% to 25%. The newer generation fibrates: gemfibrozil (3) Bezafibrate (4) (Spieker LE. *et al.* 2000), and Fenofibrate (5) afford significant protection from CHD; this might be due to the agonistic effect of PPARα that inhibits inflammatory responses at the level of the vascular wall. Finally, evidence that fibrates are able to reduce levels of plasma fibrinogen, which, in turn, reduces the likelihood of thrombogenesis (Helen *et.al.* 2002).

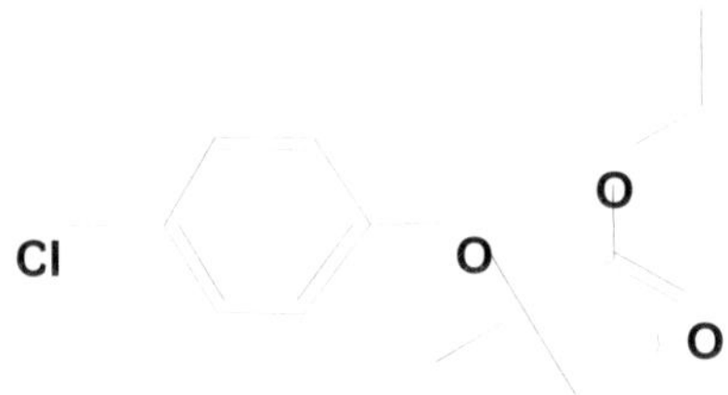

Clofibrate (2)
Ethyl 2-(4-chlorophenoxy)-2-methylpropanoic acid

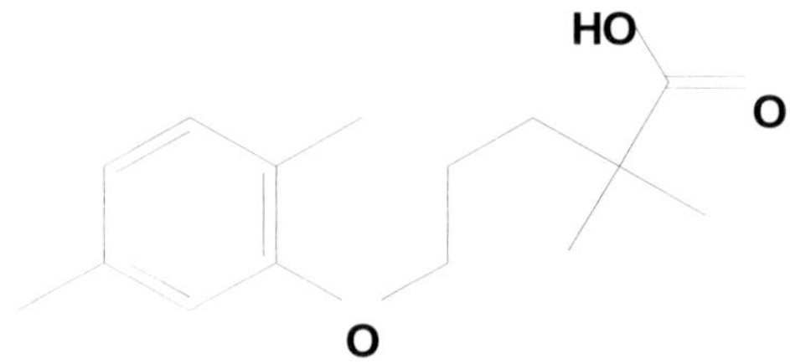

Gemfibrozil (3)
5-(2,5-dimethylphenoxy)-2,2-dimethylpentatonic acid

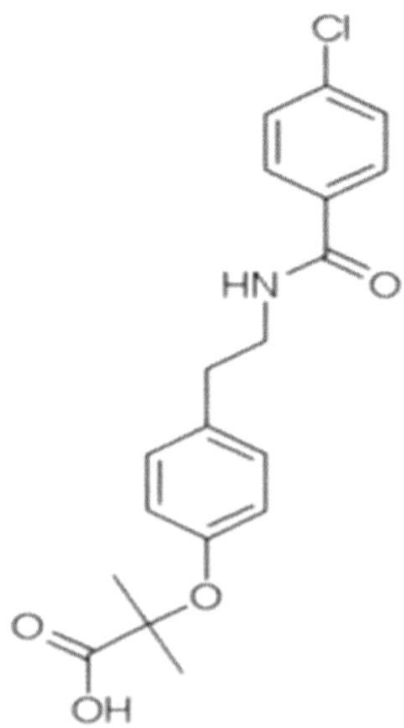

Bezafibrate (4)
2-[4-[2-[(4-chlorobenzoyl)amino] ethyl]phenoxy]-2-methylpropanoic acid

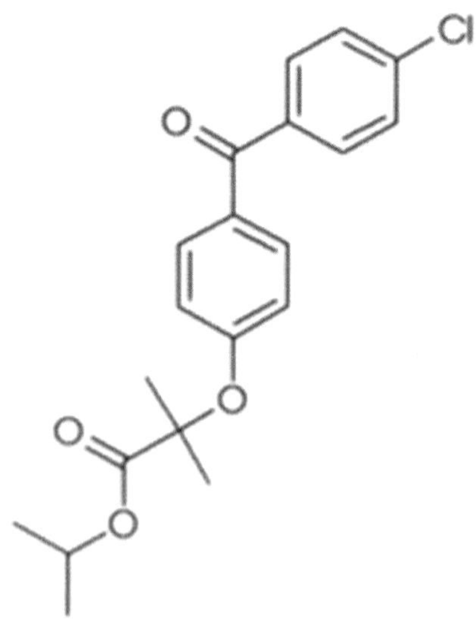

Fenofibrate (5)
Isopropyl 2-[4-(4-chlorobenzoyl) phenoxy]-2-methyl propanoate

3. **Niacin**: 3-pyridinecarboxylic acid . also know as nicotinic acid or vitamin **B3**, the name niacin was derived from nicotinic acid + vitamin, it is also referred to as "vitamin PP", a name derived from the absolute term "pellagra-preventing factor". Over the years, niacin has gained recognition as an atheroprotective agent, in part because of its capacity to lower the plasma levels of cholesterol, triglycerides by 20- 50%., and very-low- and low-density lipoproteins. It may lower LDL by 5-25% and to substantially raise high-density lipoprotein. by 15-33%..In high doses, niacin has also been reported to lower the plasma level of lipoprotein(a) (Angelo M. 2008).

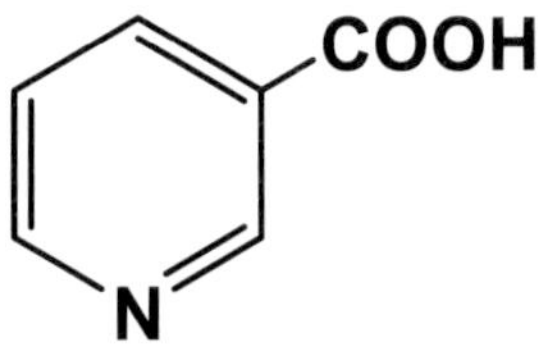

Niacin (6)
3-pyridinecarboxylic acid

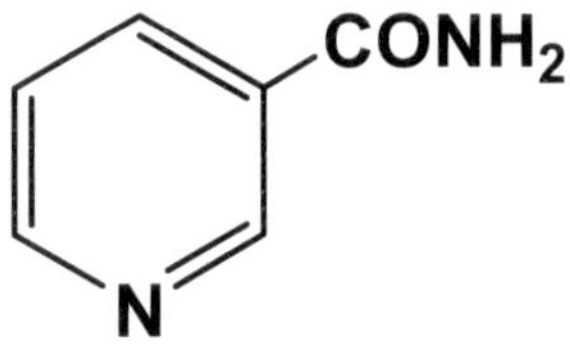

Nicotinamide (7)
3-pyridinecarboxamide

4. **Ezetimibe**: (Zetia) is a selective inhibitor of dietary cholesterol absorption. In addition to this decreased cholesterol absorption leads to an increase in LDL-cholesterol uptake into cells, thus decreasing levels in the blood plasma (Rossi S, 2006).

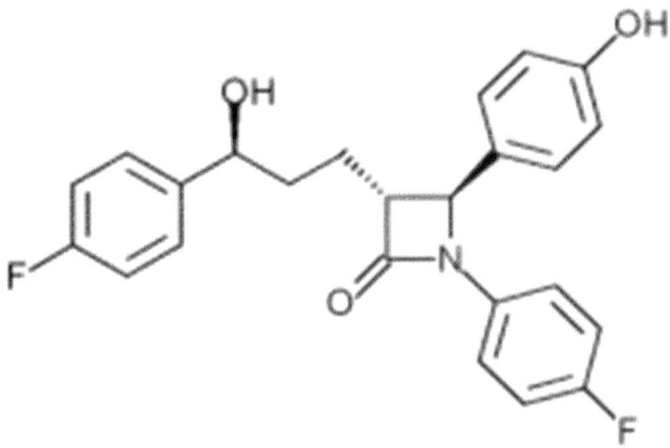

Ezetimibe (8)
(3*R*, 4S)-1-(4-fluorophenyl)-3- ((3*S*)-3-(4-fluorophenyl)-3-hydroxypropyl)-4-(4-hydroxyphenyl)-2-azetidinone

5. **Bile acid sequestrants**: e.g. **Colesevelam hydrochloride** (WelChol -- Sankyo) is a nonabsorbed, polymeric, lipid-lowering agent that binds with bile acids in the intestine and significantly reduces their reabsorption. As the bile acid pool becomes depleted, there is an increased conversion of cholesterol to bile acids, thereby reducing cholesterol concentrations. The mechanism of action of colesevelam is similar to that of cholestyramine (e.g., Questran) and colestipol (Colestid). However, the new drug has a greater binding affinity for bile acids, permitting the use of a lower dosage, and appears to have a lower incidence of gastrointestinal (GI) adverse events and a lower potential

for drug interactions. Colesevelam is indicated for use, alone or in combination with a hydroxymethyl-glutaryl-coenzyme A (HMG-CoA) reductase inhibitor (a "statin"), as adjunctive therapy to diet and exercise for the reduction of elevated low-density lipoprotein cholesterol (LDL-C) in patients with primary hypercholesterolemia (Fredrickson Type IIa). In the clinical studies, colesevelam reduced LDL-C concentrations by 15% to 18%, and increased high-density lipoprotein cholesterol (HDL-C) concentrations by 3%. There were small increases in triglyceride concentrations, but these were not statistically different from the results in those receiving placebo.

6. **Phytosterols**: have cholesterol-lowering properties; reducing cholesterol absorption in intestines, and may act in cancer prevention. Phytosterols naturally occur in small amount in vegetable oils, especially soybean oil. Sterols can reduce cholesterol in human subjects by up to 15% (Rossi S, 2006).

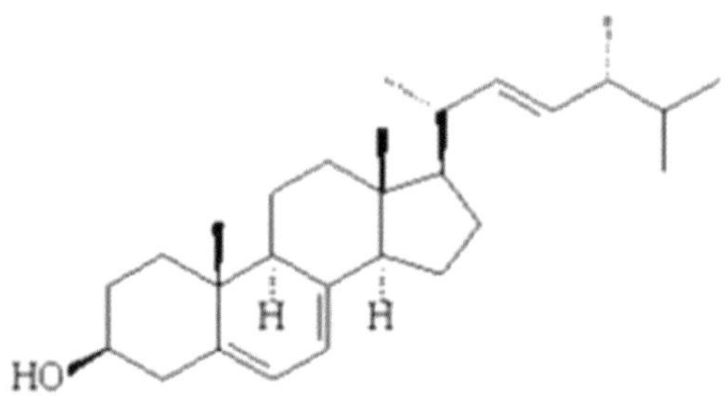

Ergosterol (9)

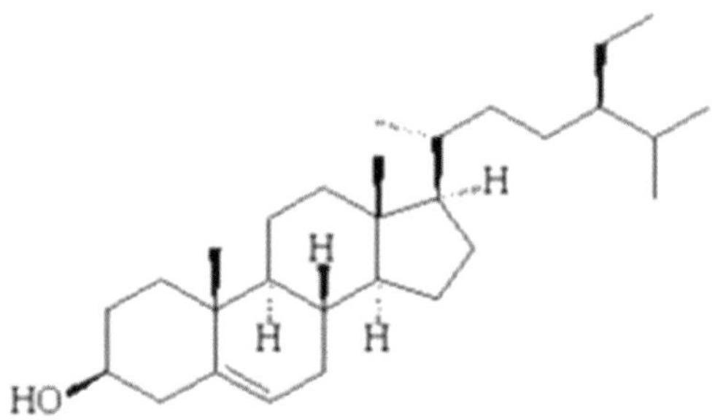

β-Sitosterol (10)

7. **Thiazolidinediones**: TZDs are now seen to fight several aspects of metabolic disease within Type II diabetes. They reduce blood glucose while enhancing insulin sensitivity, and also have a profound effect on lipid metabolism. Patients with Type II diabetes commonly present with elevated plasma levels of TGs and low HDLs. TZDs increase TG lipolysis in VLDLs, reducing the level of TGs and increasing HDLs. TZDs increase TG lipolysis in VLDLs, reducing the level of TGs and increasing HDLs and have also been shown to inhibit the progression of atherosclerosis in animal models (Schoonjans & Auwerx, 2000).

The mechanism of thiazolidinediones (TZDs) drugs by which the change in serum lipid profile occurs is not clear, but may involve increases in serum lipoprotein lipase and increased lipid uptake by adipocytes and skeletal muscle (Burant and Park). It is also possible that it results from direct effects of the drug acting on PPARα (Smith, 2001). It is not clear, especially in humans, if PPARγ promotes lipid clearance in the liver in a manner similar to PPARα.

9. Synthetic hypolipidemic agents

A continued research effort has been underway over the past several years in the area of the development of hypolipidemic agents (Chapman JM. et al. 1979&,1983 & Wyrick SD. et al. 1984).

Chapman and co-workers initially reported the hypolipidemic activity of **phthalimides** and **N-substituted phthalimides** including alkyl, methyl ketone, carboxylic acids, and acetate esters of varying chain length were synthesized and tested for hypolipidemic activity in mice, compounds **(1), (2), and (3)** were found to afford the most significant reduction in serum cholesterol and triglyceride levels. Phthalimides, the parent compound, decreased serum cholesterol and triglyceride levels by 43% and 56% respectively, in mice after 16 days of dosing at an optimum dose of 20mg/kg/day (Chapman JM. et al. 1979)

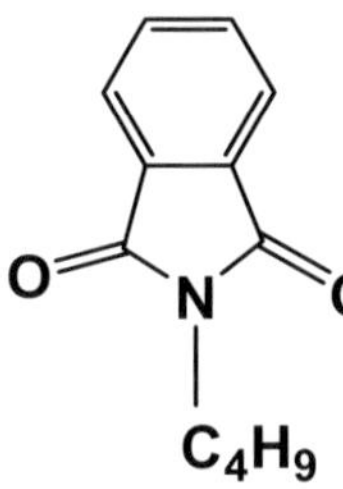

(1)

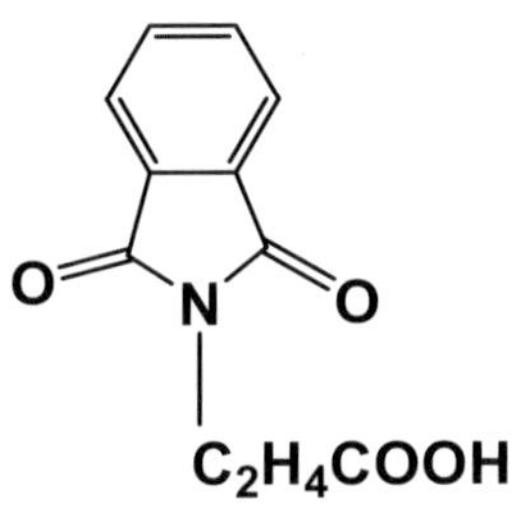

(2)

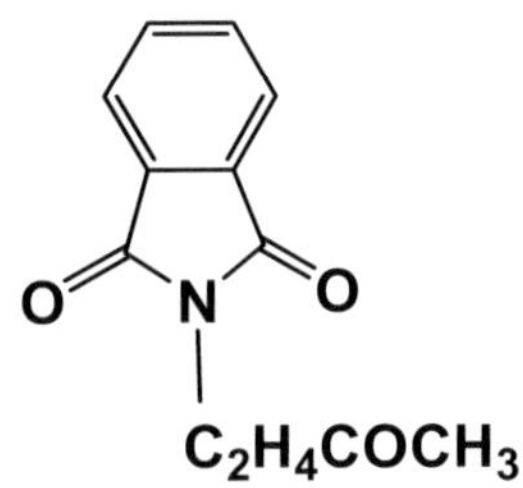

(3)

The hypolipidemic effects of aromatic versus non aromatic imides were investigated. Thus, a number of N-substituted phthalimides **(4)**,1,8-naphthalimide **(5)**, succinimide **(6)**, and glutarimide **(7)** derivatives demonstrated significant hypolipidemic activity at 20 mg/kg/day in male mice (~25gm) after16 days of intrapretonially dosing. The dose of 20 mg/kg/day was selected for structure activity relationship SAR study because this dose proved to be the optimum dose when testing phthalimides and 3-N-(1,8-naphthalimide)propionic acid. Most of the derivatives at 20mg/kg/day demonstrated improved activity over clofibrate at 150mg/kg/day. In general, 1,8-naphthalimide and glutarimide derivatives appeared to be less active than phthalimides and succinimide. Removal of phenyl ring of phthalimides resulting in succinimide led to less hypolipidemic activity in general. The loss of aromatic system of 1,8-naphthalimide resulting in glutarimide led to a slight loss of anticholesterolemic activity and only α-phenylglutarimide show slight improvement of antitriglyceridemic activity (Chapman JM. et al. 1984).

The importance of rigid imide ring system for hypolipidemic activity was determined. Therefore, two series of cyclic imides; diphenimide **(8)** and its open acyclic imides; dibenzimide **(9)**, and succimide **(10)**, and diacetimide **(11)** were examined for hypolipidemic activity in mice.

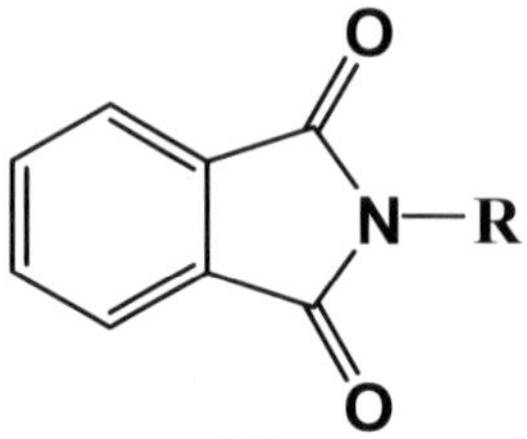

(4)

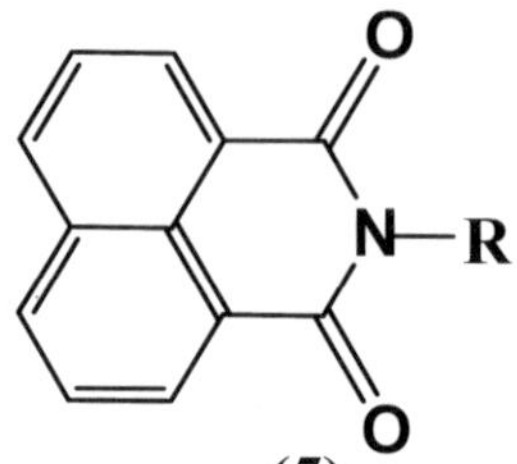

(5)

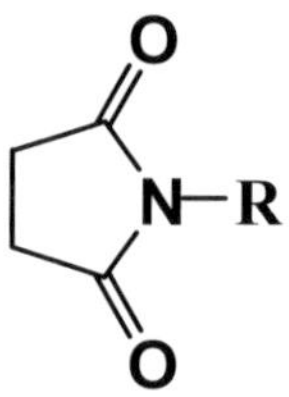

(6)

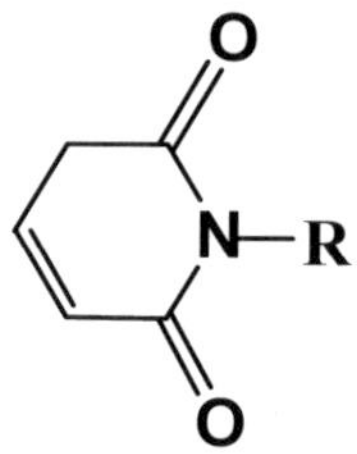

(7)

R = H
n-C_4H_9
n-C_5H_{11}
CH_2CH_2-COOH
CH_2CH_2-CO-CH_3

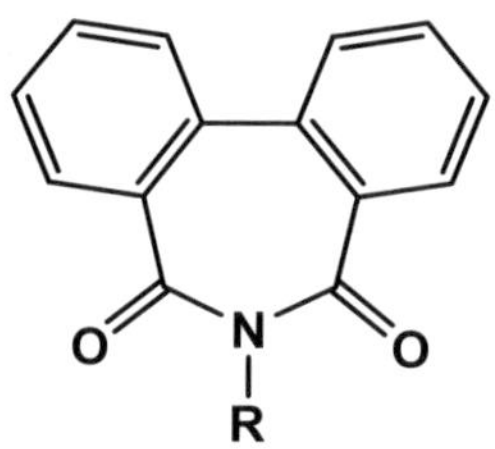

(8)

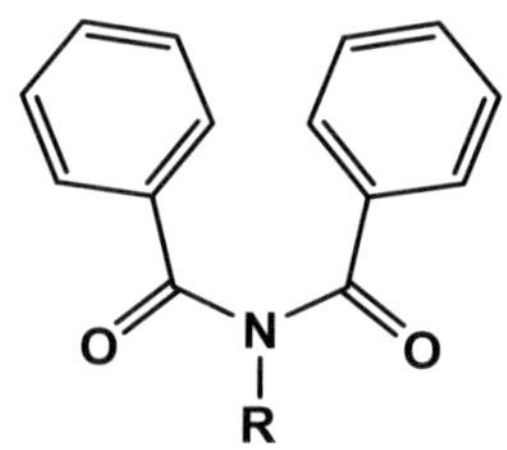

(9)

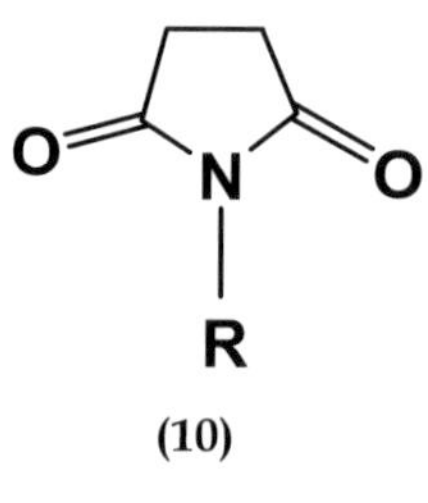

(10)

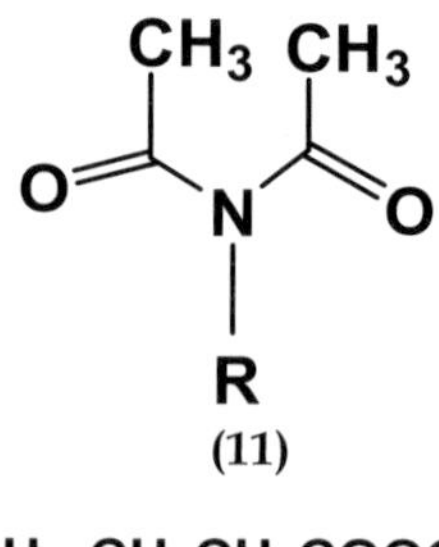

(11)

R = C_4H_9 , $CH_2CH_2COCH_3$, CH_2CH_2COOH , $CH_2CH_2COOC_2H_5$

It was shown that the rigid imide ring system was not necessary for hypercholesterolemia activity. However, the cyclic imide's structure was a necessary requirement for a good hypotriglyceridemic activity (Voorstad. et.al. 1985).

A series of nitrogen substituted N-butan-3-one derivatives of cyclic imides; such as phthalimides **(12)**, *o*-benzosulphimide **(13)**, 1,8-naphthalimide **(14)**, and diphinimide **(15)** were prepared (Chapman JM. et al. 1990).

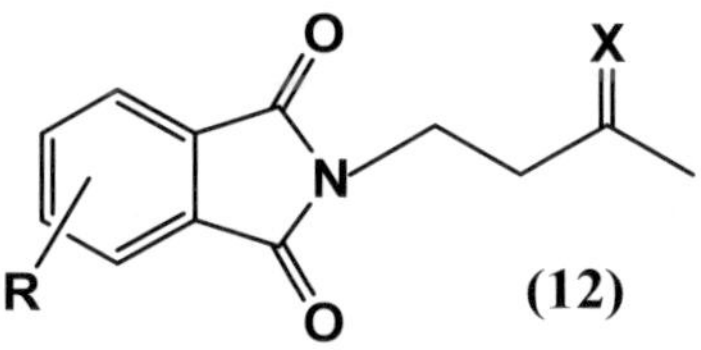

(12)

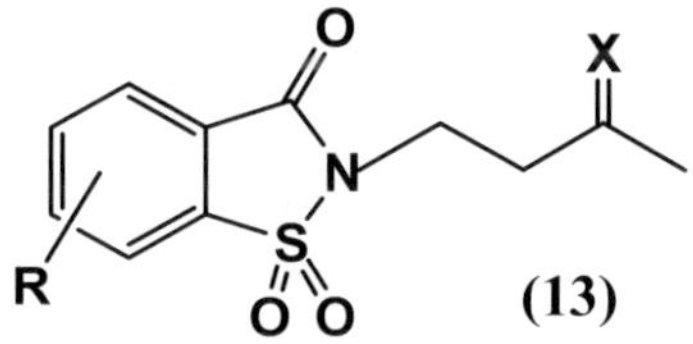

(13)

R = H, Cl, CH_3, NO_2

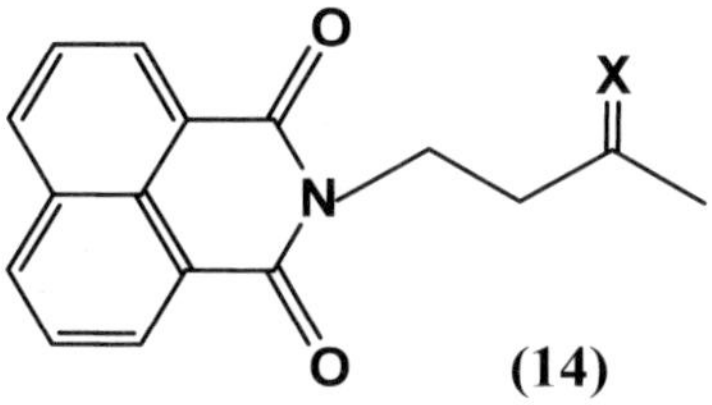

(14)

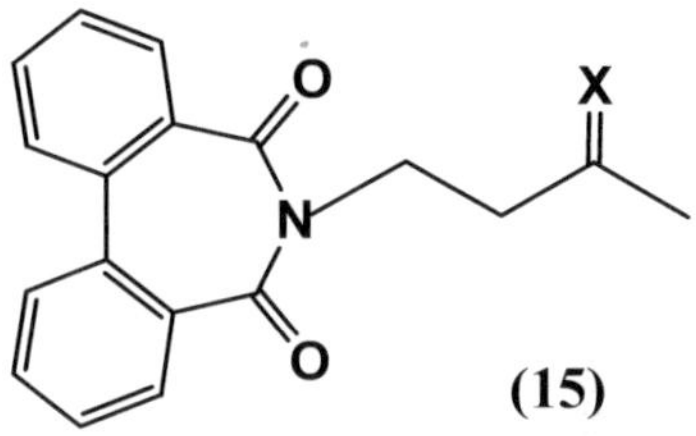

(15)

X= a) NNH-CO-NH_2, b) NNH-CS-NH_2, c)NNH-CO-CH_3

Molecular modeling programs were used to compare the **3D** structures of the some derivatives of some cyclic imides with the already known Clofibrate **(2)** (ethyl ester of 2,2-dimethylphenoxyacetic acid), These overlays were made with the aid of computer **Accelry's soft wares** at the Computer laboratory, Faculty of Pharmacy, KAU, KSA.

The Changes in the structure of phthalimide involving the imide's ring system led to the preparation of new compounds with potent and significant antihyperlipidemic effect; this is due to the good efficacy of their binding to the fatty acid receptor sites (Hall IH *et al.* 1986).

The promising hypolipidemic activity of certain cyclic imides derivatives in experimental animals strongly potentiate and recommend more researches in this area (El-Zahabi MA *et al.* 2010). Moreover; the newly synthesized compounds may be useful in the prevention of cardiovascular disease in a growing population suffering from lifestyle-induced metabolic dysfunction (Project 040/1428 H, Gad L M. *et al.*;funded by the Deanship of Scientific Research, King Abdulaziz University, KAU, Jeddah, KSA).

10. References

[1] Anderson KM, Castelli WP and Levy D (1987). Cholesterol and mortality. 30 years of follow-up from the Framingham study. *JAMA* 257: 2176–2180. Abstract-MEDLINE

[2] Anderson KM, Wilson PW, Odell PM and Kannel WB (1991). An updated coronary risk profile. A statement for health professionals. *Circulation* 83: 356-362

[3] Assmann Gerd, Paul Cullen, Helmut Schulte (2002). Clinical Investigation and Reports, Simple Scoring Scheme for Calculating the Risk of Acute Coronary Events Based on the 10-Year Follow-Up of the Prospective Cardiovascular Münster (PROCAM) Study . *Circulation* 105:310

[4] Barter PJ and Rye KA (1994). High-density lipoproteins and coronary heart disease. *J Cardiovasc Risk* 1: 217–221.

[5] Berliner JA, Navab M, Fogelman AM, Frank JS, Demer LL, Edwards PA, Watson AD and Lusis AJ (1995). Atherosclerosis: basic mechanisms. Oxidation, inflammation, and genetics. *Circulation* 91:2488–2496.

[6] von Birgelen C, Hartmann M, Mintz GS, et al. (2004) Relationship between cardiovascular risk as predicted by established risk scores versus plaque progression as measured by serial intravascular ultrasound in left main coronary arteries. *Circulation* 110:1579-1585

[7] Boden WE (2000). High-density lipoprotein cholesterol as an independent risk factor in cardiovascular disease: assessing the data from Framingham to the Veterans Affairs high-density lipoprotein intervention trial. *Am J Cardiol* 86: 19L–22L. Abstract MEDLINE

[8] Barooah N, Tamuly C, Baruah J. (2005) Synthesis, characterisation of few N-substituted 1,8-naphthalimide derivatives and their copper(II) complexes *J. Chem. Soc.* 117(2):117.

[9] Chapman JM, Cocolas GH, and Hall IH (1979) Hyperlipidemia activity of phthalimides derivatives. 1. *N*-Substituted Phthalimide derivatives. *J. Med. Chem.* 22: 1399.

[10] Chapman JM, Voorstad PJ, Cocolas GH, and Hall IH (1983). Hypolipidemic activity of phthalimide derivatives. 2. *N*-Phenylphthalimide derivatives. *J. Med. Chem.* 28: 237-243

[11] Chapman JM, Cocolas GH, and Hall IH (1983). Hypolipidemic activity of phthalimide derivatives, IV: Further chemical modification and investigation of the hypolipidemic activity of N-substituted imides. *J. Pharm. Sci. 72*: 1344-7

[12] Chapman JM, Wyrick SD, Maguire JH, Cocolas GH, and Hall IH (1984). Hypolipidemic Agents of Phthalimide Derivatives, 6. Effect of Aromatic vs. Non-Aromatic Imides. J. *Pharm. Res.* 6: 267-269

[13] Chapman JM, DeLucy P, Wong OT, and Hall IH (1990). Structure Activity Relationship of Imido N-Alkyl Semicarbazones,Thiosemicarbazones and Acetyl hydrazones as Hypolipidemic Agents in Rodents. *J. Lipid.* 25, No.7: 391-397.

[14] Chapman JM, Wyrick SD, Voorstad PJ, Maquire JH, Cocolas GH, and Hall IH (1984). Hypolipidemic activity of phthalimide derivatives V: Reduced and hydrolytic products of simple cyclic imides. *J. Pharm. Sci.* 73,(10):1482-4.

[15] Conroy RM, Pyo¨ra¨la¨ K, Fitzgerald A et al. (2003). Estimation of ten-year risk of fatal cardiovascular disease in Europe: the SCORE project. *Eur Heart J*; 24:987–1003.

[16] The Coronary Drug Project Research Group. Clofibrate and niacin in coronary heart disease. *JAMA* (1975) 231: 360 –381.

[17] Cullen P (2000). Evidence that triglycerides are an independent coronary heart disease risk factor. *Am J Cardiol* 86: 943–949.

[18] El-Zahabi MA, Gad LM, Bamanie FH, *and* Al-Marzooki Z (2010). Synthesis of new of Cyclic Imides derivatives with potential Hypolipidemic Activity.(project 048/1426H; funded by the Deanship of Scientific Research, King Abdulaziz University, KAU) Available online 25/11/2010, *Med Chem Res* (2012) 21, issue (1):75-84.

[19] Faergeman O (2000). Hypertriglyceridemia and the fibrate trials. *Curr. Opin. Lipidol* 11: 609–614

[20] Farnier M (1998). Cerivastatin in the treatment of mixed hyperlipidemia: the RIGHT study. The Cerivastatin Study Group. Cerivastatin, Gemfibrozil, Hyperlipidemia Treatment. *Am J Cardiol* 82: 47J–51J.

[21] Feussner G, Kurth B and Lohrmann J. (1997) Comparative effects of bezafibrate and micronised fenofibrate in patients with type III hyperlipoproteinemia. *Eur. J. Med. Res.* 2: pp. 165–168. Abstract-MEDLINE

[22] Fruchart JC, Brewer HB and Leitersdorf E (1998). Consensus for the use of fibrates in the treatment of dyslipoproteinemia and coronary heart disease. Fibrate Consensus Group. *Am J Cardiol* 81: 912–917. Abstract-MEDLINE

[23] Fruchart JC, Duriez P and Staels B (1999). Molecular mechanism of action of the fibrates (French). *J Soc Biol* 193: 67–75. Abstract-MEDLINE

[24] Gad LM., El-Zahabi MA, Ginienah M M., Bamanie F H, Ghareib S A. and Al-Marzooki Z H.(2011). Synthesis of new 1,8-naphthalimide derivatives with potential antihyperlipidemic activities.(Under publication).

[25] Goldstein JL (1990). Familial hypercholesterolemia, In: Scriver CR, Beaudet AI, Sly WS and Valle D, Editors. *The Metabolic Basis of Inherited Diseases*. McGraw-Hill, New York, 1215–1250.

[26] Gordon T, Castelli WP, Hjortland MC, Kannel WB and Dawber TR (1977). High density lipoprotein as a protective factor against coronary heart disease. The Framingham Study. *Am J Med* 62: 707–714.

[27] Guay DR (1999). Micronized Fenofibrate: a new fibric acid hypolipidemic agent. *Ann Pharmacother.* 33: 1083–1103

[28] Haffner SM. (2000). Coronary heart disease in patients with diabetes. *N Engl J Med.; 342:* 1040–1042

[29] Hall IH, Murthy ARK, and Wyrick SD (1986). Hypolipidemic Activity of 6-Substituted 6,7-Dihydro-5H-dibenz[c,e]azepine and the Effects of 6,7-Dihydro-5H-dibenz[c,e]azepine on Lipid Metabolism of Rodents. *J. Pharm Sci.* 75, No.6: 622-626

[30] Helen Vosper, Guennadi A. Khoudoli, Tracey L. Graham and Colin N. A. (2002). Peroxisome proliferator-activated receptor agonists, hyperlipidaemia, and atherosclerosis. pharmacology & therapeutic 95, Issue 1: 47-62.

[31] Krauss RM, (1998). Atherogenicity of triglyceride-rich lipoproteins. *Am J Cardiol* 81: 13B–17B

[32] Larsen SD.and Spilman CH (1993). New Potential Therapies for the Treatment of atherosclerosis. *Ann. Rep. Med. Chem.* 28: 217-26.

[33] Miller M (2000). Differentiating the effects of raising low levels of high-density lipoprotein cholesterol versus lowering normal triglycerides insights from the veterans affairs high-density lipoprotein intervention trial. *Am J Cardiol* 86: 23–27.

[34] Murthy AR, Wyrick SD, Voorstad PJ, and Hall IH (1985). *Hypolipidemic activity of N-substituted diphenimides in rodents. Eur. J. Med. Chem.* 20, No.6: 547-550

[35] Napoli C, Lepore S, Chiariello P, et al. (1997) Longterm treatment with pravastatin alone and in combination with gemfibrozil in familial type IIB hyperlipoproteinemia or combined hyperlipidemia. *J Cardiovasc. Pharmacol Ther.* 2(1):17-26.

[36] Revkin JH, Shear CL, Pouleur HG, Ryder SW, and Orloff DG (2007). Biomarkers in the Prevention and Treatment of Atherosclerosis: Need, Validation, and Future. *Pharmacol Rev* 59:40–53

[37] Rossi S; editor. Australian Medicines Handbook, (2006), ISBN 0-9757919-2-3 through Wikipedia, the free encyclopedia, ONLINE.

[38] Rubins HB (2000). Triglycerides and coronary heart disease: implications of recent clinical trials. *J Cardiovasc Risk* 7:339–345. Abstract-MEDLINE

[39] Rustemeijer C, Schouten JA, Voerman HJ, Hensgens HE, Donker AJ and Heine RJ (2000). Pravastatin compared to bezafibrate in the treatment of dyslipidemia in insulin-treated patients with type 2 diabetes mellitus. *Diabetes Metab Res Rev* 16: 82–87. Abstract-MEDLINE

[40] Spieker LE, Noll G, Hannak M, and Luscher TF (2000). Efficacy and tolerability of fluvastatin and bezafibrate in patients with hyperlipidemia and persistently high triglyceride levels. *J. Cardiovasc Pharmacol,* 35: 361–365.

[41] Sprecher DL (2000). Raising high-density lipoprotein cholesterol with niacin and fibrates: a comparative review. *Am J Cardiol* 86: 46–50.

[42] Staels B, Dallongeville J, Auwerz J, Schoonjans K, Leitersdorf E, Fruchart J, (1998).Mechanism of action of fibrates on lipid and lipoprotein metabolism. *Circulation.* 98, issue 19: 2088-2093

[43] Terasaka N , Miyazaki A, Kasanuki N, Ito K, Ubukata N, Koieyama T, Kitayama K , Tanimoto T, Maeda N, Inaba T (2007). ACAT inhibitor pactimibe sulfate (CS-505) reduces and stabilizes atherosclerotic lesions by cholesterol-lowering and direct effects in apolipoprotein E-deficient mice. *Atherosclerosis* 190: 239–247

[44] Turley SD, Herndon MW, Dietschy JM (1994). Reevaluation and application of the dual-isotope plasma ratio method for the measurement of intestinal cholesterol absorption in the hamster. *J Lipid Res.* 35: 328–39.

[45] Tylor HA (1987). Lowering plasma cholesterol levels decrease risk of coronary artery disease: *An overview of clinical trials* in Hypercholesterolemia

[46] Voorstad PJ, Chapman JM, Cocolas GH, Wyrick SD, and Hall IH (1985). Comparison of the Hypolipidemic Activity of Cyclic vs. AcyclicImides. *J. Med.Chem.* 28: 9-12

[47] Wyrick SD, Voorstad PJ, Cocolas GH, and Hall IH (1984). Hypolipidemic Activity of Phthalimide Derivatives. 7. Structure-Activity Studies of Indazolone Analogues. *J. Med. Chem.* 27: 768-772.

[48] Xiang-Yang Ye a, et al., (2008), Design, synthesis, and structure–activity relationships of piperidine and dehydropiperidine carboxylic acids as novel potent dual PPAR α/γ agonists. *Bioorganic & Medicinal Chemistry Letters* 18*: 3545–3550*

[49] Zhang H et al. (2009). Design, synthesis and structure–activity relationships of azole acids as novel, potent dual PPAR α/γ agonists. *Bioorg & Med Chem Lett. 19: 1451–1456.*

[50] *J. Medicinal Biology;* 2008, JMB 27:148 –153, (Review article).

6

Pyrrolobenzodiazepines as Sequence Selective DNA Binding Agents

Ahmed Kamal, M. Kashi Reddy,
Ajay Kumar Srivastava and Y. V. V. Srikanth
Division of Organic Chemistry
CSIR-Indian Institute of Chemical Technology, Hyderabad
India

1. Introduction

The heritability of cancers is usually affected by complex interactions between carcinogens and the host's genome. New aspects of the genetics of cancer pathogenesis, such as DNA methylation, and micro RNAs are increasingly recognized as important events. Chemotherapeutic drugs interfere with cell division in different ways, e.g. with the duplication of DNA or the separation of newly formed chromosomes. Most forms of chemotherapy target rapidly dividing cells and are not specific for cancer cells, although some degree of specificity may come from the inability of many cancer cells to repair DNA damage. Hence, chemotherapy has the potential to harm healthy tissues, especially those tissues that have a high replacement rate (e.g. intestinal lining). These cells usually repair themselves after chemotherapy.[1] DNA has long been considered a favored target for cancer chemotherapeutic agents. Indeed many of the most effective clinical agents, such as alkylating and interactive agents, are DNA interactive. Achieving the desired sequence specificity with DNA-interactive agents is considered to be one of the most formidable hurdles in the development of new agents to achieve therapeutic invention.[2]

Certain structural features of the alpha helix are particularly important when considering drug-DNA interaction. Double helical DNA is not a uniform structure, there are places where the strands are further apart, and where they are closer together, these are known as major and minor grooves. In B-DNA, the major groove is wider (12 versus 6 Å) and deeper (8.5 versus 7.5 Å) than the minor groove, making it more accessible to interacting molecules. The base pair arrangement for each groove is very specific, each containing certain hydrogen bond donors and acceptors. In addition, the major groove will also contain the methyl group of thymine and drug molecules or proteins bind at these sites. More importantly the difference between the donor and acceptor groups in each groove, this makes it possible for drug molecules to selectively distinguish between the different bases as well as sequences of bases.[3,4]

2. DNA groove binders

Drugs that bind to DNA may occur on the major groove face, minor groove face or a combination. The grooves are excellent sites for sequence specific recognition since there are many potential hydrogen bond donor and acceptor atoms unique to each base pair combination along the base edges. The greater width associated with the B-DNA major groove makes the major groove a somewhat more preferable binding groove. Groove binding can be via the major or minor groove and covalently or non-covalently. Most DNA interactive proteins bind in the major groove, while small molecules of less than 1000 Da, including many antibiotics, bind in the minor groove.

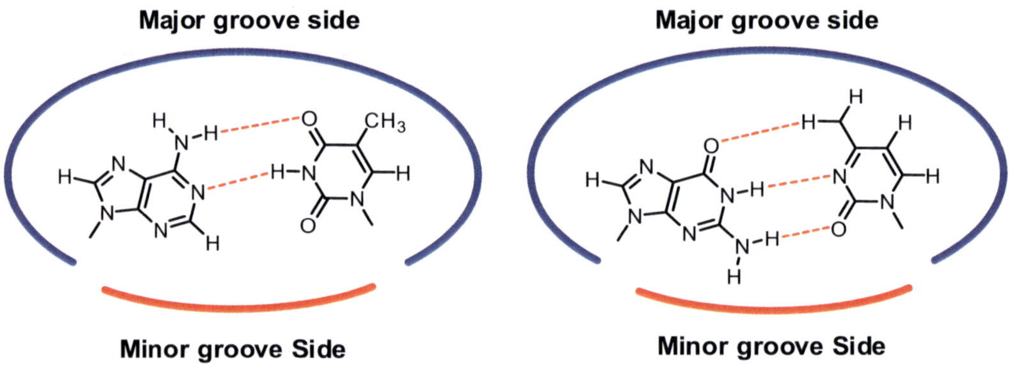

Fig. 1. Hydrogen bonding betweeb adenosine/thymine (left) and guanosine/cytosine base pairs of DNA.

The minor groove represents a vulnerable site of attack in that it is normally unoccupied, and this is presumably the reason for the evolution of antibiotics that attack the DNA of competing organisms. Thus, although at first sight minor groove binders are less attractive as probes in that they target the less information rich minor groove nevertheless, they may prove to have several advantages compared with major groove ligands. The development of sequence-specific probes based on naturally occurring DNA groove-binding agents is, therefore, an alternative and complementary approach to the antisense oligonucleotide strategy. The main motive for synthesizing a large number of analogues and conjugates of naturally occurring minor groove-binding agents, is to generate new lead compounds with potential anticancer properties and specific DNA sequence recognition.[5]

2.1 Covalent binding in the minor groove of DNA

Drugs which bind covalently to DNA are used to either add substituents onto base residues, or to form cross-links between different sections of DNA. The first mechanism results in a base-pairing mismatch during DNA replication, and the DNA is ultimately fragmented by the enzymes which try to repair it. The second mechanism binds together the two strands of DNA helix, preventing separation during the replication process. Electrophilic functional groups such as epoxides, aziridines, carbinolamines, imines and cyclopropanes are found in a variety of synthetic and natural products capable of covalent interaction with DNA; examples include mitomycin, saframycins and pyrrolobenzodiazepines (anthramycin).[6] Non-covalent binding compounds are typically isohelical with B-DNA and fits snugly within the minor groove, held in a position by a combination of hydrogen bonds, van der Waal forces and electrostatic interactions; examples include distamycin,[7] netropsin,[8] lexitropsins and bis-benzimidazole (Hoecht 33258).[9]

2.2 Pyrrolo[2,1-*c*][1,4]benzodiazepines (PBDs) as DNA binding agents

Binding of low molecular weight ligands to DNA causes a wide variety of potential biological responses. In this context pyrrolo[2,1-*c*][1,4]benzodiazepines (PBDs), a group of potent naturally occurring antitumour antibiotics isolated from various *Streptomyces* species, are one of the promising type of lead compounds. They differ in the number, type and position of substituent in both their aromatic A-ring and pyrrolidine C-ring, and in the degree of saturation of the C-ring which can be either fully saturated or unsaturated at either the C2-C3 (endocyclic) or C2 (exocyclic) positions. There is either an imine or carbinolamine methylether moiety at the N10-C11. Position, which is an elecrophilic centre responsible for alkylating DNA. To date, thirteen structures isolated, include compounds like anthramycin,[6] mazethramycin,[10] porothramycin,[11] prothracarcin,[12] sibanomycin,[13] tomaymycin,[14] sibiromycin,[15] chicamycin A,[16] neothramycin A, B[17] and DC-81[18] (Figure 2).

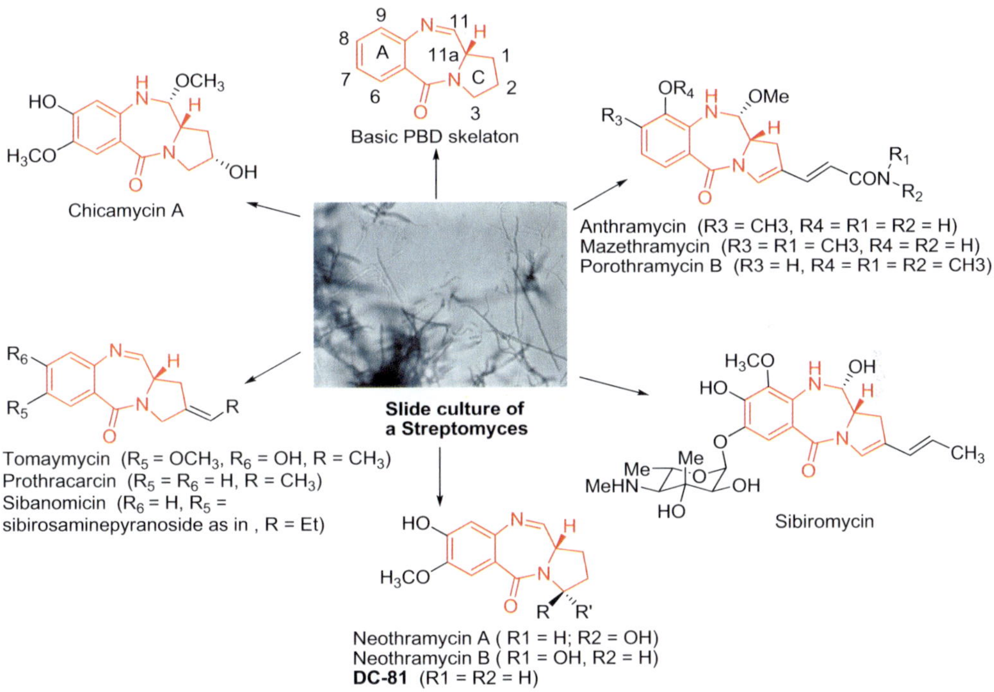

Fig. 2. Naturally occurring PBDs.

The PBD interactions with DNA are unique since they bind within the minor groove of DNA forming a covalent aminal bond between the C11-position of the central B-ring and the N2 amino group of a guanine base.[19] The cytotoxic and antitumour activity of PBDs are attributed to their ability to form covalent DNA adducts. Molecular modeling, solution NMR, fluorimetry and DNA foot printing experiments have shown that these molecules have a preferred selectivity for Pu-G-Pu sequences[14,20] that are oriented with their A-rings pointed either towards the 3' or 5' end of the covalently bonded DNA strand (as in case of anthramycin and tomaymycin). The PBDs have been shown to interfere with the action of endonuclease enzymes on DNA[21] and to block transcription by inhibiting DNA polymerase in a sequence specific manner,[22] processes which may be relevant for the biological activity.

The known PBD natural products have a (*S*) configuration at the C11a-position, which provides them with a right-handed twist when viewed from the C-ring towards the A-ring. This has given the appropriate three-dimensional shape for isohelicity with the minor groove of DNA, leading to a snug fit at the binding site. Recemization at C11a can significantly reduce both DNA binding affinity and *in vitro* cytotoxicity. A synthetic PBD with the (*R*)-configuration at C11a was shown to be devoid of both DNA binding affinity and *in vitro* cytotoxicity.[23] The N10-C11 imine moiety may exist in the hydrated form depending upon precise structure of the compound and the method of isolation or synthetic workup. Imines and methyl ether forms are interconvertable by dissolution of imine in methanol or by several cycles of refluxing the methyl ether in chloroform followed by evaporation of the solvent in vacuum (Figure 3).

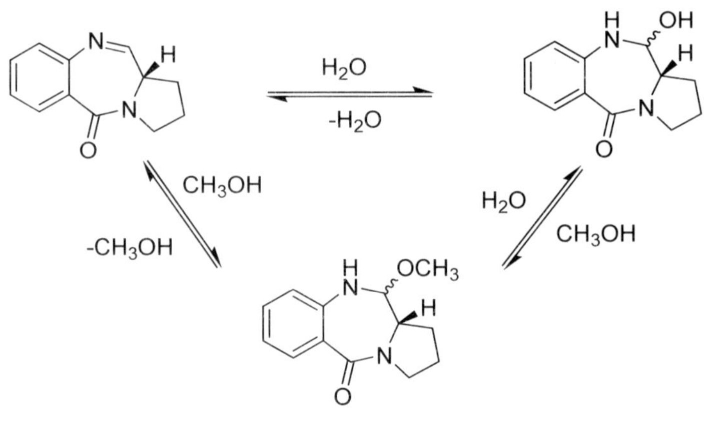

Fig. 3. Carbinolamine-methylether-imine interconversions in the PBDs.

The mechanism of action of the PBDs is associated with their ability to form, an adduct in the minor groove, thus interfering with DNA processing. After insertion in the minor groove, an aminal bond is formed through nucleophilic attack of the N2 of a guanine base at the electrophillic C11 position of PBD. X-Ray diffraction studies on crystals of anthramycin methylethers have shown that the molecule is twisted 0-50° from one end to the other along the axis, and this might fit into one of the grooves of DNA. In the CPK models, the drug fits snugly within the narrow groove without distortion of the DNA helix. The structure of the anthramycin DNA adduct was initially studied independently by Hurley and Kohn using indirect techniques,[24] but more recently fluorescence spectroscopy, high field NMR and molecular modeling have been employed (Figure 4).

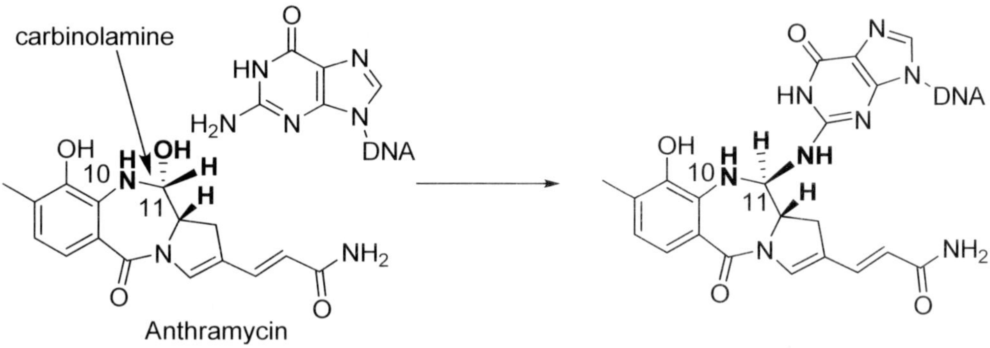

Fig. 4. Proposed mechanism for formation of the anthramycin deoxyguanosine adduct in DNA, showing formation of an aminal bond betweeb the C11 position of the PBD and exocyclic N2 of guanine base.

2.3 Preparation of PBDs

Biosynthesis of the naturally occurring PBDs have been extensively elucidated by Hurley and co-workers. The first total synthesis of a carbinolamine containing PBD of anthramycin has been reported by Leimgruber in 1968.[25] Extensive reviews of the synthetic literature of the PBDs have appeared in 1994, 1998 and 2002.[26] Various approaches to the synthesis of PBD antibiotics have been investigated, including hydride reduction of seven-membered cyclic dilactams,[27] reductive cyclization of acyclic nitroaldehydes,[28] iminothioether approach[29] cyclization of aminothioacetals,[30] deprotective cyclization of the diethylthioacetals *via* N10 protected precursors,[31] oxidation of cyclic secondary amines,[32] reductive cyclizations[33] and solid phase approaches.[34] Various synthetic methods for the synthesis of the PBDs have been reviewed extensively. The N10-C11 carbinolamine, or its chemical equivalent, is a prerequisite for antitumour activity. Several research groups have designed new PBDs with potential DNA binding affinity.[35-39]

A novel method for the oxidation of PBD secondary amine to the corresponding imines is developed in this laboratory[32]. Although PBDs with either a secondary amine or amide functionality at N10-C11 are readily synthesized, the introduction of imine or carbinolamine at this position is problematic due to the reactivity of these functional groups. As described in the literature, the cyclic secondary amine precursors have been readily prepared from corresponding nitroaldehydes. This upon oxidation with DMSO/$(COCl)_2$ or TPAP (tetra-n-propyl ammonium perruthenate) gives the corresponding imines in good yields (Scheme 1). The same group has carried out another interesting study on the enzymatic reduction of aryl azides to aryl amines by employing baker's yeast. This biocatalytic reductive methodology has been applied to the chemoenzymatic synthesis of PBDs *via* the reductive cyclization of arylazido aldehydes.[33,40]

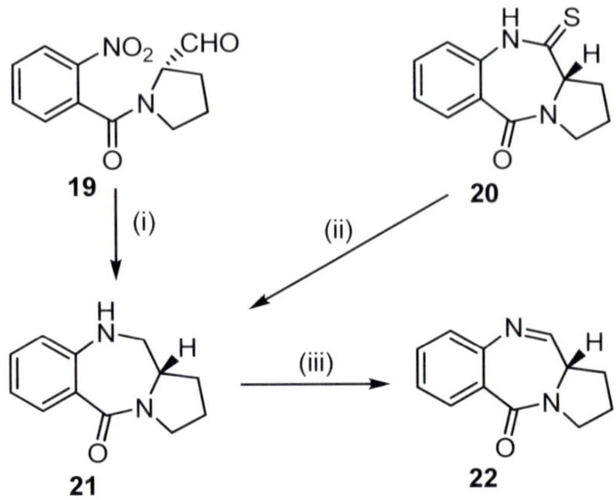

Scheme 1. Reagents and conditions: (i) Pd/C; (ii) Raney Ni; (iii) swern/TPAP.

3. Structure activity relationship studies

The naturally occurring PBDs namely anthramycin, tomaymycin, sibiromycin, neothramycin and DC-81 have different type of substitutions. The electron-donating substituents are required in the aromatic A ring for biological activity. Bulky substituent like a sugar moiety at C7 position enhances the DNA binding affinity and cytotoxicity. It is interesting to note that C ring modified PBDs appear to provide both greater differential thermal stabilization of DNA duplex and significantly enhance kinetic reactivity during covalent adduct formation. Similarly, the C2-substituted naturally occurring PBDs exhibit more cytotoxicity compared to their unsubstituted counter parts as shown in Figure 5. Based on these considerations a structure activity relationship has been derived by Thurston and co-workers.

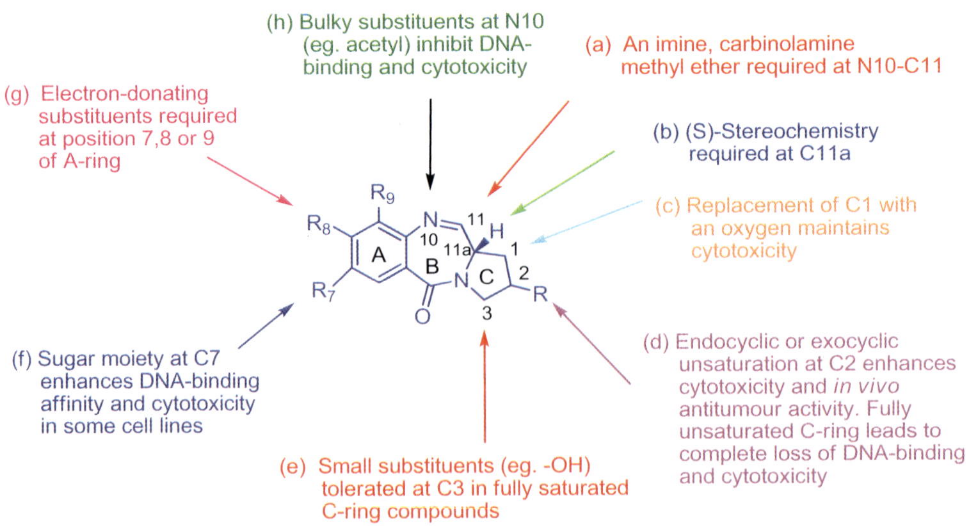

Fig. 5. Structure activity relationship of PBD ring system.

3.1 PBD A-ring modifications

Baraldi and co-workers[41] have investigated heterocyclic analogues of pyrrolo-[2,1-*c*][1,4]benzodiazepine (PBD) by replacing A ring with pyrazolo[4,3-*e*]-pyrrolo[1,2-*c*][1,4]diazepinone ring system. Some of these ring pyrazole PBD analogues exhibited interesting profile of cytotoxicity. Similarly, Thurston and co-workers[42] have synthesized some other A-ring heterocyclic PBDs and evaluated their DNA binding affinity. In this study pyrazine and pyrimidine A-ring analogues of PBDs have been prepared and evaluated for their cytotoxic potential. It is observed that the aromatic A-ring has a modest influence on thermal denaturation of DNA. They have also synthesized some tetracyclic PBD analogues like dioxolo[4,5-*h*]-pyrrolo[2,1-*c*]benzodiazepine-5-one and dieoxano[2,3-*h*]pyrrolo[2,1-*c*]benzodiazepine-5-one and they have observed that the addition of dioxazole or dioxazine rings to existing A ring of DC-81 significantly reduces DNA binding affinity (ΔT_m = 0.1 to 0.5 °C) and cytotoxicity [IC_{50} = 0.26-3.4 μM] compared to DC-81.

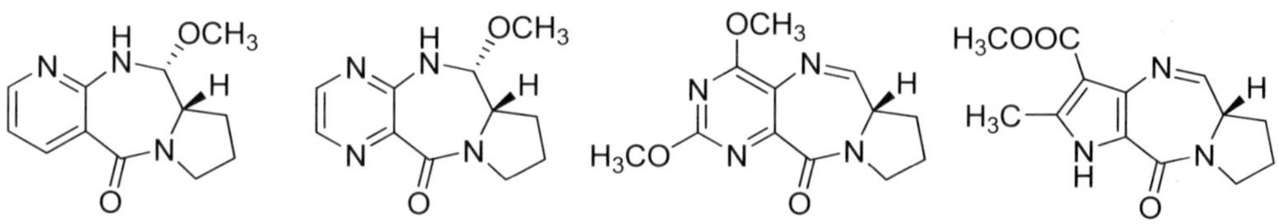

3.2 B-ring modifications

There are reports on B-ring modifications and one of them describes the synthesis and antitumour activity of pyrrolo[2,1-*c*][1,4]benzodiazepine derivatives and these compounds exhibit moderate antitumour activity. To investigate the role played by the non-covalent interactions Robba and co-workers[43] have synthesized a series of PBDs having N10-C11 amidine functionality and evaluated the DNA binding through thermal denaturation studies. It is observed that some of these compounds cause a significant increase in melting of calf thymus DNA comparable to the naturally occurring DC-81.

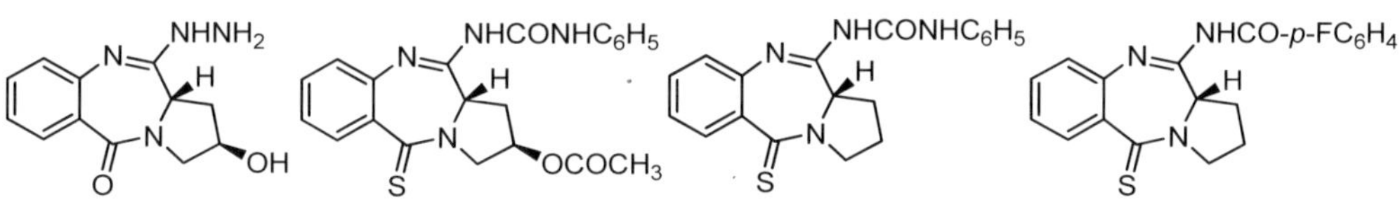

3.3 C-ring modifications

A number of naturally occurring PBDs namely anthramycin, tomaymycin, sibiromycin and neothramycin have different type of substitutions in the C ring. It is interesting to note that these C ring modified PBDs appear to provide both greater differential thermal stabilization of DNA duplex and significantly enhance kinetic reactivity during covalent adduct formation. Similarly, the C2 subistituted naturally occurring PBDs exhibit more cytotoxicity compared to their unsubstituted counter parts. Thurston and co-workers[44] have synthesized a series of C2-*exo* unsaturated PBDs, and C2-C3-*endo* unsaturated PBDs C-ring enhances both DNA-binding reactivity and *in vitro* cytotoxic potency. Recently the same group has reported the synthesis of novel C2-aryl 1,2/2,3-endo unsaturated pyrrolobenzodiazepines as potential antitumour agents and synthesized novel C2-C3 unsaturated PBD analogues containing conjugated acrylyl C2 substituents, these analogues possess not only significant cytotoxicity (in the NCI 60-cell line screen with surprisingly potency equivalent to anthramycin) but als better DNA binding ability.[45]

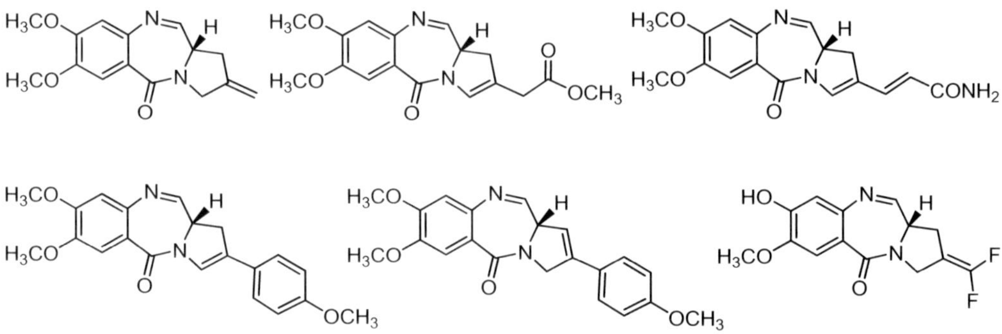

Recently, a series of C2-fluorinated PBDs[46] have synthesized and they have been screened for *in vitro* cytotoxicity against a number of cancer cell lines. The C2-fluorinated PBDs significantly increase the thermal stability of the calf thymus DNA duplex and also these compounds shows 550 fold increase in activity against the CH1 cell line when compared to the unsubstituted PBDs. A ring substituted C2-fluorinated monomers of PBD and DC-81 dimers have also been synthesized in this laboratory.[47] These compounds have shown good DNA binding ability when compared to A-ring unsubstituted C2-fluorine compounds. Moreover, such fluorinated compounds possess *in vitro* anticancer activity in a number of human cancer cell lines (Figure 6).

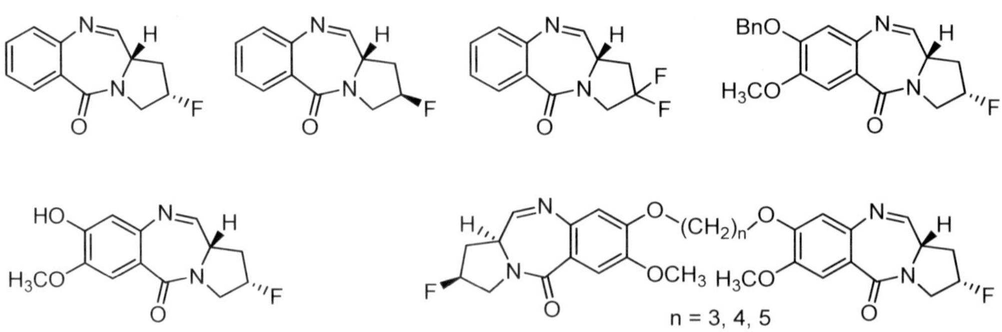

Fig. 6. Structure of fluorinated PBD monomer derivatives shown in a significant increase in melting for calf thymus dna comparable to the naturally occuring DC-81

3.4 PBD conjugates

The research of antineoplastic agents is based on the fact that a single molecule of PBD exhibits higher DNA binding affinity as well as more anticancer activity, if it contains more than one pharmacophore, each with different mode of action and capable of recognizing heterogeneous DNA sequences. For this reason, several research groups developed new PBD conjugates, such as cyclopropylbenzindole, distamycin, and netropsin. Synthesis of PBD conjugates has been carried out employing mainly pyrrolobenzodiazepine DC-81, that is linked mostly at C8 position to different moieties; rare examples of C2 linkage were described in literature these last years.[48]

The PBDs have also been used as a scaffold to attach ethylenediamine tetraacetic acid (EDTA),[49] epoxide,[50] polyamide[51] and oligopyrrole moieties[52] leading to novel hybrids of PBD, which have exhibited sequence selective DNA-cleaving and cross-linking properties. EDTA moiety has been linked to the PBD skeleton (DC-81) to study the covalent binding to DNA and its sequence selectivity.[53] Detailed analysis of the cleavage sites by laser densitometry suggested that the results are best explained by two major modes of binding/cleaving for (EDTA/DC-81)Fe^{II}. The EDTA-PBD conjugate covalently binds to DNA at 5'-PuGPu sequences leading to site specific cleavage.

Confalone and co-workers[54] have synthesized a PBD analogue with an epoxide group substituted at C11a position with the objective of producing a PBD monomer with DNA cross-linking ability, whereas no DNA binding data has been reported. Since attachment at C11a position could sterically hinder the DNA binding, interstrand guanine-guanine cross-linking C8 epoxide containing PBD has been designed and synthesized. It has been considered that the attachment of the epoxide through the C8 position could retain the isohelicity with the contour of the minor groove of the host DNA molecule.[55]

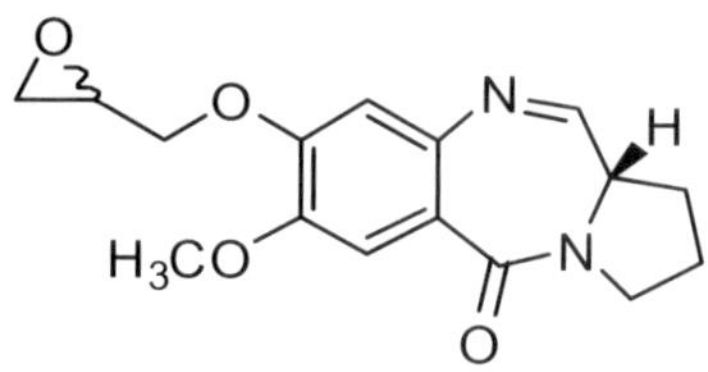

Baraldi and co-workers[56] have designed and synthesized distamycin-PBD and netropsin-PBD conjugates as novel sequence selective C8-linked PBD hybrids. These hybrids containing 1 to 4 pyrrole units have been investigated for the sequence selectivity and stability of DNA drug complexes.

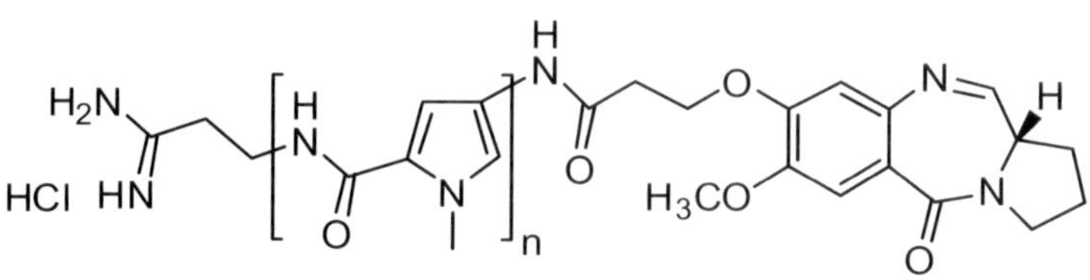

Lown and co-workers[57] have also reported the synthesis of a series of PBD-lexitropsin conjugates linked through the C8 position with a suitable linker. The conjugation has been achieved by amidic linkage to amine of the lexitropsin unit with the acid moiety of the linker attached to the PBD system. These compounds have been synthesized in view of the effect of their sequence selective binding in DNA duplex.

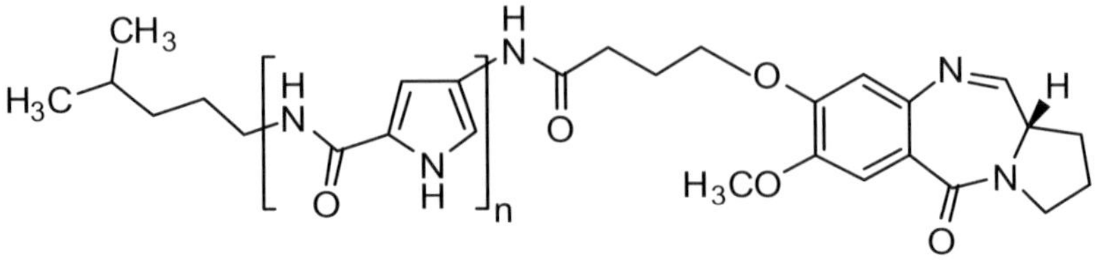

n = 1-3

Hurley and co-workers[58] have synthesized novel DNA-DNA interstrand adenine-guanine cross-linking UTA-6026 compound. Preliminary *in vitro* tests showed that UTA-6026 has remarkable potent cytotoxicity to several tumour cell lines (IC_{50} = 0.28 nM in human breast tumour cell line MCF-7, IC_{50} = 0.047 nM in colon tumour cell line SW-480 and IC_{50} = 5.1 nM in human lung tumour cell line A549).

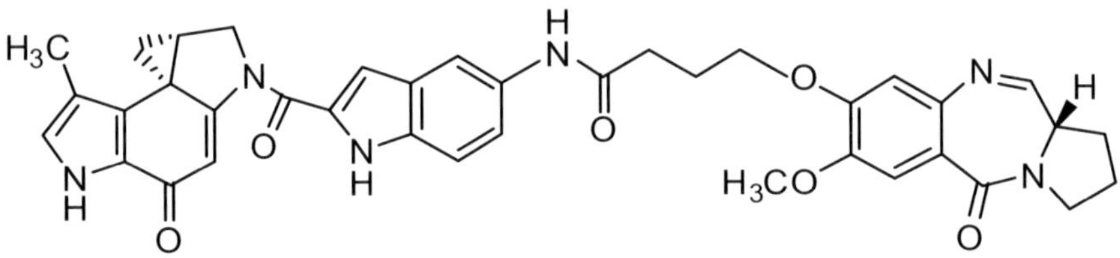

Denny and co-workers[59] have designed and synthesized unsymmetrical DNA cross-linkers by linking the *seco*-1,2,9,9a-tetrahydrocyclopropa[c]benz[e]indo-4-one (*seco*-CBI) to PBD moiety. These compounds have anticipated cross-linking between N3 of adenine and N2 of guanine in the minor groove of DNA.

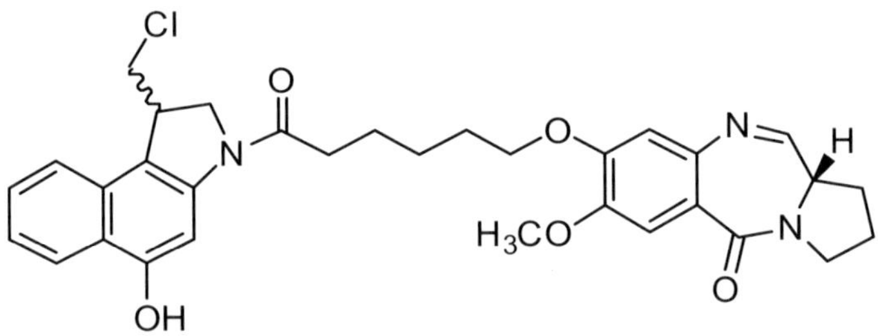

Recently, Wang and co-workers[60] have synthesized indole and enediyne PBD conjugates as potential antitumor agents and explained the correlation between antitumor activity and apoptosis.

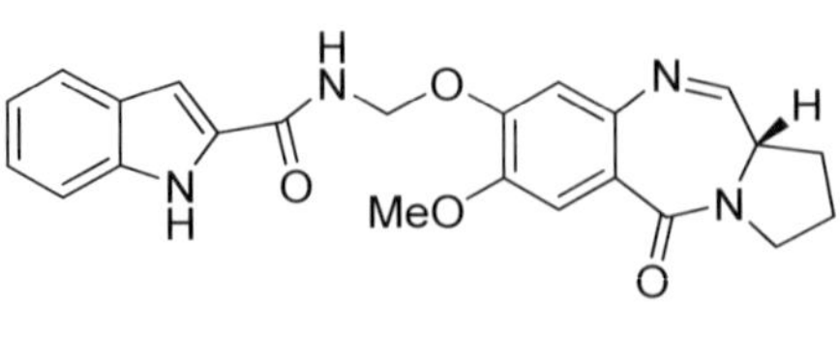

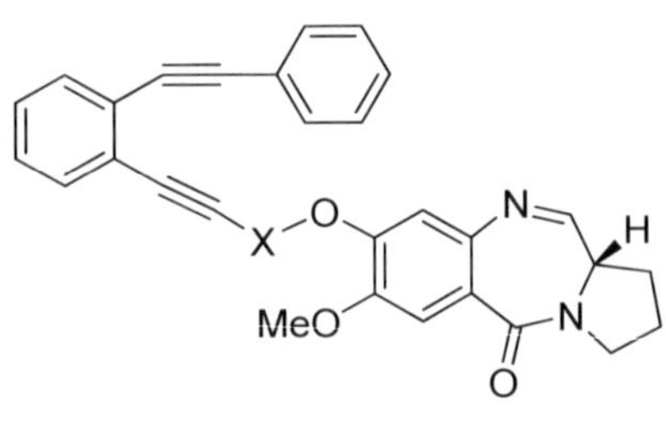

In the past few years, this research group prepared different type of conjugates, in which a known antitumor compound or some simple active moiety tethered to PBD have been designed, synthesized and evaluated for their biological activity (Figure 7).[61-73] A series of PBD conjugates by linking different DNA interacting ligands such as benzimidazoles, benzothiazoles, naphthalimides, aryl substituted naphalens, chalcones and poly-aromatic hydrocarbons (pyrene amine, chrysene amine and phenanthrinephenyl) by using varying linker length to enhance the DNA binding affinity and antitumour activity. PBD-morpholine, N-methyl piperizine and *N,N*-dimethyl amine hybrids have been prepared in an attempt to improve the water solubility and cytotoxicity of the PBD compounds.

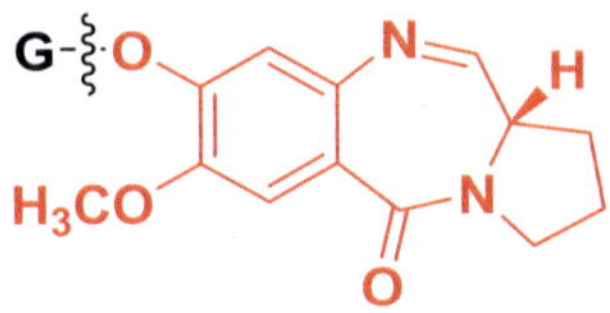

DC-81

$\Delta T_m = 0.3\text{-}0.7\ ^{\circ}C$

The DNA binding ability of these novel PBD conjugates is usually investigated by thermal denaturation studies using *calf thymus* (CT) duplex DNA at pH 7.0 employing the protocols reported in the previous studies.[67,74] All the PBD conjugates showed better melting temperature of CT-DNA compared to the naturally occurring DC-81. The DNA melting temperature studies indicate that these PBD conjugates exhibit significant DNA binding affinity. The PBD conjugates are effective as DNA binding agents particularly at G-rich sequences.[75] Additionally when the restriction enzyme digestion assay (RED assay) was carried out for some representative compounds along with the DC-81. This study clearly indicated that most of the conjugates effectively bind at G-rich region of the minor groove of DNA even at lower concentrations. These studies clearly indicate that the linking of the PBD scaffold with other conjugate partners not only enhances the binding potential significantly but also increases the base pair sequence selectivity. With regard to the PBD scaffold it is well established that it forms a covalent linkage at the N2 position of a guanine base of the DNA while the other subunit of this new conjugate is likely to interact within the DNA through the non-covalent interactions.[63,76] This aspect has been investigated in detail in case PBD–naphthalimide and benzimidazole conjugates examine their sequence selective binding ability.

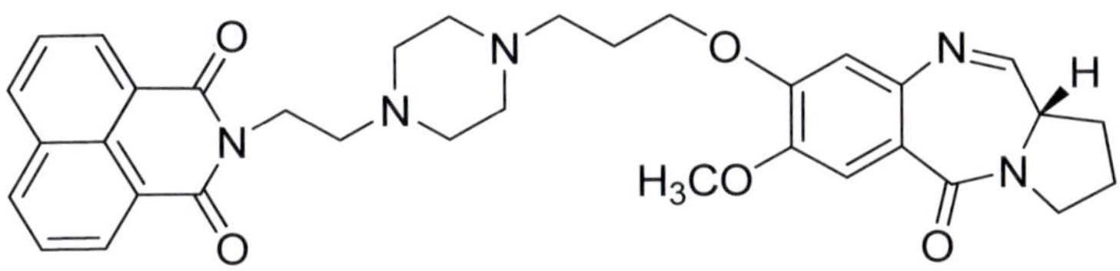

All the PBD–naphthalimide conjugates also showed promising anticancer activity with GI_{50} values of less than 0.1 to 0.5 μM against human cancer cell lines. One of the conjugate exhibited significant DNA binding affinity, that is the ΔT_m is 25.9 at 0 °C. The DNA binding of this conjugate to $d(AACAATTGTT)_2$ was studied by a combination of high-resolution ^{1}H and ^{31}P 2D NMR spectroscopy and restrained molecular dynamic calculations

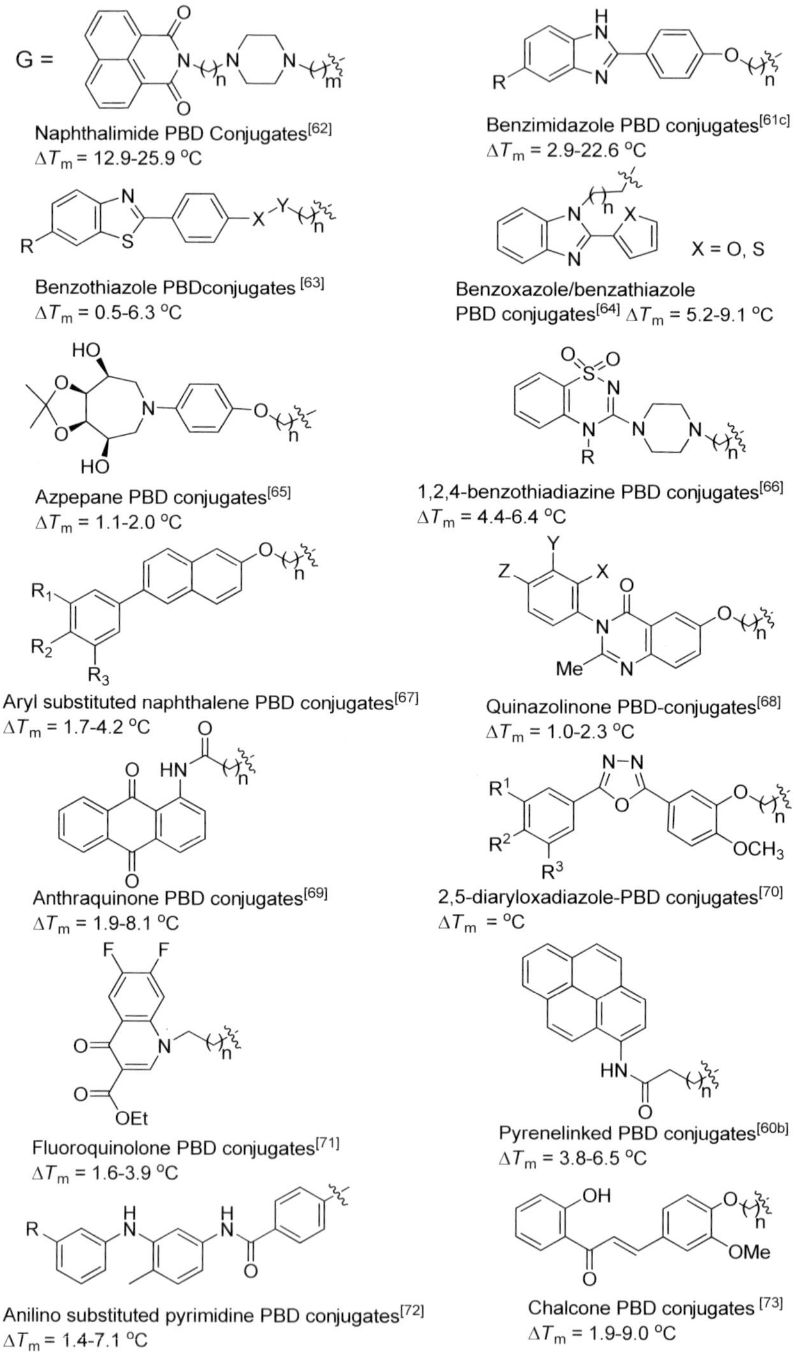

Fig. 7. Some representative PBD conjugates.

in explicit solvent. The bifunctional hybrid binds with its PBD moiety covalently linked within the minor groove to a guanine with an S stereochemistry at its covalent linkage site at C11 and a 5′-orientation of its A-ring carrying the linker with the naphthalimide ligand. The latter inserts from the minor groove between an A - A. T - T base pair step resulting in an opposite buckling of the base pairs at the intercalation site and duplex unwinding at adjacent internucleotide steps. There is NMR spectroscopic evidence that the naphthalimide undergoes a ring-flip motion with exchange rates slow to intermediate on the chemical shift time scale at ambient temperatures (Figure 8).[77]

PBD-benzimidazole conjugates also binds in the DNA minor groove with a preference for (A,T)4G sequences. Whereas the binding of both ligands is enthalpy-driven and associated with a negative entropy, the benzimidazole hybrid exhibits a less favourable binding enthalpy that is counterbalanced by a more favourable entropic term when compared to the naphthalimide hybrid.[78]

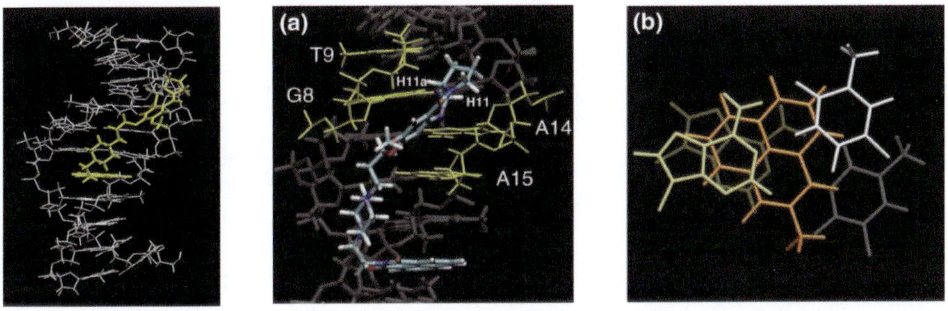

a b c

Fig. 8. a. Final energy-minimized structure of the PBD-naphthalimide-(AACAATTGTT)2 complex; view into the minor groove illustrating the position and orientation of the drug (in yellow) and the naphthalimide intercalation site. b. Close up viwe into the minor groove of the PBD-naphthalimide-(AACAATTGTT)2 complex residues G8 and T9 as well as A14 and A15 positioned on the H11a and H11 side of the covalently bound (11s, 11aS) PBD moiety are highlighted. c. Top view of the intercalation site with the naphthalimide, adenine and thymine bases colored in orange, yellow and white, repectively; base pair A5 T16 shown on top.

4. PBD dimers and trimers

A very original and interesting development for the PBD alkylating agents was obtained upon synthesis of bifunctional compounds. Suggs and co-workers have linked the two PBD moieties through the A-ring at C7/A-C7′ positions by alkanediyldioxy linker (**1**) and investigated the DNA binding properties. These molecules have been rationally designed as DNA cross-linkers and they bind reversibly to DNA and protect DNA against the action of certain restriction enzymes.[79,80] Lown and co-workers have designed and synthesized PBD dimers, joined tail to tail (C-ring) at C2 position through alkylamido linker unit (**2**). A series of these dimers have been evaluated for their cytotoxicity against 9 panels containing 60 human cell lines. It is observed that these compounds exhibited moderate to promising cytotoxic potency against different cancer cells,[81] some of the dimers are shown in Figure 9.

Thurston and co-workers have synthesized homologous series of C8 diether-linked PBD dimers (**3**, DSB-120) that span approximately six base pairs of DNA and in which sequence selectivity also increased (e.g., purine-GATC-pyrimidine).[82,83] DSB-120 exhibits potent *in vitro* cytotoxicity and enhances DNA binding affinity and sequence specificity as compared to the natural occuring DC-81. This improvement in biological activity has been attributed to the ability of these compounds to link to DNA irreversibly via guanine residues on opposite strands because of the presence of two active sites (i.e., two imine functionalities).[84] The *in vivo* studies of this compound were not encouraging, and the low therapeutic index observed was partly due to the reaction of this compound with cellular thiol-containing molecules before reacting at the tumor site.[85] Recently, another new cross-linking PBD dimer (**4**, SJG-136) having C2/C2′-exo unsaturation (that exhibits high DNA binding affinity) has been prepared by the same group.[86] This investigation has highlighted the effect of C2 unsaturation on the in vitro and in vivo cytotoxic activity. Interestingly, the comparison of this PBD dimer with its tetralactam analogue demonstrates that for maximum cytotoxicity an electrophilic imine or carbinolamine moiety is essential at the N10−C11 position of the PBD units.

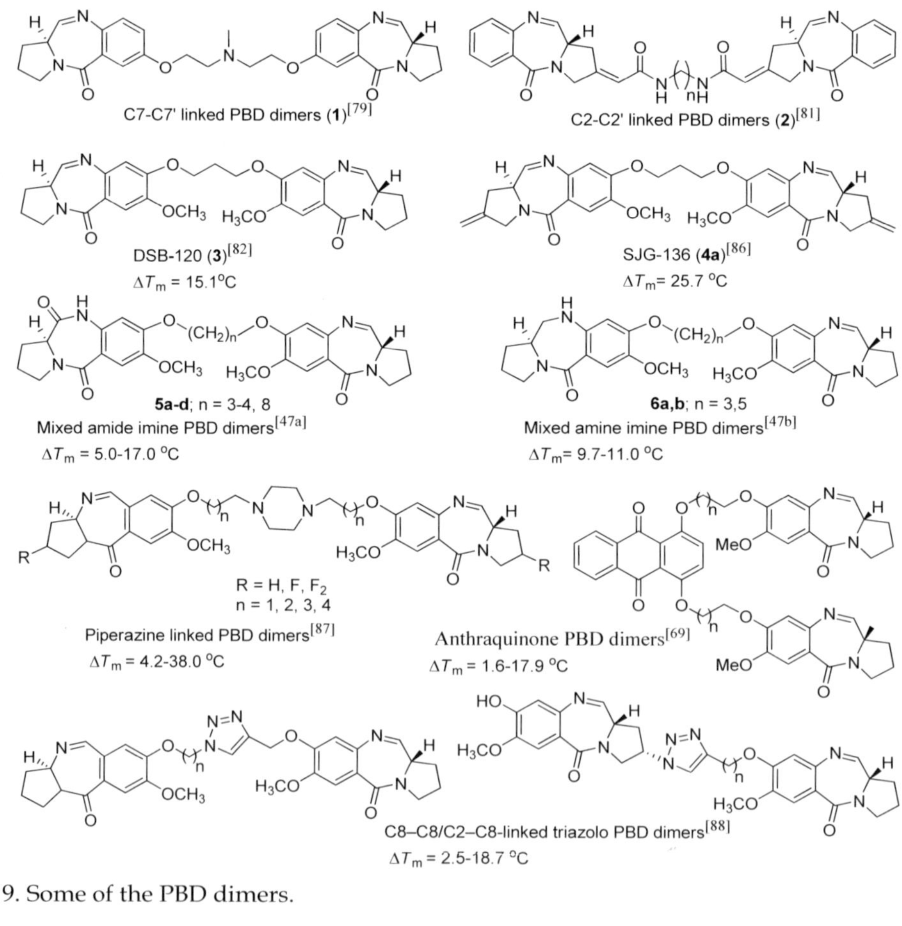

Fig. 9. Some of the PBD dimers.

SJG-136 (**4**) is a sequence-selective DNA-interactive agent that is about to enter phase II clinical trials for the treatment of malignant disease. Previous studies on the pyrrolo[2,1-c][1,4]benzodiazepine (PBD) dimers, typified by SJG-136 and DSB-120 (**3**), have shown that these planar ligands react with the exocyclic NH2 groups of two guanine bases in the base of the minor groove of DNA to form an irreversible interstrand cross-linked sequence-specific adduct. Using high-field NMR, we have characterized and modeled the previously predicted interstrand duplex adduct formed by SJG-136 with the self-complementary 5′-d(CICGATCICG)2 duplex (**4**). This SJG-136 NMR-refined adduct structure has been compared with previous high-field NMR studies of the adducts of the closely related PBD dimer DSB-120 with the same duplex and of the adduct of tomaymycin formed with 5′-d(ATGCAT)2. Surprisingly, the SJG-136 duplex adduct appears to be more closely related to the tomaymycin adduct than to that of DSB-120 adduct with respect to the orientation and depth of insertion of the ligand within the minor groove. The intrastrand duplex adduct formed in the reaction of SJG-136 with the noncomplementary 5′-d(CTCATCAC)·(GTGATGAG) duplex (**4**) has also been synthesized and modeled. In this duplex adduct, the nature of the cross-link was confirmed, the central guanines were identified as the sites of alkylation, and the stereochemical configuration at C11 at both ends of the SJG-136 molecule was determined to be S. The NMR-refined solution structures produced for the intrastrand adduct confirm the previously proposed structure (which was based solely on mass spectroscopy). Both the inter and intrastrand SJG-136 duplex adducts form with minimal distortion of the DNA duplex (Figure 10). These observations have an impact on the proposal for the mechanism of action of SJG-136 both in vitro and in vivo, on the repair of its adducts and mechanism of resistance in cells, and, potentially, on the type of pharmacodynamic assay to be used in clinical trials.[89-93]

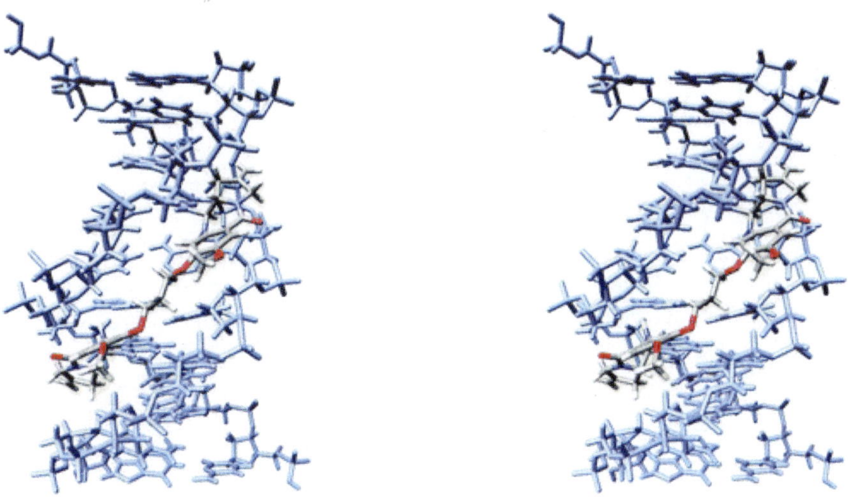

Fig. 10. Stereoview of the 5′-d(CICGATCICG)$_2$–SJG-136 intrastrand adduct. DNA strands are colored blue, and SJG-136(**4**) is shown in atom colors. Watson–Crick base pairing has been maintained, and there is minimal distortion to the β-helical structure of the DNA backbone. Models were produced in the SYBYL modeling suite and images produced using UCSF Chimera.[94]

4.1 Noncross-linking PBD dimers

This laboratory has been involved in the structural modifications of the PBD ring system and development of new synthetic strategies. It is been observed in the literature that no effort has been made to prepare and investigate PBD dimers with one imine functionality alone for exploring their cytotoxicity as noncross-linking agents (**5a-d** and **6a,b**). These type of PBD dimers were prepared to understand the contributions from the non-covalent interactions by one of the subunit in such dimers. It was observed that by incorporation of a non-covalent component surprising the DNA-binding affinity significantly enhances in such mixed type of PBD dimers.[47] One of these dimer with five alkane spacer (**5c**) elevates the helix melting temparature of CT-DNA remarkably to 17.0 °C after incubation for 18 h at 37 °C.

The binding affinity of the compounds was also measured by restriction endonuclease digestion assay based on inhibition of the restriction endonuclease *BamHI*. This study reveals the significance of noncovalent interactions in combination with covalent bonding aspects when two moieties of structural similarities are joined together. This allows the mixed imine-amide PBD dimer with a five carbon chain linker to achieve an isohelical fit within the DNA minor groove taking into account both the covalent bonding and the noncovalent binding components. This has been supported by binding studies (Figure 11), which indicate that the PBD dimer with a five carbon chain linker (**5c**) gives rise to maximum stabilization of the complex with DNA at the minor groove as compared to the other PBD dimers with three (**5a**), four (**5b**) and eight (**5d**) carbon chain linkers. The energy of interaction for all of the complexes studied was in correlation with the ΔT_m values. Mixed imine–amine pyrrolobenzodiazepine (PBD) dimers that are comprise of a DC-81 and secondary amine (N10) of DC-81 subunits tethered to their C8 positions through alkanedioxy linkers (comprised of three and five carbons) was also studied. These noncross-linking unsymmetrical PBD dimers exhibit significant DNA minor groove binding ability and one of them that was **6b** linked through the pentanedioxy chain exhibits efficient DNA binding ability (ΔT_m = 11.0 °C) in compared to naturally occurring DC-81, (ΔT_m = 0.7 °C).

4.2 PBD trimers

The unsymmetricalbis-1,2,3-triazolo-PBD trimers have been designed and synthesized by employing 'click' chemistry process. Interestingly, by using this 'click' chemistry protocol the solubility aspects have been improved that facilitated the purification and isolation of the target compounds. These new PBD trimers have shown significant DNA-binding ability. Molecular modelling studies substantiate the formation of three covalent bonds with the PBD trimer and guanine. One of the representative compound **3c** appears to be the optimal binder as further increase in linker or chain length decreases the binding strength of these compounds with DNA (Figure 12).[95]

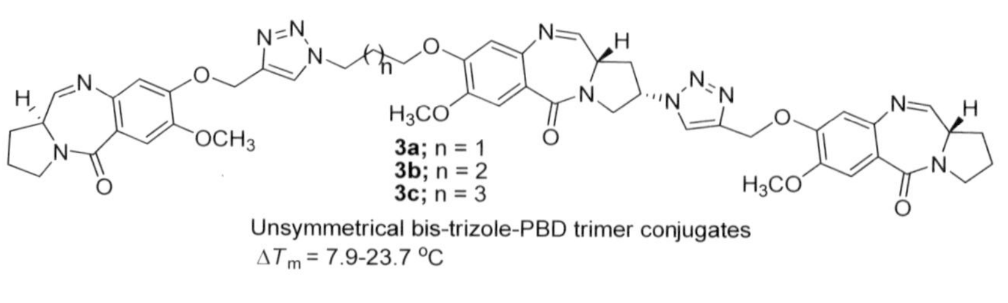

3a; n = 1
3b; n = 2
3c; n = 3

Unsymmetrical bis-trizole-PBD trimer conjugates
ΔT_m = 7.9-23.7 °C

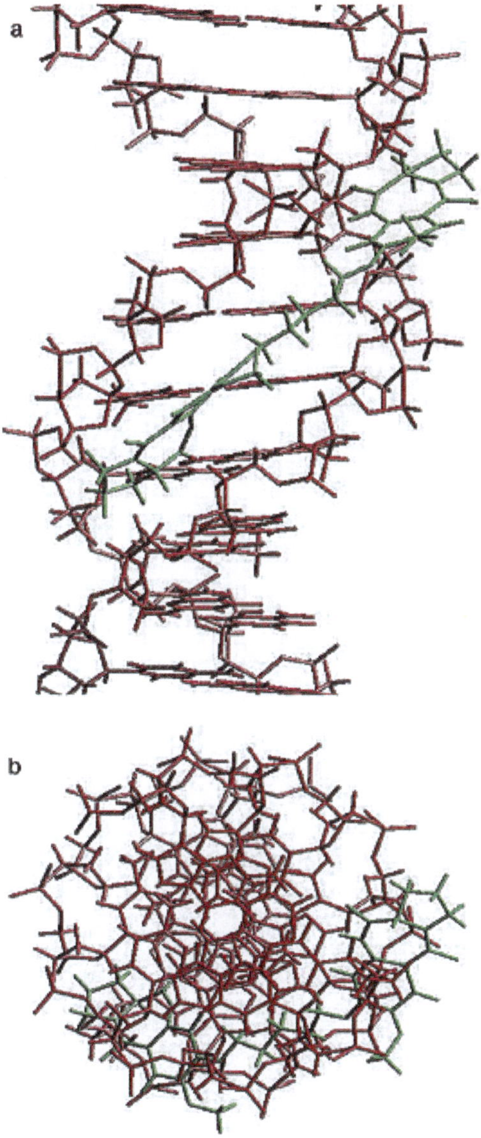

Mixed imine-amide (**5c**)

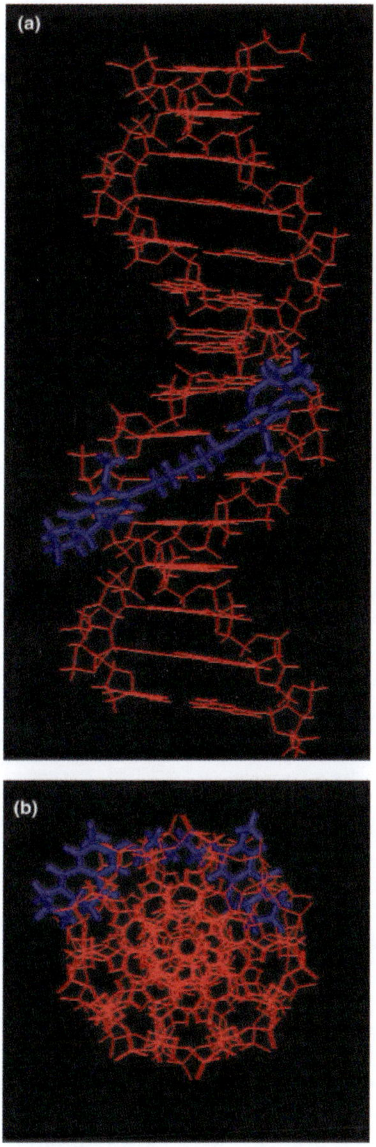

Mixed imine-amine (**6b**)

Fig. 11. Projection diagram showing the DNA-5c and 5b complexs. (a) Side on view and (b) down the helix axis.

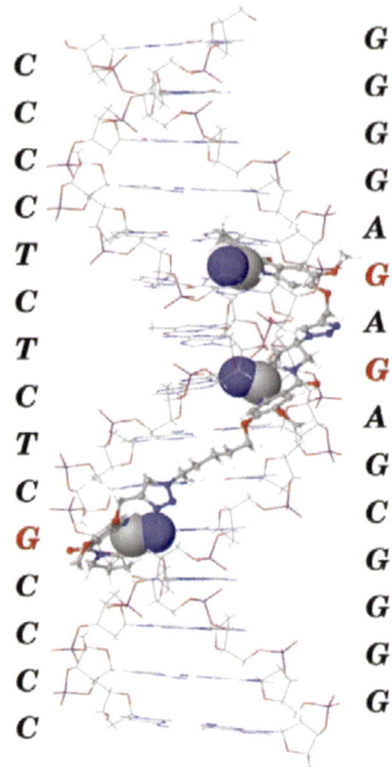

Fig. 12. Covalent bonding of PBD trimer **3c** with DNA (guanine residues involved in the bonding are written in red color, C-atom of PBD and N-atom of guanine are shown in CPK).

5. Concluding remarks

In conclusion, synthesis of imine containing pyrrolobenzodiazepines (PBDs) has often posed practical problems towards its isolation and preparation. Based on the biological importance of these pyrrolobenzodiazepines (PBDs) enhance the selectivity as well as anticancer activity. The design of hybrid ligands has provided a basis for modulating the sequence-selective binding behavior and/or tailoring the hybrid ligands for mixed-sequence recognition. This has also allowed to demonstrate that the design of such hybrids enhances anticancer activity as well as stability of drug-DNA complexes. Further some of these compounds exhibiting apoptosis inducing ability. Some of the new compounds, PBD-benzimidazole hybrids and piperazine-linked PBD dimers are undergoing preclinical studies. SJG-136 is currently undergoing Phase II evaluation in both the United States (through the NCI) and United Kingdom (through Cancer Research United Kingdom). The design of mixed dimers has allowed to illustrate the important role played by the non-covalent interactions in the enhancement of DNA-binding affinity. Interestingly, new PBD trimers have shown significant DNA-binding ability, binding and molecular docking studies substantiate the formation of three covalent bonds with the PBD trimer and guanine. Todate, a large number of PBD best molecules have been synthesized, highlighting that this area of research is extremely important for achieveing considerable importance in the recognition of DNA sequences.

However, this serch for new molecules with enhanced selectivity is in progress inorder to recognise about 15 bp for DNA sequences within the human genome.

6. Acknowledgements

The authors Kashi Reddy and Srikanth are thankful to CSIR, New Delhi, for the award of research fellowships.

7. References

[1] (a) Burke, B. M.; Wilkes, G. M.; Ingwersen, K. C. *Cancer chemotherapy. Published by Jones and Bartlett publishers*, 2001, 1; (b) Sarter, B.; Burke, B. M.; Wilkes, G. M.; Ingwersen, K. C. *Cancer chemotherapy care plans handbook, Published by Jones and Bartlett publishers*, 2001, 1.

[2] (a) Cech, T. R. *Annu. Rev. Biochem.* 1990, *59*, 543; (b) Michel, F.; Ferat, J. L. *Annu. Rev. Biochem.* 1995, *64*, 435; (c) Cech, T. R.; Gesteland, R. F.; Atkins, J. F. *Cold Spring Harbour New York*, 1993; 239.

[3] Wong, A. H. J.; Wigley, G. J.; Kolpak, F. J.; Crawfood, J. L.; Van Boom, G.; Marel. V.; Reich, A. *Nature* 1979, *282*, 680.

[4] (a) Hsiang, Y. H.; Jiang, T. B.; Lieu, L. F. *Mol. Pharmacol.* 1989, *36*, 371; (b) Pomnier, Y.; Kohn, K. W. F. L.; *CRC Pre. Inc*, 1989, 175; (c) Yamashita, Y.; Kawada, S. Z.; Nakano, H. *Biochemistry* 1991, *30*, 5838; (d) Liu, L. F. *Annu. Rev. Biochem.* 1989 *58*, 351; (e) Franklin, R. E.; Gosting, R. G. *Trans. Faraday Soc.* 1954, *50*, 298.

[5] Courtney, S. M.; Thurston, D. E. *Tetrahedron Lett.* 1993, *34*, 5327.

[6] Dwyer, P. J.; Shoemaker, D.; Zaharko, D. S.; Grieshaber, C.; Plowman, *Cancer Chemother. Pharmaco.* 1987, *19*, 6.

[7] Zimmur, C. Prog. *Nucleic Acid Res. Mol. Biol.* 1975, *15*, 285.

[8] Wartell, R. N.; Larson, J. E.; Wells, R. E. *J. Biol. Chem.* 1974, *249*, 6719.

[9] Karlovsky, P.; Decock, A. W. *Anal Biochem.* 1991, *194*, 192.

[10] (a) Kunimoto, S.; Masuda, T.; Kanbayashi, M.; Hamada, M.; Umazawa, H. *J. Antibiot.* 1980, *33*, 665; (b) Takeuchi, T.; Miyamoto, M.; Ishizuka, M.; Naganawa, H.; Kondo, S.; Hamada, M.; Umezawa, H. *J. Antibiot.* 1976, *29*, 93.

[11] Shimizu, K. I.; Kawamoto, I.; Tomita, F.; Morimoto, M.; Fuzimoto, K. *J. Antibiot.* 1982, *35*, 972.

[12] (a) Hara, M.; Tamaoki, T.; Yashida, M.; Morimoto, M.; Xlakano, *J. Antibiot.* 1988, *41*, 702; (b) Langley, D. R.; Thurston, D. E. *J. Org. Chem.* 1987, *52*, 91.

[13] (a) Itoh, J.; Watanabe, H. O.; Ishii, S.; Gomi, S.; Nagasawa, M. and Yamamoto, A. *J. Antibiot.* 1988, *41*, 1281; (b) Leber, J. D.; Hooner, J. R. C.; Holden, K. G.; Johnson, R. R.; Hed, S. M. *J. Am. Chem. Soc.* 1988, *110*, 299.

[14] Hurley, L. H.; Reck, T.; Thurston, D. E.; Langley, D. R.; Holder, K. G.; Hertzberg, R. P.; Hwover, J. R. E.; Gallegher, G.; Faucette, L. F. Jr.; Mong, S. M.; Johnson, R. K. *Chem. Res. Toxicol.* 1988, *1*, 258.

[15] Arima, K.; Kohsaka, M.; Tamura, G.; Imanaka, H.; Sakai, H. *J. Antibiot.* 1972, *25*, 437.

[16] Konishi, M.; Ohkuma, H.; Naruse, N.; Kawaguchi, H. *J. Antibiot.* 1984, *37*, 200.
[17] Tsunkawa, M.; Kamei, H.; Konishi, M.; Miyaki, T.; Oki, T.; Kawaguchi, H. *J. Antibiot.* 1988, *41*, 1366.
[18] (a) Kunimoto, M.; Masuda, T.; Kanbayashi, N.; Hamada, M.; Naganawa, H.; Miyamoto, M.; Takeuchi, T.; Unezawa, H. *J. Antibiot.* 1980, *33*, 665; (b) Thurston, D. E.; Murthy, V. S.; Langley, D. R.; Jones, G. B. *Synthesis* 1990, *1*, 81; (c) Bose, D. S.; Jones, G. B.; Thurston, D. E. *Tetrahedron*, 1992, *48*, 751.
[19] (a) Thurston, D. E. *The Macmillan Press Ltd. London, U. K.* 1993; 54; (b) Petrusek, R. L.; Uhlenhopp, E. L.; Duteau, N.; Hurley, L. H. *J. Biol. Chem.* 1982, *257*, 6207.
[20] Boyd, F. L.; Stewart, D.; Remers, W. A.; Barkley, M. D.; Hurley, L. H. *Biochemistry* 1990, *29*, 2387.
[21] Puvvada, M. S.; Hartley, J. A.; Jenkins, T. C.; Thurston, D. E. *Nucleic Acids Res.* 1993, *21*, 3671.
[22] Puvvada, M. S.; Forrow, S. A.; Hartley, J. A.; Stephenson, P.; Gibson, I.; Jenkins, T. C.; Thurston, D. E. *Biochemistry* 1997, *36*, 2478.
[23] Kopka, M. L.; Goodsell, D. S.; Baikalov, I.; Grzeskowiak, K.; Cascio, D.; Dickerson, R. E. *Biochemistry* 1994, *33*, 13593.
[24] (a) Kunitmoto, S.; Masuda, T.; Kanbayashi, N.; Hamada, M.; Nayanawa, H.; Miyamoto, M.; Takeuchi, T.; Unezawa, H. *J. Antibiot.* 1980, *33*, 665; (b) Kohn, K. W.; Speous, C. L. *J. Mol. Biol.* 1970, *5*, 551; (c) Kohn, K. W.; Gloubiger, D.; Zmijewski, M. *Biochem. Biophys. Acta.* 1974, *361*, 228; (d) Hurley, L. H.; Gairpla, C.; Smijewski, M. *Biochem. Biophys. Acta.* 1977, *475*, 521; (e) Kaplan, D. J.; Hurley, L. H. *Biochemistry* 1981, *20*, 7572; (f) Petrusek, R. L. *J. Biol. Chem.* 1981, *257*, 6207; (g) Tendler, M. D.; Korman, S. *Nature* 1963, *199*, 501.
[25] Leimgruber, W.; Batcho, A. D.; Czajkowski, R. C. *J. Am. Chem. Soc.* 1968, *90*, 5641.
[26] (a) Thurston, D. E.; Bose, D. S. *Chem. Rev.* 1994, *94*, 433; (b) Kamal, A.; Rao, M. V.; Reddy, B. S. N. *Chemistry of Heterocyclic Compounds* 1998, 1588; (c) Kamal, A.; Rao, M. V.; Laxman, N.; Ramesh, G.; Reddy, G. S. K. *Current Medicinal Chemistry–Anti-Cancer Agents* 2002, *2*, 215.
[27] (a) Kaneko, T.; Wong, H.; Doyle, T. W. *Tetrahedron Lett.* 1983, *24*, 5165; (b) Suggs, J. W.; Wang, Y. S.; Lee, K. S. *Tetrahedron Lett.* 1985, *26*, 4871.
[28] Lown, J. W.; Joshua, A. V. *Biochem. Pharmacol.* 1979, *28*, 2017.
[29] (a) Langlois, N.; Favre, F.; Rojas, A. *Tetrahedron Lett.* 1993, *34*, 4635; (b) Kaneko, T.; Wong, H.; Doyle, T. W.; Rose, W. C.; Bradner, W. T. *J. Med. Chem.* 1985, *28*, 388.
[30] (a) Langley, D. R.; Thurston, D. E. *J. Org. Chem.* 1987, *52*, 91; (b) Courtney, S. M.; Thurston, D. E. *Tetrahedron Lett.* 1993, *34*, 5327; (c) Bose, D. S.; Jones, G. B.; Thurston, D. E. *Tetrahedron* 1992, *48*, 751.
[31] Wilson, S. C.; Howard, P. W.; Forrow, S. M.; Hartley, J. A.; Adams, L. J.; Jekins, T. C.; Kelland, L. R.; Thurston, D. E. *J. Med. Chem.* 1999, *42*, 4028.
[32] (a) Kamal, A.; Rao, N. V. *Chem. Commun.* 1996, 385; (b) Kamal, A.; Howard, P. W.; Reddy, B. S. N.; Reddy, B. S. P.; Thurston, D. E. *Tetrahedron* 1997, *53*, 3223; (c) Kraus, G. A.; Melekhov, A. *Tetrahedron* 1998, *54*, 11749.
[33] Kamal, A.; Laxman, E.; Laxman, N.; Rao, N. V. *Bioorg. Med. Chem. Lett.* 2000, *10*, 2311.

[34] (a) Berry, J. M.; Howard, P. W.; Thurston, D. E. *Tetrahedron Lett.* 2000, *41*, 6171; (b) Kamal, A.; Reddy, G. S. K.; Raghavan, S. *Bioorg. Med. Chem. Lett.* 2001, *41*, 387.
[35] Fukuyama, T.; Liu, G.; Linton, S. D.; Lin, S. C.; Nishino, H. *Tetrahedron Lett.* 1993, *34*, 2577.
[36] Miyamoto, M.; Kondo, S.; Naganawa, H.; Maeda, K.; Ohno, M.; Umezawa, H. *J. Antibiot.* 1973, *30*, 340.
[37] Thurston, D. E.; Langley, D. R. *J. Org. Chem.* 1986, *51*, 705.
[38] (a) Kamal, A.; Laxman, E.; Arifuddin, M. *Tetrahedron Lett.* 2000, *41*, 7743; (b) Kamal, A.; Laxman, E.; Reddy, P. S. M. M. *Tedrahedron Lett.* 2000, *41*, 8631.
[39] (a) Kamal, A.; Reddy, G. S. K.; Reddy, K. L. *Tedrahedron Lett.* 2001, *42*, 6969; (b) Kamal, A.; Reddy, G. S. K.; Reddy, K. L.; Raghavan, S. *Tetrahedron Lett.* 2002, *43*, 2103.
[40] (a) Kamal, A.; Laxman, E.; Arifuddin, M. *Tetrahedron Lett.* 2000, *41*, 7743; (b) Kamal, A.; Laxman, E.; Reddy, P. S. M. M. *Tedrahedron Lett.* 2000, *41*, 8631.
[41] Baraldi, P. G.; Leoni, A.; Cacciari, B.; Manfreini, S.; Simoni, D.; Bergomi, M.; Menta, E.; Spinelli, S. *J. Med. Chem.* 1994, *37*, 4329.
[42] Bose, D. S.; Thompson, A. S.; Smellie, M.; Berardini, M. D.; Hartley, J. A.; Jenkins, T. C.; Neidle, S.; Thurston, D. E. *Chem. Commun.* 1992, 1518.
[43] Foloppe, M. P.; Rault, S.; Thurston, D. E.; Jenkins, T. C.; Robba, M. *Eur. J. Med. Chem.* 1996, *31*, 407.
[44] (a) Gregson, S. J.; Howard, P. W.; Corcoran, K. E.; Barcella, S.; Yasin, M. M.; Hurst, A. A.; Jenkins, T. C.; Kelland, L. R.; Thurston, D. E. *Bioorg. Med. Chem. Lett.* 1999, *10*, 1845; (b) Gregson, S. J.; Howard, P. W.; Barcella, S.; Nakamya, A.; Jenkins, T. C.; Kelland, L. R.; Thurston, D. E. *Bioorg. Med. Chem. Lett.* 1999, *10*, 1849.
[45] (a) Cooper, N.; Hagan, D. R.; Tiberghien, A.; Ademefun, T.; Matthews, C. S.; Howard, P. W.; Thurston, D. E. *Chem. Commun.* 2002, 1764; (b) Kang, G. D.; Howard, P. W.; Thurston, D. E. *Chem. Commun.* 2003, 1688; (c) Chen, Z.; Gregson, S. J.; Howard, P. W.; Thurston, D. E. *Bioorg. Med. Chem. Lett.* 2004, *14*, 1547.
[46] O'Neil, I. A.; Thompson, S.; Kalindjian, S. B.; Jenkins, T. C. *Tetrahedron. Lett.* 2003, *44*, 7809.
[47] (a) Kamal, A.; Ramesh, G.; Laxman, N.; Ramulu, P.; Srinivas, O.; Neelima, K.; Kondapi, A. K.; Srinu, V. B.; Nagarajaram, H. A. *J. Med. Chem.* 2002, *45*, 4679; (b) Kamal, A.; Ramesh, G.; Srinivas, O.; Ramulu, P.; Laxman, N.; Rehana. T.; Deepak, M.; Achary, M. S.; Nagarajaram, H. A. *Bioorg. Med. Chem.* 2004, *12*, 5427.
[48] Antonow, D.; Kaliszczak, M.; Kang, G. D.; Coffils, M.; Tiberghien, A. C.; Cooper, N.; Barata, T.; Heidelberger, S.; James, C. H.; Zloh, M.; Jenkins, T. C.; Reszka, A. P.; Neidle, S.; Guichard, S. M.; Jodrell, D. I.; Hartley, J. A.; Howard, P. W.; Thurston, D. E. *J. Med. Chem.* 2010, 53, 2927.
[49] Thurston, D. E.; Morris, S. J.; Hartley, J. A. *Chem. Commun.* 1996, 563.
[50] Wilson, S. C.; Howard, P. W.; Forrow, S. M.; Hartley, J. A.; Adams, L. J.; Jenkins, T. C.; Kelland, L. R.; Thurston, D. E. *J. Med. Chem.* 1999, *42*, 4028.
[51] Reddy, B. S. P.; Damayanthi, Y.; Reddy, B. S. N.; Lown, W. J. *Anti-Cancer Drug Des.* 2000, *15*, 225.

[52] Baraldi, P. G.; Balboni, G.; Cacciari, B.; Guiotto, A.; Manfredini, S.; Romagnoli, R.; Spalluto, G.; Thurston, D. E.; Howard, P. W.; Bianchi, N.; Rutigiiano, C.; Mischiati, C.; Gambari, R. *J. Med. Chem.* 1999, *42*, 5131.

[53] Thurston, D. E.; Morris, S. J.; Hartley, J. A. *Chem. Commun.* 1996, 563.

[54] Confalone, P. N.; Huie, E. M.; Ko, S. S.; Cole, G. M. *J. Org. Chem.* 1988, *53*, 482.

[55] Wilson, S. C.; Howard, P. W.; Thurston, D. E. *Tetrahedron. Lett.* 1995, *36*, 6333.

[56] Baraldi, P. G.; Balboni, G.; Cacciari, B.; Guiotto, A.; Manfredini, S.; Romagnoli, R.; Spalluto, G.; Thurston, D. E.; Howard, P. W.; Bianchi, N.; Rutigiiano, C.; Mischiati, C.; Gambari, R. *J. Med.Chem.* 1999, *42*, 5131.

[57] Reddy, B. S. P.; Damayanthi; Y.; Reddy, B. S. N.; Lown, J. W. *Anti-Cancer Drug Design* 2000, *15*, 225.

[58] Zou, Q.; Duan, W.; Simmons, D.; Shyo, Y.; Raymond, M. A.; Dorr, R. T.; Hurley, L. H. *J. Am. Chem. Soc.* 2001, *123*, 4865.

[59] Tercel, M.; Stribbling, S. M.; Shephard, H.; Siim, B. G.; Wu, K.; Pullen, S. M.; Bottin, K. J.; Wilson, W. R.; Denny, W. A. *J. Med. Chem.* 2003, *46*, 2132.

[60] (a) Wang, J. J.; Shen, Y. K.; Hu, W. P.; Hsieh, M. C.; Lin, F. L.; Hsu, M. K.; Hsu, M. H. *J. Med. Chem.* 2006, *49*, 1442; (b) Hu, W. P.; Liang, J. J.; Kao, C. L.; Chen, Y. C.; Chen, C. Y.; Tsai, F. Y.; Wu, M. J.; Chang, L. S.; Chen, Y. L.; Wang, J. *J. Bioorg. Med. Chem.* 2009, *17*, 1172.

[61] (a) Kamal, A.; Ramesh, G.; Ramulu, P.; Srinivas, O.; Rehana, T.; Sheelu, G. *Bioorg. Med. Chem. Lett.* 2003, *13*, 3451; (b) Kamal, A.; Ramesh, G.; Srinivas, O.; Ramulu, P. *Bioorg. Med. Chem. Lett.* 2004, *14*, 471; (c). Kamal, A.; Ramulu, P.; Srinivas, O.; Ramesh, G.; Kumar, P. P. *Bioorg. Med. Chem. Lett.* 2004, *14*, 4791.

[62] Kamal, A.; Ramu, R.; Tekumalla, V.; Khanna, G. B. R.; Barkume, M. S.; Juvekar, A. S.; Zingde, S. M.; *Bioorg. Med. Chem.* 2008, *16*, 7218.

[63] Kamal, A.; Reddy, K. S.; Khan, M. N. A.; Shetti, R. V. C. R. N. C.; Ramaiah, M. J.; Pushpavalli, S.N.C.V.L.; Srinivas, C.; Bhadra, M. P.; Chourasia, M.; Sastry, G. N.; Juvekar, A.; Zingde, S.; Barkume M. *Bioorg. Med. Chem.* 2010, *18*, 4747.

[64] Kamal, A.; Kumar P. P.; Sreekanth, K.; Seshadri, B.N.; Ramulu P.; *Bioorg. Med. Chem. Lett.* 2008, *18*, 2594.

[65] Kamal, A.; Reddy, D. R.; Reddy, P. S. M. M.; Rajendar. *Bioorg. Med. Chem. Lett.* 2006, *16*, 1160.

[66] Kamal, A.; Khan, M. N. A.; Reddy, K. S.; Ahmed, S. K.; Kumar, M. S.; Juvekar, A.; Sen, S.; Zingde S.; *Bioorg. Med. Chem. Lett.* 2007, *17*, 5345.

[67] Kamal, A.; Reddy, M. K.; Ramaiah, M. J.; Srikanth, Y. V. V.; Rajender.; Reddy, V. S.; Kumar, G. B.; Pushpavalli, S. N. C. V. L.; Bag, I.; Juvekar A.; Sen, S.; Zingde, S. M.; Bhadra M. P. ChemMedChem. 2011, *6*, 1665.

[68] Kamal, A.; Bharathi, E. V.; Ramaiah, M. J.; Dastagiri, D.; Reddy, J. S.; Viswanath, A.; Sultana, F.; Pushpavalli, S. N. C. V. L.; Bhadra M. P.; Srivastava, H. K.; Sastry, G. N.; Juvekar, A.; Sen, S.; Zingde, S. *Bioorg. Med. Chem.* 2010, *18*, 526.

[69] Kamal, A.; Ramu, R.; Tekumalla, V.; Khanna, G. B. R.; Barkume, M. S.; Juvekar, A. S.; Zingde, S. M. *Bioorg. Med. Chem.* 2007, *15*, 6868.

[70] Kamal, A.; Dastagiri, D.; M. Ramaiah, M. J.; Bharathi, E. V.; Reddy, J. S.; Balakishan, G.; Sarma, P.; Pushpavalli, S. N. C. V. L.; Bhadra M. P.; Juvekar, A.; Sen, S.; Zingde, S. *Bioorg. Med. Chem.* 2010, *18*, 6666.
[71] Kamal, A.; Devaiah, V.; Reddy, K. L.; Kumar, M. S. *Bioorg. Med. Chem.* 2005, *13*, 2021.
[72] Kamal, A.; Reddy, J. S.; Ramaiah, M. J.; E. Bharathi, E. V.; Dastagiri, D.; Reddy, M. K.; Pushpavalli, S. N. C. V. L.; Bhadra M. P. *Bioorg. Med. Chem. Lett.* 2010, 20, 5232.
[73] Kamal, A.; Shankaraiah, N.; Prabhakar, S.; Reddy, C. R.; Markandeya, N.; Reddy, K. L.; Devaiah, V. *Bioorg. Med. Chem. Lett.* 2008, *18*, 2434.
[74] Kamal, A.; Sreekanth, K.; Kumar, P. P.; Shankaraiah, N.; Balakishan, G.; Ramaiah, M. J.; Pushpavalli, S. N. C. V. L.; Ray, P.; Bhadra, M. P. *Eur. J. Med. Chem.* 2010, *45*, 2173.
[75] Puvvada, M. S.; Hartley, J. A.; Jenkins, T. C.; Thurston, D. E. *Nucleic Acids Res,* 1993, *21*, 3671.
[76] Rahman, K. M.; Vassoler, H.; James, C. H.; Thurston, D. E. *ACS Med. Chem. Lett.* 2010, *1*, 427.
[77] Rettig, M.; Langel, W.; Kamal, A.; Weisz, K. *Org. Biomol. Chem.,* 2010, *8, 3179.*
[78] Rettig, M.; Kamal, A.; Ramu, R.; Mikolajczak, J.; Weisz, K. *Bioorg. Med. Chem.* 2009, 17, 919.
[79] Farmer, J. D.; Rudnicki, S. M.; Suggs, J. W. *Tetrahedron Lett.* 1988, *29*, 5105.
[80] Farmer, J. D.; Gustafson, G. R.; Conti, A.; Zimmt, M.B.; Suggs, J. W. *Nucleic Acids Res.* 1991, *19*, 899.
[81] Reddy, B. S. P.; Damayanthi, Y.; Reddy, B. S. N.; Lown, J. W. *Anti-Cancer Drug Des.* 2000, *15*, 225.
[82] Smellie, M.; Kelland, L. R.; Thurston, D. E.; Souhami, R. L.; Hartley, J. A. *Br. J. Cancer* 1994, *70*, 48.
[83] Thurston, D. E.; Bose, D. S.; Thompson, A. S.; Howard, P. W.; Leoni, A.; Croker, S. J.; Jenkins, T. C.; Neidle, S.; Hartley, J. A.; Hurley, L. H. *J. Org. Chem.* 1996, *61*, 8141.
[84] Hartley, J. A.; Berardini, M. D.; Souhami, R. L. *Anal. Biochem.* 1991, *193*, 131.
[85] Walton, M. I.; Goddard, P.; Kelland, L. R.; Thurston, D. E.; Harrap, K. R. *Cancer Chemother. Pharmacol.* 1996, *38*, 431.
[86] Gregson, S. J.; Howard, P. W.; Hartley, J. A.; Brooks, N. A.; Adams, L. J.; Jenkins, T. C.; Kelland, L. R.; Thurston, D. E. *J. Med. Chem.* 2001, *44*, 737.
[87] Kamal, A.; Rajender, Reddy, R. R.; Reddy, M. K.; Balakishan, G.; Shaik, T. B.; Chourasia, M.; Sastry, G. N. *Bioorg. Med. Chem.* 2009, *17*, 1557.
[88] Kamal, A.; Prabhakar, S.; Shankaraiah, N.; Reddy, C. R.; Reddy, P. V. *Tetrahedron Lett.* 2008, *49*, 3620.
[89] Suzanne, R.; Thompson, S. *Biochemistry* 2011, 50, 4720.
[90] Stephen, J.; Philip W. G.; John A. H.; Natalie, H. A.; Lesley, B. J.; Terence, C. A.; Lloyd, R. J.; Thurston. D. E. *J. Med. Chem.* 2001, *44*, 737.
[91] Stephen, J.; Philip W. G.; Darren, H. R.; Hamaguchi, K.; Corcoran, K. E.; Brooks, N. A.; Hartley, J. A.; Jenkins, T. C.; Guille, S. P. M. J.; Thurston, D. E.; *J. Med. Chem.* 2004, *47,* 1161.
[92] Martin, C.; Ellis, T.; Mc Gurk, Claire J.; Jenkins, T. C.; Hartley, J. A.; Waring, M. J.; Thurston, D. E. *Biochemistry,* 2005, *44*, 4137.

[93] Smellie, M.; Bose, D. S.; Thompson, A. S.; Jenkins, T. C.; Hartley, J. A.; Thurston, D. E. *Biochemistry* 2003, *42,* 8232.

[94] Alley, M. C.; Hollingshead, M. G.; Cox, P. C. M.; Waud, W. R.; Hartley, J. A.; Howard, P. W.; Gregson, S. J.; Thurston, D. E.; Sausville, E. A. *Cancer Res*. 2004, 64, 6700.

[95] Kamal, A.; Shankaraiah, N.; Reddy, C. R.; Prabhakar, S.; Markandeya, N.; Srivastava, H. K.; Sastry, G. N. *Tetrahedron*. 2010, *66*. 5498.

7

Regulation of EC-SOD in Hypoxic Adipocytes

Tetsuro Kamiya[1,2], Hirokazu Hara[1], Naoki Inagaki[2] and Tetsuo Adachi[1]
[1]*Gifu Pharmaceutical University,*
[2]*Gifu University*
Japan

1. Introduction

Obesity is closely linked to a variety of metabolic disorders, including insulin resistance, atherosclerosis and type 2 diabetes (Eriksson, 2007). Recent studies have indicated that adipose tissue is not only an energy store but also produces and secretes various bioactive molecules called adipocytokines, such as adiponectin, tumor necrosis factor-α (TNF-α), plasminogen activator inhibitor type 1 (PAI-1) and monocyte chemoattractant protein-1 (MCP-1) (Hotamisligil & Spiegelman, 1994; Shimomura et al., 1996; Berg et al., 2002; Havel, 2004). TNF-α is a major inflammatory adipocytokine that decreases the phosphorylation of insulin receptor substrate-1 (IRS-1), and this event leads to insulin resistance (Hotamisligil et al., 1993). Moreover, because it is well recognized that TNF-α increases the adhesion molecules such as vascular cell adhesion molecule-1 (VCAM-1), intercellular adhesion molecule-1 (ICAM-1) and MCP-1, all of which are key mediators involved in atherogenesis, over secretion of TNF-α may induce and accelerate atherosclerosis. On the other hand, adiponectin is a major anti-inflammatory adipocytokine that plays a pivotal role in the improvement of glucose and lipid metabolism and the prevention of atherosclerosis and inflammation (Yamauchi et al., 2002). Further, it has been clarified that adiponectin not only increases insulin sensitivity, but also has anti-atherosclerosis properties which decrease the expression of VCAM-1 and ICAM-1 (Ouchi et al., 1999) and suppresses the proliferation of vascular smooth muscle cells (Arita et al., 2002). In patients with insulin resistance, obesity or type 2 diabetes, serum adiponectin levels are reduced (Arita et al., 1999; Hotta et al., 2000). Further, previous studies showed that TNF-α and intracellular reactive oxygen species (ROS) decrease adiponectin expression (Kim et al., 2005; Soares et al., 2005; Simons et al., 2007). On the other hand, increases in adiponectin expression have been reported during adipocyte differentiation and transcriptional factors associated with adipogenesis, including CCAAT/enhancer-binding protein-α (C/EBP-α) and peroxisome proliferator-activated receptor-γ (PPAR-γ), have been shown to up-regulate adiponectin expression (Adachi et al., 2009).

Adipose tissue has been found to suffer chronic hypoxia during the development of obesity (Brook et al., 1972; Helmlinger et al., 1997), and these conditions may lead to metabolic disorders. Hypoxic conditions can be induced by the addition of certain chemicals called 'hypoxia mimetics', such as the carcinogenic transition metal cobalt (Vincent et al., 1996). It has been suggested that cobalt stabilizes transcriptional factor, hypoxia-inducible factor-1α (HIF-1α), from proteasomal degradation by inhibiting the activity of prolyl hydroxylases (PHDs) through Fe^{2+} substitution (Schofield & Ratcliffe, 2004). In these hypoxic conditions, it has been recognized that accumulated HIF-1α increases a wide variety of genes including vascular endothelial growth factor (VEGF), heme oxygenase-1 (HO-1), erythropoietin (EPO) and cytochrome p450 (CYP) 3A6 to ensure adaptation to low-oxygen tension (Levy et al., 1995; Lee et al., 1997). On the other hand, the expression of CYP1A2, 2B and 2C are decreased by the activation of HIF-1α (Olsvik et al., 2006; Fradette et al., 2007). Further, it has been reported that both hypoxia and hypoxia mimetics increase ROS generation and dysregulate adipocytokines, and these conditions lead to and/or promote metabolic disorders (Schuster et al., 1989; Hosogai et al., 2007).

To protect cells from oxidative stress, mammalian have anti-oxidative enzymes such as superoxide dismutase (SOD), catalase and glutathione peroxidase (Amstad & Cerutti, 1990; Cerutti et al., 1994). SOD is a major antioxidant enzyme that protects cells from the damaging effects of superoxide by accelerating the dismutation reaction of superoxide by approximately 10,000 times (Faraci, 2003). As shown in Table 1, there are three SOD isozymes in mammals; copper and zinc-containing SOD (Cu,Zn-SOD), manganese-containing SOD (Mn-SOD) and extracellular-SOD (EC-SOD) (McCord & Fridovich, 1969; Keele et al., 1970; Marklund, 1982; Faraci, 2003). Among of three SOD isozymes, EC-SOD is secretory, tetrameric glycoprotein, whereas Cu,Zn-SOD and Mn-SOD are intracellular enzymes found predominantly in the cytoplasm and mitochondria, respectively. EC-SOD is a major SOD isozyme in the extracellular space but is distributed mainly in blood vessel walls (Ookawara et al., 1998). After secretion, EC-SOD slowly diffuses and binds to the heparan sulfate proteoglycans in the glycocalyx on the surface of most cell types in the vascular wall. The EC-SOD content is very low in the liver, heart, brain and other organs, with the exception of the lung, thyroid gland, and adipose tissue (Marklund, 1984). It was found that the plasma EC-SOD levels in type 2 diabetic patients were significantly and inversely related to the body mass index, homeostasis model assessment-insulin resistance index, but positively related to adiponectin levels (Adachi et al., 2004). Recently, we reported that cobalt chloride ($CoCl_2$) decreases EC-SOD in green monkey kidney COS7 cells via intracellular ROS generation and p38-MAPK, a mitogen-activated protein kinase

	EC-SOD	Cu,Zn-SOD	Mn-SOD
Molecular mass	135,000	32,000	85,000
Subunit	a4	a2	a4
Metal (atom/subunit)	1Cu, 1Zn	1Cu, 1Zn	1Mn
Rate constant ($M^{-1}s^{-1}$)	1.25×10^9	2×10^9	1.25×10^9
Location	extracell	cytoplasm	mitochondria
Carbohydrate	+	—	—
Affinity for heparin	+	—	—

Table 1. The properties of SOD isozymes

(MAPK), signaling cascade (Kamiya et al., 2008); however, the mechanisms of EC-SOD and adiponectin reductions during hypoxia remain unclear. Because the EC-SOD content in adipose tissue is comparably high, it is important to elucidate the regulation of EC-SOD may contribute to the control of cytotoxicity induced by intracellular ROS during hypoxia.

In order to address these issues, we studied the regulation of EC-SOD expression by $CoCl_2$ and examined the role of ROS, inflammatory cytokine such as TNF-α and MAPK signaling cascades in these processes. Moreover, we also studied the regulation of adiponectin expression by $CoCl_2$, because we hypothesized that the expression of EC-SOD might be co-regulated with adiponectin in 3T3-L1 cells treated with $CoCl_2$, leading to aggravate metabolic disorders.

2. Methods

2.1 3T3-L1 cell culture

3T3-L1 mouse pre-adipocytes culture and their differentiation into adipocytes were carried out as described in previous report (Adachi et al., 2009). Briefly, pre-adipocytes were maintained in Dulbecco's modified Eagle's medium (DMEM) supplemented with 10% foetal calf serum (FCS) until 2 days after confluence; then, their differentiation into adipocytes was induced by treating cells for 2 days with 5 μg/mL insulin, 0.5 μM dexamethasone and 0.5 mM isobutylmethyl-xanthine in DMEM, and then for 2 days with insulin (5 μg/mL) in the same medium. The cells were returned to the basal medium, which was replaced every other day. The effects of $CoCl_2$ and hypoxia on gene expression were investigated using 8-day differentiated adipocytes. The induction of hypoxia (1% O_2) was carried out in a culture chamber which controls O_2 concentrations by supplying N_2 gas together with 5% CO_2. After the cells were treated with $CoCl_2$ or incubated with hypoxia (1% O_2) for 24 h, RT-PCR and measurement of intracellular ROS generation were carried out.

2.2 Oil red O staining

Differentiation of 3T3-L1 mouse pre-adipocytes into mature adipocytes was confirmed by Oil red O staining as described previously (Sakaue et al., 2002). Briefly, the cells were washed twice with ice-cold PBS, and then the cells were fixed with 10% paraformaldehyde for 10 min at room temperature. After fixation, the cells were washed twice with ice-cold PBS and incubated with 60% isopropanol for 1 min followed by incubation with 1.8 mg/mL Oil red O solution for 20 min at room temperature. After the cells were washed twice with ice-cold PBS, Oil red O staining was monitored by microscope.

2.3 Measurement of cellular protein

We measured the cellular protein as an index of cell injury. After 3T3-L1 adipocytes were treated, the medium was aspirated and the cells were washed twice with ice-cold PBS and then scraped in 1 mL PBS. The cell suspension was homogenized using an ultrasonic homogenizer. The total protein in the supernatant was assayed using a Bio-Rad protein assay reagent (Bio-Rad Lab., CA, USA).

2.4 Reverse transcriptional polymerase chain reaction (RT-PCR)

After 3T3-L1 adipocytes were treated, the medium was aspirated and the cells were washed twice with ice-cold PBS. The cells were lysed in 1 mL TRIzol® reagent (Invitrogen, CA, USA). cDNA was prepared and RT-PCR performed using the methods described in our previous report (Adachi et al., 2009), with minor modifications. Densitometric analysis of the PCR products was performed with Multi Gauge V3.0 (Fuji Film, Japan).

2.5 Measurement of intracellular ROS

After the adipocytes were treated, the medium was aspirated and the cells were washed twice with PBS and incubated with fresh culture medium without serum containing 3 μM 5-(and-6)-carboxy-2',7'-dichlorodihydrofluorescein diacetate (carboxy-H_2DCFDA) for 20 min at 37°C in 5% CO_2/95% air. The cells were then washed twice with ice-cold PBS and then scraped in 1 mL PBS and centrifuged at 2,300 × g for 5 min at 4°C. The pellet was homogenized with 1 mL PBS using ultrasonic homogenizer and centrifuged at 2,300 × g for 10 min at 4°C. The DCF fluorescence of the supernatant was measured using a fluorometer (excitation at 493 nm and emission at 527 nm). Total protein concentrations were measured using a protein assay reagent.

2.6 Western blotting

Whole cell extracts were prepared in lysis buffer as described previously (Kamiya et al., 2008). Extracts containing 20 μg protein were separated by SDS-PAGE on 12% (w/v) polyacrylamide gels followed by transferring electrophoretically onto PVDF membranes. Subsequently, the membranes were incubated with the respective specific primary antibodies (C/EBP homologous protein (CHOP) and Actin). The blots were incubated with biotin-conjugated goat anti-rabbit IgG (for CHOP) or -mouse IgG (for Actin) antibody followed by incubating with ABC reagents (Vector Laboratories, Inc., Burlingame, CA, USA). Finally, the bands were detected using SuperSignal® West Pico (Thermo Scientific, Rockford, IL, USA), and imaged using an LAS-3000 UV mini (Fuji Film).

2.7 Statistical analysis

The data shown are the mean ± SD of three separate experiments. Statistical significance was estimated using ANOVA followed by *post hoc* Bonferroni tests. A *P*-value less than 0.05 was considered significant.

3. Results

3.1 Differentiation of 3T3-L1 mouse pre-adipocytes into mature adipocytes

We first investigated the differentiation of 3T3-L1 pre-adipocytes into mature adipocytes using Oil red O staining. As shown in Fig. 1A, the staining was not observed in 0 day, but observed in 8 days differentiated cells. Further, we measured the expression of adiponectin as an index of differentiation by RT-PCR. The expression of adiponectin was not observed in 0 day, but drastically increased in the 8 day differentiated-adipocytes (Fig. 1B). From these observations, we considered that the cells were differentiated into mature adipocytes, and we therefore investigated the effect of $CoCl_2$ on the expression of EC-SOD, other SOD isozymes, adiponectin and transcriptional factors.

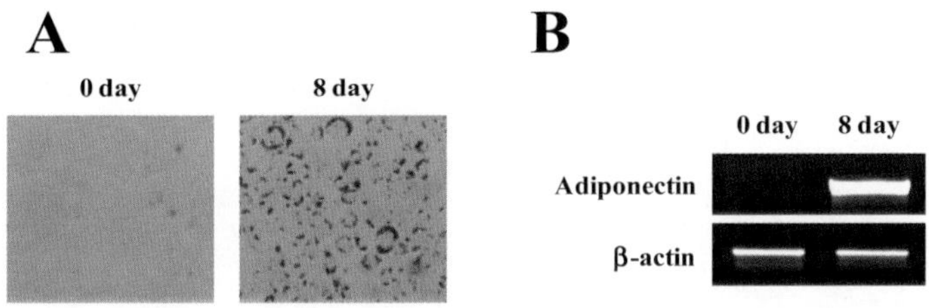

Fig. 1. Differentiation of 3T3-L1 mouse pre-adipocytes into mature adipocytes. 3T3-L1 pre-adipocytes were differentiated by the method described above. After 8 day differentiation, the differentiation degree was evaluated by Oil red O staining (A) and RT-PCR analysis (B).

3.2 Effect of $CoCl_2$ and hypoxia on the protein content

In order to elucidate the cytotoxicity of $CoCl_2$ and hypoxia (1% O_2), we measured the protein content of 3T3-L1 adipocytes treated with 0.3 mM $CoCl_2$ or incubated under hypoxia for the several hours. As shown in Fig. 2, the protein content was not affected by $CoCl_2$ and so from this we determined the concentrations of $CoCl_2$ (0 to 0.3 mM) to use in this study. Moreover, the protein content was not affected under hypoxic condition.

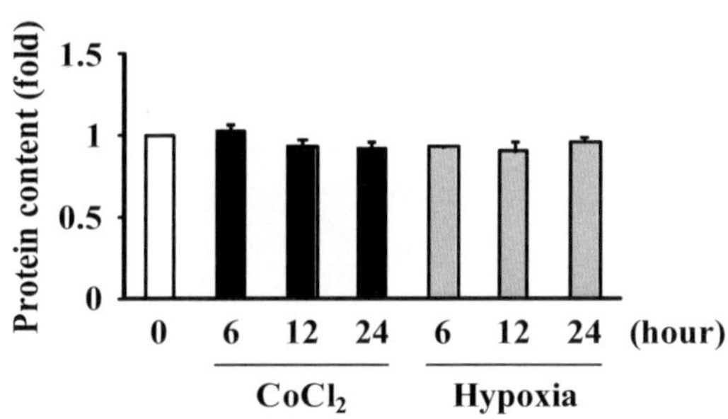

Fig. 2. Effect of $CoCl_2$ and hypoxia on the protein content. 3T3-L1 adipocytes were treated with 0.3 mM $CoCl_2$ (closed column) or incubated under hypoxia (1% O_2: gray column) for the indicated hours. After the cells were treated, protein contents were measured by using a Bio-Rad protein assay reagent.

3.3 Effect of $CoCl_2$ on the expression of SODs, adiponectin and transcriptional factors

We next investigated the effect of $CoCl_2$ on the expression of SODs, adiponectin and transcriptional factors such as C/EBP-α and PPAR-γ by RT-PCR. As shown in Fig. 3, 4, treatment with $CoCl_2$ decreased the expression of EC-SOD mRNA in a $CoCl_2$ dose- (Fig. 3) and time-dependent manner (Fig. 4). On the other hand, the other SOD isozymes (Cu,Zn-SOD and Mn-SOD) were not affected when the applied concentration of $CoCl_2$ was 0.3 mM for 24 h. It has been reported that adiponectin is suppressed in mRNA and protein levels during hypoxia; however, the expression of adiponectin during hypoxia induced by $CoCl_2$ was not fully elucidated. Treatment with $CoCl_2$ markedly suppressed the expression of adiponectin in a $CoCl_2$ dose- and time-dependent manner. Additionally, the expression of C/EBP-α and PPAR-γ, well recognized as master regulators of adipogenesis and adiponectin, was similar to that of EC-SOD and adiponectin.

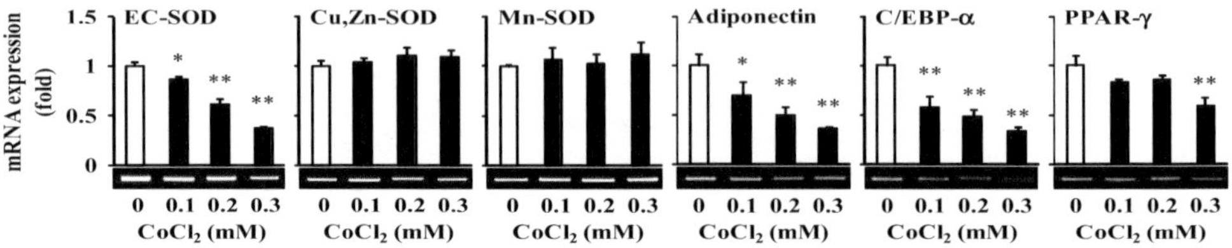

Fig. 3. Dose-dependent effect of $CoCl_2$ on the expression of SODs, adiponectin and transcriptional factors. 3T3-L1 adipocytes were treated with the indicated concentrations of $CoCl_2$ for 24 h. After the cells were treated, RT-PCR was carried out and these data were normalized using β-actin levels. (* $p<0.05$, ** $p<0.01$ vs. vehicle).

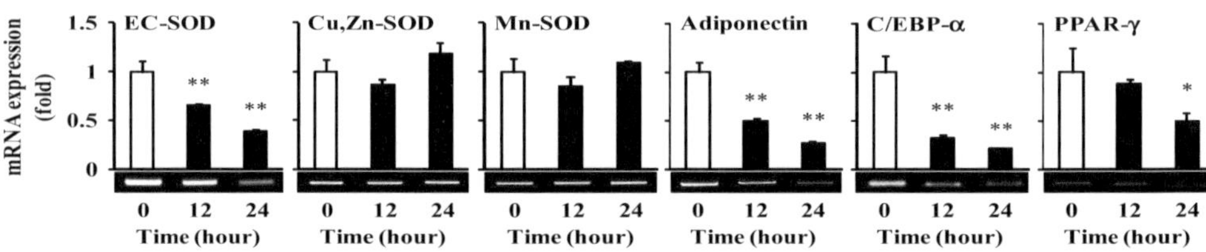

Fig. 4. Time-dependent effect of $CoCl_2$ on the expression of SODs, adiponectin and transcriptional factors. 3T3-L1 adipocytes were treated with 0.3 mM $CoCl_2$ for the indicated hours. After the cells were treated, RT-PCR was carried out and these data were normalized using β-actin levels. (* $p<0.05$, ** $p<0.01$ vs. untreated cells).

3.4 Effect of hypoxia on the expression of SODs, adiponectin and transcriptional factors

We further investigated the effect of hypoxia (1% O_2) on the expression of SODs, adiponectin and transcriptional factors. Hypoxia decreased the expression of EC-SOD, adiponectin and C/EBP-α similar to $CoCl_2$ treatment (Fig. 5); however, Cu,Zn-SOD, Mn-SOD and PPAR-γ were not changed during hypoxia.

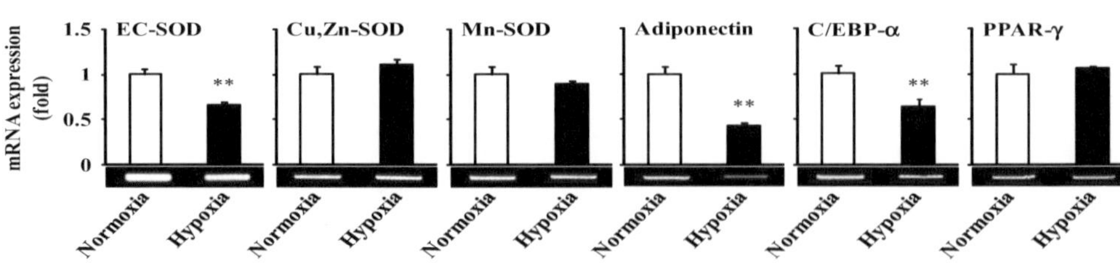

Fig. 5. Effect of hypoxia on the expression of SODs, adiponectin and transcriptional factors. 3T3-L1 adipocytes were incubated under normoxia (20% O_2: open column) or hypoxia (1% O_2: closed column) for 24 h. After the cells were treated, RT-PCR was carried out and these data were normalized using β-actin levels. (** $p<0.01$ vs. normoxia).

3.5 Involvement of ROS in $CoCl_2$-induced reduction of EC-SOD and adiponectin

We previously reported that intracellular ROS are generated under hypoxic conditions induced by $CoCl_2$ and lead to decrease the expression of EC-SOD in COS7 cells (Kamiya et al., 2008). Moreover, it has been reported that the expression of adiponectin is also decreased by the accumulation of intracellular ROS in 3T3-L1 adipocytes (Soares et al., 2005). As described in the previous reports, it was speculated that the reduction of EC-SOD and adiponectin was regulated by intracellular ROS-derived signaling. We therefore investigated the involvement of intracellular ROS in these reductions in this study. Treatment with H_2O_2 decreased the expression of EC-SOD and adiponectin, and pretreatment with antioxidant, trolox, partially, but significantly suppressed these reductions (Fig. 6A). We further investigated that generation of intracellular ROS during $CoCl_2$-treatment using carboxy-H_2DCFDA. As shown in Fig. 6B and C, treatment with $CoCl_2$ significantly increased intracellular ROS generation in a time-dependent manner and pretreatment with trolox attenuated $CoCl_2$-triggered ROS generation. However, surprisingly, pretreatment with trolox did not attenuate the reduction of EC-SOD and adiponectin (Fig. 6D), suggesting that the expression of EC-SOD and adiponectin were not regulated by intracellular ROS-derived signaling.

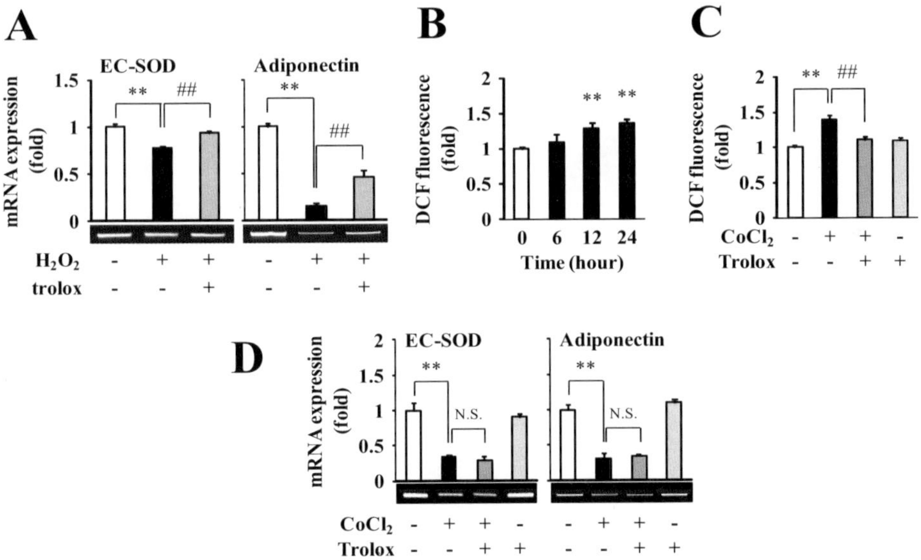

Fig. 6. Involvement of ROS in $CoCl_2$-induced reduction of EC-SOD and adiponectin. (A) 3T3-L1 adipocytes were pretreated without (–) or with (+) 0.2 mM trolox for 2 h, and then the cells were treated without (–) or with (+) 0.5 mM H_2O_2 for 24 h. (B) The cells were treated with 0.3 mM $CoCl_2$ for the indicated hours. (C, D) The cells were pretreated without (–) or with (+) 0.2 mM trolox for 2 h, and then the cells were treated without (–) or with (+) 0.3 mM $CoCl_2$ for 24 h. After the cells were treated, RT-PCR (A, D) and assay of intracellular ROS generation (B, C) were carried out. All RT-PCR data were normalized using β-actin levels. (** $p<0.01$ vs. vehicle (A, C and D) or untreated cells (B), ## $p<0.01$, N.S.: not significant vs. H_2O_2-treated cells (A) or $CoCl_2$-treated cells (C, D)).

3.6 Involvement of TNF-α in $CoCl_2$-induced reduction of EC-SOD and adiponectin

It is well recognized that the inflammatory adipocytokines including TNF-α are increased during adipocytes hypertrophy and hypoxic conditions (Ye et al., 2007). Moreover, we previously reported that exposure to TNF-α decreased EC-SOD in several kinds of cells (Adachi et al., 2006, 2009) and adiponectin in 3T3-L1 adipocytes (Adachi et al., 2009). Accordingly, we next investigated the involvement of TNF-α in the reduction of EC-SOD and adiponectin by $CoCl_2$. Treatment with $CoCl_2$ increased the expression of TNF-α at the mRNA (Fig. 7A), and pretreatment with actinomycin D, an inhibitor of mRNA synthesis, blocked the $CoCl_2$-triggered reduction of EC-SOD and adiponectin (Fig. 7B). Further, pretreatment with infliximab, a chimeric monoclonal antibody against TNF-α, partially, but significantly, suppressed the $CoCl_2$-triggered reduction of these genes (Fig. 7C), indicating that TNF-α plays an important role in the $CoCl_2$-induced suppression of EC-SOD and adiponectin.

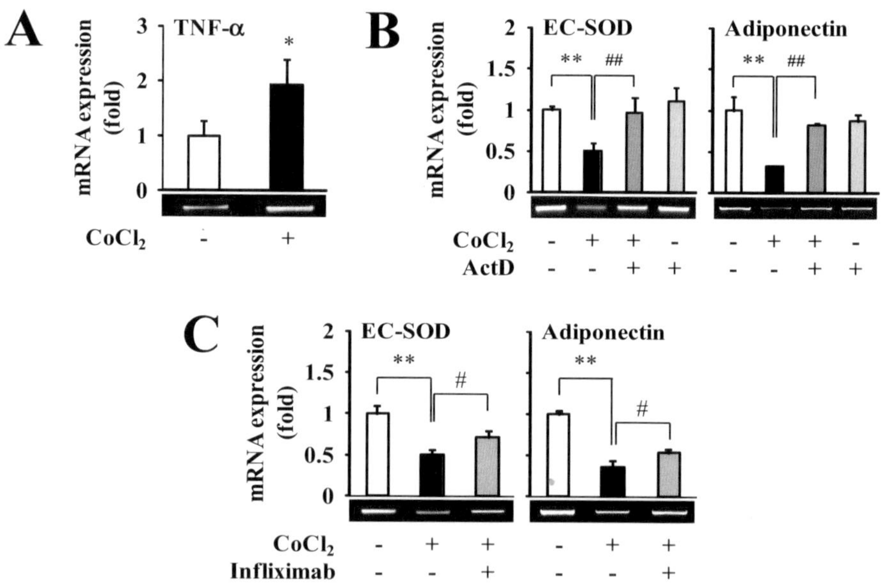

Fig. 7. Involvement of TNF-α in $CoCl_2$-induced reduction of EC-SOD and adiponectin. (A) 3T3-L1 adipocytes were treated without (–) or with (+) 0.3 mM $CoCl_2$ for 24 h. (B, C) The cells were pretreated without (–) or with (+) 1 μg/mL actinomycin D (ActD) for 1 h (B) or 10 μg/mL infliximab for 1 h (C), and then the cells were treated without (–) or with (+) 0.3 mM $CoCl_2$ for 24 h. After the cells were treated, RT-PCR was carried out. All RT-PCR data were normalized using β-actin levels. (* $p<0.05$, ** $p<0.01$ vs. vehicle, # $p<0.05$, ## $p<0.01$ vs. $CoCl_2$-treated cells).

3.7 Involvement of MAPK in $CoCl_2$-induced reduction of EC-SOD and adiponectin

In mammalian, there are three types of MAPK, such as c-jun N-terminal kinase (JNK), p38-MAPK and extracellular regulated kinase (ERK) (Kyriakis & Avruch, 2001, Pearson et al., 2001), and play several physiological roles including cell proliferation, differentiation and death. Additionally, we and others reported that activation of MAPK plays important roles in the TNF-α-induced reduction of EC-SOD in vascular smooth muscle cells (VSMCs) and adiponectin in 3T3-L1 adipocytes (Adachi et al., 2006, Kim et al., 2005). We, therefore, investigated the effect of MAPK inhibitors, such as SP600125 (for JNK), SB203580 (for p38-MAPK) and U0126 (for ERK) on the reduction of EC-SOD and adiponectin. Pretreatment with SP600125, SB203580 or U0126 did not affect the basal expression of EC-SOD and adiponectin (data not shown), and SP600125 significantly suppressed the $CoCl_2$-triggered reduction of EC-SOD and adiponectin, but others had no effects (Fig. 8), indicating that the expression of EC-SOD and adiponectin are regulated by JNK signaling cascades.

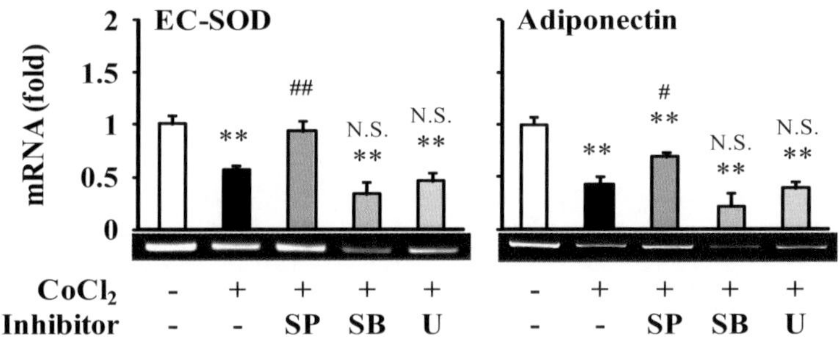

Fig. 8. Involvement of MAPK in $CoCl_2$-induced reduction of EC-SOD and adiponectin. 3T3-L1 adipocytes were pretreated without (–) or with 50 μM SP600125 (SP), SB203580 (SB) or U0126 (U) for 30 min, and then the cells were treated without (–) or with (+) 0.3 mM $CoCl_2$ for 24 h. After the cells were treated, RT-PCR was carried out. All RT-PCR data were normalized using β-actin levels. (** $p<0.01$ vs. vehicle, # $p<0.05$, ## $p<0.01$, N.S.: not significant vs. $CoCl_2$-treated cells).

3.8 $CoCl_2$ did not induce ER stress in 3T3-L1 adipocytes

It is well recognized that hypoxia is associated with endoplasmic reticulum (ER) stress, which induces metabolic disorders (Ozcan et al., 2004). Because the inhibitory effect of infliximab and actinomycin D on the reduction of EC-SOD and adiponectin by $CoCl_2$ was partial, it was speculated that the involvement of other mechanisms, such as ER stress. Therefore, we finally investigated the involvement of ER stress in the reduction of EC-SOD and adiponectin. Treatment with ER stress inducer, thapsigargin, significantly increased the expression of ER stress markers, glucose regulated-protein 78 kDa (GRP78) and CHOP; however, treatment with $CoCl_2$ did not affect the expression of these genes (Fig. 9A, B), suggesting that $CoCl_2$ decreased the expression of EC-SOD and adiponectin through ER stress-independent mechanisms.

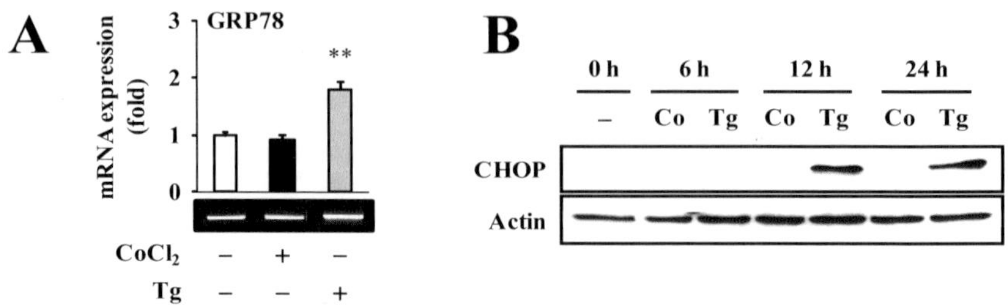

Fig. 9. Effect of $CoCl_2$ and thapsigargin on the expression of GRP78 and CHOP. (A) 3T3-L1 adipocytes were treated with 0.3 mM $CoCl_2$ or 1 μM thapsigargin (Tg) for 24 h. (B) The cells were treated with 0.3 mM $CoCl_2$ (Co) or 1 μM Tg for the indicated hours. After treatment, RT-PCR (A) and western blotting (B) were carried out. RT-PCR data were normalized using β-actin levels. (** $p<0.01$ vs. vehicle).

4. Discussion

It is well known that obesity, especially visceral fat accumulation, is closely related to a variety of metabolic disorders, including insulin resistance, atherosclerosis and type 2 diabetes (Fox et al., 2007). Further, it has been shown that inflammatory adipocytokines, such as TNF-α, interleukin (IL)-1 and IL-6, are increased, while anti-inflammatory adipocytokines, such as adiponectin, are decreased during adipocyte hypertrophy (Ye et al., 2007), all of which might lead metabolic disorder exacerbation. Additionally, it has been reported that adipose tissue suffers chronic hypoxia during above process (Brook et al., 1972; Helmlinger et al., 1997), and lead to disturb adipose homeostasis by excessive production of ROS and TNF-α, or decrease of adiponectin. In this study, chemical hypoxia mimetic, $CoCl_2$, decreased the expression of adiponectin and adipogenic master regulators, including C/EBP-α and PPAR-γ, in a $CoCl_2$ dose- and time-dependent manner (Fig. 3, 4), and these observations were similar to hypoxia (1% O_2 incubation), except for PPAR-γ (Fig. 5). From these observations and previous reports, we speculated that hypoxia mimetic decreases adiponectin via C/EBP-α and/or PPAR-γ signaling cascades, similar to hypoxia.

On the other hand, it has been well known that both hypoxia and hypoxia mimetics increase intracellular ROS generation through mitochondria-dependent and –independent mechanisms, respectively (Agani et al., 2000, Chandel et al., 1998). Similar to previous reports, we confirmed the intracellular ROS accumulation during $CoCl_2$ treatment (Fig. 6B), suggesting that hypoxic adipocytes suffered from oxidative stress. To protect cells from the damaging effect of ROS, mammalian have several kinds of anti-oxidative enzymes, such as SOD, catalase and glutathione peroxidase. EC-SOD is the major SOD isozyme in extracellular fluids and protects cells from superoxide. We previously reported that the expression level of EC-SOD through the differentiation of 3T3-L1 adipocytes changes in a similar manner to adiponectin, C/EBP-α and PPAR-γ, and down-regulation of these proteins might induce and/or promote the pathogenesis of metabolic syndrome and atherosclerosis. In fact, it was found that the plasma EC-SOD levels in type 2 diabetic patients were significantly and positively related to adiponectin levels (Adachi et al., 2004). Because, the EC-SOD content of adipose tissue was relative highly expressed compared to other organs, such as liver, heart and brain, it might be important to elucidate the regulation mechanism of that gene during hypoxia for the control of metabolic disorders. Recently, we reported that $CoCl_2$ decreases the expression of EC-SOD in COS7 cells via intracellular ROS generation. In this study, treatment with $CoCl_2$ (Fig. 3, 4), hypoxia (Fig. 5) and H_2O_2 (Fig. 6A) significantly decreased the expression of EC-SOD and adiponectin, but not of Cu,Zn-SOD and Mn-SOD. However, interestingly, an antioxidant, trolox, did not affect the reduction of EC-SOD and adiponectin by $CoCl_2$ in spite of suppressing the effect of H_2O_2 on these genes (Fig. 6A). From these observations, it is speculated that $CoCl_2$ decreases EC-SOD and adiponectin by intracellular ROS-independent, but another mechanisms.

So far, it has been reported that the expression of EC-SOD was regulated by several kinds of cytokines, such as TNF-α, transforming growth factor-β (TGF-β), IL-4 and interferon-γ (IFN-γ) (Marklund, 1992, Strålin & Marklund, 2000). Among of them, it has been well recognized that TNF-α is one of the most important adipocytokines involved in metabolic disorders, including insulin resistance, atherosclerosis and type 2 diabetes by decreasing the phosphorylation of IRS-1 and inducing adhesion molecules, such as VCAM-1, ICAM-1 and MCP-1. Moreover, we and others showed that TNF-α decreases EC-SOD and adiponectin in VSMCs and 3T3-L1 cells, respectively (Adachi et al., 2006, Kim et al., 2005). Accordingly, we investigated the involvement of TNF-α in the reduction of EC-SOD and adiponectin by the addition of $CoCl_2$. Treatment with $CoCl_2$ significantly increased TNF-α expression (Fig. 7A), and infliximab partially, but significantly, attenuated the reduction of EC-SOD and adiponectin by $CoCl_2$ (Fig. 7C). Additionally, an inhibitor of mRNA synthesis, actinomycin D, blocked the reduction of these expressions (Fig. 7B). These results suggested that $CoCl_2$ decreases EC-SOD and adiponectin via TNF-α; however, because the inhibition rate of EC-SOD and adiponectin reductions by infliximab is partial, we speculated that the mechanisms of these reductions by $CoCl_2$ involve other factors. Recently, it has been well known that hypoxia induces ER stress, which induces the apoptotic process (Kuznetsov et al., 1996). To assess the induction of ER stress by $CoCl_2$, we measured the expression of ER stress marker, GRP78 and CHOP. Treatment with ER stress inducer, such as thapsigargin, drastically increased the expression of GRP78 and CHOP at mRNA and protein levels, but treatment with $CoCl_2$ did not induce the ER stress (Fig. 9), suggesting that $CoCl_2$ decreased the expression of EC-SOD and adiponectin through ER stress-independent mechanisms.

We finally investigated the role of MAPK in the reduction of EC-SOD and adiponectin. There are three major subfamilies: JNK, p38-MAPK and ERK. Moreover, we previously reported that the expression of EC-SOD was regulated by p38-MAPK signaling cascades in $CoCl_2$-treated COS7 cells (Kamiya et al., 2008). However, in this study, pretreatment with a JNK inhibitor, SP600125, suppressed the reduction of EC-SOD and adiponectin but others, SB203580 and U0126, did not affect these reductions, indicating that $CoCl_2$ decreases EC-SOD and adiponectin through JNK signaling cascades. In our previous report, we showed the involvement of ROS and p38-MAPK in the regulation of EC-SOD in COS7 cells (Kamiya et al., 2008); however, in this study, we did not observe the involvement of intracellular ROS and p38-MAPK in the reduction of EC-SOD by $CoCl_2$. From these observations, we speculated that the difference of signal molecules leads the activation of different MAPK involved in the regulation of EC-SOD. It has been shown that the expression of mouse EC-SOD is regulated by transcriptional factors such as Sp1, Sp3, Ets, Kruppel-like and myeloid zinc finger-1 those bind to the corresponding cis-element in the promoter region (Zelko et al., 2003, 2004, 2008). According to previous reports, we hypothesized that the regulation of EC-SOD might be also mediated by these transcriptional factors.

5. Conclusion

The EC-SOD content is very low compared to other SODs in parenchymal cells. However, because it is known that adipose tissue has a moderately high content of EC-SOD, EC-SOD might have an important protective role as an anti-inflammatory factor. In this study, we demonstrated that the expression of EC-SOD was co-regulated with adiponectin through TNF-α and JNK signaling cascades. From these observations, it is speculated that the reduction of EC-SOD by hypoxic conditions is similar to adiponectin and leads to a decrease in the resistance to oxidative stress. Overall, it is speculated that the reduction of EC-SOD leads to decreased resistance to oxidative stress and accelerates ROS-derived diseases, and prevents the reduction of EC-SOD, contributing to the control of redox homeostasis under hypoxic conditions.

6. Acknowledgement

This study was supported, in part, by Grant-in-aid for Scientific Research from the Japan Society for the Promotion for Science (to TK and TA).

7. References

Adachi, T.; Inoue, M.; Hara, H.; Maehata, E. & Suzuki, S. (2004). Relationship of plasma extracellular-superoxide dismutase level with insulin resistance in type 2 diabetic patients. *J Endocrinol*, Vol. 181, No. 3, pp. 413-417, ISSN 0022-0795.

Adachi, T.; Toishi, T.; Takashima, E. & Hara, H. (2006). Infliximab neutralizes the suppressive effect of TNF-α on expression of extracellular-superoxide dismuatase *in vitro*. *Biol Pharm Bull*, Vol. 29, No. 10, pp. 2095-2098, ISSN 0918-6158.

Adachi, T.; Toishi, T.; Wu, H.; Kamiya, T. & Hara, H. (2009). Expression of extracellular superoxide dismutase during adipose differentiationin 3T3-L1 cells. *Redox Rep*, Vol. 14, No. 1, pp. 34-40, ISSN 1351-0002.

Agani, FH.; Pichiule, P.; Chavez, JC. & LaManna, JC. (2000). The role of mitochondria in the regulation of hypoxia-inducible factor 1 expression during hypoxia. *J Biol Chem*, Vol. 275, No. 46, pp. 35863-35867, ISSN 0021-9258.

Amstad, P. & Cerutti, P. (1990). Genetic modulation of the cellular antioxidant defense capacity. *Environ Health Perspect*, Vol. 88, pp. 77-82, ISSN 0091-6765.

Arita, Y.; Kihara, S.; Ouchi, N.; Takahashi, M.; Maeda, K.; Miyagawa, J.; Hotta, K.; Shimomura, I.; Nakamura, T.; Miyaoka, K.; Kuriyama, H.; Nishida, M.; Yamashita, S.; Okubo, K.; Matsubara, K.; Muraguchi, M.; Ohmoto, Y.; Funahashi, T. & Matsuzawa, Y. (1999). Paradoxical decrease of an adipose-specific protein, adiponectin, in obesity. *Biochem Biophys Res Commun*, Vol. 257, No. 1, pp. 79-83, ISSN 0006-291X.

Arita, Y.; Kihara, S.; Ouchi, N.; Maeda, K.; Kuriyama, H.; Okamoto, Y.; Kumada, M.; Hotta, K.; Nishida, M.; Takahashi, M.; Nakamura, T.; Shimomura, I.; Muraguchi, M.; Ohmoto, Y.; Funahashi, T. & Matsuzawa, Y. (2002). Adipocyte-derived plasma protein adiponectin acts as a platelet-derived growth factor-BB-binding protein and regulates growth factor-induced common postreceptor signal in vascular smooth muscle cell. *Circulation*, Vol. 105, No. 24, pp. 2893-2898, ISSN 0009-7322.

Berg, AH.; Comb, TP. & Scherer PE. (2002). ACRP30/adiponectin: an adipokine regulating glucose and lipid metabolism. *Trends Endocrinol Metab*, Vol. 13, No. 2, pp. 84-89, ISSN 1043-2760.

Brook, CG.; Lloyd, JK. & Wolf, OH. (1972). Relation between age of onset of obesity and size and number of adipose cells. *Br Med J*, Vol. 2, No. 5804, pp. 25-27, ISSN 0959-535X.

Cerutti, P.; Ghosh, R.; Oya, Y. & Amstad, P. (1994). The role of the cellular antioxidant defense in oxidant carcinogenesis. *Environ Health Perspect*, Vol. 102, Suppl. 10, pp. 123-129, ISSN 0091-6765.

Chandel, NS.; Maltepe, E.; Goldwasser, E.; Mathieu, CE.; Simon, MC. & Schumacker, PT. Mitochondrial reactive oxygen species trigger hypoxia-induced transcription. (1998). *Proc Natl Acad Sci USA*, Vol. 95, No. 20, pp. 11715-11720, ISSN 0027-8424.

Eriksson, JW. (2007). Metabolic stress in insulin's target cells leads to ROS accumulation – a hypothetical common pathway causing insulin resistance. *FEBS Lett*, Vol. 581, No. 19, pp. 3734-3742, ISSN 0014-5793.

Faraci, FM. (2003). Vascular protection. Stroke, Vol. 34, No. 2, pp. 327-329, ISSN 0039-2499.

Fox, CS.; Massaro, JM.; Hoffmann, U.; Pou, KM.; Maurovich-Horvat, P.; Liu, CY.; Vasan, RS.; Murabito, JM.; Meigs, JB.; Cupples, LA.; D'Agostino, RB., Sr. & O'Donnell, CJ. (2007). Abdominal visceral and subcutaneous adipose tissue compartments: association with metabolic risk factors in the Framingham Heart Study. *Circulation*, Vol. 116, No. 1, pp. 39-48, ISSN 0009-7322.

Fradette, C.; Batonga, J.; Teng, S.; Piquette-Miller, M. & du Souich, P. (2007). Animal models of acute moderate hypoxia are associated with a down-regulation of CYP1A1, 1A2, 2B4, 2C5, and 2C16 and up-regulation of CYP3A6 and P-glycoprotein in liver. *Drug Metab Dispos*, Vol. 35, No. 5, pp. 765-771, ISSN 0090-9556.

Havel, PJ. (2004). Update on adipocyte hormones: regulation of energy balance and carbohydrate/lipid metabolism. *Diabetes*, Vol. 53, Suppl. 1, pp. S143-S151, ISSN 0012-1797.

Helmlinger, G.; Yuan, F.; Dellian, M. & Jain, RK. (1997). Interstitial pH and pO_2 gradients in solid tumors *in vivo*: high-resolution measurements reveal a lack of correlation. *Nat Med*, Vol. 3, No. 2, pp. 177-182, ISSN 1078-8956.

Hosogai, N.; Fukuhara, A.; Oshima, K.; Miyata, Y.; Tanaka, S.; Segawa, K.; Furukawa, S.; Tochino, Y.; Komuro, R.; Matsuda, M. & Shimomura, I. (2007). Adipose tissue hypoxia in obesity and its impact on adipocytokine dysregulation. *Diabetes*, Vol. 56, No. 4, pp. 901-911, ISSN 0012-1797.

Hotamisligil, GS.; Shargill, NS. & Spiegelman, BM. (1993). Adipose expression of tumor necrosis factor-α: direct role in obesity-linked insulin resistance. *Science*, Vol. 258, No. 5091, pp. 87-91, ISSN 0193-4511.

Hotamisligil, GS. & Spiegelman, BM. (1994). Tumor necrosis factor α: a key component of the obesity-diabetes link. *Diabetes*, Vol. 43, No. 11, pp. 1271-1278, ISSN 0012-1797.

Hotta, K.; Funahashi, T.; Arita, Y.; Takahashi, M.; Matsuda, M.; Okamoto, Y.; Iwahashi, H.; Kuriyama, H.; Ouchi, N.; Maeda, K.; Nishida, M.; Kihara, S.; Sakai, N.; Nakajima, T.; Hasegawa, K.; Muraguchi, M.; Ohmoto, Y.; Nakamura, T.; Yamashita, S.; Hanafusa, T. & Matsuzawa, Y. (2000). Plasma concentrations of a novel, adipose-specific protein, adiponectin, in type 2 diabetic patients. *Arterioscler Thromb Vasc Biol*, Vol. 20, No. 6, pp. 1595-1599, ISSN 1079-5642.

Kamiya, T.; Hara, H.; Yamada, H.; Imai, H.; Inagaki, N. & Adachi, T. (2008). Cobalt chloride decreases EC-SOD expression through intracellular ROS generation and p38-MAPK pathways in COS7 cells. *Free Radic Res*, Vol. 42, No. 11-12, pp. 949-956, ISSN 1071-5762.

Keele, BB., Jr.; McCord, JM. & Fridovich, I. (1970). Superoxide dismutase from escherichia coli B. A new manganese-containing enzyme. *J Biol Chem*, Vol. 245, No. 22, pp. 6176-6181, ISSN 0021-9258.

Kim, KY.; Kim, JK.; Jeon, JH.; Yoon, SR.; Choi, I. & Yang, Y. (2005). c-Jun N-terminal kinase is involved in the suppression of adiponectin expression by TNF-α in 3T3-L1 adipocytes. *Biochem Biophs Res Commun*, Vol. 327, No. 2, pp. 460-467, ISSN 0006-291X.

Kuznetsov, G.; Bush, KT.; Zhang, PL. & Nigam, SK. (1996). Perturbations in maturation of secretory proteins and their association with endoplasmic reticulum chaperones in a cell culture model for epithelial ischemia. *Proc Natl Acad Sci USA*, Vol. 93, No. 16, pp. 8584-8589, ISSN 0027-8424

Kyriakis, JM. & Avruch, J. (2001). Mammalian mitogen-activated protein kinase signal transduction pathways activated by stress and inflammation. *Physiol Rev*, Vol. 81, No. 2, pp. 807-869, ISSN 0031-9333.

Levy, AP.; Levy, NS.; Wegner, S. & Goldberg, MA. (1995). Transcriptional regulation of the rat vascular endothelial growth factor gene by hypoxia. *J Biol Chem*, Vol. 270, No. 22, pp. 13333-13340, ISSN 0021-9258.

Lee, PJ.; Jiang, BH.; Chin, BY.; Iyer, NV.; Alam, J.; Semenza, GL. & Choi, AM. (1997). Hypoxia-inducible factor-1 mediates transcriptional activation of the heme oxygenase-1 gene in response to hypoxia. *J Biol Chem*, Vol. 272, No. 9, pp. 5375-5381, ISSN 0021-9258.

Marklund, SL. (1982). Human copper-containing superoxide dismutase of high molecular weight. *Proc Natl Acad Sci USA*, Vol. 79, No. 24, pp. 7634-7638, ISSN 0027-8424.

Marklund, SL. (1984). Extracellular superoxide dismutase in human tissues and human cell lines. *J Clin Invest*, Vol. 74, No. 4, pp. 1398-1403, ISSN 0021-9738.

Marklund, SL. (1992). Regulation by cytokines of extracellular superoxide dismutase and other superoxide dismutase isoenzymes in fibroblasts. *J Biol Chem*, Vol. 267, No. 10, pp. 6696-6701, ISSN 0021-9258.

McCord, JM. & Fridovich, I. (1969). Superoxide dismutase. An enzymic function for erythrocuprein (hemocuprein). *J Biol Chem*, Vol. 244, No. 22, pp. 6049-6055, ISSN 0021-9258.

Olsvik, PA.; Kristensen, T.; Waagbo, R.; Tollefsen, KE.; Rosseland, BO. & Toften, H. (2006). Effects of hypo- and hyperoxia on transcription levels of five stress genes and the glutathione system in liver of Atlantic cod Gadus morhua. *J Exp Biol*, Vol. 209, No. 15, pp. 2893-2901, ISSN 0022-0949.

Ookawara, T.; Imazeki, N.; Matsubara, O.; Kizaki, T.; Oh-Ishi, S.; Nakao, C.; Sato, Y. & Ohno, H. (1998). Tissue distribution of immunoreactive mouse extracellular superoxide dismutase. *Am J Physiol*, Vol. 275, No. 3, pp. C840-C847, ISSN 0002-9513.

Ouchi, N.; Kihara, S.; Arita, Y.; Maeda, K.; Kuriyama, H.; Okamoto, Y.; Hotta, K.; Nishida, M.; Takahashi, M.; Nakamura, T.; Yamashita, S.; Funahashi, T. & Matsuzawa, Y.

(1999). Novel modulator for endothelial adhesion molecules: adipocyte-derived plasma protein adiponectin. *Circulation*, Vol. 100, No. 25, pp. 2473-2476, ISSN 0009-7322.

Ozcan, U.; Cao, Q.; Yilmaz, E.; Lee, AH.; Iwakoshi, NN.; Ozdelen, E.; Tuncman, G.; Gorgun, C.; Glimcher, LH. & Hotamisligil, GS. (2004). Endoplasmic reticulum stress links obesity, insulin action, and type 2 diabetes. *Science*, Vol. 306, No. 5695, pp. 457-461. ISSN 0193-4511.

Pearson, G.; Robinson, F.; Beers, Gibson, T.; Xu, BE.; Karandikar, M.; Berman, K. & Cobb, MH. (2001). Mitogen-activated protein (MAP) kinase pathways: regulation and physiological functions. *Endocr Rev*, Vol. 22, No. 2, pp. 153-183, ISSN 0163-769X.

Sakaue, H.; Konishi, M.; Ogawa, W.; Asaki, T.; Mori, T.; Yamasaki, M.; Takata, M.; Ueno, H.; Kato, S.; Kasuga, M. & Itoh, N. (2002). Requirement of fibroblast growth factor 10 in development of white adipose tissue. *Genes Dev*, Vol. 16, No. 8, pp. 908-912, ISSN 0890-9369.

Schofield, CJ. & Ratcliffe, PJ. (2004). Oxygen sensing by HIF hydroxylases. *Nat Rev Mol Cell Biol*, Vol. 5, No. 5, pp. 343-354, ISSN 1471-0072.

Schuster, SJ.; Badiavas, EV.; Costa-Giomi, P.; Weinmann, R.; Erslev, AJ. & Caro, J. (1989). Stimulation of erythropoietin gene transcription during hypoxia and cobalt exposure. *Blood*, Vol. 73, No. 1, pp. 13-16, ISSN 0006-4971.

Shimomura, I.; Funahashi, T.; Takahashi, M.; Maeda, K.; Kotani, K.; Nakamura, T.; Yamashita, S.; Miura, M.; Fukuda, Y.; Takemura, K.; Tokunaga, K. & Matsuzawa, Y. (1996). Enhanced expression of PAI-1 in visceral fat: possible contributor to vascular disease in obesity. *Nat Med*, Vol. 2, No. 7, pp. 800-803, ISSN 1078-8956.

Simons, PJ.; van den Pangaart, PS.; Aerts, JM. & Boon, L. (2007). Pro-inflammatory delipidizing cytokines reduce adiponectin secretion from human adipocytes without affecting adiponectin oligomerization. *J Endocrinol*, Vol. 192, No. 2, pp. 289-299, ISSN 0022-0795.

Soares, AF.; Guichardant, M.; Cozzone, D.; Bernoud-Hubac, N.; Bouzaidi-Tiali, N.; Lagarde, M. & Geloen, A. (2005). Effects of oxidative stress on adiponectin secretion and lactate production in 3T3-L1 adipocytes. *Free Radic Biol Med*, Vol. 38, No. 7, pp. 882-889, ISSN 0891-5849.

Strålin, P. & Marklund, SL. (2000). Multiple cytokines regulate the expression of extracellular superoxide dismutase in human vascular smooth muscle cells. *Atherosclerosis*, Vol. 151, No. 2, pp. 433-441, ISSN 0021-9150.

Vincent, F.; Hagiwara, K.; Ke, Y.; Stoner, GD.; Demetrick, DJ. & Bennett, WP. (1996). Mutation analysis of the transforming growth factor β type II receptor in sporadic human cancers of the pancreas, liver, and breast. *Biochem Biophys Res Commun*, Vol. 223, No. 3, pp. 561-564, ISSN 0006-291X.

Yamauchi, T.; Kamon, J.; Minokoshi, Y.; Ito, Y.; Waki, H.; Uchida, S.; Yamashita, S.; Noda, M.; Kita, S.; Ueki, K.; Eto, K.; Akanuma, Y.; Froguel, P.; Foufelle, F.; Ferre, P.; Carling, D.; Kimura, S.; Nagai, R.; Kahn, BB. & Kadowaki, T. (2002). Adiponectin stimulates glucose utilization and fatty-acid oxidation by activating AMP-activated protein kinase. *Nat Med*, Vol. 8, No. 11, pp. 1288-1295, ISSN 1078-8956.

Ye, J.; Gao, Z.; Yin, J. & He, Q. (2007). Hypoxia is a potential risk factor for chronic inflammation and adiponectin reduction in adipose tissue of ob/ob and dietary obese mice. *Am J Physiol Endocrinol Metab*, Vol. 293, No. 4, pp. E1118-1128, ISSN 0193-1849.

Zelko, IN. & Folz, RJ. (2003). Myeloid zinc finger (MZF)-like, Kruppel-like and Ets families of transcription factors determine the cell-specific expression of mouse extracellular superoxide dismutase. *Biochem J*, Vol. 369, No. 2, pp. 375-386, ISSN 0264-6021.

Zelko, IN. & Folz, RJ. (2004). Sp1 and Sp3 transcription factors mediate trichostatin A-induced and basal expression of extracellular superoxide dismutase. *Free Radic Biol Med*, Vol. 37, No. 8, pp. 1256-1271, ISSN 0891-5849.

Zelko, IN.; Mueller, MR. & Folz, RJ. (2008). Transcription factors sp1 and sp3 regulate expression of human extracellular superoxide dismutase in lung fibroblasts. *Am J Respir Cell Mol Biol*, Vol. 39, No. 2, pp.243-251, ISSN 1044-1549.

8

Pattern Recognition Receptors Based Immune Adjuvants: Their Role and Importance in Vaccine Design

Halmuthur M. Sampath Kumar[1], Irfan Hyder[1] and Parvinder Pal Singh[2]
[1]*CSIR-Indian Institute of Chemical Technology, Hyderabad*
[2]*CSIR- Indian Institute of Integrative Medicine, Jammu*
India

1. Introduction

Infectious, cancer and allergic diseases have always been scourge for humans and. disease prevention through immunization has been the most cost-effective health-care intervention available. Immunization has been a great public health success story. As immunization helps to inhibit the spread of disease, many people can be protected from illness and death. It has been proved beyond doubt that with the exception of pure drinking water, no other human endeavor rivals immunization in combating infectious diseases. Millions of lives have been saved, with considerably reduced mortality rates, millions have the chance of a longer healthier life. The purpose of prophylactic vaccination is to generate a strong immune response providing long term protection against infection. Vaccines have been described as weapons of mass protection as they mainly capitalize on the immune system's ability to respond rapidly to pathogens and eliminate them. The considerable success achieved in the eradication of smallpox and the reduction of polio, measles, pertussis, tetanus and meningitis, were among the most notable achievements of the 20th century (Wack and Rappuoli 2005). Unfortunately, for today's societal dreadful diseases which are major causes of morbidity and mortality, there are no effective vaccines. Some of the existing vaccines do not induce complete protection and therefore, the development of effective vaccines towards these diseases is needed. In this chapter, an attempt has been made to explain the role of pattern recognition receptors (PRR)based immune adjuvants for the development of safe and effective vaccines. We have also discussed the recent advances in the therapeutic and prophylactic application of PRR agonist and antagonists for the treatment of infectious diseases and cancer,. This topic was extensively studied in last one decade and thousands of high quality publication and high quality reviews are reported in the literature.

2. Need for immune adjuvants

Traditional vaccines mainly consisted of live attenuated pathogens, whole inactivated organisms, or inactivated bacterial toxins. Many traditional vaccines based on pathogen whole cells often contain components that can cause toxicity related side effects. As a result of these safety limitations of conventional vaccines, several new approaches to vaccine development have emerged that may have significant advantages over more traditional approaches. These approaches include 1) recombinant protein subunits 2) synthetic peptides and 3) protein polysaccharide conjugates. By contrast, these vaccines although offering considerable advantages over traditional vaccines in terms of safety and cost of production, in most cases they have limited immunogenicity and therefore are use less as prophylactic or therapeuticvaccines on their own. These pitfalls have intensified the search of external agents that can synergistically boost the immune response of otherwise weakly immunogenic subunit vaccines. Such molecularly defined immune boosters, popularly known as *adjuvants,* ideally should constitute a non-immunogenic entities, however, able to stimulate humoral and cellular immunity in presence of a vaccine antigen and most importantly, being non toxic, suitable for animals and humans use.

3. Immune system: Innate and adaptive

The immune system in higher animals can be broadly classified into the innate and the adaptive immune systems(Janeway 2001; Janeway and Medzhitov 2002). The innate immune system was long thought to be a non-specific inflammatory response generated during exposure to foreign antigen. However, studies conducted in recent years indicate the innate immune response is able to discriminate between pathogen classes and direct innate and adaptive immune responses toward elimination of the invading pathogen(Akira, Uematsu et al. 2006; Hoebe, Jiang et al. 2006; Sansonetti 2006). The discovery of pathogen-associated molecular patterns (PAMPs) and pattern recognition receptors (PRRs) and the role they play in elimination of pathogen and activity as adjuvant has renewed interest in the importance of the innate immune system(Hopkins and Sriskandan 2005). Improved understanding of innate immunity in recent years, has led to the identification of immune pathways and adjuvant formulations more suitable for clinical advancement. The 2011 Noble Prize for Medicine was awarded to three scientists who have done more than anyone to lay bare the two-tier structure of the immune system. One area of particular interest is the discovery of agonists that target the PRRs. Adaptive immune responses are essential for the control of pathogens that escape elimination by the innate immune response(Schwartz 2000). Because of its role in immune memory, the adaptive immune systems contributions to pathogen elimination and vaccine development have been widely studied. Adaptive immunity mediates a delayed, specific response to foreign antigen while innate immunity is not antigen specific and develops immediately following exposure to immune stimuli i.e., pathogens.

4. Pattern recognition receptors

The Pattern Recognition Receptors (PRRs) of the innate immune system serve an essential role in recognition of pathogen and directing the course as well as type of innate immune response generated following exposure to foreign antigen. PRRs are differentially expressed on a wide variety of immune cells(Iwasaki and Medzhitov 2004). Engagement of PRRs invokes the cascades of intracellular signaling events that further induce many processes such as activation, maturation and migration of other immune cells and the secretion of cytokines and chemokines(Hoebe, Janssen et al. 2004; Medzhitov 2007; Kumar, Kawai et al.

2009; Blasius and Beutler 2010; Kawai and Akira 2010; Takeuchi and Akira 2010). This creates an inflammatory environment in tandem, that leads to the establishment of the adaptive immune response(Iwasaki and Medzhitov 2004). PRRs consist of non-phagocytic receptors such as **toll-like receptors** (TLRs) and **nucleotide-binding oligomerization domain (NOD) proteins** and receptors that induce phagocytosis such as **scavanger receptors**, **mannose receptors** and ***β*-glucan receptors**. In last decade, several natural, natural derived (PAMPs) and synthetic ligands of PRR belonging to the diverse structural class have been identified(Kumar, Kawai et al. 2011) and reported in the literature possessing potential immunomodulatory properties. In spite of thousand of molecules identified as potential PRR agonist properties, a hand full number of these are now in clinical or late preclinical stages of development as immune adjuvant for vaccines(Kanzler, Barrat et al. 2007; Makkouk and Abdelnoor 2009; Mbow, Gregorio et al. 2010; Basith, Manavalan et al. 2011). Various vaccine R&Ds and research group around the world are currently exploring the use of natural ligands or synthetic ligands as well-defined PRRs as adjuvants, either alone or with as formulations with other ingradients for various subunit vaccines being developed against cancers, infectious and allergic diseases. Furthermore, TLR antagonists derived from the modifications of natural ligands also appear quite promising for a number of inflammatory and autoimmune diseases.

4.1 Toll like receptors

Vaccine adjuvants are perhaps the most extensively explored applications for TLR agonists. In last decade, efforts an increasing focus has been to use natural ligands or synthetic agonists for well-defined TLRs as adjuvants, either alone or with various formulations. A number of these are now in clinical or late preclinical stages of development for multiple applications and have been the subject of research to clarify the basis of their adjuvant activity. TLR are type I membrane glycoproteins, characterized by a cytoplasmic Toll/interleukin-1 receptor homology (TIR) signaling domain and an external antigen recognition domain comprising 19–25 tandem leucine-rich repeat (LRR) motifs(Rock, Hardiman et al. 1998). TLRs were initially discovered in fruitfly, *Drosophila melanogaster*, and have been defined as factors involved in the embryonic development (Lemaitre, Nicolas et al. 1996; Hoffmann 2003)and resistance of the fly Drosophila to bacterial and fungal infection. Bieng a major component in innate immunity TLRs are known to play a significant role in innate-adaptive cross talks(Pandey and Agrawal 2006; Rezaei 2006; Kanzler, Barrat et al. 2007; Romagne 2007). First human TLR was discovered in 1997 by Medzhitov *et al.* and after that research in this filed has exploded so rapidly that all TLRs have been cloned and many of their ligands (PAMPs) and associated signaling pathways have been identified. TLRs recognize broad classes of PAMPS and are emerging as a central player in initiating and directing immune responses to pathogens. Till date, ten TLR (TLR1–10) are reported in humans and subdivided according to their localization in cell compartments. TLR1, 2, 4, 5, 6 and 10 are expressed on the cell surface and recognize PAMPs derived from bacteria, fungi and protozoa. TLR3, 7, 8 and 9 are expressed in intracellular compartments with the ligand-binding domains sampling the lumen of the vesicle and recognize nucleic acid PAMPS derived from various viruses and bacteria(Janeway and Medzhitov 2002; Akira and Hemmi 2003; Akira, Uematsu et al. 2006). Generally, natural lignads of TLR fall into three broad categories: **lipids and lipopeptides**

(TLR2/TLR1; TLR2/TLR6; TLR4), **proteins** (TLR5) and **nucleic acids** (TLR3, 7, 8, 9). TLRs forms both homo- and heterodimers to enable functioning and downstream signaling activation resulting in ligand recognition (PAMPS) of diverse structure from various sources. TLR2 preferentially forms heterodimers with either TLR1 or TLR6, whereas the other TLRs appear to associate as homodimers. Various natural (microbial) and synthetic ligands of functional TLRs as well as cellular localization of TLRs are discussed in Table 1.

PRR (Cellular localization)	**Microbial Ligands**	**Synthetic Ligands**
TLR1/TLR2 (Cell surface)	Triacyl lipopeptide (Pam3CSK4)	Pam2CSK/Pam3CSK4 analogues
TLR2/TLR6 (Cell surface)	Diacyl lipopeptides (Pam2CSK4), Lipoteichoic acid, Zymosan, porins, MALP2, Bacterial peptidoglycan, Lipoarabinomannan	Pam2CSK/Pam3CSK4 analogues
TLR3 (Endosome)	ssRNS and dsRNA virus, Respiratory syncytical virus, Mmurine cytomegalovirus	Poly I:C; poly A:U
TLR4 (Cell surface)	LPS; Mannan; Phospholipids; Envelope proteins (MMTV, RSV)	Monophosphoryl lipid A and its analogues
TLR5 (Cell surface)	Flagellin	---
TLR7 (Endolysosome)	ssRNA (viral), RNA from bacteria from group B streptococcus	GU-rich oligoribonucleotides; Loxoribin; Imiquimod; Resiquimod; Adenosine and Guanosine derivative
TLR8 (Endolysosome)	ssRNA (viral)	GU-Rich oligoribonucleotides; Adenosine and Guanosine derivative; Resiquimod
TLR9 (Endolysosome)	DNA (bacterial/viral)	Deoxynucleotides with unmethylated CpG motifs
TLR10 (Cell surface)	Unknown	----

Table 1. Pattern Recognition Receptors and their ligands

Ligand binding to TLR appears to result in conformational changes and possibly dimerization, leading to recruitment of crucial adaptor proteins. These Toll/interlukin-1 receptor homology(TIR) domain-containing molecules include myeloid differentiation primary-response protein 88 (MyD88), used by nearly all TLR, TIR domain-containing adaptor protein (TIRAP), TIR domain-containing adaptor protein inducing interferon (IFN)-β (TRIF), and TRIF-related adaptor molecule (TRAM). Engagement of these adaptors activates a series of signal transduction molecules including interleukin (IL)-1R-associated kinases (IRAKs), tumor necrosis factor receptor (TNFR)-associated factor 6 (TRAF6), transforming growth factor (TGF)-β-activated kinase (TAK1), and the inhibitor of nuclear factor-κB (IκB)-kinase complex. These events lead ultimately to activation of mitogen-activated protein (MAP) kinases and nuclear translocation of the transcription factor NF-κB, key regulators of many inflammatory response pathways. A second discrete pathway, used by intracellular TLR, leads to activation of IFN regulatory factors (IRF), particularly IRF-7, leading to high levels of type I IFN production. Differential adaptor use by different TLR and cell type-specific signaling pathways leads to many variations on this theme. Thus, the response to TLR signaling can include cell differentiation, proliferation or apoptosis, as well as induction of many secreted mediators, prominently IFNs, TNF-α, IL-1, IL-6, IL-10, IL-12, and many different chemokines. The responses produced by activation through a TLR are determined by many factors specific to individual cell types, as well as to quantitative and qualitative parameters of the TLR-ligand interaction itself.

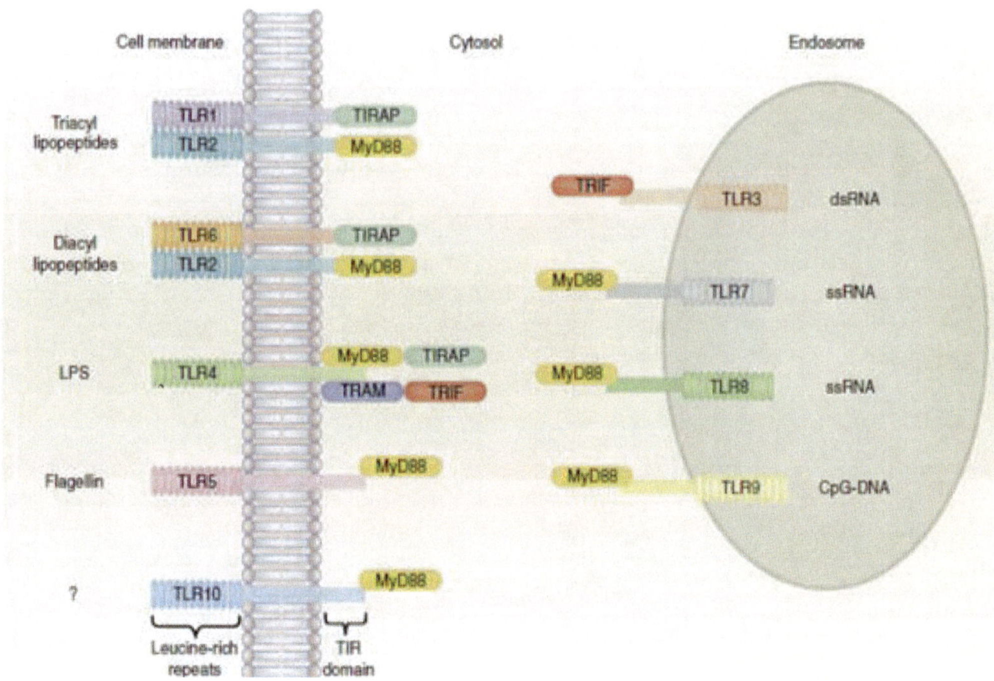

Fig. 1. Schematic diagram of human Toll-like receptors showing adaptors, cellular orientation and complimentary ligands. Source: Holger Kanzler *et al. Nature Medicine* **2007**, *13*, 552.

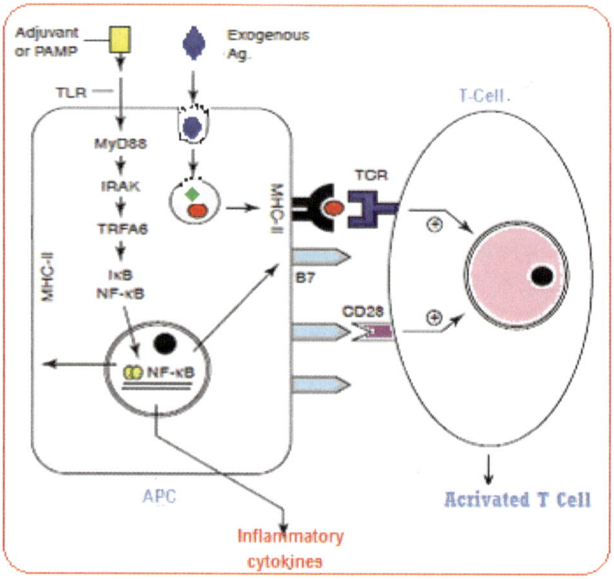

Fig. 2. Stimulation of innate immunity and induction of adaptive immunity by PAMPs or PAMP-related adjuvants.

Redundant and non-redundant functions of TLRs are responsible for the adjuvant activity required to t immune responses both in natural infection and in vaccine responses(Lien and Golenbock 2003). They have a distinct function in pathogen recognition and constitute good targets for rational adjuvant development. Table 1 shows, TLR recognize groups of widely distributed and structurally similar molecules, in contrast to the highly selective molecular-level recognition of T- and B-cell receptors. Synthetic ligands with varying degrees of similarity to natural ligands have been described for most of the TLR. Therapeutic applications to date have used either native or synthetic versions of natural TLR ligands with optimized pharmacologic properties(Kanzler, Barrat et al. 2007; Makkouk and Abdelnoor 2009; Basith, Manavalan et al. 2011).

4.2 Small molecules TLR agonists and antagonists derived from PAMPs

A number of TLR agonist and antagonists are currently under investigation are either PAMPS or PAMPS derived molecules such as DNA motifs analogs, monophosphoryl lipid A analogs, muramyl dipeptide analogs, nucleic acid analogs etc. Here, we have presented brief description of representative clinically potential agonists and antagonists and their pharmacophores responsible for stimulating immunological response.

4.2.1 Lipopolysaccharide, lipid A and monophosphoryl lipid A

The adjuvant effect of lipopolysaccharide (LPS) or endotoxin was described in 1956(Johnson, Gaines et al. 1956). LPS or endotoxin component of gram negative bacteria has a hydrophilic polysaccharide and lipophilic phospholipids which is responsible for adjuvant activity(Gupta, Relyveld et al. 1993). The active agent of LPS has been shown to be lipid A - a *disaccharide composed of two glucosamine units, two phosphate groups and five or six fatty acid chains (generally C12 to C16 in length)*. Lipid A **1** is a potent adjuvant for both protein and carbohydrate antigens, and can lead to marked increases in both humoral and cell-mediated immunity(Azuma 1992). Although LPS as a component of whole cell vaccines against pertussis, cholera and typhoid has been used in humans for many years, its extreme toxicity precludes its use as an adjuvant in humans(Johnson, Keegan et al. 1999). Attempts have been made to detoxify LPS and lipid A without affecting its adjuvanticity. The most promising derivative of lipid A is monophosphoryl lipid.

Monophosphoryl lipid A (MPLA, **Fig 3**) **1a** has been shown to exhibit potent adjuvanticity, without exhibiting significant toxicity. Structural activity relationship of the MPL shown that a hexaacylated β(1→6)-diglucosamine having three 3-n-alkanoyloxytetradecanoyl residues or six fatty acid groups is required for adjuvanticity. Careful structure examination of lipid A analogs suggests that the type and length lipid play a very crucial role in determining the activity towards stimulation (agonist) or inhibition (antagonist). Lipid A analogs having *β*-alkanoyl lipid having longer chain length shown agonist activity and lipid A analogs with shorter chain length shown antagonist activity. Both LPS and MPL exhibited adjuvant activity by triggering a signaling through TLR4(Kaisho and Akira 2002; Re and Strominger 2002), but MPLA leads to downstream signaling only through the TRIF adaptor, whereas the LPS leads to TLR4 activation through both the TRIF and MyD88 pathways, the latter pathway resulting in the high level of inflammatory cytokines, prominently TNF-α. On the other hand, MPLA activation leads to the induction of IFN-β and regulation of CD80/CD86, which is a key aspect of adjuvanticity. Three MPLA and its analog containing vaccine formulations have already been approved (Kanzler, Barrat et al. 2007; Makkouk and Abdelnoor 2009; Basith, Manavalan et al. 2011)for various diseases such as *Fendrix* (by GSK) for Hepatatis B, *Cervarix* (by GSK) for cervical cancer and *Pollinex quattro* (by Allergy Therapeutics) for allergic rhinitis and have proven to be both safe and effective. Similarly another synthetic lipid A mimetics structure known as aminoalkyl glucosaminide phosphates (AGPs) also entered clinical studies and one of the AGPs known as RC-529 (**1c**, structure shown in Fig 3) developed by Dynavax Technologies has been approved for hepatitis B vaccine *Supervax*. Similarly, CRX-675 (Aminoalkyl-glucosamine-4- posphatide of unknown structure; may be identical or similar to RC529, Table 4) developed by Corixa also find clinical application and currently in phase-I for allergen rhinitis. Other lipid A analogs as TLR4 antagonists such as CRX-526 and others are in preclinical studies for inflammatory diseases. Many lipid A analogs containing vaccine formulations are in preclinical and different stage of clinical trial for cancer, infectious and allergic diseases as given in Table 2, 3, 4. Merck has developed an innovative cancer vaccine known as *Stimuvax* containing MLP as adjuvant along with MUC1 a protein antigen to treat cancer because it is widely expressed in common cancer, and is currently undergoing phase-III clinical trial. Researcher also developed lipid A analog as TLR4 antagonists which find important application for the treatment of various autoimmune and inflammatory diseases. E-5564 (*Eritoran*) is a lipid A mimics developed by Eisai Pharmaceuticals and currently in phase-III trial for severe sepsis. From this discussion, it is evident that different lipid A analogs act differently and find useful in the treatment of hepatitis B, cancer, allergic and inflammation diseases(Kanzler, Barrat et al. 2007; Makkouk and Abdelnoor 2009; Basith, Manavalan et al. 2011).

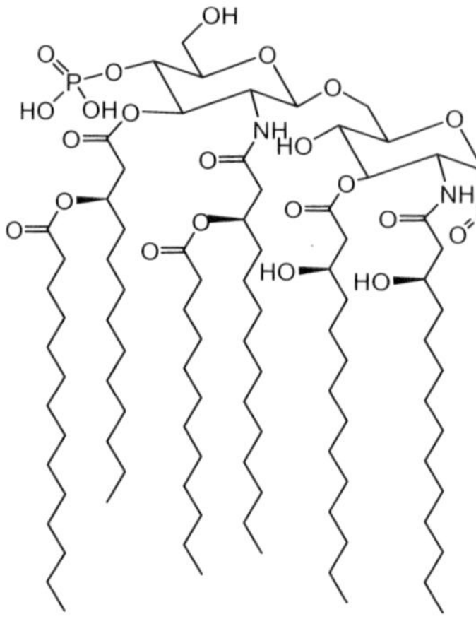

Lipid A(1)

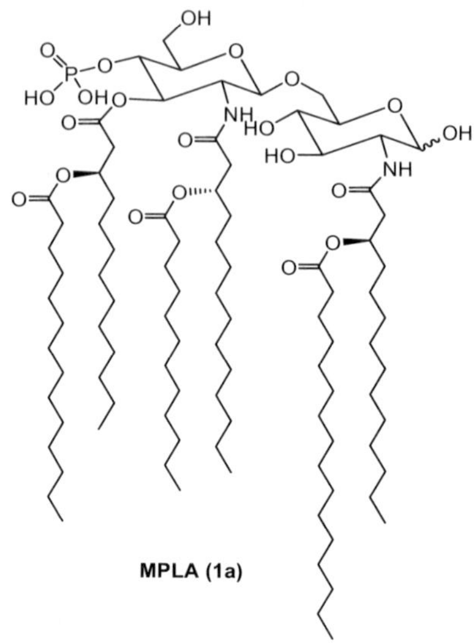

MPLA (1a)

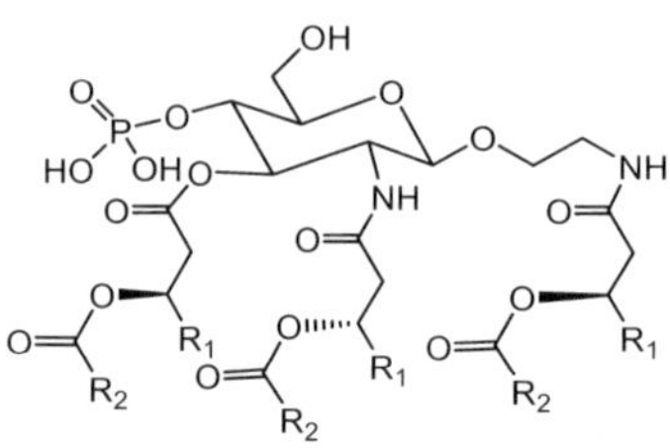

$R_1 = n\text{-}C_{11}H_{23}$: $R_2 = n\text{-}C_{13}H_{27}$

RC-529 (1b)

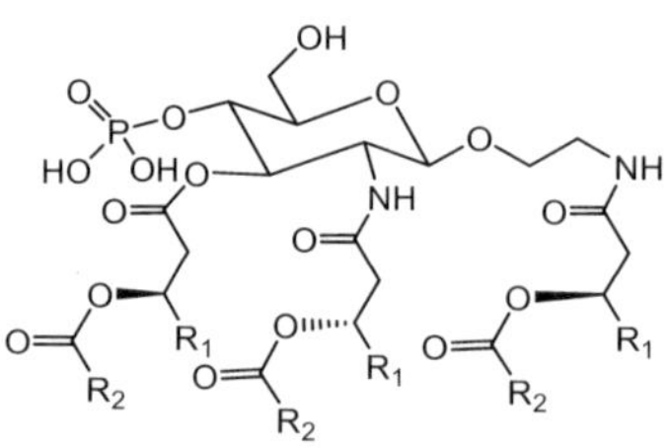

$R_1 = n\text{-}C_{11}H_{23}$: $R_2 = n\text{-}C_5H_{11}$

CRX-526 (1d)

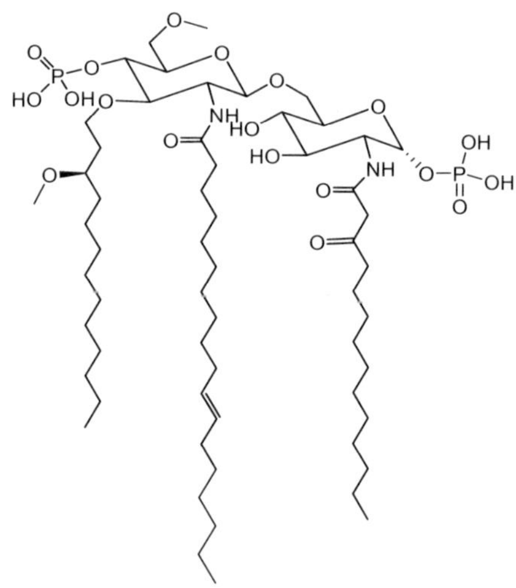

E5564 (1c)

Fig. 3. Structure of Lipid A and their synthetic analogs as TLR4 agonist and antagonists

4.2.2 Imidazoquinolines and guanosine containing compounds

Guanosine- and uridine-rich ssRNA were first identified as natural agonists for TLR7 and and 8 and because of their degradation by RNases limited their uses as immune adjuvants. In search of stable and robust small molecule TLR7 and 8 agonists lead to the discovery of imidaquinolines and guanosine and adenine analogs(Fig 4). Imidazoquinolines such as imiquimod **2a**, resiquimod **2b** are synthetic low-molecular weight TLR7/8 agonists are structural mimics of DNA or RNA oligonucleotides(Gibson, Lindh et al. 2002; Stanley 2002; Lee, Chuang et al. 2003). Imiquimod activate TLR7 while resiquimod activate either TLR7, TLR8 or both. Imiquimod represent the most promising TLR7 agoinst and 3M Pharma developed formulation containing imiquimod as 5% cream(Aldara™) approved for the treatment of genital warts, superficial basal cell carcinoma, actinic keratoses and lentigo malinga and also been used for the treatment of human papilloma virus(HPV)associated lesions and cutaneous melanoma. Another structurally related compound, R-848 (Resiquimod, 3M Pharma), is currently in Phase II (Bishop, Hsing et al. 2000)clinical study for the treatment of hepatitis C virus(HCV) and other viral infections(Pockros, Guyader et al. 2007). Similarly guanosine containing compound **2c** and other nucleoside analogs also find promising application for the number of diseases e.g., ANA975 (oral prodrug of isatoribine) was developed as an antiviral HCV treatment, shown promising activity in preliminary level but clinical studies for this were discontinued by Anadys Pharma due to indicated toxicity in the long-term animal studies(Pockros, Guyader et al. 2007).

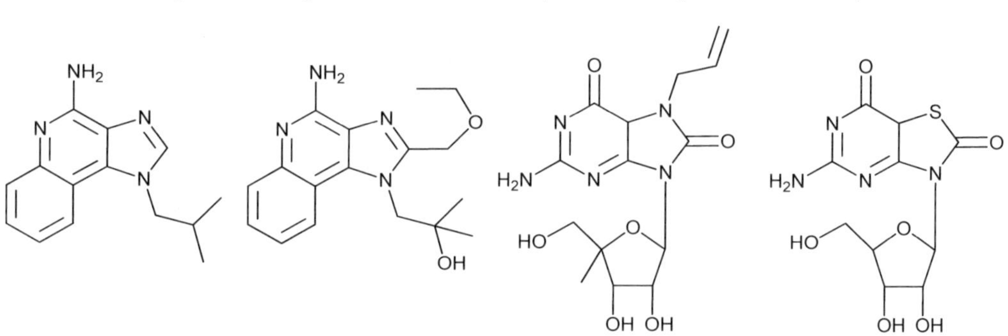

2a **2b** **2c** **2d**

Fig. 4. Structure of imidazoquinolines and other small synthetic compounds

4.2.3 Lipoproteins and lipopeptides

Lipoproteins are part of the outer membrane of gram negative bacteria, gram positive bacteria, *Rhodopseudomonas viridis* and mycoplasma. Bacterial lipoproteins have no shared sequence homology but are characterized by the *N*-terminal unusual amino acid *S*-(2,3-dihydroxypropyl)-cysteine acylated by three fatty acids. Synthetic analogues of the *N*-terminal lipopentapeptide (sLP) **3** of the lipoprotein of *E. coli* proved to be as active as the native lipoprotein(Fig 5). They activate B-cells, monocytes, neutrophils and platelets and act as potent immunoadjuvants *in-vivo* and *in-vitro(Seifert, Schultz et al. 1990; Wiesmüller, Bessler et al. 1992; Berg, Offermanns et al. 1994; Bessler, Cox et al. 1998; Hoffmann, Heinle et al. 1998).* Synthetic lipopeptides with the *RR* stereoisomer (*N*-palmitoyl-*S*-[2,3-bis(palmitoyloxy)-(2*R*)-propyl]-[*R*]-cysteine), showed higher B-cell mitogenicity and protective activity when introduced into vaccines than the mixture of other stereoisomers(Wiesmüller, Jung et al. 1989; Wiesmüller, Bessler et al. 1992).

Lipoproteins and lipopeptides induce signaling in immune cells through toll-like receptor-TLR2/TLR1 and TLR2/TLR6 heterodimers. Diacyl lipopeptides like macrophage activating lipopeptide from *Mycoplasma fermentans* (MALP-2, Pam2Cys-GNNDESNISFKEK) contain the diacylated lipoamino acid *S*-[2,3-bis(palmitoyloxy)-(2*R*)-propyl]-[*R*]-cysteine require TLR2 and TLR6 for signalling, whereas the triacylated synthetic compound like Pam3Cys-SK4 require TLR2/TLR1 heterodimers for signalling. Structure–activity relationship study supports the fact that the immune modulating activity of lipopeptides is strongly dependent on the fatty acid length and the presence of the natural amino acid S-2(*R*)-dihydroxypropyl-(*R*)-cysteine.

Lipopeptide vaccinations have been carried out in all relevant animal models and so far no toxic side effects have been observed. The safety, reproducible production and ease of storage and handling of lipopeptide vaccines suggest that they have significant potential for the development of vaccines for humans and domestic animals. Moreover, several researcher conjugated MHC class-I restricted peptides with Pam3Cys-Ser-Ser resulting in efficient priming of virus-specific cytotoxic T-cells and Tn antigen epitopes.

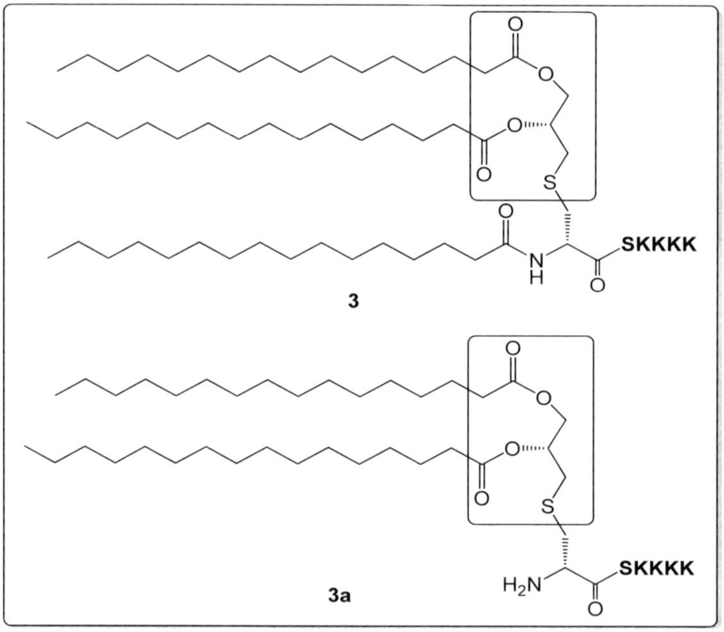

Fig. 5. Structure of lipopetides

4.3 Nucleotide-binding and oligomerization domain (NOD)-like receptor (NLR) proteins

Nucleotide-binding and oligomerization domain (NOD)-like receptor (NLRs) (Fritz, Ferrero et al. 2006; Werts, Girardin et al. 2006; Franchi, Park et al. 2008) represent another family of PRR that received great attention in recent decade and their role in linking host innate immunity to microbes and regulation of inflammatory pathways (Carneiro, Magalhaes et al. 2008)has been extensively studied. In humans the NLR family is composed of 22 intracellular pattern recognition molecules and composed of three different types of domains, a C-terminal LRR domain for ligand binding, a nucleotide binding oligomerization domain (NOD domain) and an N-terminal effector binding domain for the initiation of signaling. Among all the NLRs, NLRP, NOD1 and NOD2 were extensively studied towards their role in the treatment of inflammatory diseases and in the development of improved vaccine. PAMPs, PAMPs-derived and synthetic ligands that recognize these receptors are presented in Table 1. NOD1 recognizes a molecule called meso-DAP, that is a peptidoglycan constituent of the only gram negative bacteria(Chamaillard 2003; Girardin 2003). NOD2 proteins recognize intracellular MDP (muramyl dipeptide),]-a peptidoglycan constituent of both gram ositive and gram negative bacteria.. Whereas NALPRs have been known to detect a range of PAMPs(Hsu; Martinon, Agostini et al. 2004; Boyden and Dietrich 2006; Kanneganti 2006; Kanneganti 2006; Mariathasan 2006; Martinon, Petrilli et al. 2006; Petrilli 2007; Franchi and Nunez 2008; Li, Willingham et al. 2008)

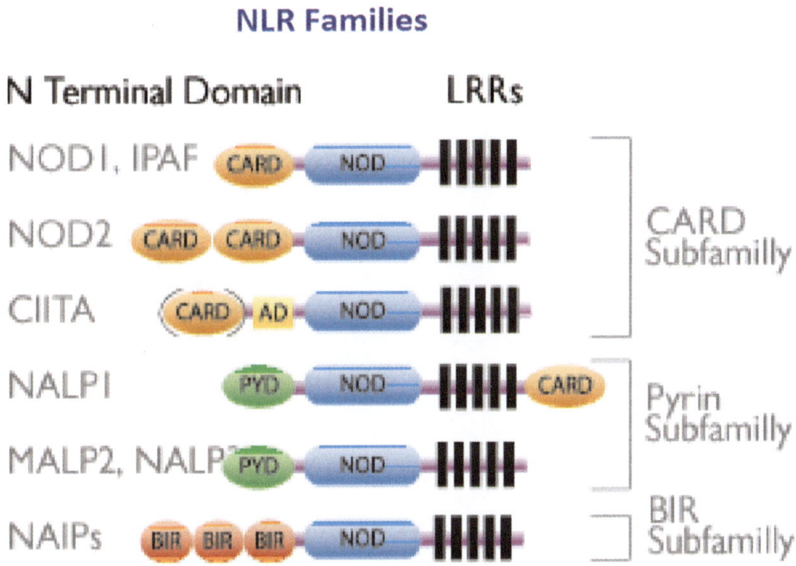

Fig. 6. Nucleotide-binding oligomerization domain (NOD) proteins receptors

4.3.1 Natural and unnatural NOD agonists/antagonists: Muramyl dipeptides

Two major class of compounds *viz.*, bacterial cell wall preparations containing peptidoglycan and inorganic crystals such as aluminium hydroxide (now identified as ligands of NLrs pathway) were extensively used for vaccination strategies throughout the twentieth century represented the strength of this pathway for vaccine and adjuvant development. Furthermore, in recent studies, it has been found that the interaction of NLRs and TLRs are crucial for the adaptive immunity and therefore researchers are looking for the combination strategy by using the ligands of two pathways for the designing of more potent and efficacious immune adjuvants for poor imunogenic vaccines. Although this area is relatively new, but many PAMPS, PAMPs derived and synthetic ligands as well as the role of their receptors in various diseases condition have been identified that will provide very useful inputs for vaccine and adjuvant development.

Eversince the identification of monomeric peptidoglycan subunits in 1970s as minimal structural responsible for the adjuvanticity of complete Freund's adjuvant (CFA) a mixture of NOD1, NOD2 and TLR ligands, which play a central role in the adjuvant action of CFA and therefore their ligands will be explored for the development of effective vaccines. Similarly, *N*-Acetyl muramyl-L-alanine-D-isoglutamine (muramyl dipeptide, MDP) **4** is another component of a peptidoglycan extracted from *Mycobacteria* possessing promising imunostimulatory properties and recently has been found to activate NOD2(Adam, Ciorbaru et al. 1974). Muramyl dipeptide (MDP) is the minimal unit of the mycobacterial cell wall complex that generates the adjuvant activity of complete Freund's adjuvant (CFA). MDP has a variety of physiological effects, including adjuvanticity, pyrogenicity and leucocytopoietic activity and extensive research has been done on these molecules to understand their role and activation pathway. Despite extensive research on MDP, the molecules was found to be pyrogenic and autoimmunogenic to be used as adjuvants in human. Furthermore, MDP have potent *in-vivo* adjuvant activity when administered as water-in oil emulsions, but MDP itself is a poor adjuvant, due to its rapid excretion in the urine when administered as an aqueous solution. Therefore, efforts towards the synthesis of less pyrogenic derivatives without compromise on their immune stimulatory activity has been attempted. . And as a result, a number of lipophilic derivatives of MDP have been prepared, and their bioactivities have been reviewed(Azuma and Seya 2001). Several MDP derivatives and related compounds such as murametide **4a**, murabutide **4b**, threonyl- MDP **4c**, murapalmintine **4d** and glycoyl-MDP **4e** have host-stimulating activities against bacterial infections in experimental models. Moreover, MDP as well as other muropeptides (tripeptides and disaccharide tripeptides and tetrapeptides) have been found to work in synergy with TLRs and enhance the effect of immunomodulatory factors such as IFNγ, IL-

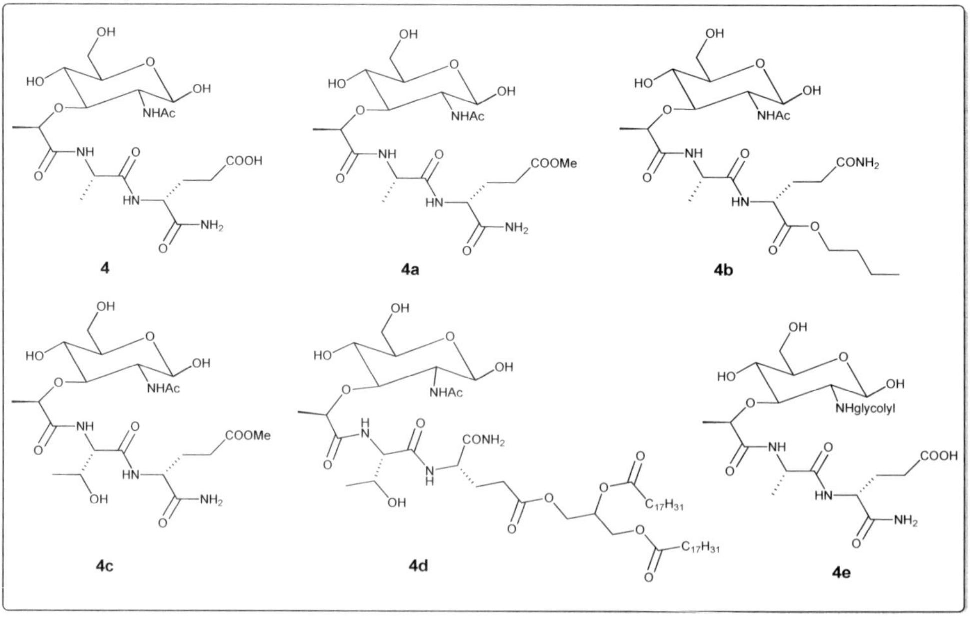

Fig. 7. Structure of MDP and its analogs

1β, IL-32 and GM-CsF. All these factors are crucial for the recruitment and activation of effector cells as well as for evoking the inflammatory processes which eventually lead to the establishment of an appropriate adaptive immune response, that leads to the increase in the therapeutic potential of NOD2 molecules(Geddes, Magalhaes et al. 2009).

On the other hand, NLRPs recognize wide range of ligands of natural sources but some recent studies shown that some NLRP particularly NLRP3 is an essential component of the inflammasome, it is possible that the activation of NLRP3 as part of the inflammosome is a common event in response to several adjuvants or more generally to particulate compounds such as chitosan (a polysaccharide derived from chitin) and Quil A (a saponin extracted from the bark of *Quillaja saponaria*) as well as silica and asbestos. However, how NLRP3 activation contributes to adjuvanticity is not fully understood. The steadily growing knowledge on NLRs will have a crucial impact on our understanding of the mechanisms of action of immune adjuvants, as well as the pathogenesiss and will help direct the development of potent and efficacious immune adjuvants in the near future(Geddes, Magalhaes et al. 2009).

4.4 Endocytic pattern-recognition receptors: Mannose receptors

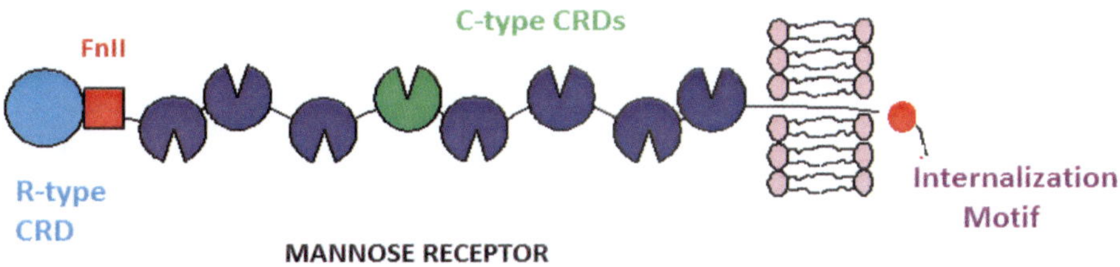

Fig. 8. Mannose receptor-A type 1 transmembrane protein

The mannose receptor (MR) is a PRR primarily present on the surface of macrophages and dendritic cells (Stahl and Ezekowitz 1998)which belongs to the multilectin receptor protein group and, provides a link between innate and adaptive immunity like the TLRs, It is a type I C-type lectin receptor with a long extracellular portion including a N-terminal cysteine-rich domain, a fibronectin type II (FNII) domain, a series of eight C-type lectin-like domains and the carbohydrate–recognition domains (CRDs), which is endowed with the capability to recognize mannosyl-, fucosyl- or N- acetylglucosamidyl-terminal glycoconjugates and sulfated sugars(Taylor and Drickamer 1993). Mannose receptor endocytoses mannosylated motifs for processing and presentation to T cells by MHC class II. Mannosylation of antigen enhances the efficiency of its presentation to T cells. In a variety f antigen delivery approches, the MR has demonstrated effective induction of potent cellular and humoral immune responses. Therefore, MR-targeted vaccines are likely to be most efficacious *in-vivo* when combined with agents that elicit complementary activation signals.

5. Importance of Th1 immune modulators

The basic knowledge of adjuvant action is very important for developing suitable vaccines for newly emerging cancer and infectious diseases. In the last one decade, much progress has been made on understanding the molecular basis for action of adjuvants, the role of cytokines and different types of cells involved in immune response and a better understanding of the correlates of immunity to various diseases(Moingeon, Haensler et al. 2001). The induction of Th1 responses is highly desirable for vaccines (Moingeon, Haensler et al. 2001)against chronic viral diseases, infections linked to intracellular pathogens such as *M.TB*, Malaria or cancer (therapeutic vaccines). This leads to the development of adjuvants, which can selectively modulate the immune response and even evoke selective T-cell response alone. Due to limitations of potential adjuvants to elicit cell mediated immune responses such as cytotoxic T-cell responses, there is a need for alternative adjuvants, particularly for diseases in which cell mediated immune responses are important for eliminating intracellular pathogens.

6. Plant based immune adjuvants

The toxicity, adverse reactions, pyrogenicity and reactogenicity associated with synthetic as well as bacterial products limited their development as immunoadjuvants and therefore, in this direction, plants can provide potent, safer and efficacious alternatives. Crude extracts derived from plants have been used as immune-potentiators from the time immemorial in various traditional medicines(Alamgir and Uddin 2010). A traditional Indian system of medicines like *Siddha* and *Ayurveda* suggested that various plants derived *Rasayanas* possess potential immunostimulatory activity(Thatte and Dahanukar 1997). The extracts and formulations prepared from Ayurvedic medicinal plants such as *Withania somnifera, Tinospora cordifolia, Actinidia macrosperma, Picrorhiza kurroa, Aloe vera, Andrographis paniculata, Asparagus racemosus, Azadirachta indica, Boswellia carterii, Chlorella vulgaris, Emblica officinalis, Morinda citrifolia, Piper longum, Ocimum sanctum* etc demonstrated significant immunostimulatory activity particularly at humoral level in experimental systems(Patwardhan 2000; Kumar, Gupta et al. (2011). QS-21 a plant based saponin present the finest example of alternate immunoadjuvants isolated from the crude extracts of *Quillaja saponaria* which was known for immunostimulatory properties(Jacobsen, Fairbrother et al. 1996). Similarly, several others single molecules based immune potentiators have been isolated and characterized from the plant sources. Even though these molecules may not operate through the similar mechanism as various PAMPS, the adjuvant effect owing to such amphilic natural products is undisputed possibly with low toxicity `unlike those derived from PAMPS. There is a major unmet need for a safe and efficacious adjuvant capable of boosting both cellular and humoral immunity. The evaluation and development of plant based immunomodulators, as the alternate adjuvants for providing maximum and lasting protective immune responses with existing vaccines, is justified due to proven safety aspects in comparison with their synthetic counterparts along with excellent tolerability, ease of manufacture and formulation.

6.1 Plant based products currently under investigation

In the last few decades, improved understanding of the mechanism of action of traditional plant based crude extracts and formulations, lead to the discovery of various class of compounds as potential immunostimulators *viz.*, alkaloids, saponins, polysaccharide, triterpenoids, iridoids, organic acids, etc(Alamgir and Uddin 2010). Several plant based products are currently under investigation for use as vaccine adjuvants. Enriched fractions of iridoid glycosides has been isolated from *Picrorhiza kurroa* (a high altitude Himalayan perennial herb) employed for medicinal purpose from time immemorial to relieve immune related diseases(Puri, Saxena et al. 1992). Several polysaccharides such as mannan and β 1-3 glucan **5** isolated from many plant sources such as *Chlorella sp, Tinospora cordifolia* etc. have been known for stimulating and targeting APCs to up-regulate Thl responses and used as vaccine adjuvants either mixed with or conjugated to immunogen. Picrosides **6** isolated from *Picrorhiza kurroa,* Cardioside **7**isolated from *Tinospora cordifolia* possesses potential immunostimulatory activity(Panchabhai, Kulkarni et al. 2008). Cannabidiol **8** and tetrahydrocannabinol **9** isolated from *Cannbis sativa* significantly attenuated the elevation of IL-2, IL-4, IL-5, and IL-13 and represent the potential therapeutic utility.

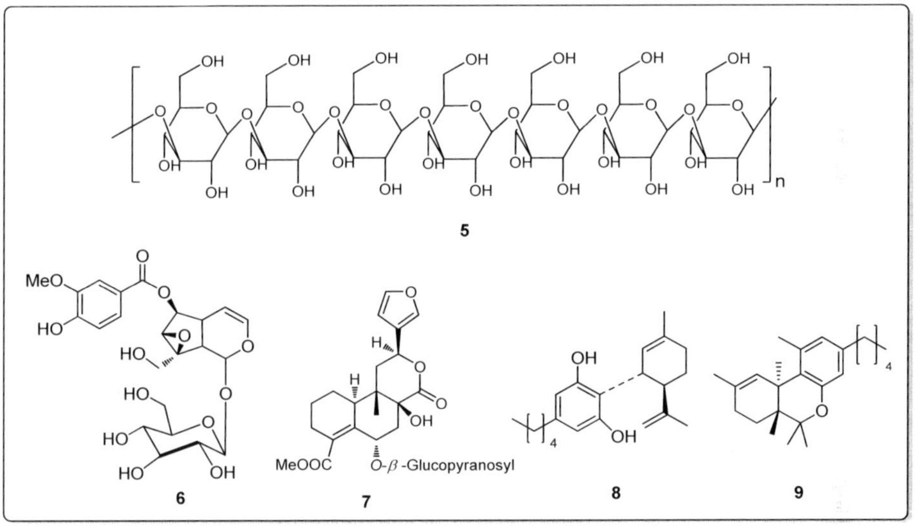

Fig. 9. Structure of plant based immunopotentiators

Despite the long term human use of secondary metabolite enriched fractions of Picrorhiza kurroa as potential immunomodulator in traditional medicines, there had been no report regarding the adjuvant activity of the molecular constituents of this valuable plant. While exploring the novel immunoadjuvants derived from *Picrorhiza kurroa* , it was found that many glycoconjugates such as picroside-I, picroside-II and catalpol, possess promising dose dependant immune potentiation ability as indicated by B and T cell proliferation. The single molecules derived from these fractions revealed varying degrees of adjuvant activity. The enriched fractions [RLJ-NE-299A, a mixture of picroside-I (PK-I) and picroside-II (PK-II)] derived from this plant exhibited promising adjuvant activity(Khajuria, Gupta et al. 2007) without significant sustained immune memory or depot formation properties, which restricted their use as plant based immune-adjuvants. In order to develop more potent, efficacious and alternate plant based immune adjuvant, recently acylated analogs of picroside-II viz. PK-II-2, PK-II-3 and PK-II-4 were synthesized and tested for immune-adjuvant activity in the presence of weak antigen ovalbumin. Among the acylated analogs PK-II-3 and PK-II-4 were found to stimulate anti-OVA IgG titer, neutralizing antibody (IgG1 and IgG2a) titer as well as the production of soluble mediators of a Th1 response (IL-2 and IFN-γ) and Th2 response (IL-4) and proliferation of T lymphocytes sub-sets (CD4/CD8).

These results support the use of acylated analogs particularly PK-II-3 and PK-II-4 as potent enhancer of antigen-specific Th1 and Th2 immune responses and thus are promising immune-adjuvant candidate for vaccines(Kumar and Singh 2010)

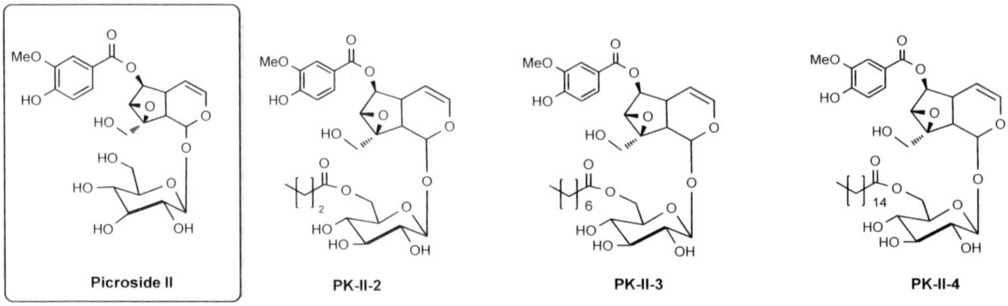

Fig. 10. Picroside II and its lipidated derivatives as immune adjuvants

Based on the traditional system of medicine, plant based products can be attractive candidates for use as safe vaccine adjuvants.

6.2 Saponins, Quil-A and QS-21

Saponins are triterpene glycosides isolated various plant sources. Crude extracts of *Quillaja saponoria* –a bark tree native of Chile, have long been known as an immunostimulator (Dalsgaard 1974). Crude extracts of plants containing saponin enhanced potency of foot and mouth disease vaccines. However, these crude extracts were associated with adverse side effects when used as vaccine adjuvants. Dalsgaard et al. partially purified the adjuvant active component from crude extracts by dialysis, ion exchange and gel filtration chromatography. The active component known as Quil A exhibited enhanced potency and reduced local reactions when compared to crude extracts.

Quil A is widely used in veterinary vaccines but its hemolytic activity and local reactions made it unsuitable for human vaccines. Further analysis and refining of Quil A by high pressure liquid chromatography (HPLC) revealed a heterogenous mixture of closely related saponins and led to discovery of QS-21(**10)** a potent adjuvant with reduced or minimal toxicity. QS-21 is a quillaic acid-based triterpene with a complex acylated 3, 28-O-bisglycoside structure (Jacobsen, Fairbrother et al. 1996). Unlike most other immunostimulators, QS-21 (**Fig 8**) is water-soluble and can be used in vaccines with or without emulsion type formulations. In a variety of animal models, QS-21 has augmented the immunogenicity of protein, glycoprotein and polysaccharide antigens (Singh and O'Hagan 1999). QS-21 has been shown to stimulate both humoral and cell-mediated Th1 and CTL responses to subunit antigens. Clinical trials are in progress with QS-21, alone or in combination with carriers and other immunostimulants for vaccines against infections including influenza, HSV, HIV, HBV and malaria and cancers including melanoma, colon and B-cell lymphoma. Several structural analogs of QS21 derived from wholly synthetic or semi synthetic route have resulted in improved understanding of the mechanism of action of this saponin molecule. Now it is imperative that the mode of action of this molecule is through the action of formyl group on the triterinoid moiety of the saponon with the T-cell receptor that leads to to strong TH_1 response. Thus it hardly needs to emphasize that development of more plant based adjuvants are highly desirable for developing vaccines against today's societal dreadful diseases like cancer and other infectious diseases.

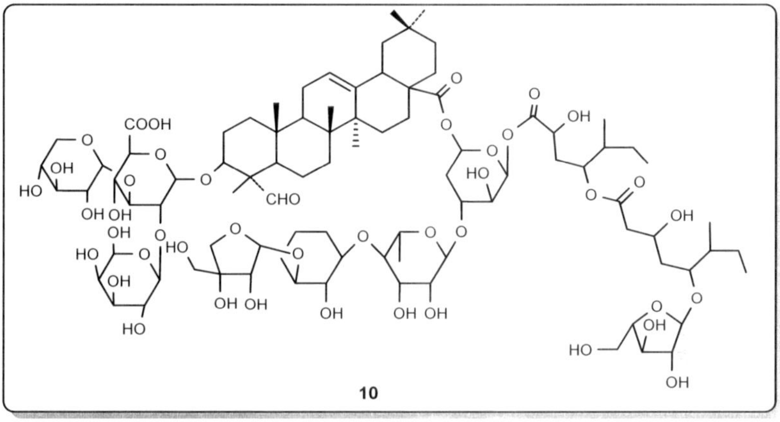

Fig. 11. QS-21, a saponin isolated from *Quillaja saponaria*

7. Current clinical status of potent immune adjuvants

As reviewed in the above sections, the use of PRR ligands particularly TLR and NLR agonists as vaccine adjuvants has been extensively explored with the new generation vaccines which contains defined antigens, These PRR ligands function as immune adjuavants and provide safe and even more effective alternate to live attenuated/dead whole organism based vaccines which induces strong Th1 and T-cytotoxic responses need to treat various cancer as well as infectious and allergic agents. In-fact, these PRR based immune adjuavnts not only enhances the immunological response of vaccine candidates/formulations but perform many functions. A number of ongoing clinical trials with PRR ligands in prophylactic as well as therapeutic vaccines against infectious agents, cancer and allergic agents are presented in Table 2, 3 and 4.

Various small molecules derived from lipid A and RNA/DNA oligonucleotides activate TLR4 and TLR7/8 respectively represents potential class of immune adjuvants and vaccine encompassing these agonists finds application in the area of infectious and allergic diseases including cancer as shown in **Table 2, 3 and 4**. As discussed in section 4.3 and 4.3.1, the discovery of and understanding of functioning of NLRs as well as identification of their ligands such as DAP-containing peptidoglycan (FK156 and FK565), MDP and its lipidated and less pyrogenic analogs, chitosan, Quil A etc. are in preclinical studies also represent important classes of future's immune adjuvants and might find clinical applications along either alone or in combination with TLRs agonist against infectious and other disease conditions. Apart from the small molecules, several proteins such as flagellin (TLR5 agonists), oligonucleotide such as polyI:poly C RNA (TLR3 agonist) and several CpG (or CpG ODN) based ligands (TLR9 agonists) also find very promising results in various phase of clinical trials. Among these three, only unmethylated cytosine-phosphate-guanine-oligodeoxynucleotides (CpG ODN) and its analogs find applications against infectious, cancer and allergic diseases as shown in **Table 2, 3 and 4**. The analogs of CPG stabilized by a phosphorothioate backbone and based on nucleotide sequence and length, CpGs are classified into class A, class B, and class C, and activate a predominantly strong Th1 response, a property which has been harnessed for oncological clinical trials (shown in Table 3). CpG ODNs can also be used as an adjuvant in vaccines and could be considered for the treatment of Th2-mediated Type I allergic disorders(Kanzler, Barrat et al. 2007; Basith, Manavalan et al. 2011) (**Table 4**).

Target	TLR agonist as adjuvants	Vaccines/antigens	Indication	Status (Company)*
TLR3	Synthetic, mismatched double-stranded **poly I:poly C RNA**	Ampligen	HIV	P-II (H)
TLR4	**MPL adjuvant**	**Fendrix**	**Hepatitis B**	**Approved in EU(GSK)**
	MPL adjuvant	**Cervarix**	**Human papillomavirus**	**Approved (GSK)**
	Synthetic MPL RC-529	**Supervax**	**Hepatitis B**	**Approved in Argentina (DT)**
TLR5	Fusion proteins of flagellin to hemaglutinin	Matrix Protein-2	Influenza	P-I (V)
TLR7/8	**Imiquimod cream 5%**	**Aldara**	**Papilloma-induced genital warts**	**Approved (3MP)**
	ANA975; oral prodrug of isatoribine (nucleotide analog)		Hepatitis C	P-I on hold (A/N)
	Resiquimod (R-848) (TLR7/8)		HCV Herpes simplex virus	P-II (3MP) P-III suspended (3MP)
	R851 (topical treatment)		Human papillomavirus	P-II (3MP/T)
TLR9	CpG-ODN 1018 ISS	Heplisav	Hepatitis B	P-III (DT) on hold
	CpG C class ODN: CpG10101,		Hepatitis C	P-II discontinued (CP)
	CpG B class ODN: CpG7909,	VaxImmune	Anthrax	P-I (CP)
	CpG-ODN	Influenza antigens	Influenza	Preclinical (DT)
	CpG-ODN	Remune (inactivated HIV-1 virus) with YB2055	Human immunodeficiency virus	P-I/II (IP/IRC)

*Full name of developing company/institutes: H – Hemispherx; GSK – GlaxoSmithKline; DT-Dynavax Technologies; V – Vaxinate; 3MP – 3M Phrama; A – Anadys; N – Novartis; CP – Coley Pharmaceuticals; IP – Idera Pharmaceuticals; IRC - Immune Response Corporation.

Table 2. TLR agonists in clinical development for infectious diseases

Target	TLR agonists as adjuvants	Vaccine/antigens	Indication	Status (Company)
TLR3	IPH 31XX (structure not disclosed)		Breast cancer	Preclinical (InP)
TLR4	MPL (enclosed in liposomal vehicle)	Stimuvax/BLP25 (Synthetic cancer-associated MUC1 protein)	Non-small-cell lung cancer	P-II (B/M)
TLR5				
TLR7/8	**Imiquimod (used as 5% cream)**	**Aldara**	**Basal cell carcinoma**	**Approved (3MP)**
	Imidazoquinoline 852A		Melanoma	P-II (3MP)
TLR9	CpG B class ODN CpG7909 or PF3512676	Along with chemotherapy	Non-small-cell lung cancer	P-III (CP/P)
	CpG B class ODN :1018ISS	Along with Rituxan	Non-Hodgkin's lymphoma	P-II (DT)
	CpG-ODN : HYB2055 or IMO-2055 or IMOxine		Renal cell carcinoma	P-II (IP)
	CpG motif containing circular ODN	dSLIM	Metastatic colorectal cancer	P-I/II (M)
	CpG B class ODN	Along with chemotherapy	Colorectal cancer	P-I (DT)
	CpG-ODN 7909 in incomplete Freund adjuvant	Melan-A peptide	Melanoma	P-I (CP/GSK)
	Immunodrug carrier QbG10	CYT004-MelQbG10 vaccine containing Melan-A/MART-1 protein	Melanoma	P-II (CB)

*Full name of developing company/institutes: InP – Innate Pharma; B – Biomera; M – Merck; P – Pfizer; M - Mologen; GSK – GlaxoSmithKline; DT-Dynavax Technologies; CB – Cytos Biotechnology; 3MP – 3M Phrama; CP – Coley Pharmaceuticals; IP – Idera Pharmaceuticals.

Table 3. TLR agonists in Clinical development for cancer

Like agonists, TLR antagonist showing promiscuous results in the clinical trial for the treatment of number of inflammatory and auto-immune diseases. These TLR antagonists have been mostly developed as structural analogs of agonists which bind to the receptor but fail to induce signal transduction, thus preventing the agonistic action of TLR ligands responsible for the induction of the inflammatory/autoimmune cascade. Two lipid A analogs such as E5564 and Tak 242 developed by Eisai and Takeda Pharma (derived from SAR studies during design of agonists) acts as potent antagonists of TLR4 and currently are in clinical trials for the treatment of sepsis or septic shock (inflammatory disorder)(Kanzler,

Barrat et al. 2007; Basith, Manavalan et al. 2011). Similarly, CpG ODN analog such as DV1079 (developed by collaborative efforts of Dynavax and GSK) act as potent TLR7/9 antagonists and is currently in preclinical study for the treatment of autoimmune disorder. Despite the development of many small immune adjuavnts, still there is a need for more efficacious and potent immune adjuavants for poorly immunogenic antigenic based vaccine, while going through the structural features of many PAMPs based and synthetic adjuvants as well as understanding their role in vacccine formulation, the molecules become ideal immune adjuavnts when they qualifies the parameters as discussed in section 9. Furthermore, while designing immune adjuvant, we should keep certain structural features in mind as discussed in section 10 which might give direction for the generation of potent, efficacious and ideal immune adjuvants. Moreover, in recent years, the co-crystal structure of PRRs(Kanzler, Barrat et al. 2007; Basith, Manavalan et al. 2011) particularly TLRs with their ligands have been identified, therefore their bio-informatics model system would be developed which further provide very useful inputs towards the designing of potent and ideal immune adjuvants.

Target	TLR agonists as adjuvants	Vaccines/antigens	Indication	Status (Company)
TLR4	**MPL**	**Pollinex Quattro (modified allergens)**	**Allergic rhinitis (multiple allergens)**	**Marketed (EU)**
	MPL	Ragweed SC/Pollinex Quatro; Ragweed/Pollinex R (ragweed pollen extract	Allergic rhinitis (ragweed)	P-II (AP)
	CRX-675	Ragweed allergen	Allergic rhinitis (ragweed)	P-I (GSK(C))
TLR9	Covalently linked CpG B class ODN: 1018 ISS	Tolamba (Amb a 1 ragweed allergen	Allergic rhinitis (ragweed)	P-II/III (DT)
	Immunodrug carrier QbG10	Allergen extract (CYT005-AllQbG10)	Allergic rhinitis (dust mite)	P-II (CB)
	CpG B ODN	Amba 1	Asthma	P-II (DT)
	Second generation CpG-ODN		Asthma	P-I (DT/AZ)
	CpG-ODN	AVE0675	Asthma	P-I (CP/SA)

*Full name of developing company/institutes: AP – Allergy Therapeutics; GSK – GlaxoSmithKline; DT - Dynavax Technologies; N – Novartis; CP – Coley Pharmaceuticals; IP – Idera Pharmaceuticals; CB – Cytos Biotechnology; AZ – Astra Zeneca; SA – Sonafi-Aventis.

Table 4. TLR agonists in clinical development for allergic diseases

Target	TLR antagonists	Indication	Status (Company)
TLR4	TAK-242	Severe sepsis	P-III (TPC)
	E5564 or Eritoran: a lipid A derivative	Severe sepsis	P-III (E)
TLR7 and TLR 9	Immunoregulatory sequence IRS 954	Lupus	Preclinical (DT)

Full name of developing company/institutes: TPC – Takeda Pharmaceutical Company; E- Eisai.

Table 5. TLR antagonists in clinical development for anti-inflammatory and auto-immune diseases

8. Role of adjuvants in the immune responses

Precisely, how adjuvants enhance the immune response is yet unknown, but they appear to exert different effects to improve the immune response to vaccine antigens, as such they:

i. *Immunomodulation*- This refers to the ability of adjuvants to activate the immune response either to Th1 or Th2.
ii. *Targeting*- Improve antigen delivery to antigen presenting cells (APCs), increase cellular infiltration, inflammation, and trafficking to the injection site.
iii. Activation of APCs by up-regulating co-stimulatory signals, major histo-compatibility complexes (MHC) expression and inducing cytokine release.
iv. *Antigen Presentation*- Enhance antigen processing and presentation by APCs and increase the speed, magnitude and duration of the immune response.
v. Antigen Depot formation
vi. *Induction of antibody*-modulation of antibody avidity, affinity as well as the magnitude, isotype or subclass induction.
vii. *Stimulate cell mediated immunity* and lymphocyte proliferation nonspecifically.

9. Characteristics of an ideal adjuvant

It is likely that the "ideal" adjuvant does not and will not exist, because each adjuvant and its targeted antigen will have their unique requirements. Nevertheless, the generic characteristics summarized below would be desirable. To date, no adjuvant meets all of these goals.

i. It must be safe, including freedom from immediate and long-term side effects.
ii. It should be biodegradable or easily removed from the body after its adjuvant effect is exhausted to decrease the risk of late adverse effects.
iii. It should elicit a more robust protective or therapeutic immune response combined with the antigen than when the antigen is administered alone.
iv. It must be defined chemically and biologically, so that there is no lot-to-lot variation in the manufactured product, thereby assuring consistent responses in vaccines between studies and over time.
v. Efficacy should be achieved using fewer doses and/or lower concentrations of the antigen.

10. Requirement for adjuvants

While going through the structure of various immune adjuvants of diverse classes, we conclude that following are few chemical traits molecules should ppossess to become more efficious and potent immue adjuvants. Furthermore, following chemical traits should also be considered for the chemical modifications of PAMPS or other natural derived molecules.

Following are the structural requirements for a molecule to act as an efficient adjuvant:

i. Hydrophilic-lipophilic balance.
ii. Presence of micellar structures to facilitate depot formation.
iii. Lipophilic structure enveloping the antigen to preserve the structure required for its immunogenicity.
iv. Lipophilic structures capable of effective cytosol trafficking.
v. Presence of functional groups to activate/substitute co-stimulatory signals for effective Th1 immunity.
vi. Overall structural design to stimulate Th1 and Th2 balance.
vii. Structure to be ligand for T cell or DC surface receptors.

11. Conclusion and future prospects regarding the use of immune adjuvants towards design of new breed potent vaccines

The literature discussed here present a wide variety of pathogen derived natural and synthetic PRR agonist and antagonists, among these some of these molecules already which find potential application as immune adjuants in various vaccine formulations to treat dreadful cancer, infectious and allergic diseases. Furthermore, various plant derived immune are also discussed here which are now in very preliminary stages and also present the potential starting points and need serious efforts first towards the understanding of their mechanism of action and further development. For TLR agonists to achieve further recognition in the clinic it will be critical to undertake side-by-side comparisons against the same antigen using selected immune monitoring assays that measure the quantity and quality of responses (e.g. avidity, memory cell generation, durability) as well as further refinement in their chemical structure (wherever need) keeping in mind the above motioned points required for molecules to become ideal immune adjuavants. Furthermore, the potential immune adjuvant candidates either in the preclinical or in various clinical phases discussed here represent only a fraction of the current efforts to clinically translate our current understanding of some of the exploited PRR and innate immunity. Many other strategies and tactics to stimulate or inhibit others PRR are being developed and these studies are just beginning. Understanding the role of different PRR for different pathological conditions are growing rapidly and this will surely continue to be more productive and fruitful field for the development of more efficacious and potent vaccine candidates for various unmet cancer and infectious diseases.

12. References

Adam, A., R. Ciorbaru, et al. (1974). "Adjuvant activity of monomeric bacterial cell wall peptidoglycans." *Biochem. Biophys. Res. Commun.* 56: 561–567.

Akira, S. and H. Hemmi (2003). "Recognition of pathogen-associated molecular patterns by TLR family." *Immunol. Lett.* 85: 85–95.

Akira, S., S. Uematsu, et al. (2006). "Pathogen Recognition and Innate Immunity." *Cell* 124: 783-801.

Alamgir, M. and S. J. Uddin (2010). "Recent advances on the ethnomedicinal plants as immunomodulatory agents." *Ethnomedicine: A Source of Complementary Therapeutics*: 227-244.

Azuma, I. (1992). "Synthetic immunoadjuvants: application to non-specific host stimulation and potentiation of vaccine immunogenicity." *Vaccine* 10: 1000-1006.

Azuma, I. and T. Seya (2001). "Development of immunoadjuvants for immunotherapy of cancer." *International Immunopharmacology* 1: 1249-1259.

Basith, S., B. Manavalan, et al. (2011). "Toll-like receptor modulators: a patent review (2006 -- 2010)." *Expert Opin. Ther. Patents* 21: 927-944.

Berg, M., S. Offermanns, et al. (1994). "Synthetic lipopeptide Pam3CysSer(Lys)4 is an effective activator of human platelets." *American Journal of Physiology* 266: C1684-1691.

Bessler, W. G., M. Cox, et al. (1998). "Synthetic lipopeptide analogs of bacterial lipoprotein are potent polyclonal activators for murine B lymphocytes." *Journal of Immunology* 135: 1900-1905.

Bishop, G. A., Y. Hsing, et al. (2000). "Molecular mechanisms of B lymphocyte activation by the immune response modifier R-848." *Journal of Immunology* 165: 5552-5557.

Blasius, A. L. and B. Beutler (2010). "Intracellular Toll-like receptors." *Immunity* 32: 305–315.

Boyden, E. D. and W. F. Dietrich (2006). "Nalp1b controls mouse macrophage susceptibility to anthrax lethal toxin." *Nature Genet.* 38: 240–244.

Byars, N. E. and A. C. Allison (1987). "Adjuvant formulation for use in vaccines to elicit both cell-mediated and humoral immunity." *Vaccine* 5: 223-228.

Carneiro, L. A., J. G. Magalhaes, et al. (2008). "Nod-like proteins in inflammation and disease." *J. Pathol.* 214: 136–148.

Chamaillard, M. (2003). "An essential role for NOD1 in host recognition of bacterial peptidoglycan containing diaminopimelic acid." *Nature Immunol.* 4: 702–707.

Chamaillard, M., M. Hashimoto, et al. (2003). "An essential role for NOD1 in host recognition of bacterial peptidoglycan containing diaminopimelic acid." *Nature Immunology* 4: 702-707.

Coulombe, F., M. Divangahi, et al. (2009). "Increased NOD2-mediated recognition of N-glycolyl muramyl dipeptide." *Journal of Experimental Medicine* 206: 1709-1716.

Dalsgaard, K. (1974). "Saponin adjuvants III. Isolation of a substance from Quitfaja saponaria Molina with adjuvant activity in foot and-mouth disease vaccines." *Arch Gesamte Virusforsch* 44: 243-254.

Franchi, L. and G. Nunez (2008). "The Nlrp3 inflammasome is critical for aluminium hydroxide-mediated IL-1â secretion but dispensable for adjuvant activity." *Eur. J. Immunol.* 38: 2085–2089.

Franchi, L., J. H. Park, et al. (2008). "Intracellular NOD-like receptors in innate immunity, infection and disease." *Cell. Microbiol.* 10: 1–8.

Fritz, J. H., R. L. Ferrero, et al. (2006). "Nod-like proteins in immunity, inflammation and disease." *Nature Immunology* 7: 1250–1257.

Geddes, K., J. G. Magalhaes, et al. (2009). "Unleashing the therapeutic potential of NOD-like receptors." *Nat. Rev. Drug Discov* 8: 465-479.

Gibson, S. J., J. M. Lindh, et al. (2002). "Plasmacytoid dendritic cells produce cytokines and mature in response to the TLR7 agonists, imiquimod and resiquimod." *Cell Immunology* 218: 74-86.

Girardin, S. E. (2003). "Nod1 detects a unique muropeptide from gram-negative bacterial peptidoglycan." *Science* 300: 1584–1587.

Girardin, S. E. (2003). "Nod2 is a general sensor of peptidoglycan through muramyl dipeptide (MDP) detection." *J. Biol. Chem.* 278: 8869–8872.

Gupta, R. K., E. H. Relyveld, et al. (1993). "Adjuvants-a balance between toxicity and adjuvanticity." *Vaccine* 11: 293-306.

Hoebe, K., E. Janssen, et al. (2004). "The interface between innate and adaptive immunity." *Nat Immunology* 5: 971–974.

Hoebe, K., Z. Jiang, et al. (2006). "TLR signaling pathways: opportunities for activation and blockade in pursuit of therapy." *Curr Pharm Des* 12: 4123-34.

Hoffmann, J. A. (2003). "The immune response of Drosophila." *Nature* 426: 33–38.

Hoffmann, P., S. Heinle, et al. (1998). "timulation of human and murine adherent cells by bacterial lipoprotein and synthetic lipopeptide analogues." *Immunobiology* 177: 158-170.

Hopkins, P. A. and S. Sriskandan (2005). "Mammalian Toll-like receptors: to immunity and beyond." *Clinical Experimental Immunology* 140: 395-407.

Hsu, L. C. "A NOD2–NALP1 complex mediates caspase-1-dependent IL-1â secretion in response to Bacillus anthracis infection and muramyl dipeptide." *Proc. Natl Acad. Sci. USA* 105: 7803–7808.

Inohara, N. (2003). "Host recognition of bacterial muramyl dipeptide mediated through NOD2. Implications for Crohn's disease." *J. Biol. Chem.* 278: 5509–5512.

Iwasaki, A. and R. Medzhitov (2004). "Toll-like receptors control of the adaptive immune responses." *Nature Immunology* 5: 987-995.

Jacobsen, N. E., W. J. Fairbrother, et al. (1996). "Structure of the saponin adjuvant QS-21 and its base-catalyzed isomerization product by 1H and natural abundance 13C NMR spectroscopy." *Carbohydrate Research* 280: 1-14.

Janeway, C. A. J. (2001). "How the immune system works to protect the host from infection: a personal view." *Proceedings of the National Academy of Science USA* 98: 7461-7468.

Janeway, C. A. J. and R. Medzhitov (2002). "Innate immune recognition." *Annual Review Immunology* 20: 197-216.

Johnson, A. G., S. Gaines, et al. (1956). "Studies on the 0 antigen of Salmonella typhosa V. Enhancement of antibody response to protein antigens by the purified lipopolysaccharide." *Journal of Experimental Medicine* 103: 225-246.

Johnson, D. A., D. S. Keegan, et al. (1999). "3-O-Desacyl monophosphoryl lipid A derivatives: synthesis and immunostimulant activities." *Journal of Medicinal Chemistry* 42: 4640-4649.

Kaisho, T. and S. Akira (2002). "Toll-like receptors as adjuvant receptors." *Biochimica. Biophysica Acta* 1589: 1-13.

Kanneganti, T. D. (2006). "Bacterial RNA and small antiviral compounds activate caspase-1 through cryopyrin/Nalp3." *Nature* 440,: 233–236.

Kanneganti, T. D. (2006). "Critical role for Cryopyrin/Nalp3 in activation of caspase-1 in response to viral infection and double-stranded RNA." *J. Biol. Chem.* 281: 36560–36568.

Kanzler, H., F. J. Barrat, et al. (2007). "Therapeutic targeting of innate immunity with Toll-like receptor agonists and antagonists." *NATURE MEDICINE* 13: 552-559.

Kawai, T. and S. Akira (2010). "The role of pattern-recognition receptors in innate immunity: Update on Toll-like receptors." *Nat Immunology* 11: 373–384.

Khajuria, A., A. Gupta, et al. (2007). "RLJ-NE-299A: A new plant based vaccine adjuvant." *Vaccine* 25: 2706-2715.

Kumar, H., T. Kawai, et al. (2009). "Pathogen recognition in the innate immune response." *Biochem J* 420: 1–16.

Kumar, H., T. Kawai, et al. (2011). "Pathogen Recognition by the Innate Immune System." *International Reviews of Immunology* 30: 16–34.

Kumar, H. M. S. and P. P. Singh (2010). "Development of Novel Lipidated Analogs of Picroside as Vaccine adjuvants: Acylated analogs of Picroside II elicit strong Th1 and Th2 response to Ovalbumin in mice." *Vaccine* 28: 8327-8337.

Kumar, S., P. Gupta, et al. ((2011). "A review on immunostimulatory plants." *Journal of Chinese Integrative Medicine* 9: 117-128.

Lee, J., T. H. Chuang, et al. (2003). "Molecular basis for the immunostimulatory activity of guanine nucleoside analogs: activation of Toll-like receptor 7." *Proceedings of the National Academy of Sciences USA* 100: 6646-6651.

Lemaitre, B., E. Nicolas, et al. (1996). "The dorsoventral regulatory gene cassette spatzle/Toll/cactus controls the potent antifungal response in Drosophila adults." *Cell* 86: 973–983.

Li, H., S. B. Willingham, et al. (2008). "Cutting edge: inflammasome activation by alum and alum's adjuvant effect are mediated by NLRP3." *J. Immunol.* 181: 17–21.

Lien, E. and D. T. Golenbock (2003). "Adjuvants and their signaling pathways: beyond TLRs." *Nature Immunology* 4: 1162-1164.

Makkouk, A. and A. M. Abdelnoor (2009). "The potential use of toll-like receptor (TLR) agonists and antagonists as prophylactic and/or therapeutic agents." *Immunopharmacology and Immunotoxicology* 31: 331–338.

Mariathasan, S. (2006). "Cryopyrin activates the inflammasome in response to toxins and ATP." *Nature* 440: 228–232.

Martinon, F., L. Agostini, et al. (2004). "Identification of bacterial muramyl dipeptide as activator of the NALP3/cryopyrin inflammasome." *Curr. Biol.* 14: 1929–1934.

Martinon, F., V. Petrilli, et al. (2006). "Gout-associated uric acid crystals activate the NALP3 inflammasome." *Nature* 440: 237–241.

Mbow, M. L., E. D. Gregorio, et al. (2010). "New adjuvants for human vaccines." *Current Opinion in Immunology* 22: 411–416.

Medzhitov, R. (2007). "Recognition of microorganisms and activation of the immune response." *Nature* 449: 819–826.

Migliore-Samour, D. (1979). "Immunostimulating and adjuvant activities of a low molecular weight lipopeptide." *C R. Seances Acad. Sci. D(in French)* 289: 473–476.

Moingeon, P., J. Haensler, et al. (2001). "Towards the rational design of Th1 adjuvants." *Vaccine* 19: 4363-4372.

Panchabhai, T. S., U. P. Kulkarni, et al. (2008). "Validation of Therapeutic Claims of Tinospora cordifolia:A Review." *Phytotherapy Research* 22: 425-441.

Pandey, S. and D. K. Agrawal (2006). "Immunobiology of toll-like receptors:Emerging trends." *Immunol. Cell Biol.* 84: 333–341.

Parant, M., G. Riveau, et al. (1984). "Inhibition of endogenous pyrogen-induced fever by a muramyl dipeptide derivative." *American Journal of Physiology* 247: 169-174.

Patwardhan, B. (2000). "Ayurveda: the designer medicine: review of ethnopharmacology and bioprospecting research." *Indian Drugs* 37: 213- 227.

Petrilli, V. (2007). "Activation of the NALP3 inflammasome is triggered by low intracellular potassium concentration." *Cell Death Differ.* 14: 1583–1589.

Pockros, P. J., D. Guyader, et al. (2007). "Oral resiquimod in chronic HCV infection: safety and efficacy in 2 placebo-controlled, double-blind phase IIa studies." *J Hepatol* 47: 174-82.

Puri, A., R. P. Saxena, et al. (1992). "Immunostimulant activity of Picroliv, the iridoid glycoside fraction of Picrorhiza kurroa, and its protective action against Leishmania donovani infection in Hamsters." *Planta Medica* 58: 528-532.

Re, F. and J. L. Strominger (2002). "Monomeric recombinant MD-2 binds toll-like receptor 4 tightly and confers lipopolysaccharide responsiveness." *Journal of Biological Chemistry* 277: 23427-23432.

Rezaei, N. (2006). "Therapeutic targeting of pattern-recognition receptors." *Int. Immunopharmacol.* 6: 863–869.

Rock, F. L., G. Hardiman, et al. (1998). "A family of human receptors structurally related to Drosophila Toll." *Proc Natl Acad Sci USA* 95: 588-93.

Romagne, F. (2007). "Current and future drugs targeting one class of innate immunity receptors: The toll-like receptors." *Drug Discov. Today* 12: 80–87.

Sansonetti, P. J. (2006). "The innate signaling of dangers and the dangers of innate signaling." *Nat Immunology* 7: 1237-42.

Schwartz, R. S. (2000). "Advances in Immunology-A New Series of Review Articles." *New England Journal of Medicine* 343: 61.

Seifert, R., G. Schultz, et al. (1990). "Activation of superoxide formation and lysozyme release in human neutrophils by the synthetic lipopeptide Pam3Cys-Ser-(Lys)4. Involvement of guanine-nucleotide-binding proteins and synergism with chemotactic peptides." *Biochemical Journal* 267: 795-802.

Singh, M. and D. O'Hagan (1999). "Advances in vaccine adjuvants." *Nature Biotechnology* 17: 1075-1081.

Stahl, P. D. and R. A. Ezekowitz (1998). "The mannose receptors is a pattern recognition receptor involved in host defence." *Current Opinion in Immunology* 10: 50-5.

Stanley, M. A. (2002). "Imiquimod and the imidazoquinolones: mechanism of action and therapeutic potential." *Clinical and Experimental Dermatology* 27: 571-577.

Takeuchi, O. and S. Akira (2010). "Pattern recognition receptors and inflammation." *Cell* 140: 805–820.

Taylor, M. E. and K. Drickamer (1993). "Structural requirements for high affinity binding of complex ligands by the macrophages mannose receptors." *Journal of Biological Chemistry* 268: 399-404.

Thatte, U. M. and S. A. Dahanukar (1997). "The 'Rasayana' Concept: Clues from Immunodulatory Therapy. In: upadhyay S. (ed); Narosa Publishing House, New Delhi." *Immunomodulation*: 141-148.

Wack, A. and R. Rappuoli (2005). "Vaccinology at the beginning of the 21st century." *Current in Opinion Immunology* 17: 411-418.

Werts, C., S. E. Girardin, et al. (2006). "TIR, CARD and PYRIN: three domains for an antimicrobial triad." *Cell Death Differ.* 13: 798–815.

Wiesmüller, K.-H., W. G. Bessler, et al. (1992). "Solid phase peptide synthesis of lipopeptide vaccines eliciting epitope-specific B-, T-helper and T-killer cell response." *International Journal of Peptide Protein Research* 40: 255-60.

Wiesmüller, K.-H., G. Jung, et al. (1989). "Novel low-molecular-weight synthetic vaccine against foot-and-mouth disease containing a potent B-cell and macrophage activator." *Vaccine* 7: 29-33.

9

Development of an Ultrasensitive CRP Latex Agglutination Reagent by Using Amino Acid Spacers

Tomoe Komoriya[1], Kazuaki Yoshimune[1], Masahiro Ogawa[2], Mitsuhiko Moriyama[2] and Hideki Kohno[1]
[1]*College of Industrial Technology, Nihon University, Nerashino, Chiba*
[2]*School of Medicine, Nihon University, Chiyoda-ku, Tokyo*
Japan

1. Introduction

William S. Tillett (1930) discovered that C-Reactive Protein (CRP) is an acute-phase serum protein that reacts with the C polysaccharide of *Pneumococcal cell wall*. CRP is present in human serum and its level increases during systemic inflammation. Therefore, CRP represents a sensitive marker of systemic inflammation and tissue damage; precise determination of CRP levels has proven to be useful in the screening of various diseases, monitoring treatment response, and detection of concomitant infections[1)].

In recent years, studies have indicated that arteriosclerosis may be due to vascular inflammation, and that CRP concentration in the blood correlates with the degree of functional disorder of the vascular endothelium. High CRP serum levels have been shown to be a risk factor for anginal damage or myocardial infarction-induced stroke[2-4)]. Therefore, a highly sensitive and accurate method of measuring CRP is clinically significant.

We conducted a sensitive quantification of CRP concentration using latex turbidimetric immunoassay (LTIA). This method measures turbidity changes in the latex immunoagglutination reaction using a latex reagent containing an antibody or antigen conjugated to latex particles[5-8)]. LTIA is a simpler, more rapid, and more highly sensitive assay of CRP compared with radioimmunoassay (RIA) and enzyme immunoassay (EIA). LTIA can measure CRP concentrations at levels between 10^{-10}–10^{-11} mol/l of serum, and can be performed using automated systems for high throughput immunoassay analysis.

In this study, we investigated a latex reagent containing an amino acid spacer to measure high-sensitivity CRP. We measured serum CRP levels in healthy individuals, people with liver disease, and diabetics. We report that this method is highly useful and clinically beneficial.

2. Materials and methods

2.1 CRP antigens

We used two kinds of whole CRP and five forms of CRP fragments. The first C-Reactive Protein High Control (human serum), termed Human CRP, was purchased from Dako

(Glostrup, Denmark) for use as an immunogen and standard. The second whole CRP protein, termed recombinant CRP (rCRP), was purchased from Oriental Yeast (Tokyo, Japan). This was used in the screening of hybridoma cells for the production of monoclonal antibodies. Five CRP fragments were prepared by the production of recombinant CRP fragments a method described below for epitope analysis.

2.2 Production of monoclonal antibodies (MoAbs)

Two 6 to 8-week-old BALB/c female mice (Oriental Yeast) were immunized biweekly with Human CRP. The CRP was injected in complete Freund's adjuvant (Sigma-Aldrich, St.Louis, MO) or incomplete Freund's adjuvant (Sigma-Aldrich) and sterile saline subcutaneously at multiple sites on the ventral area of the mouse. One week following the fifth booster immunization, tail blood was collected, and the ability of the antibody present in the serum to bind rCRP was determined by ELISA. Splenocytes were prepared 3 d after final immunization, and were used in cell fusion experiments.

The cell fusion experiments were described previously.[9] Briefly, immune spleen cells and a 1:5 ratio of P3U1 myeloma cells cultured in RPMI 1640 medium (Invitrogen, Carlsbad, CA) supplemented with 10% v/v FetalClone II (Thrmo Fisher Scientific, Waltham, MA) were fused using 50% w/v polyethylene Glycol 1500 in 75 mM Hepes (pH 8.0; Roche, Basel, Switzerland). The fused cells were then suspended in RPMI 1640 medium containing HAT Supplement (HAT medium, Invitrogen), and cultured in 96-well plates (10 cells/100 μl/well) under standard 5% CO_2 culture conditions at 37°C. After approximately 10 d in culture, the hybridoma supernatants were screened by ELISA. Antibody-secreting hybridomas were then expanded in HAT medium, cloned by limiting dilution, and cultured for a further 10 d. The hybridomas were then subjected to two further rounds of selection by ELISA screening and cloning by limiting dilution. Selected hybridomas were cultured in RPMI 1640 medium. The resulting supernatants were used in MoAb characterization. MoAbs were isotyped using the IsoStrip Mouse Monoclonal Antibody Isotyping kit (Roche). Antibodies were also prepared on a large scale, as ascitic fluid, by inoculating the relevant hybridoma cells into 10-week-old pristane-treated male BALB/c mice. The MoAbs included in the ascitic fluid were purified by ammonium sulfate precipitation at 50% and by protein A or protein G chromatography.

Care and treatment of the experimental animals conformed to the Nihon University guidelines for the ethical treatment of laboratory animals.

2.3 Detection of antibodies in serum and culture medium by enzyme-linked immunosorbent assay (ELISA)

rCRP diluted in 100 mM carbonate buffer (pH 9.6) was added to 96-well plates and incubated for 2 h at 25°C. After three washes with phosphate-buffered saline (PBS) containing 0.05% v/v Tween 20 (PBS-T), the wells were blocked for 1 h at 25°C with 5.0% w/v skim milk (Becton, Dickinson, Franklin Lakes, NJ) in PBS, and washed 3 times with PBS-T. The antibody diluted in mouse serum or hybridoma supernatant was appropriately diluted in PBS and added to the wells, and this was incubated for 1 h at room temperature. PBS in place of the antibody solution served as a negative control. After three washes in PBS-T, 100 μl of HRP-conjugated goat anti-mouse IgG secondary antibody (diluted 1:4,000 in phosphate buffer) was then added to the wells, and this was incubated for 1 h at room temperature. The wells were then washed with TBS-T, and peroxidase activity was measured colorimetrically using 100 μl of substrate solution containing 0.4% *o*-phenylenediamine dihydrochloride (Sigma-Aldrich) in a solution of 0.1% citric buffer (pH 5.0), and H_2O_2 added at a final concentration of 0.015% immediately prior to use. Following incubation for 20 min at room temperature, the reaction was stopped by the addition of 2N H_2SO_4, and the absorbance at 492 nm was determined using a microplate reader (Spectra Max M2, Molecular Devices, Ontario, Canada).

2.4 Production of recombinant CRP fragments

2.4.1 Amplification of the CRP gene

Genomic DNA was extracted from whole blood using the GFX Genomic Blood DNA Purification kit (GE healthcare, Buckinghamshire, England). Using the extracted genomic DNA as template, seven forward primers containing the CACC sequence and one reverse primer (Table 1) were used to amplify five different *CRP* gene fragments, named CRP 01, CRP 02, CRP 03, CRP 04, CRP 05, CRP a F, CRP a F and CRP b R, CRP b R by polymerase chain reaction (PCR).

Primer	Sequence (5′→3′)	Tm (°C)	Length (bp)
CRP-01	5′-CACCATGTCGAGGAAGGCTTTTG-3′	70.5	612
CRP-02	5′-CACCTCGTATGCCACCAAGAGACA-3′	71.1	465
CRP-03	5′-CACCAGGGTGAGGAAGAGTCTGAAG-3′	70.1	276
CRP-04	5′-CACCGAAGGAAGCCAGTCCCT-3′	76.6	183
CRP-05	5′-CACCACCATCTATCTTGGCGGG-3′	71.3	105
CRP-R	5′-TCAGGGCCACAGCTGGGGTTT-3′	73.9	-
CRP-a-F	5′-CACCGACATGTCGAGGAAG-3′	64.5	300
CRP-a-R	5′-TCAGGACTCCCAGCTTGTACA-3′	64.7	-
CRP-b-F	5′-CACCGGGTACAGTATTTTC-3′	56.9	375
CRP-b-R	5′-TCAGTTAATCTCATCTGGTGA-3′	57.2	-

Table 1. Forward and Reverse primers for Recombinant CRP

2.4.2 Expression of recombinant CRP fragments

Amplified *CRP* gene fragments were separated by agarose gel electrophoresis containing 0.8 μg/ml of crystal violet. Separated DNA fragments were then extracted and purified using WizardSV GEL and PCR Clean-up System (Promega, Madison, WI).

pET100/D-TOPO vector (Invitrogen) was used to express the *CRP* fragments. pET100/D-TOPO vector and purified DNA were mixed, and the mixture incubated for 5 min at room temperature to complete ligation. *Escherichia coli* TOP10 competent Cells (Invitrogen) were then added to the mixture on ice, which was incubated for 15 min and transformed by the heat-shock treatment method for 30 s at 42°C. Transformed colonies were then identified by colony PCR. The recombinant plasmids were purified using the Wizard SV GEL and SV

Miniprep DNA Purification Systems (Promega), and were transformed into *E. coli* BL21 Star (DE3) (Invitrogen) by heat-shock treatment for 30 s at 42°C . S.O.C. medium (Super Optimal broth with Catabolite repression) containing 2% Tryptone, 0.5% Yeast Extract, 10 mM sodium chloride, 2.5 mM potassium chloride, 10 mM magnesium chloride, 10 mM magnesium sulfate, and 20 mM glucose was then added, the mixture was incubated for 1 h, and the culture solution was transferred to Luria-Bertani broth containing ampicillin (100 μg/ml) and cultured for a further 20 h at 37°C. When an optical density (O.D, λ = 600 nm) of 0.7 was achieved, isopropyl β-D-1-thiogalactopyranoside (IPTG) was added to a final concentration of 1.0 mM. Following 1.5 h incubation, the cells were separated from the culture supernatant by centrifugation (5 min at 14,000 × *g*) and the *E. coli* pellet was lysed with lysis buffer containing 3 mM potassium dihydrogenphosphate, 47 mM dipotassium hydrogenphosphate, 0.4 M sodium chloride, 0.1 mM potassium chloride, 10% v/v glycerine, 0.5% v/v Triton X-100, and 1 mM Imidazole. The suspension was then subjected to three rounds of freeze-thawing, and was divided into soluble and insoluble fractions by centrifugation (5 min at 14,000 × *g*). The proteins in each fraction were then analyzed by sodium dodecyl sulphate-polyacrylamide gel electrophoresis (SDS-PAGE).

2.5 Epitope analysis by western blotting

Expressed CRP fragments were separated by SDS-PAGE on a 12.5% acrylamide gel and transferred to PVDF membrane (Bio-Rad Laboratories, Hercules, CA) using the iBlot Gel Transfer Device and iBlot Transfer stacks mini (Invitrogen) at 20 V for 6 min. A PVDF membrane was then submerged in methanol and ultra pure water and sandwiched in the iBlot Transfer stack mini system. The membrane was blocked for 1 h at 25°C in 5.0% w/v skim milk in PBS-T and washed 3 times in PBS-T. The membranes were then incubated with 4 MoAbs, numbered 4, 5, 7, and 8, for 1 h at room temperature, followed by alkaline phosphatase (AP)-conjugated goat anti-mouse IgG for 1 h at room temperature. Finally, protein bands were visualized using a substrate solution prepared by diluting BCIP/NBT (Moss, Pasadena, MD) 1:10 in buffer (pH 9.8) containing 50 mM 2-amino-2-hydroxymethyl-1,3-propanediol, Tris, 50 mM sodium chloride, and 25 mM magnesium chloride hexahydrate.

2.6 Preparation of anti-CRP latex reagents using monoclonal antibodies (MoAbs)

The binding of antibody to latex particles was performed using the water-soluble carbodiimide (WSC) method[10)] with 1-ethyl-3-(3-dimethyl-aminopropyl) (EDAC; Dojindo Laboratories, Kumamoto, Japan). In this method, carbodiimide activation of carboxylate groups on the surface of latex particles (under acidic conditions) produces an unstable reaction intermediate, O-acylisourea. O-acylisourea subsequently reacts with N-hydroxysuccinimide (NHS; Acros Organics, Antwerp, Belgium) to produce a stable NHS ester (Fig. 1).

Briefly, 0.1 ml of 10% polystyrene latex particles, 0.225 mm in diameter (G1225; JSR, Tokyo, Japan), was added to 1.9 ml of buffer A containing 0.05 mol/l 2-morpholinoethanesulfonic acid monohydrate (MES) buffer (pH 5.6). The mixture was then centrifuged at 22,600 × g for 20 min, and the precipitate was resuspended in 1.0 ml of buffer A. This suspension was then added to 2.0 ml of 20 mg/ml EDAC and 0.23 ml of 50 mg/ml NHS, both dissolved in buffer

A; the mixture was stirred for 30 min at room temperature to form the NHS ester. After production of the NHS ester, the suspension was washed twice with buffer A and the precipitate was resuspended in 1.0 ml of buffer A. The suspension was then added to 2.0 ml of 0.133 mmol/ml amino acid, and the mixture was stirred for 30 min at 37°C and centrifuged at 22,600 × g for 20 min. The precipitate was then washed with buffer A by centrifugation. Similarly, anti-C-reactive protein (anti-CRP) antibody (100 μg/ml in 1.0 ml of buffer A) (Immuno Probe, Saitama, Japan) was conjugated to the latex particles with an amino acid spacer. The latex-conjugated anti-CRP antibody was resuspended in 1.0 ml of buffer A, and the suspension was added to 1.0 ml of 1.0% w/v denatured bovine serum albumin (dnBSA). The suspension was then stirred for 30 min at 25°C and washed with buffer B, containing 0.1 mol/l Tris buffer (pH 8.2) by centrifugation at 22,600 × g for 20 min. The precipitate was then suspended in buffer B.

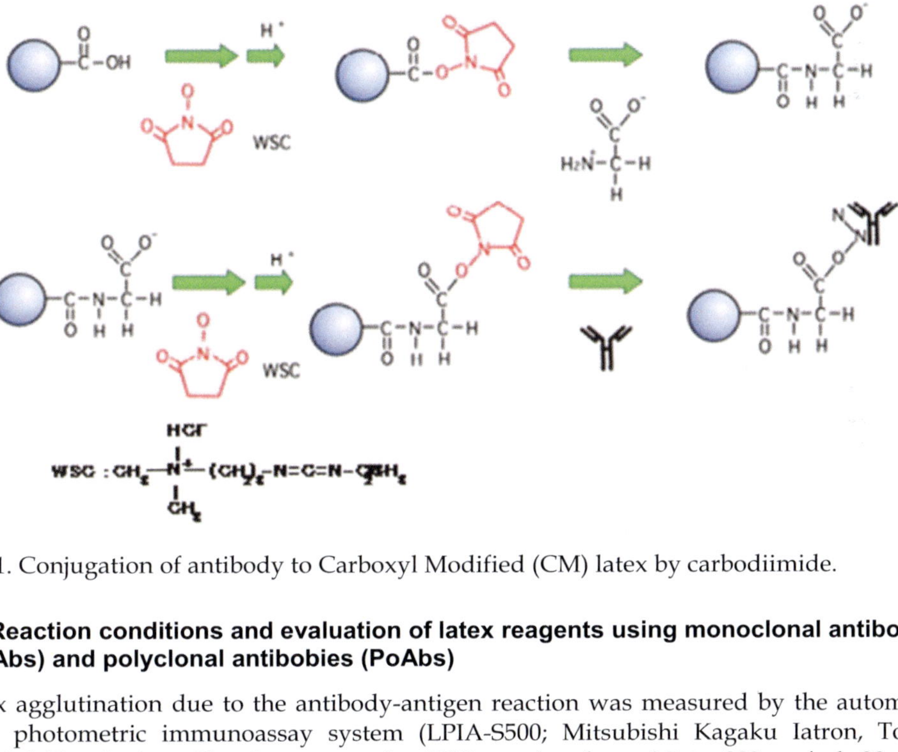

Fig. 1. Conjugation of antibody to Carboxyl Modified (CM) latex by carbodiimide.

2.7 Reaction conditions and evaluation of latex reagents using monoclonal antibodies (MoAbs) and polyclonal antibobies (PoAbs)

Latex agglutination due to the antibody-antigen reaction was measured by the automated latex photometric immunoassay system (LPIA-S500; Mitsubishi Kagaku Iatron, Tokyo, Japan).[6] To obtain calibration curves for CRP ranging from 0.5 to 200 ng/ml, 30 μl of standard CRP solution at various concentrations was diluted with 0.1 M Tris-BSA buffer (pH 8.2) containing 0.1 M Tris, 0.1% w/v EDTA•2Na, 0.8% w/v sodium chloride, 1% w/v BSA, and 0.1% w/v sodium azide following the manufacturer's directions. Thirty μl of sample and 50 μl of 0.1 M Tris-BSA buffer (pH 8.2) were then transferred to a plastic cuvette, and 40 μl of 0.25% latex reagent solution and 180 μl of 0.1 M Tris-BSA-PEG buffer (pH 8.2) containing 1% w/v PEG20000 were added. The rate of the latex agglutination was calculated by recording the absorbance at 800 nm at 12-s intervals, as reported previously.[6] Latex reagents prepared using the 4 MoAbs were evaluated for sensitivity, linearity, and stability of latex agglutination. Specimens were properly diluted and measured for CRP concentration.

2.8 Anti-CRP polyclonal antibody and the F(ab')$_2$ fragment

Anti-CRP polyclonal antibody was produced by Immuno Probe (Saitama, Japan) The specific F(ab')$_2$ fragment was prepared by pepsin digestion, as previously described.[11)]

2.9 Clinical samples

We tested CRP levels in serum samples of 62 healthy individuals, 263 patients with liver disease, and 230 diabetic patients. Fifty diabetic patients had type 2 diabetes and were not under insulin treatment. All patients were examined in the Surugadai Nihon University Hospital, Tokyo, between April 2005 and March 2007. The study was approved in advance by the Ethics Committee of the hospital, and was conducted in accordance with the Helsinki Declaration. All study participants provided written informed consent prior to participation in this study.

3. Result and discussion

3.1 Characterization of monoclonal antibodies produced by established hybridomas

MoAbs produced from hybridoma cells were screened by ELISA, and seven MoAbs were subsequently established as stable hybridoma cells. Examination of MoAb reactivity revealed that hybridoma clone 5 had the highest sensitivity. Clonal sensitivity was ranked in the following order: clone 5 > clone 8 > clone 7 > clone 9 > clone 3 > clone 4 > clone 1. These isotypes and subclasses were then analyzed using the IsoStrip kit. The MoAb 1 produced from hybridoma clone 1 and clones 3, 5, 7, 8, and 9 were IgG1κ, while clone 4 was IgG2aκ. In addition, the specificity of the MoAbs was confirmed by western blotting using Human CRP. The MoAbs recognized a protein band at a molecular weight of approximately 11,500 Da. These results suggest that the MoAbs reacted specifically with CRP.

3.2 Epitope analysis

Protein epitopes are generally present in the areas of a protein that exhibit specific characteristics, including hydrophilicity,[12,13)] solvent accessibility,[14)] mobility,[15,16)] and the presence of protrusions.[13)] In addition, epitopes are commonly 5–10 amino acid residues containing loops and/or protruding regions.[17,18)] The hydrophilicity plot for the prediction of protrusions from the protein sequences can be measured by a simple method.[13)] Hydropathy analysis of CRP in this study was performed by the SOSUI system WWW-based tool (http://bp.nuap.nagoya-u.ac.jp/sosui/),[19)] since it was anticipated that hydrophilic epitopes would be present in CRP.

We mapped epitope locations using the seven CRP fragments. CRP-01 was 203 amino acid residues in length and was translated from the second exon (amino acid sequence positions 4 to 206); CRP-02 was 155 amino acid residues in length (amino acid sequence positions 52 to 206); CRP-03 was 91 amino acid residues in length (amino acid sequence positions 116 to 206); CRP-04 was 60 amino acid residues in length (amino acid sequence positions 147 to

206); CRP-05 was 34 amino acid residues in length (amino acid sequence positions 173 to 206); CRP-a was 100 amino acid residues in length (amino acid sequence positions 4 to 103). and CRP-b was 125 amino acid residues in length (amino acid sequence positions 49 to 173). The seven recombinant CRP peptide fragments were then expressed in *E. coli* and their relative molecular weights were observed by SDS-PAGE and Coomassie Brilliant Blue staining (Fig. 2). In each case, the relative molecular weight corresponded to the predicted size of the recombinant peptide fragments.

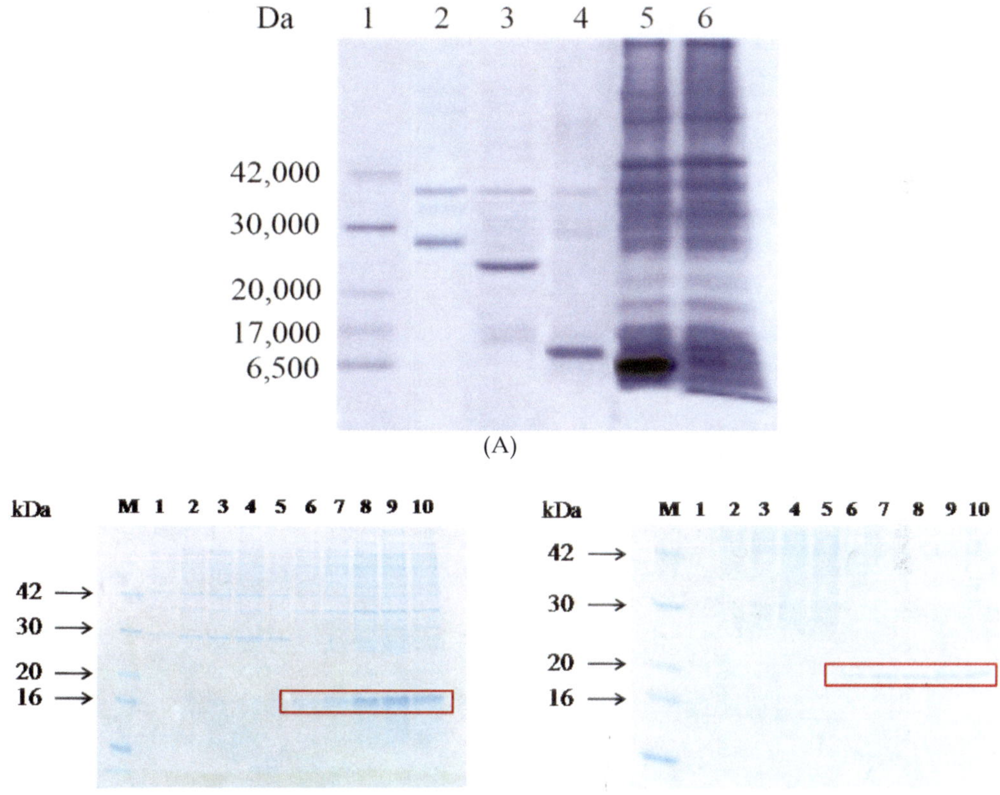

(A) Molecular weight marker (lane 1), CRP-01 of recombinant CRP fragment (lane 2), CRP-02 (lane 3), CRP-03 (lane 4), CRP-04 (lane 5), and CRP-05 (lane 6) were separated by SDS-PAGE and stained with Coomassie Brilliant Blue. Recombinant CRP fragments for CRP-01, CRP-02, CRP-03, CRP-04, and CRP-05 correspond to molecular weights of 26.3, 19.9, 11,7, 6.8, and 4.0 kDa respectively. (B) Recombinant protein CRP-a, Lane 1-5: Add IPTG to culture pellet 0-5h, Lane 6-10: Culture pellet 0-5h. (C) Recombinant protein CRP-b, Lane 1-5: Add IPTG to culture pellet 0-5h, Lane 6-10: culture pellet 0-5h. M: Low range molecular weight marker (Wako Pure Chemical Industries)

Fig. 2. SDS-PAGE Analysis of Recombinant CRP Fragments Expressed in *E. coli*.

The results of epitope analysis using Western blot are presented in Table 2. MoAbs 4, 7, and 8 were found to react with all fragments, while MoAb 5 reacted with CRP-01, CRP-02, CRP-

03, and CRP-04. This suggests that the C-terminal fragment (positions 173 to 206, Fig. 3B) contains the epitope for MoAbs 4, 7, and 8 while the fragment containing amino acid residues 147 to 172 (Fig. 3A) contains the epitope for MoAb 5. It is not a hydrophilicity epitope. However, these epitope regions include helix and loop structures, and there have been only a few reports of cross-reaction with these epitopes.[20,21] Hence, we hypothesized that these epitopes represent specific antigen sites.

Monoclonal antibody	Isotype	Reactivity with Recombinant CRP						
		CRP-01	CRP-02	CRP-03	CRP-04	CRP-05	CRP-a	CRP-b
No. 4	IgG2aκ	+	+	+	+	+	+	+
No. 5	IgG1κ	+	+	+	+	–	+	+
No. 7	IgG1κ	+	+	+	+	+	+	+
No. 8	IgG1κ	+	+	+	+	+	+	+

Table 2. Reactivity of the Anti-CRP Monoclonal Antibody with CRP Fragments by Western Blot Analysis

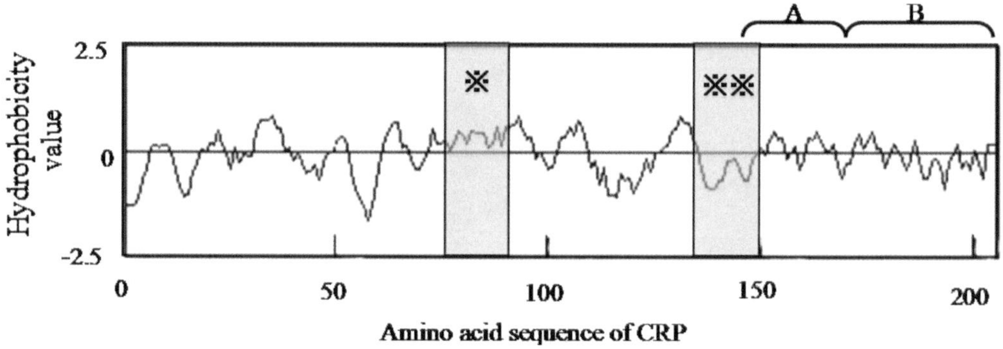

The C-terminal fragment from positions 173 to 206 (B) might contain the epitopes for MoAbs 4, 7, and 8, while the fragment spanning positions 147 to 172 (A) is thought to contain the epitope for MoAb 5.
※Cross-reactive site with heat shock protein 60.[20]
※※ Site similar to pentraxins in other species.[21]

Fig. 3. Hydrophobicity Plot of the CRP Amino Acid Sequence.

3.3 Reactivity of anti-CRP latex reagents using polyclonal antibody (PoAb)

3.3.1 Optimization of amino acid spacer concentration

First, bond concentrations of the amino acid spacers were examined. Preparation of latex reagent with amino acid spacers was synthesized using glycine at concentrations of 1.0–20 mg/ml, and the reagent produced binding antibody using latex synthesized at each glycine concentration. The examination of reactivity was performed to react CRP antigen with the binding antibody using the synthesized reagent. As seen in Fig. 3, the examination of reactivity improved as glycine concentrations increased. The optimum glycine concentration was 10 mg/ml, and the excess glycine bond was decreased by the reactivity of latex reagent. Thus, latex responsiveness was improved by the combination of the amino acid and latex at a concentration of 0.26 mmol.

The result of each reagent using glycine (Gly), alanine (Ala), valine (Val), leucine (Leu), and peptide synthesized by Fmoc solid phase (5 molecule bond of glycine: Gly5) are shown in Fig. 4. The rank order of reactivity was Gly5 > Gly > Ala > Leu > Val. Each amino acid produced a gentle sloping curve, and Gly5 produced a good reaction curve.

The accuracy of each amino acid is shown in Table 3. CV was about 0.5 or less and the stabilizing reagent was synthesized. Gly sensitivity is shown in Fig. 5. We demonstrated that it was possible to measure up to 500 ng/dl by calculating mean ± 3 SD values.

This study demonstrates that a latex reagent made by using 5 types of amino acid spacer molecules increased reactiveness by 40% as compared to using only 1 glycine molecule. It is possible that the long amino acid spacer reduces steric hindrance in the antigen-antibody reaction with the latex and thus reactiveness to the antibody is increased. Because the reactiveness is examined by using the amino acid, the position of the carboxyl group is the same as the amino group necessary for the peptide bond formation. Therefore, the length of the latex particle and antibody is constant. Because the alkyl group of the amino acid used is aliphatic, the hydrophobe of the amino acid, and the volume of the molecule are chiefly different (Table 4), the difference in reactiveness may be due to the side chain of the amino acid. As seen in Fig. 6, there was a 70% or greater increase in reactivity for all amino acids when the bonding amounts of the amino acid were compared, and a significant difference was not seen in the amount of antibody binding. Therefore, it is suggested that the reactiveness is due to the interaction of the aliphatic amino acid spacer with the hydrophobe.

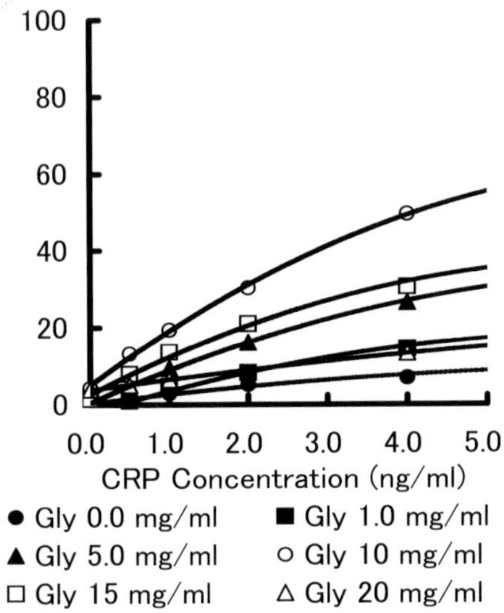

Fig. 4a. Comparison of reactivity in various concentration of glycine spacer

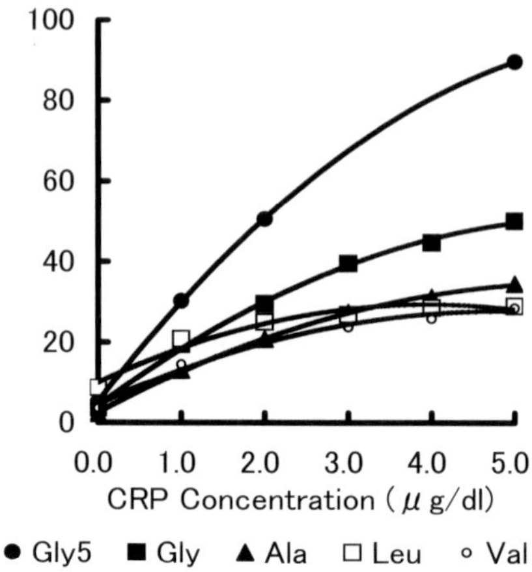

Fig. 4b. Comparison of reactivity in various types of amino acid spacers

Glycine						
Concentration (μg/dl)	0	1.0	2.0	3.0	4.0	5.0
Mean (absorbance)	0.058	0.288	0.430	0.481	0.542	0.583
SD	0.007	0.009	0.022	0.018	0.029	0.015
CV(%)	12.70	3.22	5.18	3.68	5.40	2.56
Alanine						
Concentration (μg/dl)	0	1.0	2.0	3.0	4.0	5.0
Mean (absorbance)	0.021	0.107	0.171	0.224	0.258	0.288
SD	0.010	0.012	0.021	0.030	0.033	0.041
CV(%)	49.44	11.24	12.26	13.53	12.92	14.06
Valine						
Concentration (μg/dl)	0	1.0	2.0	3.0	4.0	5.0
Mean (absorbance)	0.070	0.268	0.380	0.446	0.380	0.446
SD	0.006	0.016	0.022	0.026	0.022	0.026
CV(%)	8.74	5.89	5.85	5.81	5.85	5.81
Leucine						
Concentration (μg/dl)	0	1.0	2.0	3.0	4.0	5.0
Mean (absorbance)	0.191	0.389	0.515	0.550	0.604	0.603
SD	0.029	0.064	0.069	0.078	0.080	0.089
CV(%)	15.18	16.54	13.33	14.10	13.22	14.81
Gly5						
Concentration (μg/dl)	0	1.0	2.0	3.0	4.0	5.0
Mean (absorbance)	0.051	0.302	0.505	-	-	0.896
SD	0.05	0.081	0.083			0.093
CV(%)	15.54	10.95	7.32			7.96

Table 3. With in-run precision

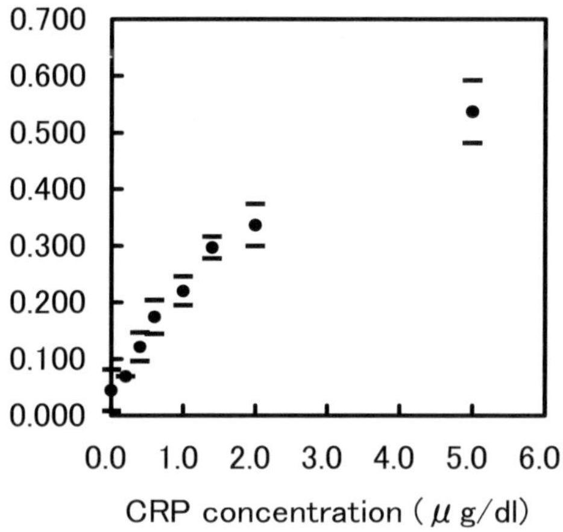

Fig. 5. Detection sensitivity

Amino acid	MW	pI	The solubility of amino acid in H_2O	
Glycine	75.07	5.97	14.18	(0°C)
			24.99	(25°C)
Alanine	89.09	6.00	12.73	(0°C)
			16.51	(25°C)
Valine	117.15	5.96	—	(0°C)
			8.34	(25°C)
Leucine	131.18	5.98	2.27	(0°C)
			2.19	(25°C)

Table 4. Amino acid spacers

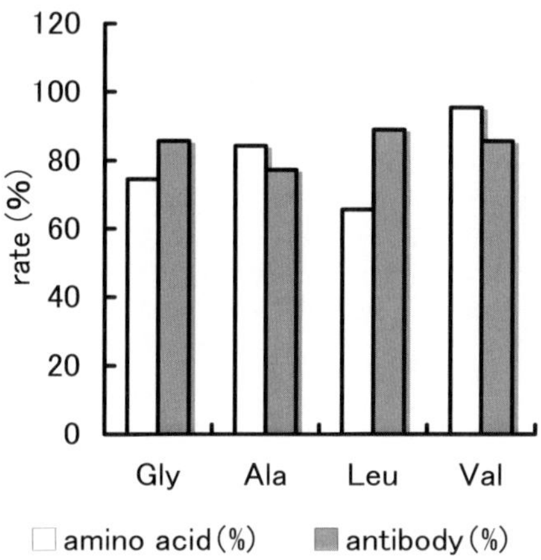

Fig. 6. Amount of conjugated amino acid and antibody

3.3.2 Immunoreactivity of prepared latex reagent

The latex reagent was produced by the method previously described using $F(ab')_2$ antibody, and the reactivity was compared with the conventional reagent. The $F(ab')_2$ reagent and conventional reagent were used to draw calibration curves from standard CRP samples and CRP levels derived from the 263 clinical samples from patients with liver disease. As seen in Fig. 7, the $F(ab')_2$ reagent correlated with a conventional reagent ($r^2 = 0.746$, $y = 0.4879$, and $x + 1.77$). Moreover, when CRP concentration was between 0.030 and 2.0 mg/dl, the correlation was $r^2 = 0.829$, $y = 0.909$, and $x + 0.6073$, indicating that there was a significant correlation at low concentrations. However, at high latex concentrations, this method was less sensitive.

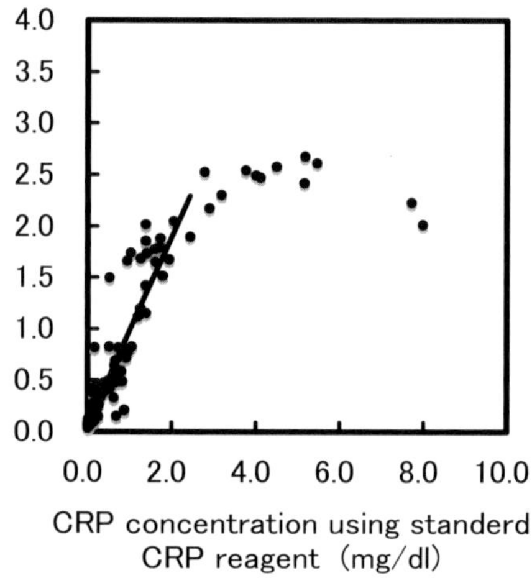

Fig. 7. Comparative study of CRP latex reagent

3.3.3 LTIA for titration of the MoAb and oligoclonal antibody

Three latex reagents with MoAb were used to quantify the CRP antigen by LTIA. The immunoreactivity curve of the latex agglutination rates using the various antibodies is shown in Fig. 8. We found that the reaction rates increased with the concentration of CRP antigen in an approximately linear fashion. The reactivity of these reagents was ranked in the following order: MoAb 5 > MoAb 8 > MoAb 7. This order of reactivity observed for the latex agglutination tests was found to be the same as that for the ELISA tests. The detection limit, which was calculated as the concentration equivalent to 3 standard deviations above the mean signal from 10 replicates of the zero standard, was calculated at 10 ng/ml.

Further, we prepared two types of latex reagent. First we mixed the two above-mentioned latex reagents together to form "mixed latex reagents," and combined these suspensions with CRP (Fig. 9). Then latex reagents were prepared using two MoAbs at a total antibody concentration of 100 μg/ml, and the latex reagent with two antibodies as the oligoclonal antibody were reacted with the CRP antigen (Fig. 10). The sensitivity of the latex reagents containing MoAb 5 was found to be the highest, and the latex reagents with the oligoclonal antibody were more sensitive than the mixed latex reagents. The lower limit of CRP antigen

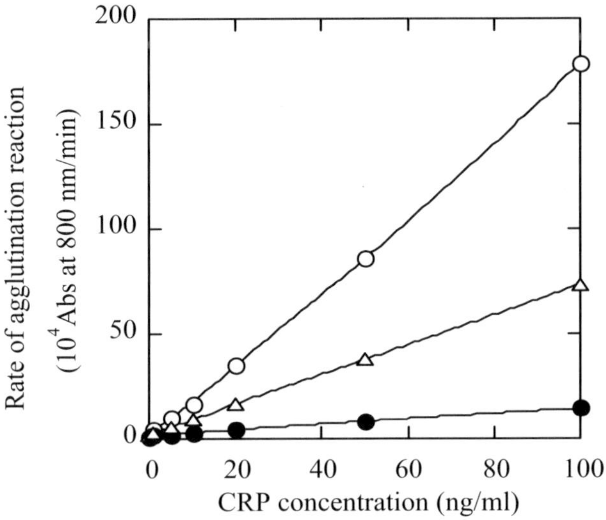

The latex reagent containing MoAb 5 (○) was found to have the highest activity, while the latex reagent containing MoAb 7 (●) was found to have the lowest activity. The latex reagent containing MoAb 8 (△) was found to have an intermediate level of activity.

Fig. 8. Comparison of Reactivity between Latex Reagents.

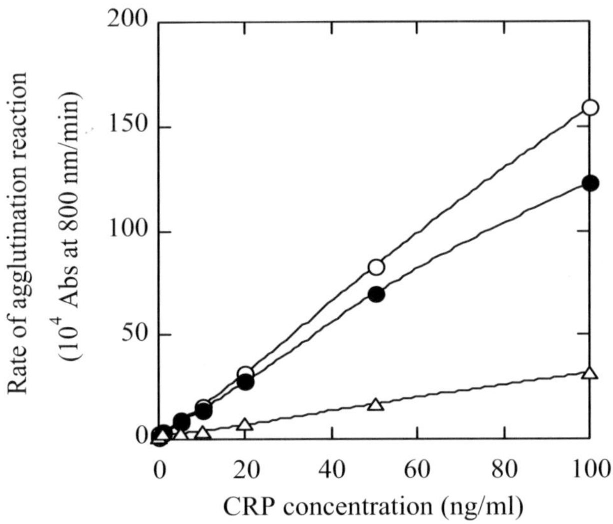

Three types of mixed latex reagents were prepared using MoAb 5 latex reagent and MoAb 7 latex reagent (○), MoAb 5 latex reagent and MoAb 8 latex reagent (●), and MoAb 7 latex reagent and MoAb 8 latex reagent (△). The mixed latex reagents containing MoAb 5 were found to have higher activity than the others.

Fig. 9. Comparison of Latex Reagent Reactivity Following Mixing of Two Types of Latex Reagents Containing Different MoAbs.

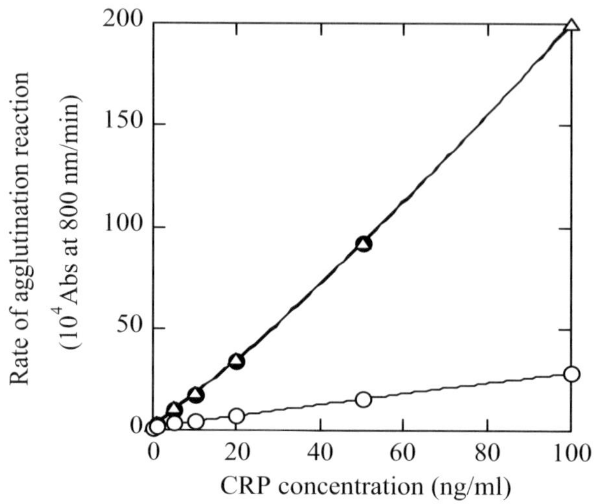

Three types of latex reagents with oligoclonal antibody were prepared with a combination of MoAb 5 and 7(●), MoAb 5 and 8(△), and MoAb 7 and 8(○). Two types of latex reagents sensitizing MoAb 5 were found to have higher sensitivity than the rest.

Fig. 10. Comparison of Reactivity Among Latex Reagents Containing Two Kinds of MoAbs.

detection, which was defined by the mean ± 3 SD method, was calculated as 10 ng/ml for the mixed latex reagents and 5 ng/ml for the latex reagent containing the oligoclonal antibody. When MoAbs for two different epitopes were used, the resulting latex reagent exhibited higher sensitivity than the MoAbs for two nearby epitopes. We suggest that latex reagents can be further increased in sensitivity through the use of MoAbs directed against remote epitopes.

3.4 Examination of clinical significances for quantification of CRP level in normal, hepatic disease, and diabetic subjects

The CRP level of sera in normal, hepatic disease, and diabetic subjects were measured by latex reagents prepared using glycine spacers (Fig. 11). Normal subjects (n = 62) showed a CRP average value of 0.03 mg/dl (maximum, 0.12 mg/dl; minimum, 0.01 mg/dl). These CRP levels in sera were 0.02 mg/dl lower than reference healthy individuals .

Patients with liver disease (n = 263) caused by hepatitis B and C had an average CRP level of 0.14 mg/dl (maximum, 2.7 mg/dl; minimum, 0.04 mg/dl) in sera.

Type 2 diabetes mellitus subjects (n = 230) had an average CRP level of 0.07 mg/dl (maximum, 1.9 mg/dl; minimum, 0.01 mg/dl).

Furthermore, CRP level in hepatitis B and C patients sera was compared with hepatic disease subjects classified as having hepatitis, hepatic cirrhosis, and hepatic cancer (Fig. 12). CRP levels tended to increase with the advancement of the disease.

This new method of assaying CRP, which uses a latex reagent made with a glycine spacer, shows that there is a tendency for CRP levels to increase with age. We were able to get CRP readings at low concentrations (0.020 mg/dl) in a subset of healthy volunteers (n = 63) who were between 20–30 years of age. This method was also used to measure CRP levels in patients with liver disease, and the levels were correlated with disease advancement. In traditional CRP assays, small changes are not usually detected owing to viral infection. Moreover, because the liver produces CRP, the decrease of CRP production has been linked to hepatic infection. However, the change in such CRP level due to liver disease was confirmed by this new highly sensitive CRP density measurement. Our data indicate that CRP is produced by the inflammatory response of the liver in patients with hepatitis B and C.

We also measured CRP levels in patients with diabetes. Chronic high blood sugar in diabetic patients increases the risk of arteriosclerosis. Recent studies indicate that insulin-resistant diabetes is especially correlated with arteriosclerosis and that heightened level of CRP in type 2 diabetes may be a sensitive marker of arteriosclerosis.

This study indicates that CRP levels are not only elevated in people with particular infectious diseases, cardiac infarction, and arteriosclerosis, but also in the sera of people with liver disease and diabetes. These findings indicate that assaying CRP level will become more important for diagnosing multiple diseases and may be used to measure the effectiveness of therapies for patients with liver disease. Additionally, this newly developed method can detect even small changes in CRP levels and thus is much more sensitive than traditional methods.

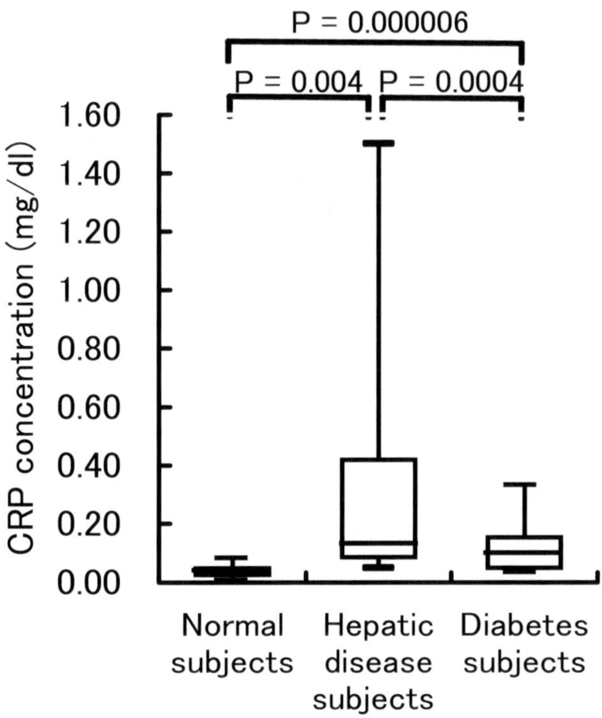

Fig. 11. Box and whisker plots in CRP measurement of normal subjects and patients

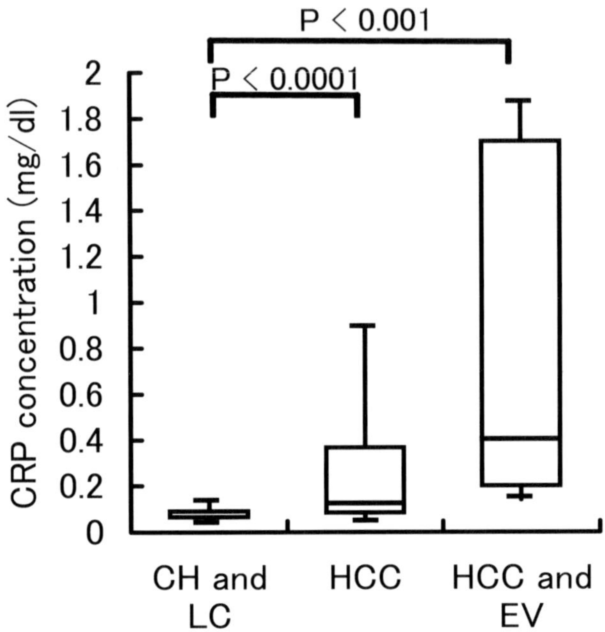

Fig. 12. Box and whisker plots in CRP measurement of various types of hepatic disease

4. Conclusion

We developed four novel MoAbs directed against CRP (MoAb 4, 5, 7, and 8), and classified these antibodies into two major groups. The epitopes for MoAbs 4, 7, and 8 were located between the amino acids residing at positions 173 to 206 of the CRP sequence. The epitope for MoAb 5 was located between the amino acids residing at positions 147 to 172 of the CRP sequence. These MoAbs were used in the preparation of latex reagents. The latex reagents constructed using these MoAbs were found to be highly sensitive. Moreover, the latex reagents, containing a cocktail of MoAbs specific for different epitopes, were also found to be highly sensitive. The lower limit of detection of CRP antigen, which was defined using the mean ± 3 SD method, was calculated to be 5 ng/ml for the latex reagents containing oligoclonal antibodies. Furthermore, the latex reagents that were prepared using three kinds of MoAbs reacted specifically with CRP-present patients with type-2 diabetes. In Fig. 12, the obtained CRP value, appear to be indicated the hepatitis disease situation with the extreme increased of CRP values in transition of disease phase from the point of these clinical evaluations. We concluded that high sensitive CRP measurement should be usable in the diagnosis of metabolic syndrome, such as diabetes and cardiac disease, early prediction of infection disease, and clinical follow-up of infection of neonates that show low concentrations of CRP.

We suggest that latex reagents can be increased in sensitivity and specificity through the use of MoAbs directed against remote epitopes. The results from this study might also prove to be applicable to additional substances such as interleukin, *etc.*

This study presents a new CRP reagent with an amino acid spacer. In this method, the latex particles contain a glycine spacer, the anti-CRP antibody can be supported, and the orientation can be given to the antibody. As compared with other methods, this method allows for quick, efficient, and highly sensitive measurement of CRP levels even in low concentrations.

Additionally, we determined the serum CRP levels in a clinical sample of healthy subjects, people with liver disease, and diabetic subjects to be 0.1374 mg/dl, 0.0332 mg/dl, and 0.0704 mg/dl, respectively. There was a significant difference in the CRP levels between patients with type B and type C hepatitis. We also detected small differences in CRP levels between type 1 and 2 diabetic patients.

5. References

[1] Hirschfield GM and Pepys MB, *Q. J. Med.*, 96,793-807(2003).
[2] Ridker PM, Glynn RJ, and Hennekens CH, *Circulation*, 97, 2007-2011 (1998).
[3] Ridker PM, Cushman M, Stampfer MJ, Tracy RP, and Hennekens CH, *N. Engl. J. Med.*, 336, 973-980 (1997).
[4] Ridker PM and Cook N, *Circulation*, 109, 1955-1959 (2004).
[5] Sudo T, Satoshi, Tsutsui M, Ito S, Morita S, and Sawai M, *Kitasato Arch. Exp. Med.*, 53, 55-68 (1980).
[6] Kawaguchi H, *Prog. Polym. Sci.*, 25, 1171-1210 (2000).
[7] Borque L, Bellod L, Rus A, Seco ML, and Galisteo-GonZalez F, *Clin. Chem.*, 46, 1839-1842 (2000).
[8] Kohno H, Akihira S, Nishino O, and Ushijima H, *Pediatr. Int.*, 42, 395-400 (2000).
[9] Köhler G and Milstein C, *Nature*, 256, 495-497(1975).
[10] Komoriya T, Ito I, Nemoto H, Nakagawara H, Sagawa C, Okamoto M, Ogawa M, Arakawa M, and Kohno H, *Japanese Journal of Clinical Laboratory Automation* (in Japanese), 33, 14-20 (2008).
[11] Porter RR, *Science*, 180, 713-716(1973).
[12] Hopp TP and Woods KR, *Proc. Natl. Acad. Sci. USA*, 78, 3824−3828 (1981).
[13] Thornton JM, Edwards MS, Taylor WR, and Barlow DJ, *EMBO J.*, 5, 409-413 (1986).
[14] Lee B and Richards FM, *J. Mol. Biol.*, 55, 379-400 (1971).
[15] Novotný J, Handschumacher M, Haber E, Bruccoleri RE, Carlson WB, Fanning DW, Smith JA, and Rose GD, *Proc. Natl. Acad. Sci. USA*, 83, 226-230(1986).
[16] Westhof E, Altschuh D, Moras D, Bloomer AC, Mondragon A, Klug, A, and van Regnmortel MH, *Nature*, 311, 123-126 (1984).
[17] Barlow DJ, Edwards MS, and Thornton JM, *Nature*, 322, 747-748 (1986).
[18] Huang J and Honda W, *BMC Immunol.*, 7:7, doi:10.1186/1471-1272-7-7 (2006).

[19] Hirokawa T, Boon-Chieng S, and Mitaku S, *Bioinformatics*, 14, 378-379 (1998).
[20] Udvarnoki K, Cervenak L, Uray K, Hudecz F, Kacskovics I, Spallek R, Singh M, Füst G, and Prohászka Z, *Clin. Vaccine Immunol.*, 14,335-341(2007).
[21] Ying SC, Marchalonis JJ, Gewurz AT, Siegel JN, Jiang H, Gewurz BE, and Gewurz H, *Immunology*, 76, 324-330 (1992).

10

Microarray Analysis in Drug Discovery and Biomarker Identification

Yushi Liu[1] and Joseph S. Verducci[2]
[1]*Lovelace Respiratory Research Institute*
[2]*The Ohio State University*
USA

1. Introduction

1.1 Motivation of microarray development

Microarrays play important roles in Medicinal Chemistry and Drug Discovery. In the Pre-microarray era, scientists used to study one gene at a time. This approach is costly and time consuming. Quite often, many genes that interact with each other would be ignored. Therefore, the discovery of candidate drug targets is challenging, requiring the rapid development of techniques to identify the difference genomic profiling in disease and normal conditions, which will facilitate the understanding of the disease mechanism and the development of potential drugs for disease treatment.

1.2 Examples of microarray in biomarker identification

Microarray has been successfully applied to the comparison of genomic profiling for human tissues. One advantages of microarray is that it can find some potential drug targets which have been ignored previously. The example for this is the study by Heller *et al* in rheumatoid tissues. (Heller et al, 1997) They found around 100 genes known to be involved in inflammation. (Heller et al, 1997) However, additional genes such as interleukin-6 and matrix metallo-elastase are also found to be overexpressed remarkably, which is not anticipated *a priori,* since matrix metallo-elastase is thought to be distributed only within alveolar macrophages and placental cells.(Debouck and Goodfellow, 1999). Beside human, microarray has also been successfully applied to model organisms such as mouse. (Debouck and Goodfellow, 1999) Animal models play important roles in discovering therapeutic targets and potential drug development. Although the genome for the animals does not agree completely with the human genome, they are more easily to be manipulated. By careful design of the experiments, the treatment effect can be seen more clearly with less noisy background. Moreover, genes can be either knocked down or overexpressed to study the influence on phenotype. People used to use techniques such as differential display PCR to discover genes that are differentially expressed in the animal models and achieved some success. (Wang et al, 1995) However, this technique is much slower compared with microarray.

Quite often, drugs can bind to specific targets within cells and potentially influence different pathways.(Windle & Guiseppi-Elie, 2003) The genes that are differentially expressed between drug-treated and untreated conditions are typically known as biomarkers. Such biomarkers not only help to identify patients at risk, but they also may lead to breakthroughs in understanding the mechanism for different diseases.(Ko et al., 2005)An example is the review by Chen that summarized the recent microarray research in biomarker identification in atherosclerosis and in-stent stenosis.(Chen et al., 2011)

1.3 Diagnosis using microarray

Microarray has greatly advanced the biology field and the biomarkers identified can be further used to form classifiers for prediction in clinical studies. For example, Gulob *et al* used the gene expression pattern from microarrays to classify acute myeloid leukaemia (AML) and acute lymphoblastic leukaemia (ALL) without other information. (Gulob et al, 1999) Therefore, this field draws the attention not only from biologists but also statisticians and bioinformaticians. Through their collaborative efforts, there are many successful instances. We will introduce some of them in section two later.

The rapid development of this technique also resulted in several FDA approved test. AmpliChip CYP450 test is a clinical test to find specific genetic variation of two cytochrome P450 genes CYP2D6 and CYP2C19 genes including deletion and duplications. (de Leon, 2006) These two enzymes account for the variability of drug metabolism for each patient and offers enriched information for the doctors during prescription of psychiatric drugs. (de Leon, 2006) CYP2D6 can be divided into four categories: Poor Metabolizer, Intermediate Metabolizer, Extensive Metabolizer, and Ultrarapid Metabolizer. (de Leon, 2006) Similarly, for CYP2C19, only two categories are found: Poor Metabolizer and Extensive Metabolizer. (de Leon, 2006) The assay works as follows: First, the gene is amplified by PCR and then the amplified product will be fragmented and labelled. Subsequently, these fragments will be hybridized to the microarray chip and the chip is scanned for further analysis. (de Leon, 2006) For further information of this FDA approved test, please see the website at http://molecular .roche.com/assays/Pages/AmpliChipCYP450Test.aspx.

Another FDA approved diagnosis test is MammaPrint to assess the risk of breast tumor and this will help to decide the effectiveness of chemotherapy on the patients. (van't Veer et al, 2002) The assay uses the fresh tissue to study the Amsterdam 70-gene breast cancer gene signature by microarray analysis. (van't Veer et al, 2002) Readers interested in this test can also obtain more information about the MINDACT trial (Microarray In Node negative and 1-3 positive lymph node Disease may Avoid Chemo Therapy) in the paper by Cardoso et al.(Cardoso et al, 2008)

In general, identification of biomarkers by microarray greatly speeds the progress of research by enabling the simultaneous monitoring of the expression of thousands of genes. However, there are many potential pitfalls in analyzing the output from these arrays. (Verducci, et al., 2006) Due to importance of proper analysis, we will give a brief introduction to the statistical methodology underlying proper analysis.

2. Mechanisms and processing of microarrays

Medicinal chemistry has increasingly employed microarrays to identify both key target genes and gene networks that can regulate the effectiveness of drugs. The basic scheme is illustrated in Figure 1.1. Two cell strains (one is drug treated and one is non-treated) are harvested and the whole RNA from each strain is then extracted. This is followed by reverse transcription of RNA and the resulted cDNA is labelled with either of the two fluorescence dyes (Cys-3 or Cys-5). Then the mixed cDNA from both samples is hybridized to the probesets on the microarray chip. The probesets are the small oligonucleotides that have the complementary sequence of the cDNA attached to the array at each spot. After intensive washing, the intensity from the fluorescence of the dye labelled on cDNA at each spot is measured and recorded. These data will be used for further analysis.

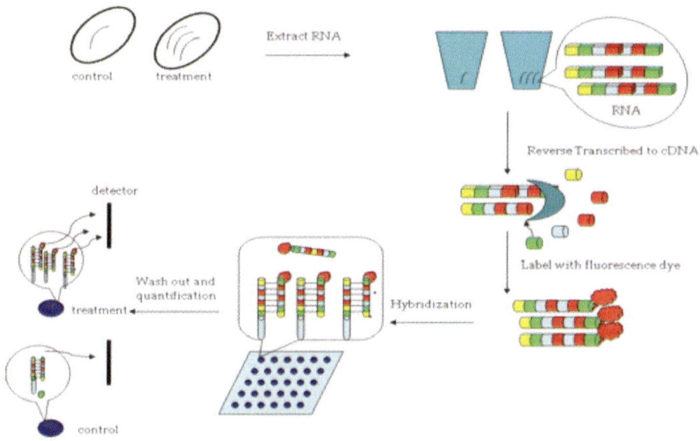

Fig. 1. Illustration of the microarray process. RNA is extracted from treated (treatment) and untreated (control) cell lines, followed by reverse transcription. The reversely transcribed cDNA is then labelled with the fluorescence dye and hybridized to the probes containing complementary fragments. After unbounded cDNA is washed away, the binding at each probe is then quantified based on the fluorescence intensity of the bounded cDNA.

The above method is referred to as a two channel array because a mixture of cDNA from two treatments is measured directly. In contrast, a one channel array will only have cDNA from one sample to be hybridized to the probesets. In this case the fluorescence intensity from each sample is measured separately. For either type of array, processing and analyzing the data present both statistical and biological challenges. Fortunately, many such approaches have been integrated in the freely distrubuted statistical software R (http://www.r-project.org/) and the software Bioconductor (http://www. bioconductor. org/). Typically the data processing step includes four steps: image analysis, quality assessment, pre-processing and statistical inference.(Tibshirani et al., 2005)

2.1 Image analysis and quality assessment

In the image analysis step, each spot is quantified and then converted to intensity afterwards. The method of quantification depends on the brand of the arrays. Quality assessment is usually performed at two levels: array level and probe level. On the array level, fingerprint smudges or washed out corners, are generally recognized. Other problems such as defects of the array, errors in RNA extraction also belong in this category. One common criterion is that if the percentage of spots without any signal is higher than 30%, the expression array will fail in the quality control step.(Tibshirani et al., 2005) Poor quality at probe level will include errors like faulty printing, uneven distribution, contamination, or poor level of signal to noise ratio. In addition, several parameters can be used to determine the quality of the array: uniformity, which is minimal variation in pixel intensity within a spot; and the brightness, which is the foreground to background ratio.(Tibshirani et al., 2005) Normally, researchers will ignore the spots of poor quality in subsequent analysis.

2.2 Pre-processing

Two types of errors usually happen at this stage: (1) systematic error, which influences all measurements within one microarray chip with similar effect -- this error may be corrected by estimation; and (2) random error that cannot be explained or corrected, which is typically known as noise. Such errors are totally stochastic and have different influence on different probes.(Tibshirani et al., 2005) Typically, the pre-processing stage contains three steps: background correction, normalization and summarization. For the widely used Affymetrix chips, many Bioconductor routines are available in R for pre-processing. These require creation of an *AffyBatch* object based on raw Affymetrix data (in a .cel file). The first step is the background adjustment. In this step, one tends to subtract the control intensity from the treatment, to 'denoise' the intensity. However, direct subtraction of uncertain quantities can increase the level of noise and possibly result in negative intensity values for certain spots. Various methods to circumvent these problems are available as *method* parameters in the *bg.correct* function in *R*:

a. *RMA method*: which is based on the assumption that the observed signal is a mixture of Gaussian background noise (N) with mean μ variance σ^2 and exponential signal (S) with mean a. Thus the fluorescence intensity O we observe is the addition of the signal and noise. Assuming the above, $E(S|O)$, which is the conditional expectation of the signal based on the observed intensity will be used as the background corrected values. However, the disadvantages for this are: only the PM(perfect match) values are used and MM(mismatch) values, which contains useful information for background noise are discarded.(Tibshirani et al., 2005) and the results may not be robust if there are gross deviations from the model assumptions. These assumptions may be checked visually via different plotting methods.
b. *MAS 5.0 method*: due to the above disadvantages, *RMA* may not produce optimal result. Therefore, *MAS 5.0* is sometimes used instead. Here, the whole array can be partitioned as k rectangular grids.(Tibshirani et al, 2005) The probeset, with lowest intensity for the grid, is used as the noise value to calculate the background corrected intensity within a particular rectangle. The intensities of these probes are further adjusted according to the weighted average of the background intensity of all grids according to the following formula:

$$W_{k(x,y)}=1/(d^2_{k(x,y)}+S_0) \tag{1}$$

In the above formula, the weight is determined by the Euclidean distance from (x,y) to the centroid of the space k and the smoothing coefficient represented by d^2_k and S_0, respectively.(Tibshirani et al, 2005) Irizarry *et al.* (2003) compare *RMA* and *MAS 5.0* in detail.

c. *Ideal mismatch*: Neither of the above methods uses mismatch information. Although direct subtraction of the mismatch intensity from the perfect match intensity creates the problems of added noise and negative intensity, *ideal mismatch* adjusts the observed mismatch so that it will never be higher than the PM intensities. The detailed formula of this is available in (Tibshirani et al., 2005) for further reading.

The next step is normalization of scores across different microarrays so that they can be compared fairly with each other. A variety of methods available in the *normalize* function of Bioconductor will be introduced:

a. *Scaling normalization*: All the arrays are normalized using the same selected baseline. This is almost identical to fitting linear regression without the intercept.(Tibshirani et al., 2005)
b. *Non-linear transformations*: Although linear regression is simple and easy to implement, in microarray study, the relationship may be more complicated and thus non-linear methods are developed including include cross-validated splines and loess smoothers.(Yang et al., 2001) The "invariantset" method developed by Li and Wong is very robust and is thus recommended.(Li & Wong, 2001) First an "invariantset" is identified. This gene set is composed of non-differentially expressed genes (sometimes called "household function genes) across the arrays and the expression values (or the rankings) of these genes can be used to construct the baseline for normalization (Li & Wong, 2001) However one challenge for this method is the identification of the "invariantset", which may not be available *a priori*.
c. *Quantile normalization*: The purpose of this method is to adjust the empirical distribution on all arrays so that they could be the same. The algorithm in *R* works as follows: First the columns of expression data matrix *X* are properly ranked (dimension $p \times n$, p: number of the genes on the array; n: the number of the arrays). Suppose v is the p-dimensional vector of row means of the sorted data matrix and V is the $p \times n$ matrix whose columns are all equal to v, sort each column of V by the inverse permutation. The obtained matrix is then quantile normalized.(Tibshirani et al., 2005) The basis for this method is that the total energy that cells exert for gene expression remains fairly constant, although the choice of which genes get expressed may differ widely.
d. *Cyclic loess normalization*: An MA plot is used for this normalization procedure: M (which stands for "multiple") is the difference of two log intensities, while *A* is the average of the two log intensities. Subsequently, a loess curve is fitted for the MA plot and M is predicted by this curve.(Tibshirani et al., 2005) Each intensity value is adjusted based on the difference between the real and predicted M value. The process is iterated until all the arrays or probesets converge. However, the drawback of this method is that it is computationally expensive and time consuming.(Tibshirani et al., 2005) In *R*, the above two steps can be integrated. It has advantages like using all the information across arrays for normalization, and is thus, theoretically, more reliable. The "*vsn*" package in *R* is a representative and can perform the above two steps seamlessly.(Tibshirani et al., 2005)

The final step of preprocessing step is the summation, which is trying to integrate intensity values from multiple probes of a particular gene and obtain its expression value. The R routines *expresso* and *threestep* offer great flexibility in deciding how much to weight each probe. (Tibshirani et al., 2005) Summation completes the pre-processing step, and we are now ready to begin proper analysis.

2.3 Statistical methods for biomarker identification in microarray analysis

2.3.1 Introduction to basic microarray analysis

Since microarray can be viewed as high-dimensional dataset with fewer replicates. Traditional variable selection procedures like stepwise selection cannot identify the biomarkers effectively; modifications or new procedures are developed to accommodate this.

a. *Shrinkage Methods*: One particular drawback from stepwise selection of genes that distinguish treatment from control is its poor performance when the variables (gene expression levels) are highly correlated. However, this is exactly what happens on for microarray data since many genes on the array typically are involved in the same pathway. This inspired the development of the shrinkage methods, which can be viewed as constrained optimization. One advantage of shrinkage methods is they are more continuous than the subset selection and do not exhibit high variance. (Hastie et al., 2001) Theoretically, shrinkage methods do not minimize the residual sum of squares; instead, they impose a penalty on the residual sum of squares. Nowadays, different forms of penalty are proposed and some of the most commonly used ones are introduced here.

Ridge Regression: Ridge regression introduces a penalty on the size of the coefficients, thus leading to the shrinkage of the regression coefficients.(Hastie et al., 2001) Mathematically, $\tilde{\beta}^{ridge}$ solves the following:

$$\tilde{\beta}^{ridge} = \underset{\beta}{\arg\min}\{\sum_{i=1}^{N}(y_i - \beta_0 - \sum_{j=1}^{p} x_{ij}\beta_j)^2 + \lambda\sum_{j=1}^{p}\beta_j^2\} \tag{2}$$

Here, λ (the regularization parameter) is greater than or equal to zero and controls the amount of shrinkage towards zero. When the regularization parameter is zero, this approach is converted back to ordinary least square (OLS) estimation. The penalized formulation (2) has an equivalent formulation in terms of constrained optimization, which may be achieved using convex programming methods:

$$\tilde{\beta}^{ridge} = \underset{\beta}{\arg\min}\sum_{i=1}^{N}(y_i - \beta_0 - \sum_{j=1}^{p} x_{ij}\beta_j)^2$$
$$\sum_{j=1}^{p}\beta_j^2 \le s \tag{3}$$

Ridge estimation is suitable for situations when many correlated variables are present in the model.(Hastie et al., 2001) In these cases, the least squares estimator may be poorly determined, since the large positive coefficients may cancel out the negative coefficients on the correlated variables.(Hastie et al., 2001) Ridge regression can effectively prevent this from happening. As the unique solution to (2), the ridge estimator has explicit form:

$$\tilde{\beta}^{ridge} = (X^tX + \lambda I)^{-1}X^tY \tag{4}$$

where I is the identity matrix. Hence, adding a positive constant to the diagonal of X^tX allows a singular matrix to be inverted, effectively reducing the dependencies among the estimated coefficients. This was the original motivation. (Hoerl & Kennard, 1970)

Lasso Regression: Lasso regression is similar to ridge regression, simply replacing the L_2 norm ridge penalty in (2) by an L_1 norm penalty. The lasso form of (3) becomes

$$\tilde{\beta}^{lasso} = \arg\min_{\beta} \sum_{i=1}^{N} (y_i - \beta_0 - \sum_{j=1}^{p} x_{ij}\beta_j)^2 \qquad \sum_{j=1}^{p} |\beta_j| \le t \tag{5}$$

Changing from an L_2 to an L_1 penalty results in a estimator that is nonlinear in y.(Hastie et al., 2001) In this case, nonlinear programming is needed to get the lasso solution iteratively.(Hastie et al., 2001) The algorithms of the least angle regression (LARS) can be simply modified to implement the lasso.(Bradley et al., 2004) A special feature of the lasso is the "sparseness" of the solution: some of the coefficients become exactly zero the constraint *t* becomes sufficiently small. If t is large enough, then no shrinkage is performed. For the case of orthonormal columns of X, the lasso has a simple form in terms of the OLS coefficients and the penalty γ:

$$sign(\hat{\beta}_j)(|\hat{\beta}_j| - \gamma)_+ \tag{6}$$

Bridge Regression: Both ridge and lasso regressions are very popular. They can be generalized to bridge regression to achieve the some of the benefits of both.(Ildiko & Friedman, 1993) In bridge regression, people try to find β that satisfies the following, where $1 \le q \le 2$:

$$\tilde{\beta} = \arg\min_{\beta} \sum_{i=1}^{N} (y_i - \beta_0 - \sum_{j=1}^{p} x_{ij}\beta_j)^2 \qquad \sum_{j=1}^{p} |\beta_j|^q \le s \tag{7}$$

SCAD Regression: Despite the good theoretical properties lasso/ridge regression, these penalties do not achieve the following desired properties simultaneously: unbiasedness (the estimator is close to the true parameter when the true parameter is large), sparseness (irrelevant predictors are automatically removed), and continuity (estimator is continuous, preventing the instability of hard thresh holding estimators).(Fan & Li, 2001) The new penalty is defined for a parameter θ as

$$p'_\lambda(\theta) = \lambda \left\{ I(\theta \le \lambda) + \frac{(a\lambda - \theta)_+}{(a-1)\lambda} I(\theta > \lambda) \right\} \tag{8}$$

This penalty, known as the Smoothly Clipped Absolute Deviation (SCAD) penalty (Fan & Li, 2001) helps to improve the properties of L_1 and hard thresh holding penalties such

$p_\lambda(\theta) = \lambda^2 - (|\theta| - \lambda)^2 I(|\theta| < \lambda)$. The SCAD penalty can also be viewed as a quadratic spline function, with knots at λ and $a\lambda$.(Fan & Li, 2001) Also, it does not extremely penalize large values of θ and the solution is continuous.(Fan & Li, 2001) Fan gave the solution to SCAD in the context of wavelets.(Fan, 1997) The SCAD estimator has the following form:

$$\begin{aligned} &\hat{\theta} = sign(z)(|z| - \lambda)_+ \quad when\ |z| \le 2\lambda \\ &\hat{\theta} = \{(a-1)z - sign(z)a\lambda\} / (a-2) \quad when\ 2\lambda < |z| \le a\lambda \\ &\hat{\theta} = z \quad when\ |z| > a\lambda \end{aligned} \tag{9}$$

One feature of this penalty is the oracle property: when some variables are not present in the true model, these corresponding coefficients tend to be estimated as zero when the sample size gets large.(Fan & Li, 2001) Asymptotically, it provides as good estimation of the coefficients as if the underlying model were known beforehand.(Fan & Li, 2001) Selection and estimation of the variable coefficients is automatic and simultaneous.(Fan & Li, 2001) Among the many instances where SCAD has been applied to microarrays for biomarker selection, the study by Wang *et al.* (2007) successfully discovered 71 potential transcriptional factors (TF) in the cell cycle of yeast. These included 19 out of 21 known and experimentally verified TFs related to the cell cycle. Additional TFs showed periodic transcriptional effects and thus were biologically important and worth further study.(Wang et al., 2007)

b. *Methods Involving Derived Inputs: Principal Components Regression:* When a large number of correlated inputs (e.g. potential biomarkers) are available, instead of keeping all these inputs in a regression model, it may be beneficial to consider just a few linear combinations of them. A logically justifiable choice for the coefficients used in the linear combination is the normalized vector a that gives the largest sample variance of all possible normalized linear combinations of the input variables. (Hastie et al., 2001) This is called the first principal component. The first p principal components are found sequentially, with each successive component maximizing input variation subject to being orthogonal to previous ones. When all the principal components are used, the method becomes the usual least square estimation. However, when fewer principal components are used, this method is similar to ridge regression.(Hastie et al., 2001) As an example, Tan *et al.* (2005) used total principal component regression to classify the tumors into different categories.

Partial Least Squares: In contrast to principal component regression, which uses linear combination only of the input variables, partial least square(PLS) also allows for some information from the response variable y in the linear combinations.(Hastie et al., 2001) The algorithm is as follows: Assume y is centered and each x_j is properly standardized. PLS first regresses y on each x_j to obtain the corresponding coefficient $\hat{\varphi}_{1j}$. Subsequently, we can define the first partial least square direction as $z_1 = \sum \varphi_{1j} x_j$. (Hastie et al., 2001) Then Y is regressed on z_1 to obtain the corresponding coefficients which is followed by orthogonalizing $x_1 \ldots x_p$ in reference to z_1.(Hastie et al., 2001) This process is repeated until the desired number of directions is reached. As with principal component regression, using all p directions results in the usual least square estimation.(Hastie et al., 2001) Differently from principal component regression, PLS seeks input that is in the direction of high variation and high correlation with y.(Hastie et al., 2001) In addition, when the inputs are orthogonal to each other, the PLS will coincide with the least square estimates after the 1st step, setting the coefficients to be zero for the subsequent steps.

Because of its good properties with small sample sizes and many predictors, PLS has been applied to high-dimensional genomic data.(Boulesteix & Strimmer, 2006; Aaroe, *et al.*, 2010) Moreover, PLS regression can also be used to impute missing data. For example, Bras and Menezes (2006) impute missing values using PLS regression with all the genes as predictors. Huang *et al.* (2004) use a penalized version of PLS, which removes genes with poor power of prediction, in order to predict LVAD (left mechanical ventricular assist device) support time. In this case, the shrinkage parameter and the number of latent components are obtained using cross-validation. After proper shrinkage, some genes have coefficient zero, thus removing them from the model.(Huang et al., 2004) This reduces the complexity of the model, and serves as an example for combining both shrinkage and PLS.

c. *Bayes Variable Selection Methods:* Bayesian approaches use knowledge across genes for further inference.(Nott et al., 2007) For example, George and Foster (2000) adopted a binomial prior for the number of the differentially expressed genes (i.e. biomarkers) and a normal prior for their corresponding coefficients, assuming known and constant variance parameter. With informed choice of the hyperparameters, the authors ranked the genes according to the posterior probability that the gene belonged to the differentially expressed gene set or not. Interestingly, the gene ranking agreed with the ranking obtained by other criteria such as AIC (Akaike, 1973) or BIC (Schwartz, 1979; Nott *et al.*, 2007) When the variance parameters were unknown, different priors were assumed for effects of the genes and variance of the genes. Lonnstedt and Speed used a normal prior for effects of the differentially expressed genes and an inverted gamma prior for the corresponding variance.(Lonnstedt & Speed., 2002) Thus, after choosing the hyperparameters properly, people derived an explicit expression for the log odds of differentially expressed genes, which was known as B-statistic. (Lonnstedt & Speed, 2002) In contrast, Nott *et al* considered a double tailed exponential prior for effects of the differentially expressed genes and an inverted gamma for the corresponding variance.(Nott et al., 2007) The motivation was that double tailed exponential was heavier on the tails and was related to lasso.(Nott et al., 2007) The proposed linear model was as follows:

$$M_{gj}=\mu_g+\varepsilon_{gj} \tag{10}$$

M_{gj} is the expression value of gene g for array j. μ_g is the gene specific mean expression value. ε_{gj} is $N(0, \sigma_g^2)$ where σ_g^2 is the gene specific variance. All the σ_g^2 are independent. Except the situation where we have infinite sample size, we can only conclude gene g is differentially expressed when $|\mu_g|>k$ and gene g is not differentially expressed when $|\mu_g|\leq k$.(Nott et al., 2007) As a predefined cutoff value, k depends on the purpose of the experiment and other conditions. Correspondingly, B-statistic is then defined as follows to explore whether gene g belongs to the set of differentially expressed gene or not:

$$B(k)=\log\frac{\Pr\left(\left|\mu_g\right|>k\middle|M\right)}{\Pr\left(\left|\mu_g\right|\leq k\middle|M\right)} \tag{11}$$

The above represents the log odds ratio of the posterior probability given the data M. To implement this hierarchical Bayes procedure, calculation of the posterior probability is necessary. A modified version of MCMC (Markov Chain Monte Carlo) algorithm was proposed, and details of the computation of the above *B*-statistic when the prior distributions are given is discussed by Nott et al. (2007). When k is chosen to be 0 and a proper prior allows μ_g to be exactly 0, an explicit form of B(0) can be developed accordingly.(Lonnstedt & Speed., 2002) People usually use this statistic to rank genes instead of making inferences.(Nott et al., 2007; Lonnstedt & Speed., 2002)

d. *Hypotheses Testing as a Variable Selection Methods:* The t-statistic has already been widely used for hypothesis testing for a long time. Therefore, people try to apply this to microarray study to select appropriately biomarkers on microarray. However, the traditional t-statistic will not work in this situation due to the following reasons: First, hundreds or thousands hypotheses are being tested simultaneously; therefore, the multiple comparison issue exists. However, Bonferroni correction is too conservative and sometimes no gene can pass this vigorous criterion. Thus, suitable adjustment methods need to be developed to further control the overall error. Second, during the microarray analysis, large outliers are frequently observed, and they tend to drive the t-statistic to be large. Similarly, due to large number of tested genes and small number of replicates, the estimated variance for each gene is usually small, which tends to drive the t-statistic to be large.

To meet the first challenge, a new method known as false discovery rates (FDRs) has been proposed. (Benjamini & Hochberg, 1995; Tusher et al., 2001) False discovery rate is defined as the expected proportion of type I error using the available decision rule.(Benjamini & Hochberg, 1995) This method, readily available in *R*, is especially useful for microarray study, since it is easy to compute and not as overly conservative as is Bonferroni adjustment.

The second challenge requires a robust modification to the current version of t-statistic. One of them is known as *ad hoc* modification, which defines the modification by the data. Efron's 90% rule is in this category.(Efron et al., 2000) The modification is to add a constant term to the denominator to prevent the variance in the t-statistic from being too small.(Efron et al., 2001) The constant a_0 is defined as the 90th percentile of all the standard errors of the genes.(Efron et al., 2000) Thus the ordinary t-statistic has the following format:

$$S_g = M_{g.} / (s_g + a_0) \tag{12}$$

$M_{g.}$ denotes the average expression value for gene g, and s_g denotes the corresponding standard deviation. Another example belonging to *ad hoc* modification is the SAM (Significance Analysis of Microarrays).(Tusher et al., 2001) For each gene, the SAM method assigns a score relative based on the changes in expression relative to the standard deviation for the repeated experiments. For genes with scores higher than certain thresholds, a permutation distribution is used to estimate the FDR.(Tusher et al., 2001) This method may be viewed as an empirical Bayes procedure, simply adding a constant each set of genes levels when estimating individual variances. This avoids difficulties when variances are computed from a small number of observations for each gene.(Tusher et al., 2001) This method showed great improvement in gene identification both FDR-wise and fold-wise in terms of the human cell response to the ionizing radiation.(Tusher et al., 2001) Despite of its robustness to individual outliers, the use of this *ad hoc* modification is still limited, and it is challenging to derive and study its theoretical properties.

Accordingly, a penalized likelihood version of t-statistic has been proposed and implemented. For example, Wu (2005) proposed another modified t-statistics, taking advantage of both SAM and lasso methods. The method works as follows: assume the linear regression situation,

$$x_{ij}=\beta_0+ y_j+\varepsilon_j \tag{13}$$

where x_{ij} represents the expression of gene i on array j; y_j is the indicator, whether the jth sample belongs to the control or treatment group. A t-statistic or F-statistic can be developed.(Wu, 2005) The test statistic involves ordinary between/within group sum of squares, both of which can be penalized like in lasso regression.(Wu, 2005) The test statistic in this scenario can be derived as:

$$t_i^* = sign(\bar{x}_{i1} - \bar{x}_{i2})\frac{\left(|\bar{x}_{i1} - \bar{x}_{i2}| - \lambda\right)_+}{\sqrt{n/(n_1n_2)s_i^2 + \lambda^2/(n-2)}} \tag{14}$$

$$F_i^* = \frac{(|\bar{x}_{i1} - \bar{x}_{i2}|^2 - \lambda^2)_+}{n/(n_1n_2)s_i^2 + \lambda^2/(n-2)} \tag{15}$$

Tusher's SAM statistic is as follows:

$$d_i = \frac{\bar{x}_{i1} - \bar{x}_{i2}}{s_0 + s_1\sqrt{n/(n_1n_2)}} \tag{16}$$

Comparing the formulas (14—16), we can see that the penalized F or t statistic can be viewed as a special version of SAM, since the term $\lambda^2/(n-2)$ coincides with the constant s_0 in SAM statistic, which helps to stabilize the variance.(Wu, 2005) Furthermore, Wu showed that FDR can be calculated by permutation and then a cutoff can be put on the test statistic.(Wu, 2005) What makes the penalized SAM statistic superior to the ordinary SAM statistic is that penalized SAM statistic is derived rigorously from the situation of linear model and thus easier to develop its theoretical properties.(Wu, 2005) Through applications, this statistic also shown good performance.(Wu, 2005)

Another modified t-statistic is refined for a statistical model assuming both multiplicative and additive errors.(Ideker et al., 2000) The parameters within the model are subsequently estimated using maximum likelihood method with all the observations.(Ideker et al., 2000) Subsequently, a traditional maximum likelihood ratio test for each individual gene is carried out to identify the significance of the intensities.(Ideker et al., 2000) In some examples, this method can be shown superior to the simple fold approach.(Ideker et al., 2000) However, this method is naïve and has potential limitation as follows: first, the author does not use any multiple comparison adjustment techniques when performing multiple tests on thousands of genes simultaneously; this may be corrected by introducing the traditional FDR. Second, the author used chi-square as the distribution of -2*ln(likelihood ratio), which may not hold for small sample size.(Ideker et al., 2000) A more suitable distribution needs to be derived accordingly.

One more example of a "modified" t-statistic is derived from a Bayesian approach, which has become popular in statistics. For example, the B-statistic, the log odd ratio of the posterior probability can be viewed as a Bayesian version of t-statistic.(Lonnstedt & Speed, 2002) Another example of "moderated" *t*-statistic is proposed by Smyth.(Smyh, 2004) It assumes a scale inverse chi square prior for the variances of the genes.(Smyh, 2004) Additionally, the parameters can be estimated using Bayesian method and the 'moderated' t statistic is obtained by substituting the corresponding variance with their estimate.(Smyh, 2004) Cui *et al* propose another modified t-statistic using similar approach.(Cui et al., 2005) First, they performed a simulation from a chi-square distribution, whose degrees of freedom depends on the sample size to estimate the variance. Then they derive a bias-corrected Stein estimator on the log scale.(Cui et al., 2005) Thus, this estimator is more robust since the shrinkage in the variance makes the estimator of variance more robust.

As we can see, the main drawback of "moderated t" is that it depends on a particular type of distribution. When the distribution assumption is not satisfied, these estimators will be inefficient and often lead to false inferences. This inspires the birth of the distribution free 'shrinkage t' statistic.(Opgen-Rhein & Strimer, 2007) The main idea behind this is shrinking the empirical variance of each gene towards the common median of all the variance.(Opgen-Rhein & Strimer, 2007) For each group, the ordinary variance is replaced by the corresponding shrinkage variance in the test statistic:

$$t_k^* = \frac{\overline{x}_{k1} - \overline{x}_{k2}}{\sqrt{\frac{v_{k1}^*}{n_1} + \frac{v_{k2}^*}{n_2}}} \tag{17}$$

For the above formula, n_1 and n_2 are sample size for group 1 and 2, respectively. v^* stands for the corresponding shrinkage variance estimator. Here, each empirical variance is shrinking towards the median, which is shown to be more efficient or robust than shrinking towards the mean or zero.(Opgen-Rhein & Strimer, 2007) We can also view the "shrinkage t" as a combination of a standard t statistic and the fold change statistic.(Opgen-Rhein & Strimer, 2007) Another feature is that the "shrinkage t" belongs to the James-Stein estimator, not relying on any explicit prior distribution assumption and its theoretical property will be easily derived. Furthermore, this method is computationally efficient and the corresponding gene ranking is consistent with other tests.(Opgen-Rhein & Strimer, 2007)

Shrunken centroid method and SCOOP: From a different point of view, Tibshirani developed the shrunken centroid method for biomarker identification.(Davies & Bromage, 2002; Tibshirani et al., 2005) For each gene within each group (i.e. treatment group or control group), the overall mean and the group means are calculated. The group means are shrunk toward the overall mean iteratively for each gene.(Davies & Bromage, 2002; Tibshirani et al., 2005) The shrunken values are used to rank the genes and the cutoff is chosen by cross-validation. (Davies & Bromage, 2002; Tibshirani et al., 2005) The shrunken values can be also used to form a classifier and the authors used this method to classify the cancer conditions. (Davies & Bromage, 2002; Tibshirani et al., 2005) Despite the successes this method has achieved, it has one potential drawback: information about correlation among genes is distorted or lost during successive shrinkage, and, therefore, the identified genes may appear falsely to be independent of each other. Based on this method, Liu *et al.* (2009) developed an improved version of shrinkage centroid method: SCOOP (**S**hrunken **C**entroid **O**rthogonal **O**rdering **P**rojection) to extend to the cases with correlation variables. Instead of shrinking along the natural axes (Tibshirani et al., 2005), which ignores the potential linkage between variables, SCOOP rotates the axis and shrinks the group means in the direction preserving the least correlation information of variables. The algorithm of SCOOP is as follows: With the input of group information and the gene expression values from microarrays, two matrices are further identified: Between Epoch Covariance Matrix, containing all the variation between different groups, and Within Epoch Covariance Matrix, containing the variation originating from replication. Then, the eigenvalues and eigenvectors for both Between Epoch Covariance Matrix and Within Epoch Covariance Matrix are calculated by spectral decomposition. Since we have small number of samples and large number of variables (i.e. the genes) for microarray studies, both Between Epoch Covariance Matrix and Within Epoch Covariance Matrix are going to be highly singular. The union of the eigenvectors of the Between Epoch Covariance Matrix and Within Epoch Covariance Matrix with nonzero eigenvalues will form the basis functions of the new space (known as the Augmented Discriminant Space). For each gene, the group mean expression is shrunk towards the overall mean along the direction orthogonal to the Augmented Discriminant Space until the group means coincide, at which point that gene is eliminated from consideration. The amount of shrinkage needed for each gene is considered as its measure of importance. The above algorithm is carried out individually for each gene, producing a ranking of genes according to the importance measure. SCOOP has been successfully applied to identify biomarkers responsible for female rainbow trout reproductive cycle.(Liu, 2009, 2011)

2.3.2 Introduction to basic microarray time course analysis

Due to the decreasing cost of microarrays, their use in time course analysis has become ever more popular. The corresponding analysis is more challenging statistically than the two sample microarray situation. The time course may be longitudinal (where the mRNA samples for different time points are taken from the same individual), or cross-sectional (where the mRNA samples are extracted from different individual).(Tai & Speed, 2005) As a result, gene expression tends to be correlated for the longitudinal study or a design used for the cross-sectional study using a common reference. In addition, usually only 5-10 time points are available. Therefore, the traditional time series model cannot deal with such small series. This will require the development of new methods for analysis.

Typically, researchers are interested in identifying the genes whose expressions change over time. In the one-sample problem, some genes' patterns vary according to a common pattern. In the two-sample problem, we need to identify genes whose temporal changes differ under two or more biological conditions.(Tai & Speed, 2006)

One popular method typically used is a regression model. As an example, maSigPro belongs to this category and is available in *R*. (www.bioconductor.org) To find significantly different genes for two or more biological conditions, maSigPro first builds a global regression model with different experiment conditions acting as dummy variables.(Conesa et al., 2006) Then the significance of the estimated parameters in the model was tested to assess the significant differences between gene time course profiles.(Conesa et al., 2006)

Another method for microarray time course analysis is via ANOVA and the F-statistic. The classical ANOVA and mix-effect ANOVA models are used for cross-sectional and longitudinal study, respectively.(Diggle et al., 2002; Neter et al., 1996; Tai & Speed, 2005) For the one-sample problem, time is treated as one factor. Thereafter, the corresponding F-statistic is calculated.(Tai & Speed, 2005) Moreover, this method can be extended to the situation with multiple experiment conditions. Time, experiment condition and potentially their interaction are included for this model. An example of the classical ANOVA in time course study is available in (Wang & Kim, 2003). Also the multiple comparison adjustment for testing error is discussed for this method.(Ge & Speed, 2003)

Later, a robust version of ANOVA approach was proposed by Park *et al*, since it does not require the normality assumption.(Park et al., 2003) Similar to a two-way ANOVA model which includes time, biological conditions and their interaction as factors, genes that are concluded insignificant in this model will be reanalyzed in the same ANOVA model without the interaction term. (Park et al., 2003) Genes that are concluded significant in both models are chosen.(Park et al., 2003) Another modified ANOVA method is the ANOVA-SCA (analysis of variance-simultaneous component analysis), which takes into consideration about the correlation structure of the measured variables.(Nueda et al., 2007) Basically, principle component analysis is used to the estimated parameters of each source of variation in the ANOVA model.(Nueda et al, 2007) One advantage of this method is that it utilizes information from the experiment design and takes into consideration about correlation among the each source of variability associated with experimental factors. To identify the differentially expressed genes, the authors proposed another criterion for ANOVA-SCA: the mixture of leverage and SPE (square prediction error).(Nueda et al., 2007) Leverage quantifies how much a particular gene contributes to the multivariate ANOVA-SCA model, while SPE evaluates the goodness of fit of the model to a particular gene.(Nueda et al., 2007) The potential test statistic is and its p-value are obtained with reference to a weighted χ^2 distribution.(Box, 1954) Nonetheless, the drawback of this method is that it does not use the actual time scale and direct smoothing cannot be applied. Besides, this method cannot be used when the time course points are irregular.

In summary, the ANOVA and the corresponding modified versions offer substantial advantages: they can separate variation due to each different factor, therefore, removing the non-random effects and reducing the potential noise within the data.(Box, 1954) However, there are two innate limitations: First, it assumes independent among different time points ignoring the potential correlation; second, the small number of replicates leads to unstable estimation of gene-specific variance, leading to big value of within time F-statistics even for genes with just small amount of changes. This leads to high false positive rates.(Tai & Speed, 2005) In addition, some differentially expressed genes may have outliers which tend to cause low F-statistic, resulting in false negative rates.(Tai & Speed, 2005) Thus, the idea of moderation is introduced.

To reduce the false positive rate or false negative rate, the gene-specific variance is shrinking towards a common value estimated from the whole gene set, known as moderation.(Tai & Speed, 2005) One example about the application of moderation to microarray time course is performed by Tai and Speed.(Tai & Speed, 2006) They derived the *MB*- and $\tilde{T}^2$-statistic for one-sample or two-sample problem in the scenario of longitudinal microarray time course study, taking into consideration about the correlation across times. In detail, *MB*-statistic is the log 10 of the posterior odds whether the null or alternative hypothesis is true. When the number of replicates is equal for all genes, the *MB*-statistic under the null hypothesis is supposed to have the expected profile equal to 0 in one-sample case or equal expected profiles in two-sample scenario.(Tai & Speed, 2006) Then the form of *MB*-statistic becomes a monotonic increasing function in $\tilde{T}^2$. $\tilde{T}^2$-statistic is $\tilde{t}'\tilde{t}$ where $\tilde{t}$ is the moderated multivariate t-statistic in the form of $\tilde{t} = n^{1/2}\tilde{S}^{-1/2}\overline{X}$.(Tai& Speed, 2006). $\tilde{S} = \frac{(n-1)S + \nu\Lambda}{n-1+\nu}$

where S represents the gene-specific variance-covariance matrices, $\overline{X}$ is the gene-specific average time course vector. n represents the number of replicates. The other two parameters v and Λ can be estimated from all the genes. Both of the two statistic are derived when we assume independent and identical inverse Wishart priors to the gene-specific covariance matrices.(Tai & Speed, 2006) The advantage of this method comes from the incorporation of the information about the correlation structure, moderation and replication.(Tai & Speed, 2006) In addition, this statistic outperforms the ordinary F-statistic, due to moderation in empirical Bayes framework.(Tai & Speed, 2006) This procedure is shown to be very effective in false positive or negative rate reduction.(Tai & Speed, 2005) Thus, this procedure is incorporated in the Bioconductor "timecourse" package in *R*. (http:/ /www. bioconductor.org/packages/2.3/bioc/vignettes/timecourse/inst/doc/timecourse.pdf). The drawback of this method is modeling each gene independently, ignoring the latent genes pathway network and making no use of the actual time scale.

Another method that is used similar idea to estimate the unstable variance robustly and incorporate correlation in the study is based on the likelihood-based approach. Guo *et al.* develop a test based on the Wald statistic for one-sample longitudinal data.(Guo et al., 2003) This method adds a positive number to each diagonal element in the denominator matrix to incorporate the idea of moderation and stabilize the estimation of the variance.

$$w(i) = [L\hat{\beta}(i)]^T [L\hat{V}_s(i)L^T + \lambda_\omega I_{r\times r}]^{-1}[L\hat{\beta}(i)] \qquad (18)$$

In the above formula, L represents a matrix with dimension r X p, $\hat{\beta}$ represents the p X 1 regression parameters estimation and $\hat{V}s$ is the corresponding estimated variance-covariance matrix. λ_ω is an estimated positive scalar to prevent inverting a highly singular matrix.(Guo et al., 2003) However, the limitation of this method is that it is only suitable for one-sample problem and using the asymptotic theory will not be suitable for small number of replicates.

Despite of the popularity of the above method, they all ignore one important fact in time course study: They do not make use of the time points dynamically. This is the reason to introduce B-splines or wavelets to model the gene temporal expression profiles. Natural B-splines are piecewise cubic polynomials, which are smoothly connected at knots. It can describe the complicated gene expression patterns over time, since the linear combination of a series of basis functions can mimic any temporal profiles for genes. Each basis function can be thought as the potential expression pattern locally (i.e. the basis function will be zero outside certain time range). Comparing with methods that do not utilize time scale directly, B-splines have many advantages: reduce the noise, assuming only smoothing changes occur with time; use the actual time taken for the samples, easy to adapt for schedules with irregular time points; As an example, Bar-Joseph *et al.* present an algorithm to characterize the expression pattern of each gene by a continuous curve fitted by B-splines.(Bar-Joseph et al., 2003) They constrain the spline coefficients of genes within the same class so that their expression profiles can vary similarly. Thus, the gene expression pattern can be viewed dynamically. Comparing with previous methods, the reconstruction of the gene timecourse has 10-15% less error for those points that are not observed.(Bar-Joseph et al., 2003) Another approach proposed by Hong and Li is to solve the two-sample problem with B-splines adaption.(Hong & Li, 2006) In details, to identify biomarkers whose expression profiles are different under multiple biological conditions, linear combinations of basis functions are used to create smooth gene expression timecourse. The Markov chain Monte Carlo EM algorithm (MCEM) can be used to estimate the gene-specific parameters and hyperparameters from the hierarchical model. The genes are chosen using the empirical Bayes log posterior odds and the posterior probability based FDR.(Hong & Li, 2006) As a result, this method outperforms the traditional ANOVA model and is suitable for long time course data. Another example developed by Storey *et al.* and denoted as EDGE (**E**xtraction of **D**ifferential **G**ene **E**xpression) is also widely used for microarray timecourse study.(Storey et al., 2005) It estimates the coefficients of a B-spline function to fit the timecourse for each gene, and test whether all the coefficients are zero or not by an F-statistic. If all the coefficients are zero, the genes are not differentially expressed. Q-value based on false discovery rate(FDR) is calculated for each individual gene to offer a suitable cutoff value.(Storey et al., 2005) This method is an example to combine B-splines with the hypothesis testing, using FDR to control the error rate. Therefore, this method is superior to other methods. However, this method does not use the correlation information between variables (i.e. genes) and needs improvement. Thus SCOOP in combination with B-spline offers an alternative for biomarker identification for microarray timecourse study. (Liu, 2009, 2011)

When the situation of multiple biological condition in microarray timecourse study is encountered, Yuan *et al.* develop a hidden Markov model approach.(Yuan & Kendziorski, 2006) For this method, the authors consider all possibilities of equality and inequality for all the means among the different biological conditions and the expression pattern process is modelled as a Markov chain.(Yuan & Kendziorski, 2006) These biological conditions are referred as states. Thus, the observations are conditionally independent given the state of the chain. In summary, this method can monitor the expression pattern for each gene and the observations at different time points may be dependent on each other. The differentially expressed genes are then selected based on the posterior probabilities of states of interest.(Yuan & Kendziorski, 2006) Moreover, it is suggested that the associated posterior probability is useful to cluster genes.(Yuan & Kendziorski, 2006)

2.3.3 What is next?

Although the microarray technology has lead to big breakthroughs in biology, there is one innate drawback in this technique: since all the sequence information about genes incorporated into the probes needs to be known *a priori*, the microarray can only obtain fixed and partially information about gene variants within the cell. This limitation requires the development of new techniques to gain the information for all the gene alleles simultaneously. Therefore, the next generation sequencing technique gains popularity and may be consequently lead to more informative microarrays. The first generation sequencing is accredited to Frederick Sanger in 70s. (Sanger et al, 1977) Before the development of Sanger's chain-terminator method, Maxam and Gilbert used toxic chemicals to modify the bases, inferring the sequence of DNA fragment.(Maxam & Glibert, 1977) Sanger's chain-terminator method gained popularity since the method involved less toxicity. The key of the chain-terminator method is the dideoxynucleotide triphosphates(ddNTPs) to terminate the DNA chain elongation. To sequence a particular DNA fragement, the DNA template, primer, DNA polymerase and deoxynucleotidephosphates(dNTPs) is split into four separate reactions with the addition of only one of the four radioactively or fluorescently labelled dideoxynucleotides (ddATP, ddGTP, ddCTP or ddTTP) in the four reactions.(Sanger et al., 1977) Therefore, during the elongation, ddNTPs are incorporated into some of the strands, leading to DNA fragments that have varying length. These fragments can be separated using gel electrophoresis and the relative position of the band on the gel be used to determine the base identity.(Sanger et al., 1977)

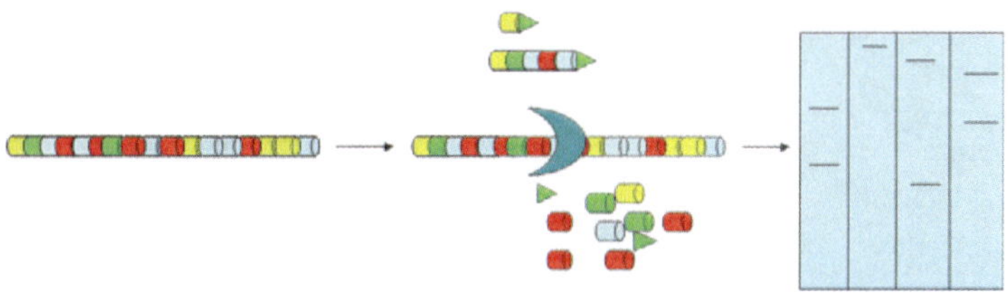

Fig. 2. The Sanger's chain-terminator method. For a fragment of DNA, the sample is split into four reactions containing dNTP, polymerase. Each reaction is supplemented with one type of ddNTP, serving as the chain terminator. In the above figure, we show only one reaction: the dNTP is depicted as tubes and ddCTP is depicted as triangles. The ddCTP terminates the reaction upon the addition of the ddCTP. The other three reactions form similar ladders and the sequences can be detected based on their relative position on the gel after gel electrophoresis.

In recent years, instead of using one fluorescence dye and four reactions, four different fluorescence dyes with unique emission wavelength will be used in a single reaction. Then the dye reader can automatically read the base identity after capillary electrophoresis. Readers interested in this technique can read the user's manual for ABI PRISM® 373 DNA Sequencer manual available at http:/ /www3.appliedbiosystems.com /cms/groups/ mcb_support/documents/generaldocuments/cms_041831.pdf.

Therefore, the previous sequencing technique is laborious and time consuming. The current biological studies require more efficient ways to sequence. This is the motivation for next generation sequencing development.

The first step for the high-throughput sequencing is to prepare a template. In this step, genomic DNA is randomly split into small pieces to construct fragment template.(Metzker, 2010) When the genomic DNA is first circularized by ligation and then split into small fragments, this is known as mate-pair template, which has advantages over fragment template in alignment.(Metzker, 2010) However, due to the reason that single fluorescence event is hard to detect, the templates need to be amplified. Emulsion PCR by Roche and bridge PCR by illumina are introduced here. The sheared genomic DNA will be ligated with adaptors containing the same fragment.(Metzker, 2010) This allows the amplication of the DNA fragment using common PCR primer. For emulsion PCR, the water droplet containing the bead-DNA complex, primer, polymerase, and dNTP will be used to perform PCR amplification. Numerous droplets are created by emulsifying the oil-aqueous mixture, allowing all the genomic DNA fragments to be amplified simultaneously.(Metzker, 2010) Another popular amplification method is bridge PCR. Bridge PCR has two steps: initial priming and extension of the template. The genomic DNA fragments with adaptors at both ends will be immobilized and bent over to form a bridge. Subsequently, the DNA molecules will be amplified to form clusters.(Metzker, 2010) Despite the great success, the amplification procedure is time consuming and complicated. Moreover, AT or GC-rich sequences may be biased during the amplification. (Metzker, 2010) Therefore, single-molecule templates technique which involves the immobilization of primer, template, or polymerase has become popular.(Metzker, 2010) The readers interested in this can obtain more details about this technique in Metzker 2010.

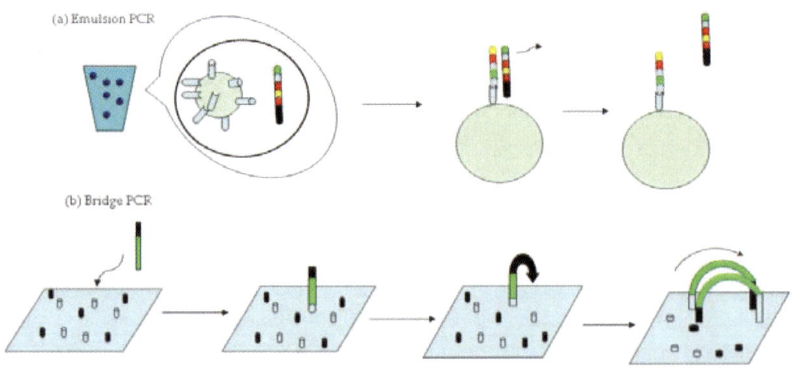

Fig. 3. The illustration of the emulsion PCR and bridge PCR. For emulsion PCR, the aqueous droplets can be created by emulsion in the oil water mixture. Then the template can be amplified with the primers within the bead. In the end, thousands of DNA fragments containing identical sequences to the template will be available within one bead for each aqueous droplet. For bridge PCR, the template is immobilized and bridge amplified to form a cluster.

Sequencing and imaging step follows the above amplification step. The four colour reversible termination method by illumina is introduced here. Right after the template clusters are obtained, the four nucleotides labelled with distinct fluorescence dye will be incorporated according to the template sequence and the elongation step halts upon the addition of fluorescence labelled nucleotide. Upon total internal reflection fluorescence imaging, TCEP (tris(2-carboxyethyl)phosphine) will be used to cleave the fluorescence dye and 3′-inhibitor to allow the next cycle of elongation. This process is iterated until the identities of all the nucleotides are known.(Metzker, 2010) The sequencing process for Roche/454 is called pyrosequencing, which uses a different mechanism for sequencing: following the emulsified PCR, the DNA-amplified beads are loaded into PTP (PicoTiterPlates) wells. Subsequently, this method allows the polymerase to add only one particular type nucleotide with the release of pyrophosphate. The pyrophosphate will then be converted with the emission of light by a series of reactions.(Ronaghi et al., 1998) This is further recorded by a charge-coupled device camera. The order of the light emission will be used to induce the sequence. This mechanism is totally different from the reversible termination method and it does not require the use of modified dNTP to halt the elongation process.(Metzker, 2010)

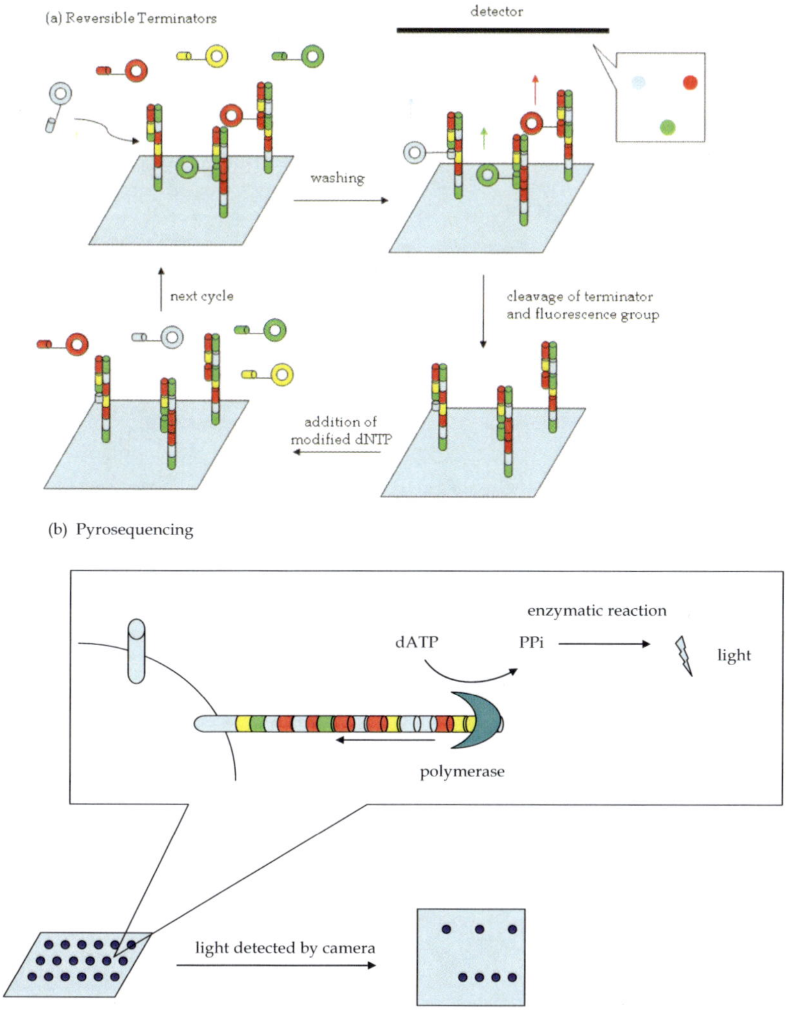

Fig. 4. The illustration of the reverse terminator sequencing and pyrosequencing. For reverse terminator sequencing, different dNTP is labelled with different fluorescence dye. Upon addition of each dNTP, the reaction halts and the fluorescence is the recorded. Then the terminator and fluorescence dye of dNTP is cleaved. Subsequently, the next dNTP is incorporated and the whole process is iterated. For pyrosequencing, one single dNTP flows through with the addition of the nucleotide in the corresponding position. The release of the pyrophosphate will undergo enzymatic reaction to produce light. Therefore, the camera will record which of the fragments has this dNTP at its current position.

The next generation sequencing reads will subsequently need to be aligned to the reference genome or assembled *de novo*.(Chaisson et al., 2009; Pop & Salzberg, 2008; Trapnell & Salzberg, 2009) There are several challenges for the genome assembly and alignment besides cost and effort: First, some reads may not be aligned to reference genome due to the structural variant (e.g. deletion or insertion).(Metzker, 2010) Second, some reads are difficult to align to the highly repetitive regions.(Metzker, 2010) *de novo* assembly will be complicated for large genome although some successes are reported.(Butler *et al*, 2008; Hernandez et al., 2008; Zerbino & Birney, 2008)

Although there are so many challenges, this field is still undergoing rapid development and will play a main role in the personal genome era and personalized medicine field. The gigantic information from the next generation sequencing studies will require the collaboration between biologists, bioinformaticians, and biostatisticians. What we envision are more and more big breakthroughs in the field of life science.

3. Conclusion

In summary, we presented a detailed overview of microarray studies. We introduced the mechanism, the associated statistical analysis, and the potential substitution for microarray-next generation sequencing. Several examples of microarray studies to identify biomarkers are also presented. We hope this chapter can serve as a guide for beginners in the field of biomarker identification and drug discovery.

4. Acknowledgment

The authors thank NCI NIH HHS for the support of Grant R01 CA095568/ and NSF for the support of Grant DMS-0540693. The authors also thank the editor and reviewers for their constructive comments.

5. References

Aarøe, J.;Lindahl, T.; Dumeaux, V.; Sæbø, S.; Tobin, D.; Hagen, N.; Skaane, P.; Lönneborg, A.; Sharma, P.; & Børresen-Dale, A-L. (2010). Gene Expression Profiling of Peripheral Blood Cells for Early Detection of Breast Cancer. *Breast Cancer Research,* Vol. 12, R7.

Akaike, H. (1973). Information Theory and an Extension of the Maximum Likelihood Principle. *Second International Symposium on Information Theory*, pp. 267-281.

Bar-Joseph, Z.; Gerber, G.; & Gifford, D. K. (2003). Continuous representations of time-series gene expression data. *Journal of Computational Biology,* Vol. 10, pp. 341-356

Benjamini, Y.; & Hochberg, Y. (1995). Controlling the False Discovery Rate: A practical and Powerful Approach to Multiple Testing. *Journal of The Royal Statistical Society,* Vol. Ser B 57, pp. 289-300.

Boulesteix, A.; & Strimmer, K. (2006). Partial Least Squares: a Versatile Tool for the Analysis of High-dimensional Genomic Data. *Briefings in Bioinformatics,* Vol.8, pp. 32-44.

Box, P. (1954). Some theorems on quadratic forms applied in the study of analysis of variance problems: effect of inequality of variance in one way classification. *Ann. Math.Stat.,* Vol. 25, pp. 290-302.

Bras, L.P.; & Menezes J.C. (2006). Dealing with Gene Expression Missing Data. *IEE Syst Biol,* Vol. 153, pp. 105-119.

Butler, J.; MacCallum, I.; Kleber, M.; Shlyakhter, I.A.; Belmonte, M.K.; Lander,E.S.; Nusbaum, C.; & Jaffe, D.B. (2008). ALLPATHS: de novo assembly of whole-genome shotgun microreads. *Genome Res.,* Vol. 18, pp. 821-829.

Cardoso, F.; Van't Veer, L.; Rutgers, E.; Loi,S.; Mook, S.; & Piccart-Gebhart, M.J. (2008) Clinical application of the 70-gene profile: the MINDACT trial. *J. Clin. Oncol.,* Vol. 26, pp. 729-735.

Chaisson, M.J.; Brinza, D.; & Pevzner, P. A. (2009). De novo fragmentassembly with short mater-paired reads:does the read length matter? *Genome Res,* Vol. 19, pp. 336-346.

Chen, J.; Traci, T. G; Brigitta, C. B.; Li, J.; Spencer, B. K.; Nicolas, C.; Jiang, H.; & Hou, D. (2011). Microarray Applications in Occlusive Vascular Disease. *Cardiovascular & Hematological Agents in Medicinal Chemistry,* Vol.9, pp. 84-94.

Conesa, A.; Nueda, M.; Ferrer, A.; & Talon M. (2006). maSigPro: a method to identify significantly differential expression profiles in time-course microarray experiments. *Bioinformatics,* Vol. 22, pp. 1096-1102.

Cui, X.; Hwang, J.T.G.; Qiu, J.; Blades, N.J.; & Churchill G.A. (2005). Improved statistical tests for differential gene expression by shrinking variance components estimates. *Biostatistics,* Vol. 6, pp. 59-75.

Davies, B.; & Bromage, N.(2002). The effects of fluctuating seasonal and constant water temperatures on the photoperiodic advancement of reproduction in female rainbow trout, Oncorhynchus mykiss. *Aquaculture,* Vol. 205, pp. 183-200.

Debouck C.; & Goodfellow P.N. (1999). DNA microarrays in drug discovery and development. *Nature,* Vol 21, pp. 48-50.

de Leon J.(2006)AmpliChip CYP450 test: personalized medicine has arrived in psychiatry. *Expert Rev Mol Diagn,* Vol. 6 pp. 277-286.

Diggle,P.J.; Heagerty, P.; Liang, K.-Y.; & Zeger S.L. (2002). *Analysis of Longitudinal Data* (2nd ed.). New York: Oxford University Press.

Efron, B.; Tibishirani, R.; Goss. V.; & Chu, G. (2000). *Microarrays and Their Use in a Comparative Experiment. Technical Report,* Vol. 213, Stanford Univeristy, Available from
http://statistics.stanford.edu/~ckirby/techreports/GEN/2000/2000-37B.pdf

Efron, B.; Hastie, T.; Johnstone I.; & Tibshirani, R. (2004). Least Angle Regression. *Ann. Statist.,* Vol.32, pp. 407-499.

Efron, B.; Tibishirani, R.; Storey, J.; & Tusher, V. (2001). Empirical Bayes Analysis of a Microarray Experiment. *Journal of the American Statistical Association,* Vol. 96, pp. 1151-1160.

Fan J. (1997). Comments on 'Wavelet in Statistics: A Review' by A. Antoniadis. *Journal of the Italian Statistical Association,* Vol. 6, pp. 131-138.

Fan, J.; & Li. R. (2001). Variable Selection via Nonconcave Penalized Likelihood and its Oracle Properties. *Journal of the American Statistical Association,* Vol. 96, pp. 1348-1359.

Ge, Y.; Dudoit, S.; & Speed, T. (2003). Re-sampling based multiple testing for microarray data analysis. *Test,* Vol.12, pp. 1-77.

Gentleman, R.; Carey V.J.; Huber, W.; Irizarry, R.A.; & Dudoit, S. (2005). *Bioinformatics and Computational Biology Solutions Using R and Bioconductor*:(1st ed.) Springer, New York.

George, E.I.; & Foster, D.P. (2000). Calibration and Emprical Bayes Variable Selection. *Biometrica,* Vol.87, pp. 731-747.

Golub, T.R.; Slonim, D.K.; Tamayo, P.; Huard, C.; Gaasenbeek, M.; Mesirov, J.P.; Coller, H.; Loh, M.L.; Downing, J.R.; Caligiuri, M.A.; Bloomfield, C. D.;& Lander E. S.(1999) Molecular Classification of Cancer: Class Discovery and Class Prediction by Gene Expression Monitoring. *Science*, Vol. 286, pp. 531-537.

Guo, X.; Qi, H.; Verfaillie, C.M.; & Pan, W. (2003). Statistical significance analysis of longitudinal gene expression data. *Bioinformatics,* Vol. 19, pp. 1628-1635.

Hastie, T.; Tibshirani, R.; & Friedman, J. (2001). *The Elements of Statistical Learning* (1st ed.). Springer, New York.

Hernandez, D; Francois, P.; Farinelli, L.; Osteras, M.; & Schrenzel, J. (2008). *De novo* bacterial genome sequencing: millinos of very short reads assembled on a desktop computer. *Genome Res,* Vol. 18, pp. 802-809.

Heller, R.A.; Schena, M.; Chai, A.; Shalon, D.; Bedilion, T.; Gilmore, J.; Woolley, D. E.; & Davis, R. W. (1997) Discovery and analysis of inflammatory disease-related genes using cDNA microarrays. *Proc. Natl. Acad. Sci.,* Vol. 94, pp.2150-2155.

Hoerl, A.E.; & Kennard, R. (1970). Ridge Regression:Biased Estimation for Nonorthogonal Problems. *Technometrics,* Vol. 12, pp. 55-67.

Hong, F.; & Li, H. (2006). Functional Hierarchical Models for Identifying Genes with Different Time-Course Expression Profiles. *Biometrics,* Vol. 62, 534-544.

Huang, X.; Pan, W.; Park, S.; Han, X.; Miller L. W.; & Hall, J. (2004). Modeling the Relationship between LVAD Support Time and Gene Expression Changes in Human Heart by Penalized Partial Least Squares. *Bioinformatics,* Vol. 20, pp. 888-894.

Ideker, T.; Thorsson, V.; Siegel, A.F.; & Hood L.E. (2000). Testing for Differentially-Expressed Genes by Maximum-Likelihood Analysis of Microarray Data. *Journal of Computational Biology,* Vol. 7, pp. 805-817.

Ildiko, E. F.; & Friedman, J. H. (1993). A statistical view of some chemometrics regression tools. *Technometrics,* Vol. 35, pp. 109-135.

Irizarry,R. A.;. Bolstad, B. M; Collin, F.; Cope, L. M.; Hobbs, B.; & Speed, T. P. (2003). Summaries of Affymetrix GeneChip probe level data. *Nucleic Acids Research,* Vol.31 pp. e15 doi:10.1093/nar/gng015

Ko, D.; Xu, W.; & Windle, B. (2005). Gene Function Classification Using NCI-60 Cell Line Gene Expression Profiles. *Computational Biology and Chemistry,* Vol. 29, pp. 412-419.

Li, C.; & Wong, W. H. (2001). Model-based analysis of oligonucleotides arrays: model validation, design issues and standard error application. *Genome Biology,* Vol. 2, pp. research 0032.

Liu, Y.; Verducci, J.; Nagler, J.; Schultz, I.; Hook, S.; Cracium, G.; Sundling K.; & Hayton, W. (2009). Time Course Analysis of Microarray Data for the Pathway of Reproductive Development in Female Rainbow Trout *Statistical Analysis and Datamining,* Vol. 2, pp. 192-208

Liu, Y. (2011). *Properties of the SCOOP method of selecting gene sets. OhioLink,* Ph.D. dissertation, Dept. of Statistics,The Ohio State University, Columbus.

Lonnstedt, I.; & Speed, T.P. (2002). Replicated Microarray Data. *Statist. Sinica,* Vol. 12, pp. 31-46.

Nott, D. J.; Yu, Z.; Chan, E.; Cotsapas, C.; Cowley, M.J.; Pulvers, J.; Williams, R.; & Little, P. (2007). Hierarchical Bayes variables selection and microarray experiments. *Journal of Multivariate Analysis,* Vol. 98, pp. 852-872.

Nueda, M.J.; Conesa, A.; Westerhuis, J.A.; Hoefsloot, H.C.; Smilde, A.K.; Talón, M.; & Ferrer, A. (2007). Discovering gene expression patterns in time course microarray experiments by ANOVA-SCA. *Bioinformatics,* Vol. 23, pp. 1792-1800.

Maxam, A.M.; & Gilbert, W. (1977). A new method for sequencing DNA. *Proc Natl Acad Sci,* Vol. 74, pp. 560-564.

Metzker, M.L. (2010). Sequencing technologies--the next generation. *Nature Reviews,* Vol. 11, pp. 31-46.

Neter, J.; Kutner, M.H.; Wasserman, W.; & Nachtsheim, C. (1996). *Applied Linear Statistical Models* (4th ed.). Irwin: McGraw-Hill.

Opgen-Rhein, R.; & Strimer, K. (2007). Accurate Ranking of Differentially Expressed Genes by a Distribution-Free Shrinkage Approach. *Statist. Appl. Genet. Mol.Biol.,* Vol.6, pp. article 9.

Park, T.; Yi, S-G.; Lee, S.; Lee, S. Y.; Yoo, D-H.; Ahn, J-I.; & Lee Y-S. (2003). Statistical tests for identifying differentially expressed genes in time-course microarray experiments. *Bioinformatics,* Vol. 19, pp. 694-703.

Pop, M.; Salzberg S.L. (2008). Bioinformatics challenges of new sequencing technology. *Trends Genet.,* Vol. 24, pp. 142-149.

Ronaghi, M.; Karamohamed, S.; Pettersson, B.; Uhlen, M.; & Nyren, P. (1998). Real-time DNA sequencing using detection of pyrophosphate release. *Anal. Biochem.,* Vol. 242, pp. 84-89.

Sanger, F., Nicklen, S.; & Coulson, A.R. (1977). DNA sequencing with chain-terminating inhibitors. *Proc. Natl. Acad. Sci. USA,* Vol. 74, pp. 5463-5467.

Schwartz, G. (1979). Estimating the Dimension of a Model. *Ann. Statist.,* Vol. 6, pp. 461-464.

Smyh, G.K. (2004). Statistical Application in Genetics and Molecular Biology. *Statist. Appl. Genet. Mol.Biol.,* Vol. 3, pp. article 3.

Storey, J.D.; Xiao, W.; Leek, J.T.; Tompkins, R.G.; & Davis, R.W. (2005). Significance analysis of time course microarray experiments. *Proc. Natl. Acad. Sci,* Vol. 102, pp. 12837-12842.

Tai, Y.C.; & Speed, T.P. (2005). Statistical Analysis of Microarray Time Course Data. Available from *http://www.ds.unifi.it/StatGen2005/works/day4/speed_latest.pdf.*

Tai, Y.C.; & Speed, T.P. (2006). A multivariate empirical Bayes statistic for replicated microarray time course data. *Ann. Statist.,* Vol. 34, pp. 3287-2412.

Tan, Y.; Shi, L.; Tong W.; & Wang, C. (2005). Multi-class cancer classification by total principal component regression (TPCR) using microarray gene expression data. *Nucleic Acids Research,* Vol. 33, pp. 56-65.

Tibshirani, R.; Hastie, T.; Narasimhan, B.; & Chu, G. (2005). Diagnosis of multiple cancer types by shrunken centroids of gene expression. *Proc. Natl. Acad. Sci,* Vol. 99, pp. 6567-6572.

Trapnell, C.; & Salzberg, S.L. (2009). How to map billions of short reads onto genomes. *Nature Biotech,* Vol 27, pp. 455-457.

Tusher, V.; Tibishirani, R.; & Chu, C. (2001). Significance Analysis of Microarrays Applied o Transcriptional Response to Ionizing Radiation. *Proc. Natl. Acad. Sci,* Vol. 98, pp. 5116-5121.

van't Veer, L.J.;Dai, H.; van de Vijver, M.J.; et al. (2002) Gene expression profiling predits clinical outcome of breast cancer. *Nature,* Vol. 415, pp. 530-536.

Verducci, J., Melfi, V., Lin, S., Roy, S and Sen, C. (2006) Microarray Analysis of Gene Expression: Considerations in Data Mining and Statistical Treatment *Physiological Genomics* 25(3):355-63.

Wang, L.; Chen, G.; & Li, H. (2007). Group SCAD Regression Analysis for Microarray Time Course Gene Expression Data. *Bioinformatics,* Vol. 23, pp. 1486-1494.

Wang, J.; & Kim, S.K. (2003). Global analysis of dauer gene expression in Caenorhabditis elegans. *Development,* Vol. 130, pp. 1621-1634.

Wang, X.; Yue, T.L.; Barone, F.C.; White, R. F.; Clark, R. K.; Willette, R. N.; Sulpizio, A. C.; Aiyar, N. V.; Ruffolo Jr, R. R.; & Feuerstein G. Z. (1995). Discovery of adrenomedullin in rat ischemic cortex and evidence for its role in exacerbating focal brain ischemic damage. *Proc. Natl. Acad. Sci.,* Vol. 92, pp.11480-11484.

Windle, B. & Guiseppi-Elie, A. (2003). Microarrays and Gene Expression Profiling Applied to Drug Research in: *Burger's Medicinal Chemistry and Drug Discovery* (6th ed.). John Wiley and Sons, Inc. Hoboken, New Jersey.

Wu, B. (2005). Differential Gene Expression Detection Using Penalized Linear Regression Models: the Improved SAM Statistics. *Bioinformatics,* Vol. 21, pp. 1565-1571.

Yang, Y.H.; Dudoit, S.; Luu P.; & Speed, T.P. (2001). *Normalization for cDNA Microarray Data.* San Jose, California. Available from http://www.stat.berkeley.edu/users/terry/zarray/TechReport/589.pdf

Yuan, M.; & Kendziorski, C. (2006). Hidden Markov Models for Microarray Time Course Data in Multiple Biological Conditions. *Journal of the American Statistical Association,* Vol. 101, pp. 1323-1332.

Zerbino, D.R.; & Velvet, B.E. (2008). algorithms for de novo short read assembly using de Bruijin graphs. *Genome Res.,* Vol. 18, pp. 821-829.

11

Effective Kinetic Methods and Tools in Investigating the Mechanism of Action of Specific Hydrolases

Emmanuel M. Papamichael*, Panagiota-Yiolanda Stergiou, Athanasios Foukis, Marina Kokkinou and Leonidas G. Theodorou
University of Ioannina, Department of Chemistry, Ioannina
Greece

1. Introduction

1.1 The idea of the reaction mechanism

The idea of mechanism of a catalyzed (e.g. enzymatic) and/or uncatalyzed reaction requires understanding and enough experience on the reaction intermediates, their sequence, structures and energetic interactions in drawing all necessary kinetic steps without chemical ambiguity. (Knowles, 1976).

1.2 How essential is the investigation and identification of a reaction mechanism?

The investigation and identification of a reaction mechanism is essential in the sense that it provides information as to the molecular species of the reaction, and it is strongly based on the number and types of the phases involved; however, this discrimination is not always sharp (Vaimakis & Papamichael, 2002). Additionally, the kinetic mechanisms of enzymatic reactions provide evidence of how these biocatalysts could bind with their substrates to accomplish catalysis; thus the molecular machinery of enzyme action can be explained (Papamichael & Theodorou, 2005).

1.3 The importance of an enzymatic hydrolysis mechanism in science and technology

The importance of an enzymatic hydrolysis mechanism in science and technology is now well documented. The third class of enzymes plays an important role in the enzymatic scientific and industrial processes so far, as about 80% of the working enzymes are hydrolases catalyzing the cleavage of C-O, C-N, C-C and some other bonds, including P-O bonds in phosphates (Liese et al., 2000). Numerous hydrolases are now known, and they have been classified into many sequentially and structurally unrelated clans and families. Hydrolases are found in all living organisms, performing functions from simple digestion to regulation of the immune response, blood coagulation and glucose homeostasis (Bachovchin, 2001). Most of hydrolases are used in processing reactions, degrading proteins, carbohydrates and lipids in

---

* Corresponding Author

many scientific and industrial disciplines. "How these enzymes work?" is a question that has attracted big attention over past decades (Henrissat, 1991, 1995).

1.4 Enzyme kinetics

The section of biochemistry, which deals with enzymes, is termed "Enzymology", whose a branch is known as "Enzyme kinetics" relevant to the study of enzyme mechanisms, their reaction rates and the conditions which affect these rates. Enzyme kinetics is a particular case of chemical kinetics as enzymes are acting as catalysts, i.e. they increase the rate of a reaction without modifying its overall standard Gibbs-energy change (NC-IUB, 1983). The rate of an enzymatic reaction is expressed as the change in concentration of one of its substrates or products versus time, and it may be the function of several parameters including enzyme and substrate concentrations, time, pH-value and temperature of the reaction medium, as well as of others, affecting the reaction rate. The study of various kinds of models of enzymatic reactions attain of great interest in research, as well as in industrial applications of these biocatalysts, enhancing our knowledge about these processes and/or estimating the values of useful variables and parameters of these systems (Hogan & Woodley, 2000). The rate equation of an enzymatic reaction is a mathematical expression illustrating the catalysis in terms of rate constants and reactant concentrations, and it should best fit the experimental data. Additionally, an enzymatic kinetic mechanism provides evidence of how enzymes and their substrates could be combined in order to accomplish catalysis, as well as it explains the molecular machinery of enzyme action; its knowledge is required in order to be understood how enzymes perform catalysts as well as how their catalytic function could be regulated, and thus to provide information on the nature of the transition states, the geometry of the enzyme's active site, the substrate specificity, the acidic and/or basic groups associated with catalysis, the possible allosteric properties, the mode of regulation, etc.

2. Prerequisite knowledge

2.1 Catalysis by proteases, amylases, lipases, and their generally accepted mechanisms

2.1.1 Catalytic motifs and sequences of two, three, etc, subsites, substrate specificity, example mechanisms and oxyanion hole

Although the catalytic motifs of several specific hydrolases, which are discussed in this context, may be regarded as generally being similar in structure, however a deeper observation reveals that their functional reality is unambiguously completely different, even though similar groups of two, three, etc residues constitute their catalytic sites. Moreover, with respect to catalysis by hydrolases, the term "subsite" was largely brought into general use from proteases (Schechter & Berger, 1967) whose substrates are composed by amino acid residues whose side chains is assumed to interact with specific subsites, i.e. parts of the active site of protease. The conceptual idea of subsite as fundamental mechanistic feature of the enzymatic hydrolysis originated from glucoamylases; quantitative theoretical and experimental kinetic measurements were applied firstly in *Rhizopus* glucoamylases whose binding modes of substrates and their analogues, as well as the subsite interactions were elucidated and important parameters were estimated and reported in a series of inspired works (Hiromi, 1983). But, how subsites could function? Dynamic and mechanistic manipulations take place within the active sites due to the reorganization of important residue side chains related to the structures of subsites (Buckle & Fersht, 1994). An enzymatic active site comprises a dual role, i.e. the binding of substrate onto subsite, and the reaction performed by the catalytic residues, while the effectiveness of these roles determines the specificity of enzyme towards its substrate. Let's start this journey with proteases (EC 3.4.x.x), which are distinguished in endopeptidases or proteinases (EC 3.4.11-99.x) and exopeptidases (EC 3.4.21-99.x) (Rawlings & Barret, 1994). The most of endopeptidases are classified into four groups: serine proteases (EC 3.4.21.x), cysteine proteases (EC 3.4.22.x), aspartic proteases (EC 3.4.23.x), and metalloproteases (EC 3.4.24.x) (Rawlings & Barrett., 1993). Furthermore, glycosidases hydrolyze the glycosidic bonds; the enzymes of α-amylase, α-(1→4)-D-glucan-4-glucanohydrolase, family catalyze the hydrolysis and/or trans-glycosylation at the α-1,4- and α-1,6-glucosidic linkages. Furthermore, lipases (triacylglycerol acylhydrolases, EC 3.1.1.x) have not completely defined, as lipolysis takes place at the lipid–water interface of biphasic systems. The example in figure 1 represents the active site of a papain.

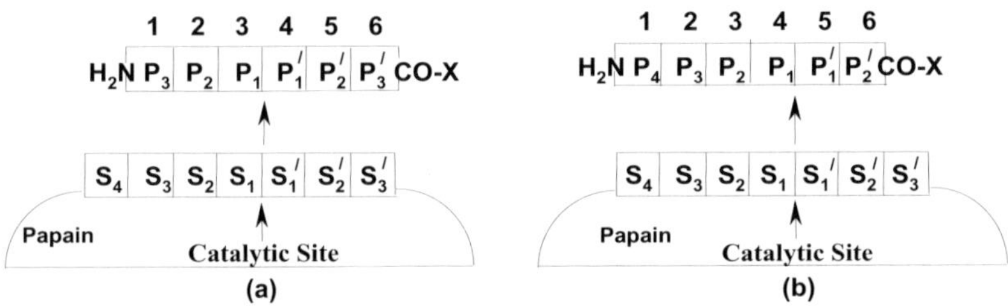

Fig. 1. Illustration of papain catalytic site, which is composed of seven "subsites" i.e. $\mathbf{S_1}$ - $\mathbf{S_4}$ and $\mathbf{S_1}'$ - $\mathbf{S_3}'$, located on its both sides; positions **P**, on substrate are numbering similarly as the subsites that they occupy, and are counted from the point of cleavage. When a hexapeptide binds onto papain, then, in **(a)** are formed two tripeptide molecules, while in **(b)** one tetrapeptide and another dipeptide are formed (modified from Schechter &. Berger, 1967).

Additional examples could be referred about the subsites of trypsin where an aspartyl-carboxylate group improves the binding of a lysine side chain. More specific examples of subsites could be found in matrix and other Zn^{2+}-dependent metalloproteinases, whose subsite function is facilitated by three histidines chelating the metal cation; the metal cation behaves as oxyanion hole where a glutamate residue ($\mathbf{E^{202}}$ - thermolysin numbering) resembles to a subsite as appeared in figures 2(a) and 3(b) (Auld, 1997; Pelmenschikov & Siegbahn, 2002).

It has been reported that the active site of α-amylases comprises 5–11 subsites, each interacting with one glucose unit of the substrate, and they were designated from **A** to **K**, while the reducing end of the α-glucose chain is located towards **K** subsite (Muralikrishnaa & Nirmala, 2005). However, in amylase-like glycosidases, we should understand a subsite noticeably differently, as these enzymes break more than one glycoside bond without dissociation of the **E-S** complex due to multiple or repetitive attack mechanism, where the enzyme is moving along the polysaccharide chain (sliding), as illustrated in figure 3 (Muralikrishnaa & Nirmala, 2005; Mazur & Nakatani, 1993).

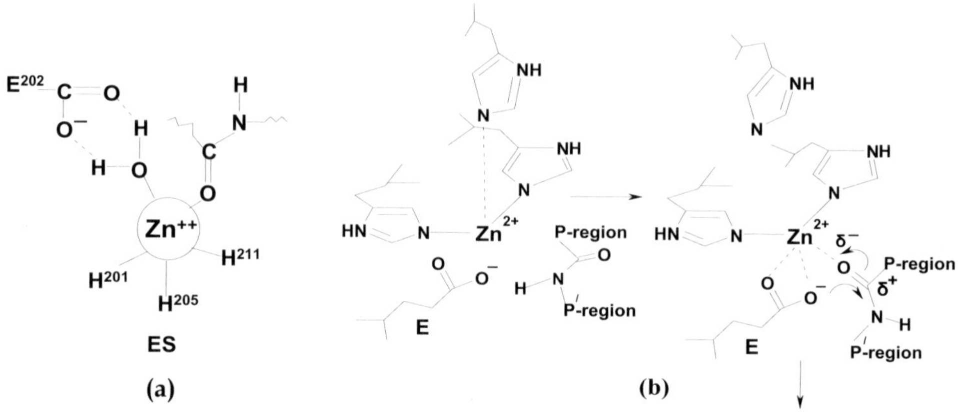

Fig. 2. Catalytic motifs of thermolysin-like metalloproteases: (a) a H_2O chelates Zn^{2+} as part of the catalytic motif, (b) no H_2O participate in the catalytic motif (modified from Auld, 1997, and Pelmenschikov & Siegbahn, 2002, respecively).

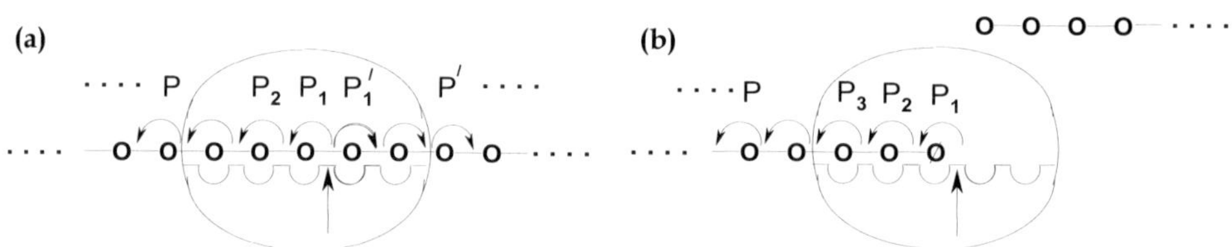

Fig. 3. Complexes of α-amylase with a polysaccharide substrate: (a) is the initial and (b) the same complex after a bond break (**O** and **Ø** are glucose and reduced glucose residues, respectively) (modified from Mazur & Nakatani, 1993).

The catalytic motifs of lipases are similar to those of serine proteases, and are expected analogous effects in the case of subsites. Although this is true, however it should be taken into account that: (a) the natural substrates of lipases are lipids, (b) lipolysis takes place at the water/lipid interface of biphasic (heterogeneous) systems, and (c) lipases should be equipped with the appropriate structural tools as it is the lid domain which plays an essential role in substrate selectivity towards triglycerides, and along with other structural features of lipases undergo a local reorganization to allow free access of substrate onto the subsites. Hence, in heterogeneous reaction media, where a physical adsorption of enzyme on the lipid interface occurs including activation by the lid opening, lipases catalyze reactions by different enzyme-substrate binding modes (Van Tilbeurgh et al., 1993). It should be underlined that the hydrolytic effectiveness of catalytic motifs varies among hydrolases even within the same family. On the other hand, a huge variety of substrates have been synthesized for hydrolases providing complete maps specificity and allowing the detection of interactions between substrate subsites; casual examples of synthetic substrates for different hydrolases can be found in the literature (Gosalia et al., 2005; Papamichael et al, 1999; Dune et al, 1986; Ohtaki et al, 2001).

An enzymatic reaction proceeds to its accomplishment through several sequential steps comprising the formation of intermediates; this course of action could be designated as a mechanism. The series of sequential step-reactions is likely to be accelerated by the functional groups found in the active site of enzymes. Thus, in enzymatic reactions, the catalysis is moved on due to conformational changes in the enzyme and/or the substrate molecule (Palfey, 2004); during the catalysis, hydrolases change the molecularity of the reaction, which although starts with two reactants (E and S, i.e. bimolecular), however, after the formation of the ES-complex, the reaction continues as unimolecular (Buckle & Fersht, 1994). Fundamental in serine proteases (chymotrypsin-like) is that they maintain one serine (**S**) residue in their catalytic motif which is commonly complemented by two more residues (aspartic acid **D**, and histidine **H**). It is generally accepted that the alcoholic oxygen of **S** plays the role of nucleophile. A functional example could be the triad $\mathbf{D^{102}}$, $\mathbf{H^{57}}$, and $\mathbf{S^{195}}$ (chymotrypsin numbering) (Auld, 1997; Bachovchin, 2001). In cases of more specific substrates a negative charge is spread all over the catalytic motif of these enzymes, designated as "Charge Relay System", whose a structural characteristic is the uncharged imidazole aromatic ring of the catalytic **H**. In cases of less specific substrates, the negative charge is localized on the alcoholic oxygen of $\mathbf{S^{195}}$ (the nucleophile) while the imidazole ring of catalytic **H** remains positively charged (general acid-base catalysis) (Hunkapiller et al.,1976); in both cases the development of an "oxyanion hole" is a prerequisite for catalysis by serine proteases. At a first glance, cysteine proteases perform catalysis similarly as serine proteases do, while one cysteine (**C**) residue is fundamental in their catalytic motif; regularly, cysteine (**C**) residue forms an ion-pair along with a histidine (**H**) residue ($\mathbf{C^{25}\text{-}S^{-}/H^{159}\text{-}Im^{+}H}$ - Papain numbering ion-pair) (Rawlings & Barret, 1993,1994). In cysteine proteases, acylation proceeds through the formation of an anionic tetrahedral adduct, the enzyme-substrate (**ES**) complex, while an oxyanion hole may be developed although it is not a prerequisite for catalysis by these enzymes (Theodorou et al., 2001). However, cysteine proteases do not perform catalysis via a catalytic dyad but through more complicated ways whose the main feature is the development of a hydrogen bond (Theodorou et al, 2007a). These latter are shown in figure 4.

Aspartic proteases (EC 3.4.23.x) have a long and perplexed history in Enzymology; the most of aspartic proteases perform catalysis by means of two eponymous aspartyl residues, which are found in opposite states of protonation. Both catalytic aspartyl residues are located in deep clefts formed at the interface of two lobes (e.g. porcine pepsin) (Polgár, 1989). It has been reported that a water molecule attacks the carbonyl carbon of the scissile bond, serving as a third catalytic component along with the active aspartic carboxyl groups, in the catalysis by aspartic proteases (Rebholz & Northrop, 1991); two catalytically active aspartate residues are in either a right or wrong protonic state, involving general base-catalyzed attack by a water molecule on the carbonyl carbon of the scissile bond. Recent ab-initio molecular dynamics simulations on HIV-1 protease were focused on the catalytic $\mathbf{D^{25}}$ and $\mathbf{D^{25\prime}}$, and resolved all the uncertainties within a unifying hypothesis, as illustrated in figure 5 (Piana & Carloni, 2000).

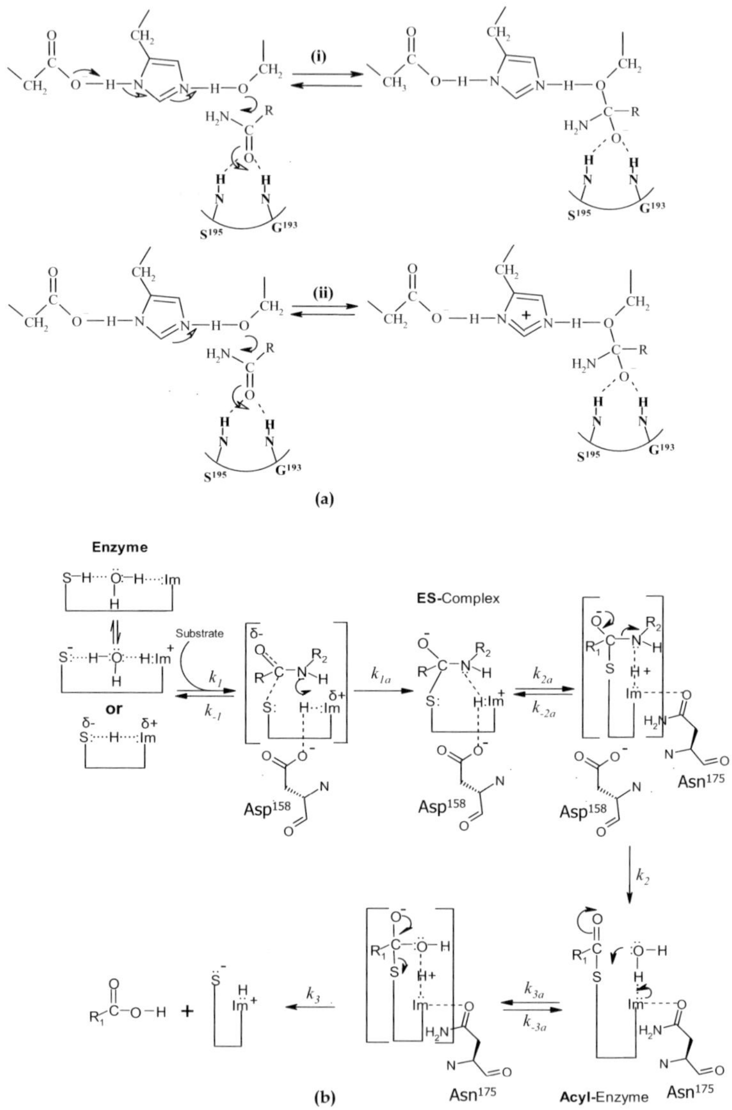

Fig. 4. **(a)** dual function of catalytic triad in serine proteases, where catalysis is performed: (i) by the charge relay system, and (ii) by general acid-general base (the oxyanion hole is formed by **G193** and **S195** residues), **(b)** function and role of the catalytic residues **C25**, **H159**, **D158** and/or **N175** (in bromelain) in cysteine proteases of papain family; a hydrogen bond necessary for efficient catalysis is developed between $D^{158}_{COO^-}$ and/or $N^{157}_{O^{\delta 1}}$, and the positively charged **H159**.

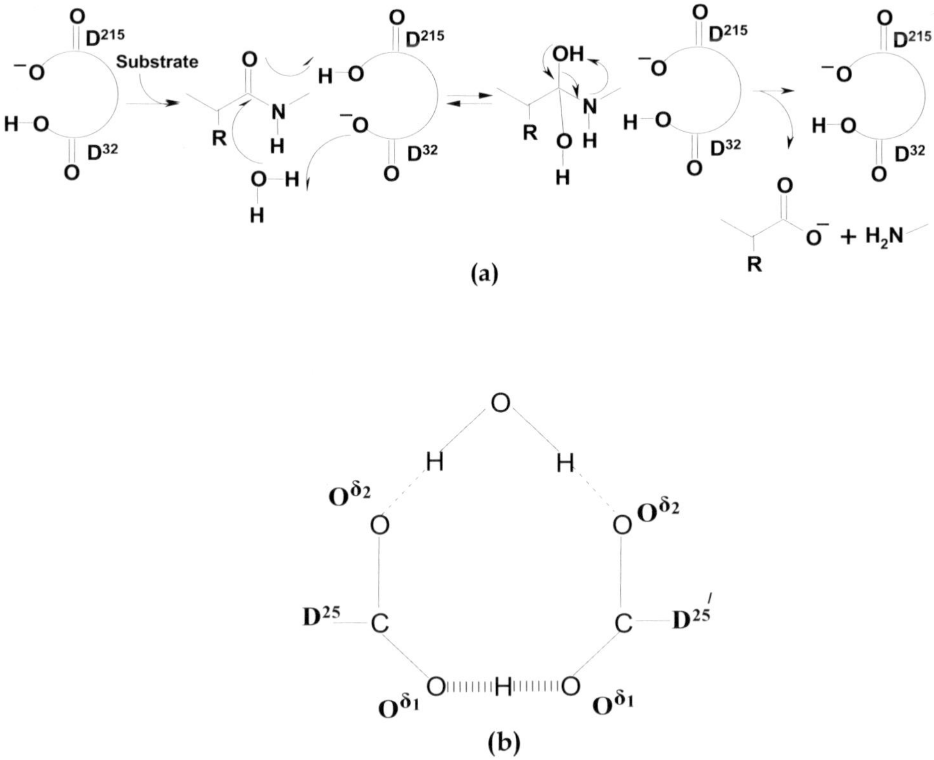

Fig. 5. (a) illustration of the catalysis by pepsin, where **D**^{32} was protonated before first turnover, while one proton is transferred from **D**^{215} to **D**^{32}; (b) the catalytic aspartates of HIV-1 protease in a coplanar arrangement where a LBHB joins the $\mathbf{O}^{\delta 1}$ oxygens and the H_2O and the $O^{\delta 2}$ oxygens are normally hydrogen bonded (modified from Northrop, 2001).

A variety of methods were applied in studying zinc or other matrix thermolysin-like metalloproteases (**EC 3.4.24.x**), focusing on how protein modulates the properties of zinc cation to achieve specificity and catalytic efficiency. It is well known that bivalent zinc allows many ligands and coordination geometries, and it is unaffected by oxidant or reductive reagents. Nitrogen, oxygen and/or sulfur donors form complexes with the zinc cation; additional ligand to the catalytic zinc cation may be considered one water molecule whose ionization and polarization provides hydroxide ions at neutral pH, while its displacement leads to acid catalysis by the zinc cation (Auld, 1997; Pelmenschikov & Siegbahn, 2002). By means of molecular dynamics, a novel catalytic mechanism has been reported for the metalloproteases, as based on the formation of an anhydride intermediate where a **E**-residue, also, chelates the zinc cation as part of the catalytic motif of these enzymes. Both cases are illustrated in figure 6. The important with metalloproteases is that although two apparently contradicting mechanisms have been suggested, however, both they share common features; the zinc cation is penta-coordinated and it behaves also as the oxyanion hole (Manzettia et al, 2003; Pelmenschikov & Siegbahn, 2002).

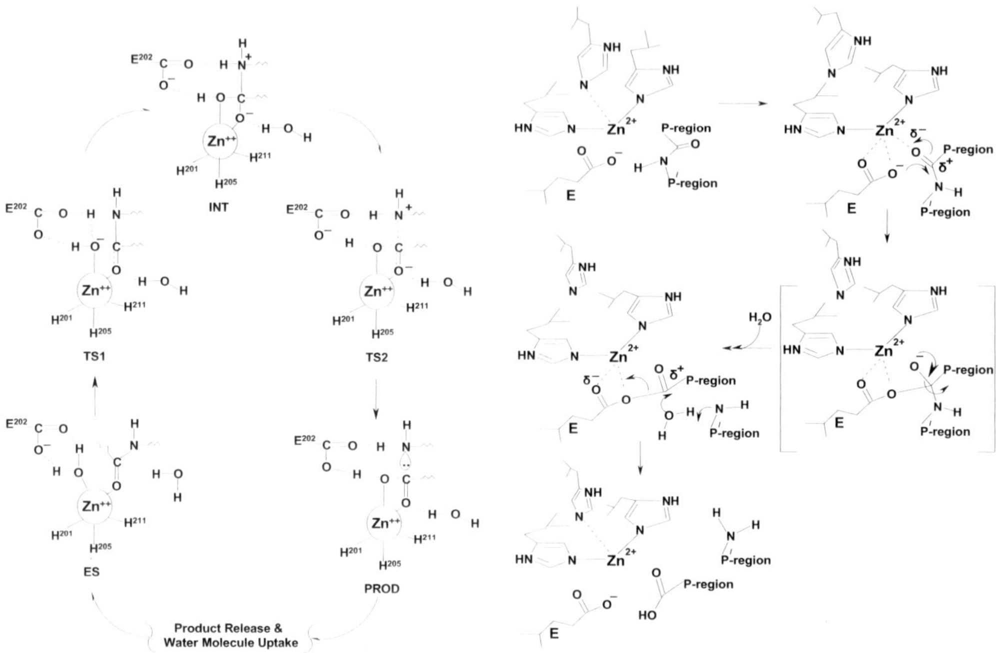

(a) (b)

Fig. 6. Matrix metalloproteases: initially, **Zn**$^{2+}$ is three-coordinated and continues as penta-coordinated either (a) with three **H**$^{\varepsilon 2}$-nitrogens, the $P_{1'}$-carbonyl oxygen and one H_2O-oxygen or (b) with two **H**$^{\varepsilon 2}$-nitrogens, the $P_{1'}$-carbonyl oxygen and two oxygens of catalytic **E**-residue (modified from Pelmenschikov & Siegbahn, 2002).

Amylase-like glycosidases perform catalysis by hydrolyzing glycosidic bonds either with net inversion of the α-anomeric configuration or with net retention. Glycosidases, either retaining or inverting, catalyze the same overall reaction both by employing acid-base catalysis while the former employ also the covalent catalysis; they are equipped with four highly conserved sequence regions containing all the catalytic residues and most of the substrate binding sites. Although retaining glycosidases perform catalysis by either a glutamate or aspartate, functioning as possible nucleophiles (Svensson, 1994), however, another set of catalytic residues is found in α-amylases, and other related enzymes. It is a triad of carboxylic acids (**D**^{197}, **E**^{233}, **D**^{300} - porcine pancreas α-amylase numbering) (Qian, 1994), where two of them (**E**^{233}, **D**^{300}) are most probably involved in acid catalysis and **D**^{197}, the putative nucleophile providing further electrostatic stabilization of the transition state (Mc Carter &Withers, 1994). In more details, the hydrolysis of glycosidic bonds by glycosidases proceeds by means of a general acid catalysis requiring a proton donor (electrophile) and a nucleophile (the base). In both cases the position of the electrophile is closer to the glycosidic oxygen, and although the nucleophile is closer to the anomeric carbon, in the retaining mechanism, however, it is more distant in the inverting mechanism (Davies & Henrissat, 1995). Oxyanion holes have not been identified in the mechanism of action in these enzymes, so far. Examples of the retaining and inverting mechanisms are shown in figure 7 (Kirby, 2001).

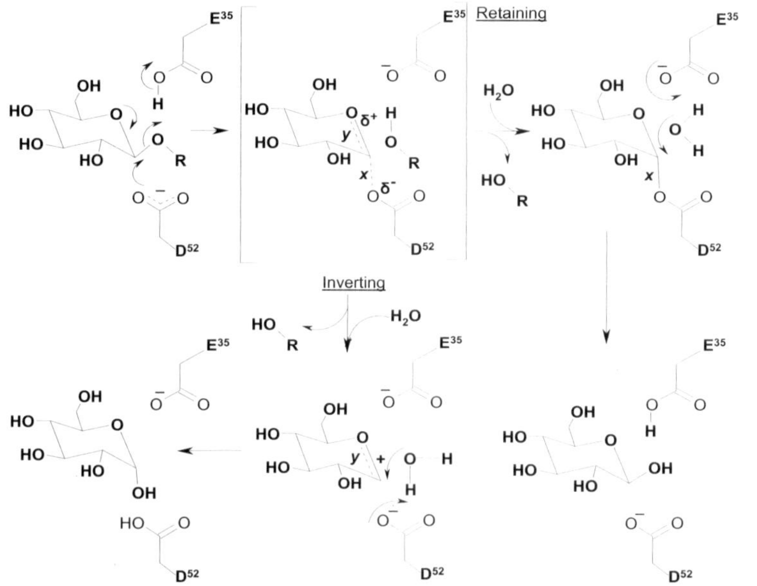

Fig. 7. Retaining and inverting mechanisms of glycosidases: Only one of the dashed bonds (*x* or *y*) of the intermediate (in brackets) actually occurs and defines the mechanism, i.e. *x* occurs with the retention mechanism, while *y* occurs with the inversion mechanism (modified from Kirby, 2001).

Lipases hydrolyze carboxylic ester bonds, and mainly convert tri-glycerides into di-glycerides or mono-glycerides, and fatty acids and glycerol. Additionally, lipases behave as esterases catalyzing also esterification, interesterification and transesterification reactions in nonaqueous media. The reaction course followed by a lipase in its catalytic function depends on the medium (aqueous or nonaqueous) in which reaction takes place. In media of low water content or in non-aqueous systems, lipases catalyze synthetic reactions (e.g. esterification etc) provided that water should be continually removed (Salleh et al, 2006). It is generally accepted that lipases carry out catalysis via a catalytic triad consisting of the residues $\mathbf{S}^{162}$, $\mathbf{H}^{263}$ and $\mathbf{D}^{176}$ (porcine pancreas lipase numbering) (De Caro et al, 1981), though there are cases where an **E** has replaced the **D** residue. Although, there is little homology among the known sequences of lipases, however, there are evidences indicating the convergent nature of the catalytic motifs of serine proteases and lipases (Ollis et al, 1992). Another feature of lipases which has been identified as essential for hydrolysis in nonaqueous media, is a surface loop, the lid domain, which covers the active site of lipases (Aloulou et al, 2006). Mechanistic features, similar to those of serine proteases, have been reported also for lipases, as it is the oxyanion hole, although its development differs in these enzymes due to their structural particularities (Aloulou et al, 2006). Recently, a full mechanism of action for the lipase from bovine pancreas (PPL) has been reported and it is analogous to this reported for serine proteases (figure 4a) (Kokkinou et al., 2011). However, it is essential to show that the mechanism of fatty acid ester hydrolysis by lipases in micelles, small aggregates or emulsion particles is noticeably different. It should be emphasized that Michaelis-Menten kinetics is applied only in isotropic reaction media, and thus alternative models have been suggested comprising two steps, i.e., a physical adsorption of lipase at the aqueous/lipid interface leads to its activation (opening of the lid) and the formation of the enzyme-substrate complex, and then, the hydrolytic reaction give the products and the adsorbed free enzyme (Aloulou et al, 2006; 1994; Verger & de Haas, 1976). Actually, a two-dimensional Michaelis-Menten catalytic step occurs when the soluble lipase (**E**) is adsorbed on the aqueous/lipid interface (**E***) and binds a substrate molecule resulting the development of the **E*S** complex; then, the soluble product **P*** is immediately diffused in the water layer (**P**). All these are illustrated in figure 8.

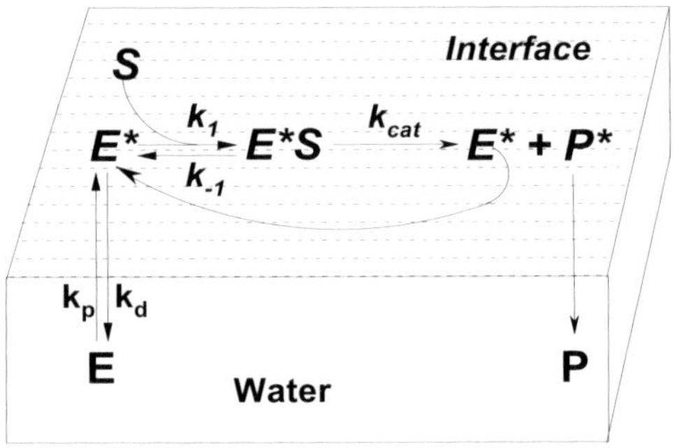

Fig. 8. Illustration of a water soluble lipase catalyzing an interfacial reaction, acting on an insoluble substrate; the asterisk denotes species onto the lipid/water interface, and **E**, **S**, **E*S**, and **P** are the free enzyme, free substrate, enzyme-substrate complex and product, respectively, while $\mathbf{k_p}$ and $\mathbf{k_d}$ are constants associated with the adsorption/desorption of enzyme between aqueous and lipid/water interface (modified from Aloulou et al, 2006).

Overall, the concept of the catalytic motif was not presented as a steady but rather as a dynamic ontologic entity in this context, independently of the number of contributing residues. Thereupon, it seems as more accurate that serine as well as cysteine proteases perform catalysis not by means of the routinely known catalytic triad and or dyad but through extraordinary manipulation of up to five catalytic residues. A similar treatment is worth for aspartic proteases and metalloproteases (Auld, 1997; Rawlings & Barret, 1994; Rebholz & Northrop, 1991; Svensson, 1994) showing that in general, the viewing of an enzymatic mechanism should not be focused only on the markedly referred catalytic residues. The concept of the catalytic sequence gets of special interest, when we have to do with α-amylase-like enzymes as it is illustrated in figures 3(a) and (b), where what extraordinary happens is that each monomer of polymeric substrates acts as catalytic residue! Is not it amazing?

2.1.2 Intermediates and acyl-enzymes

A significant selection of reports has been published, which deals with the mechanisms of action of specific enzymes. The idea of an enzymatic reaction mechanism has been already introduced, herein, where the knowledge of possible intermediates, their sequence, and structure was underlined. Therefore, understanding enzymatic catalysis it means to predict pathways and rates of enzyme-catalyzed reactions, i.e. to study reaction intermediates and to investigate enzyme structures. Enzymatic reactions which can be described by the Michaelis-Menten model equation they can be also properly divided into steps. For example, in homogeneous reactions at least three main steps may be distinguished, i.e. enzyme-substrate binding, main reaction, and splitting to products and free enzyme; within the latter may occur more than one elementary steps proceeding by means of additional intermediates. Therefore, the term "intermediate" does not comprise a unique notion, and some examples have been already given within this text. An inspection in figures 3 - 7 is enough to show a diversity of **ES** intermediates and structures; anionic intermediates are shown in figures 3(a,b) which are breaking down through transition states, where heavy atom reorganizations and proton transfers occur, and/or covalent intermediates precede the formation of the reaction products in figures 6 and 7. In case of glycosidases (figure 8), the intermediates have the form either of complicated covalent molecular species or of cationic structure (Hiromi, 1983; Ishikawa et al, 2007). By taking into account the concept of the intermediate, it is easier to understand the importance of acyl-enzymes and how these molecular species contribute in the overall catalysis. Nevertheless, an acyl-enzyme is developed, and destroyed (within an enzymatic mechanism) through a nucleophilic attack in most cases, and this is a matter of specific treatment comprising complicated series of extraordinary techniques (Papamichael et al.,2009; Theodorou,2001,2007a).

2.1.3 The low-barrier hydrogen bond (LBHB)

Before closing this topic, an emphasis should be given in the important role and the catalytic contribution of hydrogen bonding within the mechanism of action, in all cases of hydrolytic enzymes, which should provide optimization of the binding energy in the transition state; this latter can be achieved by hydrolases through their functional groups which extend ionic, hydrogen-bond and other interactions. Hydrogen atoms that are bonded to heavy electronegative atoms, being at a short distance from a Lewis-base, may form hydrogen bonds which are mostly ionic in character (Gosalia et al, 2005). Generally, there are certain structural and environmental prerequisites for the development of a hydrogen bond; indicative examples could be (a) the shell of solvent-water, which surrounds and stabilizes the bio-molecules in aqueous solutions, (b) subtle conformational changes due to enzyme-substrate binding interactions, (c) interactions between catalytic residues (e.g. between $\mathbf{C}^{25}$ and $\mathbf{H}^{159}$ in papain-like proteases), which form nucleophilic species, (d) significantly altered $\mathbf{p}K_a$-values of side chains of important residues, and so forth. Nevertheless, the dominant characteristics of a hydrogen bond depend upon the corresponded $\mathbf{p}K_a$s of the electronegative atoms sharing the hydrogen and some structural examples could verify the previous sentences (Northrop,2001); a network of hydrogen bonding is contributing significantly in the catalysis either by proteases and lipases, in figure 5, 6(b), 7(a), and 8, including the development of the oxyanion hole, whose hydrogen bonds are stabilized due to a short-lived negative charge on the carbonyl oxygen of the substrate. However, an outstanding type among hydrogen bonds is the low-barrier-hydrogen-bond (LBHB) which has been proved a useful tool in understanding enzymatic catalysis. LBHBs in transition-states or in transient intermediates are originating form ground state weak hydrogen bonds, while the energy released in forming a LBHB is used to help the reaction to be accomplished by lowering its activation barrier (Cleland, 2000).

2.2 Inhibition and enzymatic inactivation

2.2.1 Transition-state analogues

It is generally accepted that the completion of a chemical reaction is passing through unstable short-lived structures, the so-called transition states, whose structures are balanced between ground and product states, while their lifetimes equal approximately that for a single bond vibration (Schramm, 1998). Enzymatic reactions are chemical catalytic reactions which take place in the microenvironment of the enzyme-substrate complex, and hence, our understanding of the enzymatic catalysis should take into account both the structure of the unbound enzyme and its complexes with substrates, inhibitors, intermediates and products; enzymes alter the electronic structure of these latter reactants by protonation, proton abstraction, electron transfer, geometric distortion, hydrophobic partitioning, and interaction with Lewis acids and bases (Schramm, 1998). Herein, we have already commented the substrate binding onto enzymes, as well as the structural role of subsites in the catalysis by specific hydrolases. The transition state inhibitors support the transition state stabilization hypothesis in enzymatic catalysis, and this information helps in comparing transition states, in design transition state inhibitors, as well as in providing a basis for predicting the affinity of enzymatic inhibitors. However, transition state properties cannot always be predicted, as direct information on their structure is available from kinetic isotope effect studies. In this way, enzyme and inhibitor, and/or other transition state analog ligand, should share geometric and electronic similarity as both being necessary in order to provide correct distance to the catalytic site, and to correct hydrogen or ionic and/or hydrophobic bonding in the transition state interactions. The reversible inhibitors are analogs with some minimum structural features of substrates, and thus they get of great theoretical importance in the elucidation of enzyme mechanisms. At least some serious chemical insight into the catalytic mechanism of the enzymatic reaction, and substantial skill, is required for the design and identification of reliable inhibitors. Similar and useful phenomena are the substrate inhibition and activation whose systematic study may identify more pathways and complexes; but it should pointed out that these phenomena are not due to multiple active sites and/or cooperativity effects (Taylor, 2004). In figure 9 are illustrated three hypothetical free energy diagrams corresponding to three distinct cases of reactions, one non-catalyzed and two catalyzed by an enzyme, where **$\Delta G^{\ddagger}$, $\Delta G^{\ddagger}_{uncat}$, $\Delta G^{\ddagger}_{cat}$, $\Delta G^{\ddagger}_{M}$, E, ES**, and **P** are the free energy of activation of an uncatalyzed or catalyzed reaction, their free energy difference, the free enzyme, the enzyme-substrate complex, and the products.

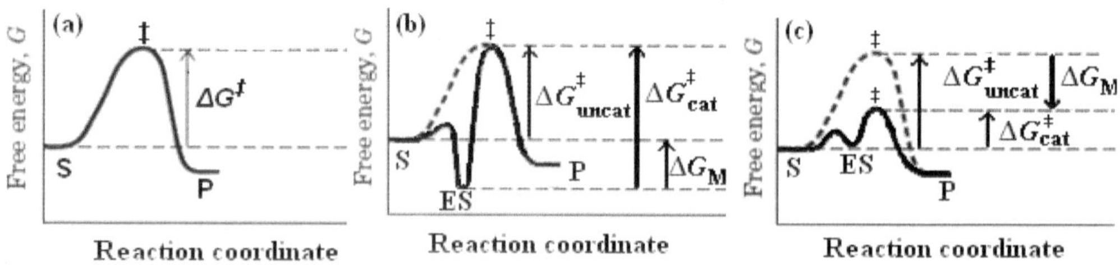

Fig. 9. (a) Non enzymatic reaction, (b) enzymatic reaction where enzyme is complementary to substrate, and (c) enzymatic reaction where enzyme is complementary to transition state. When enzyme is complementary to the substrate (b), the **ES** complex is more stable, resulting an increase in the energy of activation (modified from Taylor, 2004).

2.2.2 Stable acyl-enzymes

It has been reported that stable peptidyl acyl-enzymes of elastase may be formed at low pH, while the carbonyl oxygen of the scissile bond occupies the oxyanion hole; moreover, the tetrahedral adduct has a planar structure in the case of ester substrates. The stability of these acyl-enzymes is more likely due to the protonation of $\mathbf{H}^{57}$ at low pH-values of the reaction medium (Wilmouth et al, 2001). On the other hand, numerous compounds can be found which inactivate hydrolases through the development of stable acyl-enzyme intermediates; this latter stability is owed to several factors. Firstly, an intrinsic reactivity of the acyl group is experimentally obvious and for ester substrates (especially in proteases and lipases) is reduced due to an increased electron density of the carbonyl group of the scissile bond as substituents become more and more electron-donating; similar effect has been reported in cases where heteroatoms have substituted α-carbons of the amino acid residues of synthetic substrates (e.g. azapeptides) (Gupton et al, 1984). Besides, leaving groups of synthetic substrates, as it is *p*-nitrophenol could be offset the effects on acylation. A second reason contributing in the stability of acyl-enzyme intermediates is that they do not interact with the oxyanion hole (conversion of $3sp^2$ hybridized carbonyl carbon to $4sp^3$ in the tetrahedral intermediate) (Wilmouth et al, 2001), while a third explanation could be the protonation of $\mathbf{H}^{57}$ which disrupts the catalytic triad and cannot activate the nucleophilic water. More reasons of the stability of acyl-enzymes have been reported and they are related to reversible inhibitors, as transition state analogs. More examples could be those reported on the synthesis and the effectiveness of specific peptide reversible inhibitors and/or peptide "sticky" substrates, as useful probes for the investigation of the mechanism of action of particular hydrolytic enzymes (Bieth et al, 1989; Papamichael & Lymperopoulos, 1998).

2.3 Issues in the function of the catalytic motifs

2.3.1 Particular role of several catalytic residues, and one-proton vs. two-proton mechanisms

As we have previously discussed, the active sites of enzymes are equipped with a number of amino acid residuals whose side chains can act as both proton donors and acceptors, allowing proton transfers, and providing catalysis; proton transfers are the most common biochemical reactions. In this section we will be concentrated on the catalytic residues of the enzymes under consideration, and let it be as first example the charge relay system encountered for serine proteases, and under certain circumstances for lipases; the general features of the charge relay system are widely accepted, although the issue of whether the proton is located on the $\mathbf{H}^{57}$ or $\mathbf{D}^{102}$ (chymotrypsin numbering) has been particularly arguable. Proton transfers have been reported from $\mathbf{S}^{195}$ to $\mathbf{H}^{57}$ and from $\mathbf{H}^{57}$ to $\mathbf{D}^{102}$ involving a tetrahedral intermediate formation, as well as neutral $\mathbf{D}^{102}$ and $\mathbf{H}^{57}$; this latter requires a two-proton-transfer mechanism which in turn demands that the pK_a of $\mathbf{H}^{57}$ should be lower than that of $\mathbf{D}^{102}$, as it is depicted in figure 5(a) (Bieth,1978). In this way, a different mechanism designated as "His flip" has been proposed in an attempt to resolve the problem "one or two protons are transferred" during the acylation process in serine proteases (Bieth, 1989); according to "His flip" mechanism, after the formation of the tetrahedral intermediate, the positively charged histidine flips and place its $\mathbf{N}^{\delta_1}$ proton near to the leaving group, although it seems quite unlikely because it violates the principle of least motion (Kidd, 1999). Additional experimental results showed that the charge relay system operates most likely through the mechanism of figure 4(a,i), in cases of more specific substrates (tetrapeptides or larger) occupying more subsites in the active site of the hydrolase under consideration (Stein et al, 1987; Theodorou et al, 2007a,2007b). Different kinds of ambiguities have been brought up in the case of cysteine proteases, mainly arguing both on the number of catalytic residues, and on how catalysis is accomplished. In conclusion, cysteine proteases are equipped with four catalytic residues, i.e. $\mathbf{C^{25}}$, $\mathbf{H^{159}}$, $\mathbf{D^{158}}$/$\mathbf{N^{157}}$ and $\mathbf{N^{175}}$ (papain/bromelain numbering - bromelain lacks a $\mathbf{N^{175}}$ residue vs. papain), which may be regarded as a "double catalytic triad", as appeared in figure 4(b). The mechanism of action of cysteine proteases, of the papain family, has been most likely completely elucidated and all uncertainties have been resolved (Theodorou et al, 2001,2007a). The proposed catalytic mechanisms for aspartic proteases comprises two catalytically competent carboxyl groups constituting a functional unit which transfers one proton from the attacking water molecule onto the nitrogen atom of the leaving group. The main issue of these mechanisms requires a coplanar arrangement of the catalytic aspartates where a LBHB joins their $O^{\delta 1}$ oxygens, and it involves proton transfer from the water onto aspartic dyad which is followed by another proton transfer from the dyad onto carbonyl oxygen of the scissile bond; then, the formed intermediate breaks down to products by concerted general acid-base catalysis (Northrop, 2001). Then again in the case of metalloproteases there are certain ambiguities, since two main mechanisms of action have been suggested comprising similarities as well as differences. The similarities include a penta-coordinated $\mathbf{Zn^{++}}$ cation, linked with two $\mathbf{H^{\varepsilon 2}}$-nitrogens and one $P_{1'}$-carbonyl oxygen of the scissile amide bond, while among differences should be mentioned a third $\mathbf{H^{\varepsilon 2}}$-nitrogen ligand, two oxygen atoms of a catalytic **E**-residue, and that no water is present in the transition state, as they are depicted in details in figure 6. Despite the differences between retaining and inverting mechanisms it is noteworthy that both of them employ a pair of carboxylic acids at the active site with different roles; additionally, both classes of these enzymes operate via transition states with substantial oxocarbenium ion character. A variation on the retaining mechanism involves an ion pair rather than a covalent intermediate (McCarter & Withers, 1994). A general acid, in inverting enzymes, provides one proton for the leaving glycoside oxygen, while a general base supports the nucleophilic attack by a water molecule; on the contrary, in retaining glycosidases a covalent glycosyl intermediate is formed (figure 7).

2.3.2 The hydrolytic water

So far in this text, it has been obvious to a certain extent that water molecules play important roles in the catalysis performed by the hydrolytic enzymes. The hydrolysis of synthetic peptide substrates by serine proteases offers informative examples; the hydrolytic water molecule seems that approaches the acyl-enzyme from the leaving group side and although it should be hydrogen bonded to $\mathbf{H^{57}}$, however it is found in an unfavorable angle relatively to the carbonyl carbon of the scissile bond (Dixon & Matthews, 1989). Inverse solvent isotope effects, found for the reaction governed by the k_{cat}/K_m parameter when several proteases catalyze the hydrolysis of synthetic peptide substrates, seems more likely that they originate from two contributing exchangeable hydrogenic sites in the ground and the transition state. A working example is referred in papain, whose reactive thiolate-imidazolium ion-pair is likely to be in equilibrium with its tautomer neutral thiol-imidazole form, or alternatively, a low barrier hydrogen bond (LBHB) may exist between them; both of these latter hypotheses are equally likely displaying an effective ground state as a value of $\phi^G = 0.17$ was found by proton inventories (figure 4b) (Theodorou et al, 2001). Similar results were found for the ground state of free enzyme and substrate in case of thiolsubtilisin (Papamichael et al, 2004), and although similar proton inventories were obtained in the case of PPL, in hydrolyzing the ester substrate p-nitrophenyl laurate (L-p-ONP) in aqueous media, however, the value of ϕ^G was found greater than 0.2 arguing for a different way of E-S binding mode. However, in glycosidases the catalytic role of water is profoundly different between retaining and inverting mechanisms, while its effect depends strongly on the ionization of the catalytic acidic residues of the enzyme (figure 7).

3. A step-by-step procedure

3.1 Synthetic part

The art to design and synthesize either a particular single substrate or a series of specific and/or non-specific substrates possessing special binding or interaction properties, it is based on the knowledge of the specificity of subsites, of the enzymes under consideration; as a matter of fact we are dealing with a feedback procedure, where it dominates the logic of "trial and error". In this field of research it could be an advantage the working with proteases; their synthetic substrates are peptides, whose synthesis has found an increased interest due to their huge applications. For example, it has been reported that the active site of papain comprises seven subsites, where the interactions of the $\mathbf{S_1'}$ - $\mathbf{P_1'}$ and $\mathbf{S_2}$ - $\mathbf{P_2}$ character have been found as the more important ones (Kim et al, 1992; Patel et al,1992). Later, by based on the previous experience, the S_1 - P_1 and S_3 - P_3 interactions between purified papain and four newly synthesized peptide substrates were investigated (Papamichael et al, 1999; Theodorou et al, 2001). The logic behind this research was based on the need to elucidate the mechanism of action of cysteine proteases of the papain-C1 family, and although the common substrate Cbz-FR-pNA was convenient for activity assay measurements however, it was experienced as insoluble at higher concentrations so that its Michaelis-Menten parameters were always estimated without reaching the saturation of the used enzyme; the latter is unacceptable by enzyme kineticists, and therefore novel substrates should be synthesized. Finally, we synthesized the substrates X-FY-pNA/ONPh/NMec, where X={Suc, Pht, Cbz} and Y={F, R}. More instructive examples and practices will be provided, herein, which they are referred to different needs and experimental conditions, as well as to the synthesis of both substrates and transition state analog reversible inhibitors for serine proteases (elastase from porcine pancreas – PPE). The conception behind these synthetic probes was based on the need of a serious contribution to the elucidation of mechanism of action of serine proteases; our first results were from suitable **^{13}C** NMR studies on the side chain motions of three specifically **^{13}C**-labeled trifluoro-acetyl peptide reversible inhibitors bound on PPE (e.g. the CF_3CO|U-^{13}C|-AA-m-Ph-CF_3) (Dimicoli et al, 1987). Later, and in this way we synthesized more series of substrates and transition state analog reversible inhibitors for PPE, which were found suitable also, for other serine proteases. Although the most of substrates showed Michaelis-Menten kinetics, however some of them showed substrate inhibition and others substrate activation and along with the synthetic inhibitors led to significant contribution in the elucidation of the mechanism of action of PPE (de la Sierra et al, 1990).

3.2 Computing part: Specific non-linear algorithms and computer programs for experimental data fitting, and suitable tools for statistical analysis (parametric, non-parametric, and experimental design)

It is always the case among enzyme kineticists to have to fit their experimental data with a mostly nonlinear model equation in order to both optimize experimental procedures and to estimate the values of precious parameters (Papamichael, 1987). These procedures may be carried out by using specific nonlinear curve fitting packages, usually equipped with gradient algorithms and requiring from the experimenter a set of initial parameter guessing values; then the package either converges or not, depending on certain factors, whose more important is the continuity of the parameter derivatives, the awkwardness of the model equation, the presence of outliers, and the choice of the fitting algorithm and criterion of convergence (Cornish-Bowden, 1995). In many cases the response of an enzymatic reaction is described by a multi-parametric model-equation which may possesses a more or less awkward character (e.g. multi-substrate kinetics, equations of non competitive and/or substrate inhibition, the Hill equation, etc). Furthermore, the discontinuity of the parameter derivatives of model-equations, which are commonly encountered in enzyme kinetics, is another annoying difficulty, though the relatively high incidence of outliers constitutes a real problem when only few replicates could be obtained as it is the common practice in enzyme kinetic measurements; this latter strongly affects also the choice of the criterion of convergence, as influencing the error distribution (Mannervik, 1982). Therefore, a number of solutions could be suggested to overcome these problems which may include the use of search algorithms instead of the gradients ones, where no need of parameter derivatives is required, as well as non-parametric curve fitting methods where initial parameter guessing values are not required. Likewise, a variety of search algorithms and non-parametric curve fitting methods have been reported, and more or less have been employed successfully (Fletcher, 1965; Papamichael & Evmiridis,1988,2000) on the other hand it is not surprising that enzyme kineticists were involved in such a kind of research trying to provide reasonable solutions to intrinsic problems which often are raised in enzyme kinetics. Independently of the employed algorithm and/or the curve fitting method further robust statistical analysis is necessary for accomplishing a best fit of any nonlinear multi-parametric equation to a series of experimental data (Cleland, 1979). Thus, three additional issues should be taken into account namely the errorless and unbiased estimation of the involved parameter values, as well as the application of suitable information criteria for the discrimination among model-equations, which in several situations employ the same number of parameters (Cleland,1979); the third issue is due to the inborn problem of enzyme kinetics where statistically few experimental data supplied with few replicates impose for an optimal experimental design in order to minimize error and maximize the precision of the parameter estimates (Box, 1971, Kafarov, 1976). Then again, a variety of relative works and methods may be suggested whose application will surmount these three additional requirements (Evmiridis &. Papamichael, 1991; Papamichael, 1995; Comish-Bowden & Eisenthal, 1974).

3.3 Experimental – Kinetic part

3.3.1 Evidence for Michaelis-Menten and/or other type of kinetic behavior

Mathematical model-equations along with computer techniques are valuable tools in searching for optimal experimental conditions and effective enzymatic action. The study of various model-equations incorporates the information concerning each particular enzymatic reaction or system, it attains of great interest in the basic research and applications of these biocatalysts and they have been proved as effective tools in estimating the process variables. The rate equation of an enzymatic reaction illustrates the catalytic process in terms of rate constants and reactant concentrations; the initial rate of an enzymatic reaction is directly proportional to the concentration of enzyme preparation, and it is increased nonlinearly with increasing the substrate concentration up to a limiting maximum value. The well know Henri-Michaelis-Menten equation (1) is based on reasonable assumptions associated with the quasi-steady-state approximation (QSSA) (Michaelis & Menten, 1913), where the relations $[E]_t=[E] + [ES]$ and $[S]_t \approx [S]$ are valid ($[E]_t$, $[E]$, $[S]_t$, and $[S]$, are the total and free enzyme, and the total and free substrate concentrations, respectively); the physical meaning of its two parameters V_{max} and K_m is familiar among enzymologist. Currently, any non-linear model equation as the Henri-Michaelis-Menten (H-M-M) one can be used for fitting enzymatic experimental data and obtaining parameter estimates due to the available computers and software. Not often, the H-M-M equation cannot fit experimental data from enzymatic reactions; then, it is not uncommon to assume some reasonable modifications of equation (1) to succeed the best fit. It is recommended to use rational equations having the general form of equation (2), where $\mathbf{n} \geq \mathbf{m}$, whereas the meaning of parameters $\mathbf{a_1}$, $\mathbf{a_2}$,...$\mathbf{a_n}$, and $\mathbf{b_1}$, $\mathbf{b_2}$,...$\mathbf{b_m}$, depends on the reaction itself and the experimental conditions (NC-IUB, 1983). A specific case of equation (2) is equation (3) known as the Hill equation (Hill, 1913), and it is valid when polymeric enzymes extend positive cooperativity, consisting of more than one subunits, comprising n equivalent binding sites (a single substrate molecule is bound per subunit). In equation (3), the parameter K_H no longer equals the substrate concentration that yields half-maximal velocity except for $n = 1$. In equation (3) $\alpha = -\ln(K_H)$, $\beta = n$ (n is the Hill coefficient and K_H is the Hill parameter which is similar to K_m), and $x = \ln([S])$.

$$v = \frac{k_p [E]_t [S]}{K_S + [S]} = \frac{kp\,[E]_t\,[S]}{[S] + \dfrac{(k_{-1} + k_p)}{k_1}} = \frac{V_{max}\,[S]}{[S] + K_m} \quad (1)$$

$$v = \frac{a_1[S] + a_2[S]^2 + a_3[S]^3 + ... + a_n[S]^n}{1 + b_1[S] + b_2[S]^2 + b_3[S]^3 + ... + b_m[S]^m} \quad (2)$$

$$v = \frac{V_{max}\,[S]^n}{K_H + [S]^n} = \frac{V_{max}\dfrac{[S]^n}{K_H}}{1 + \dfrac{[S]^n}{K_H}} = \frac{V_{max}\,e^{a+\beta x}}{1 + e^{a+\beta x}}, \text{ and } \ln[\frac{[S]^n}{K_H}] = n\ln[S] - \ln(K_H) = a + \beta x \quad (3)$$

The rate of any reaction, including the enzymatic ones, depends on the number of contacts between the different kinds of molecules, and in isotropic systems is proportional to the product of concentrations of reactants. When the reactive species belong to macromolecular systems, as they are the enzyme molecules, the evaluation of the average number of their contacts should take into account all different conformations of these macromolecules. This latter is rarely taken into account in enzymatic reactions, which are handled as homogeneous because experimenters use to keep always valid the relation $[S]_t >> [E]_t$ (Segel, 1975). In this way, and in order to describe different behaviors in enzyme kinetics, a variety of multi-parametric nonlinear equations have been proposed whose parameters are surprisingly complicated functions of individual rate constants. Attempts to counterbalance this situation led a number of authors to present alternative mathematical formulations in enzyme kinetics; characteristic examples may be equations (4) and (5), where D, V^{eff}_{max} and K^{eff}_{m} are the fractal dimension and the effective individual H-M-M parameters, while A_2, A_3, etc. are the equivalent virial coefficients, respectively (Lymperopoulos et al., 1998; Savageau, 1998). Equations (4) and (5) offer appreciable economy in numerical treatment of enzyme kinetic experimental data, as compared with the conventional equations, allowing an overall view of the complexity of the reaction path of enzymatic catalysis; when $D = 1$ equation (4) takes on the form of H-M-M equation, and V^{eff}_{max}, and K^{eff}_{m} receive their ordinary meaning. In the case of equation (5) we should recall the QSSA condition on which it was based on the development of the H-M-M equation and where $\left(-\frac{d[ES]}{dt}\right) = (k_{-1} + k_p)[ES] = \left(+\frac{d[ES]}{dt}\right) = k_1[E][S]$; instead, it can be written that $k_1[E][S] = C(E,S)$ i.e. the average number of contacts between the two reactants, which in turn depends on the kind of more complicated contacts between **S** and **E**, and leads to a complicated dependence on **[S]**, i.e. $C(E,S) = [E][S](1 + A_2[S] + A_3[S]^2 + A_4[S]^3 + \ldots)$. Moreover, virial coefficients can be positive or negative expressing positive or negative contributions to $C(E,S)$ from pairs, triples etc. of **S** in the neighborhood of **E**. Both equations (4) and (5) can fit a variety of experimental data (Lymperopoulos et al., 1998; Savageau, 1998).

$$v = \frac{V^{eff}_{max}\,[S]^{2-D}}{[S] + K^{eff}_{m}} \tag{4}$$

$$v = \frac{V_{max}\,[S](1 + A_2[S] + A_3[S]^2 + \ldots)}{K_m + [S](1 + A_2[S] + A_3[S]^2 + \ldots)} \tag{5}$$

3.3.2 Experimental design – Factorial experimentation

In a previous section we referred and explained a number of reasons on the necessity of use the experimental design, as an essential method for the minimization of time, cost, and the wasting of valuable and expensive reagents; now we ought to describe how this could be done in the course of enzyme kinetics. Any general procedure in obtaining experimental design for nonlinear multi-parametric equations should take into account the range where its independent variable is defined, as well as the insurmountable occurrence of experimental errors, and it comprises the following: (a) establishment of a model-equation which best fits the experimental points, (b) choice of the optimality principle, (c) reasonable parameter estimates for the model-equation, (d) validation of the performance of the optimal-design experimental points. Herein, we will adopt the **D**-optimality principle in finding the required optimal experimental points and obtain parameter estimates of the chosen model-equation with the maximum possible precision. We will focused to multi-parametric nonlinear model equations with one independent variable i.e. $y = \mathbf{f}(x;\theta_1,\theta_2 \dots \theta_r) = \mathbf{f}(x;\theta_p)$ with p parameters ($p = 1,2 \dots r$), where $\theta_1,\theta_2 \dots \theta_r$ are the parameter estimates, while the experimental series are defined by the column vector $D = \{x_i\}$. Then, we have to choose a set of $\mathbf{x_i}$ values ($i = 1,2 \dots n$), in order to observe the response y; so that from these observations to estimate the p parameters as precisely as possible; n is the number of trials, i.e. the optimal-design experimental points. In such a case, for single independent variable equations, the column vector $D = \{x_i\}$ is identical with the design matrix which is replaced by the *Jacobian matrix* **F*** for nonlinear multiparametric model-equations (Papamichael et al, 1995). The partial derivatives of a multi-parametric nonlinear model-equation with respect to the $\mathbf{r^{th}}$ parameter θ_r for each optimal-design experimental x_i point are $f_{ir}^* = \dfrac{\partial f(x_i;\underline{\theta})}{\partial \theta_r}$, and $\underline{\theta} = \begin{bmatrix} 1^* \\ 2^* \\ \cdot \\ r^* \end{bmatrix}$ is a set of parameters obtained by preliminary curve fitting ($i = 1,2 \dots n$, and $r = 1,2, \dots r$), and considered to be very close to the true parameters. The $n \times p$ dimensional matrix $\mathbf{F^*} = \{ f_{ir}^* \}$ is usually chosen to have $n = p$ and accordingly the relation $\left|F^{*T} \bullet F^*\right| = \left|F^*\right|^2$ is valid; then, the procedure is an attempt to maximize the modulus of the determinant $\left|F^*\right|$, or to minimize its inverse $\mathbf{1}/\left|F^*\right|$, while when $n > p$ the alternative is to maximize $\left|F^{*T} \bullet \mathbf{F}^*\right|$ or to minimize its inverse. The experimenter should proceed by drawing a diagram having common abscissa the independent variable of its model-equation, and as ordinates the partial derivatives of the model-equation with respect to each single parameter, i.e. $\partial y/\partial\theta_1, \partial y/\partial\theta_2, \dots \partial y/\partial\theta_r$; then, as optimal points are selected these ones where the abscissa values of the partial derivatives present minima or maxima, or even approached and/or are removed each other. Furthermore, it is recommended to ultimate the optimization studies by taking into account both cases $n = p$ and $n > p$, and then to consult the inverse correlation ($\mathbf{R}^{-1}$) and the hat (**H**) matrices (Papamichael et al, 1995).

There are many procedures, where the experimenter is concerned with the effect of a series of parameters on certain estimated attributes. In such cases factorial analysis is a key method, where "factors" are variable parameters to be considered in the experiment, and are distinguished in either quantitative (varied continuously) or qualitative (cannot be varied continuously) ones. Typically, the experimenter, should assign the values of quantitative factors at pre-determined levels (e.g. low, medium, high), while this is not requisite for the qualitative factors. The collection of levels of all employed factors in a given trial has been designated as the "treatment"; this latter provides a full description of the experimental conditions which affect the studied factors and where the term "experiment" refers to the whole collection and not to an individual trial. Then, the numerical result per trial, based on a given treatment, has been designated as "response", which is the attribute we measure. Normally, the value of a response is varied as the factor level is varied, whereas factors are regarded as independent variables and responses as dependent variables. In order to determine the effects of one or more factors on a specific chemical feature we should carry out one or more experimental trials with each of the possible combinations of the levels of the factors, and that is the so-called "factorial experiment". Factorial experiments may be performed from the simplest case at two levels up to more composite and of higher difficulty combinations. A factorial experiment at two levels may involving two factors A (e.g. temperature) and B (e.g. feed rate of a reactor). In order to find the effect of A on B, a first trial with A at T_1=50°C and B at Fr_1 = 50 ml/h, and a second trial with A at T_2=150°C and B at Fr_2 = 75 ml/h, were performed to find the effect of temperature; then a third trial at T_1=50°C and B at Fr_2 = 75 ml/h as well as a fourth trial at T_2=150°C and Fr_2 = 75 ml/h were performed in order to find the effect of the feed rate. From these data it could be defined an effect due to variation in factor A as follows i.e. effect of A = (33 - 27 = 6), and effect of B = (8 - 27 = -19). In each of these effects they were used only two of the three observations, and while the observation T_1=50°C and Fr_1 = 50 ml/h was used twice, while the rest two observations were used only once. Moreover, by varying one factor at a time we cannot comment the possibility of interaction between these two factors; the fourth trial may give the solution. Both A and B should be increased for higher yield, i.e. the effect of A at B-first level equals to 33 - 27 = 6, and the effect of A at B-second level = 70 - 8 = 62 (Davies & Henrissat, 1995).

3.3.3 Detailed analysis of the experimental data from pH and temperature profiles, of the Michaelis-Menten parameters, and estimation of useful constants and/or relations

It is common to assign **p*K*a** values on free enzyme (**E**) from k_{cat}/K_m vs pH profiles, by based on the ambiguous assumptions that proton transfers to and from **E** and **S** are much faster than formation and breakdown of the **E-S** complex; similarly common is to assume that productive binding is allowed only to a single protonic state of the enzyme. However, both assumptions are valid in cases of sticky substrates i.e. in cases where substrates dissociate from the active site of enzyme at a rate comparable to or slower than that at which the **ES** complex reacts to form product (Cleland, 1977); the stickiness of a substrate is proportional to the ratio k_2/k_{-1} (Theodorou et al, 2001). Nevertheless, in a general point of view the profiles of the dependencies of Michaelis-Menten parameters vs. pH show many reactive hydronic states, comprising equal number of pK_a values and equal or less number of pH-independent rate constants. In order to determine such parameters as they are the values of **p*K*a**s and of rate constants, it is necessary to plan and employ appropriate equations derived by using models in which enzyme and substrate ionizations are considered to be at QSSA (Brocklehurst et al, 1979). The following reaction figures 10 along with equation (6) it may be an instructive example. However, the experimental data from Michaelis-Menten parameters vs. pH dependencies profiles should normally described by the general equation (7), where k_{obs} is the estimated value of the rate constant, $(k)^{lim}$ is its marginal maximum value for the hydronic state EH_{i-1}, n is the number of reactive hydronic states, B_{ij} is a description of the form $K_{XHp}[H^+]^m$, while m and p are elements of two matrices **I** and **II**, corresponding to i and j indices, respectively.

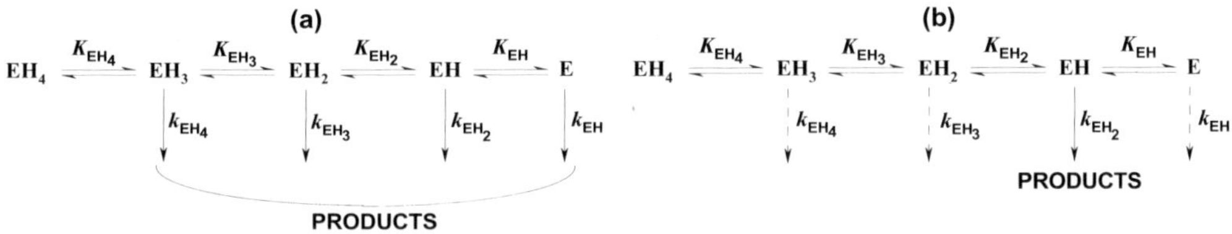

Fig. 10. (a) reaction scheme involving four reactive hydronic states from **E** to $\mathbf{EH_3}$ and one $\mathbf{EH_4}$ not reactive, characterized by four macroscopic acid dissociation constants and four pH-independent rate constants, (b) similar reaction scheme where only one hydronic state designated as **EH** is reactive and characterized by four macroscopic acid dissociation constants and only one pH-independent rate constant; this latter is a particular case of (a).

$$k_{obs} = \frac{(k_{EH})^{lim}}{1 + 10^{pK_{EH_4} + pK_{EH_3} + pK_{EH_2} - 3pH} + 10^{pK_{EH_3} + pK_{EH_2} - 2pH} + 10^{pK_{EH_2} - pH} + 10^{pH - pK_{EH}}} \quad (6)$$

$$k_{obs} = \sum_{i=1}^{n} \frac{k_i^{lim}}{\left(1 + \sum_{j=1}^{n} B_{ij}\right)} \quad (7)$$

Matrix I

	j=1	2	3	4	5	6...n
i=1	1	2	3	4	5	6...n
2	-1	1	2	3	4	5...n-1
3	-2	-1	1	2	3	4...n-2
4	-3	-2	-1	1	2	3...n-3
5	-4	-3	-2	-1	1	2...n-4
6	-5	-4	-3	-2	-1	1...n-5
...	...	...	...	...	...	...
n	1-n	2-n	3-n	4-n	5-n	6-n...1

Matrix II

	j=1	2	3	4	5	...n
i=1	-1	-1.2	-1.2.3	-1.2.3.4	-1.2.3.4.5	...-1.2.3...n
2	1	-2	-2.3	-2.3.4	-2.3.4.5	...-2.3.4...n
3	1.2	2	-3	-3.4	-3.4.5	...-3.4.5...n
4	1.2.3	2.3	3	-4	-4.5	...-4.5.6...n
5	1.2.3.4	2.3.4	3.4	4	-5	...-5.6.7...n
6	1.2.3.4.5	2.3.4.5	3.4.5	4.5	5	...-6.7.8...n
...	...	...	...	...	...	...
n	1.2.3..n	2.3.4..n	3.4.5..n	4.5.6..n	5.6.7..n	...-n

The thermal variation of enzymatic reaction rate constants conform to the well known Arrhenius equation: $k = A\ e^{-E/RT}$, where A, **E**, **R** and **T** represent the frequency factor, the activation energy, the gas constant and the absolute temperature, respectively; k may be any one of the Michaelis-Menten and/or other enzymatic mechanism rate constants, and thus its value could be generally evaluated. The thermo stability of enzymatic activity is a prerequisite and it should be tested by incubating enzyme preparations for sufficient time at as possible high and/or low temperatures, and then by measuring their activity at the optimum temperature (Papamichael, & Theodorou, 2010). By integrating the Arrhenius equation, the temperature dependence of enzymatic rate constants can be found and illustrated in equation (8), assuming constant activation energy; in equation (9) k_j, $k_{j,0}$, E_j, R, T_0 and T, are the rate constant under consideration at different temperatures, its value at the reference absolute temperature, the activation energy associated with the rate constant, the gas constant, and the reference absolute temperature, and the independent variable of equation (Papamichael et al, 2010). When k_j equals to either k_{cat}/K_m or k_{cat}, then equation (8) is transformed to equation (9) or (10), where E_a=E_{-1}-E_2, and a=k_2/k_{-1}, and are referred to the well known "three-step mechanism": $E + S \underset{k_{-1}}{\overset{k_1}{\rightleftharpoons}} ES \xrightarrow{k_2} E\text{-}S^* \xrightarrow{k_3} E + P$ (Wang et al, 2006). In homogeneous reactions and in terms of the transition state theory (TS) the activation energy $E_a = \Delta H^\ddagger + RT$ can be evaluated as it has been formulated by the Eyring equation ($k = (k_B/\hbar)Te^{-\Delta G\ddagger/RT} = (k_B/\hbar)T\ e^{-\Delta H\ddagger/RT}\ e^{-\Delta S\ddagger/R}$). Therefore, the study of rate constants as function of the absolute temperature provides thermodynamic data on the TS (Papamichael, & Theodorou, 2010).

$$k_j = k_{j,0}\ \text{Exp}\left[-\frac{E_j}{R}\left(\frac{1}{T}-\frac{1}{T_0}\right)\right] \tag{8}$$

$$\frac{k_{cat}}{K_m} = \frac{k_{1,0}\ a_0 \text{Exp}\left[\frac{E_a}{R}\left(\frac{1}{T}-\frac{1}{T_0}\right)\right]}{1+a_0\text{Exp}\left[\frac{E_a}{R}\left(\frac{1}{T}-\frac{1}{T_0}\right)\right]}\ \text{Exp}\left[-\frac{E_1}{R}\left(\frac{1}{T}-\frac{1}{T_0}\right)\right] \tag{9}$$

$$k_{cat} = \frac{k_{2,0}\ k_{3,0}\text{Exp}\left[-\frac{E_2+E_3}{R}\left(\frac{1}{T}-\frac{1}{T_0}\right)\right]}{k_{2,0}\ \text{Exp}\left[-\frac{E_2}{R}\left(\frac{1}{T}-\frac{1}{T_0}\right)\right]+k_{3,0}\text{Exp}\left[-\frac{E_3}{R}\left(\frac{1}{T}-\frac{1}{T_0}\right)\right]} \tag{10}$$

4. Application of several effective methods and tools

4.1 Kinetic and thermodynamic methods

4.1.1 H/D solvent isotope effects, and proton inventories, on constants and parameters

The light hydrogen isotope protium (H) can be replaced by deuterium (D) in the hydrogenic sites of the water species (i.e. HOD, D_2O, $H^+{}_3O$, $H^+{}_2OD$, $D^+{}_2OH$, $D^+{}_3O$, etc), under certain circumstances, and as a consequence deuterium may replace protium into some sensitive positions of enzymes and substrates; these replacements have been designated as solvent isotope effects (SIE) and usually they affect the kinetic and equilibrium constants associated with the enzymatic reactions. Obviously, these SIE are related to the isotopic solvents and thus should disturb rate and/or equilibrium constants, and influence both initial (ground) and final (transition or product) states. In the course of the development of an enzymatic reaction mechanism, it is commonly required to identify isotope effects for individual hydrogenic sites, where the notion of the isotopic fractionation factors is used. Furthermore, the hydrogenic sites are classified into these established in the structural framework of the solutes (internal ϕ-sites), as well as to those found in the isotopic water molecules (external ϕ-sites) which strongly interact with the solutes. It is a mechanistic affair to distinguish between ϕ-sites and it is based on information arose from solvent isotope-effect data. Based on the above concepts new extra methods can be originated, which are useful in enzyme kineticists. One of them is the "proton inventories", which seems more likely that they constitute reliable tools in investigating enzymatic mechanisms (Theodorou et al, 2007b); this method comprises kinetic studies of SIE in a series of mixtures of H_2O and D_2O, while the reaction parameters are expressed as $\boldsymbol{k_n(n)}$ functions of deuterium atom fraction $\boldsymbol{n = [D_2O]/\{[H_2O]+[D_2O]\}}$ present in the isotopic solvent, according to equation (11). In equation (11) $\boldsymbol{k_0}$ is a reaction rate in H_2O, and ϕ_i^T and ϕ_j^G are the isotopic fractionation factors of **ith** transition state, and of **jth** ground state protons, respectively; the values ϕs, as well as the shape of the $\boldsymbol{k_n(n)}$ functions, and the number of the transferred protons are diagnostic of the reaction mechanism (Theodorou et al, 2001). Gross and co-workers had published a series of papers on phenomena in mixtures of isotopic solvents, where they introduced a critical assumption for the easy use of solvent isotope effects. Accordingly, the relative abundances of all probable species in isotopic waters could be determined solely by statistics and by the ratio of protium to deuterium in the medium, with the additional assumption that deuterium rather than protium occupies the hydronic sites of enzyme and/or substrate independently of whether deuterium or protium is already found onto that site. This assumption is currently known as the Rule of the Geometric Mean, and led both Gross and Butler to a particularly clear algebraic formulation of the dependence of the reaction rate on $\boldsymbol{n}$. To determine the significance of parameters of the Gross-Butler-Kresge equation (11), all previous theoretical approaches should be used in order to formulate simplified forms of this equation capable to best fit the available series of the experimental data; a variety of simplified forms of equation (11) have been already published and can be easily incorporated into any curve fitting program and/or algorithm.

$$k_n = k_0 \frac{\prod_{i=1}^{\mu} (1 - n + n\phi_i^T)}{\prod_{j=1}^{v} (1 - n + n\phi_j^G)} \tag{11}$$

4.1.2 Determination of kinetic isotope effects via NMR studies (^{1}H v.s. ^{2}H NMR spectroscopy and NMR-Proton inventories for intramolecular/intermolecular hydrogen transfer reactions)

NMR spectroscopy is one among many probes that have been reported for the evaluation of kinetic isotope effects. Several NMR methods, as analogs of previous proton inventory techniques involving classical kinetic methods were reported, involving line-shape analyses and polarization transfer experiments on the exchanging protons or deuterons and/or on the remote spins as functions of the deuterium atom fraction $\boldsymbol{n}$ in the mobile proton sites. Moreover, the kinetic isotope effects and the number of transferred protons originating from the NMR spectra were developed both in theory and praxis by the application of a specific technique. The theory was based on the study of kinetic isotopic exchange reactions (e.g. for two molecules **AH** and **AD**, there is the option of performing experiments either on the **A** spins, the **H** and/or **D** spins), where the obtained various experimental kinetic quantities depend on which nuclear spins are chosen for the experiments. In following, the relation between rate constants of intermolecular H/D transfer reactions and inverse lifetimes measured by NMR spectroscopy were estimated. These theoretical description may be more comprehensible if the features of NMR spectroscopy will be demonstrated by considering a simple equilibrium $i \rightleftarrows j$, which is described by the constant $K_{ij} = k_{ij}/k_{ji} = [j]/[i]$. Generally, any NMR experiment is performed under equilibrium, and the NMR line-shapes depend on the inverse lifetimes, according to equation (12), where $\mathbf{d}[i \rightarrow j]/\mathbf{dt}$ is the number of molecules per volume leaving from the environment i to j during time **dt**. A first approach to a more skilled and profound knowledge on these methods and techniques is the excellent work of H-H. Meschede and Limbach (1991), where is given a theoretical background of dynamic NMR spectroscopy in the presence of kinetic isotope effects, as well as applications and selected examples (Meschede & Limbach, 1991).

$$\tau_{ij}^{-1} = k_{ij}.= -[i]^{-1} \times \mathrm{d}[i \rightarrow j]/\mathrm{dt} \quad (12)$$

4.1.3 CD-stopped flow spectroscopy

In order to examine early events during a reaction it is necessary to employ rapid mixing and detection system, such as that provided by stopped-flow apparatus including the stopped flow CD techniques and devices. Moreover, stopped flow CD has been used extensively in kinetic measurements of conformational transitions in proteins and in protein folding studies on a millisecond time scale, allowing the collection of time-resolved CD spectra. The changes in ellipticity in both the far and near UV give information about the regain of secondary and tertiary structure respectively, providing valuable information on the mechanism of protein folding (Kelly & Price, 2000). The limitation of stopped-flow CD is the "dead-time" of the mixing process which is typically almost more than 2 milliseconds (Clarke & Jones, 1999).

4.1.4 Substrate assisted catalysis

The classic is that all necessary groups which are essential for catalysis are provided by the enzyme to convert substrates into products; however, there are some exceptions in this rule, where the substrate may provide also functional groups which will participate in the catalytic reaction course. This phenomenon has been reported in either case of native enzymes or engineered mutants, and it is designated as "substrate-assisted catalysis" (SAC). Several enzymes namely serine proteases, GTPases, type II restriction endonucleases, lysozyme and hexose-1-phosphate uridylyl-transferase have been shown as susceptive for substrate assisted catalysis. As examples of SAC in naturally occurring enzymes may be the type II restriction endonucleases, while examples of engineered enzymes may be serine proteases; in that latter case a functional group from a substrate can substitute a catalytic residue of enzyme which has been replaced by site-directed mutagenesis. SAC, in serine proteases, is mainly used in order to modify specific sites for proteolytic cleavage, and it may provide strategies for change of the catalyzed reaction. In the point of view of an enzymologist, SAC may contribute significantly to the activity of some enzymes representing functional intermediates in the evolution of catalysis. In figure 11 is given an example of substrate assisted catalysis (Dall'Acqua & Carter, 2000).

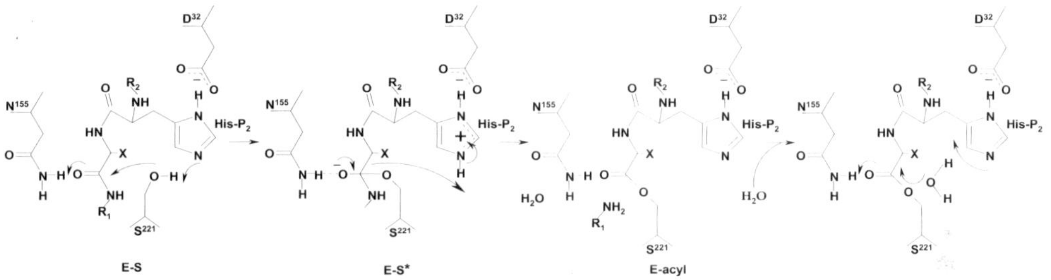

Fig. 11. The H64A subtilisin BPN9 mutant with a peptide substrate containing a histidine residue at the P_2 position, where the mutated catalytic residue has been omitted for clarity (modified from Dall'Acqua & Carter, 2000).

4.1.5 Detecting the rate-limiting step (R.L.S.) and identifying the kinetic (hydrolytic) mechanism

Usually the terms (a) rate-limiting step, (b) rate-determining step, and (c) rate-controlling step are regarded as synonymous; however, other meanings that have been given to them should be mentioned, as it is necessary to be aware of them in order to avoid confusion. The term rate-determining step is mostly used as special case of rate-controlling step, being assigned only to an initial slow step which is followed by rapid steps. Therefore, in an enzymatic reaction, the rate-limiting step is generally the stage that requires the greatest activation energy or the transition state of highest free energy. The idea of a rate-limiting step is a fundamental concept for understanding reaction rates. Thus, the slowest step of a multi-step reaction is often called the rate-limiting or rate-determining step. An approach to finding the rate-limiting step is based on locating the transition state of highest energy. However, this method may fail for irreversible reactions where intermediates more stable than the reactants usually occur; another approach which has been used in the kinetic mechanism of cysteine proteases, and it could found more general usages, is the application of the PI method along with pH and absolute temperature profiles in a attempt to estimate the individual rate constants.

4.1.6 Distinguishing between concerted and stepwise mechanisms

In this section we would like to approach what it concerns the general acid-base catalysis and its associated proton transfer. For example, what determines whether a reaction proceeds by stepwise acid-base catalyzed or concerted reaction mechanisms?, or does catalysis take place in such a way as to avoid the most unstable intermediate?, etc. Answers to these queries may be found in a rule which states that: "Concerted general acid-base catalysis of complex reactions in aqueous solution can occur only (a) at sites that undergo a large change in **pK_a** in the course of the reaction, and (b) when this change in **pK_a** converts an unfavorable to a favorable proton transfer with respect to the catalyst; i.e., the **pK_a** of the catalyst is intermediate between the initial and final **pK_a** values of the substrate site"; however, "the rule does not apply to certain diffusion-controlled reactions in which separate proton transfer steps are not possible. It does apply to the separate steps of reactions proceeding through intermediates so long as these intermediates have a significant lifetime; if there are no such intermediates it should be applied to the overall reaction" (Jencks, 1972). It is commonly the case that a reported enzymatic mechanism seems more or less as incomplete in that the structures of its transition states are not defined in terms of bond orders, atomic charges and/or other features. This can be achieved by specifying the degree of proton transfer (PT), from a nucleophilic reagent onto an electrophilic one, as well as the degree of heavy atom reorganization (HAR); this latter corresponds to the extent of bond breaking and/or making to heavy atoms. Usually, a transition state structure could be described by a diagram of two dimensions relating HAR to PT. Therefore, appropriate experimental data from proton inventories and rate constant vs. pH profiles are prerequisite in order to draw a HAR/PT diagram for enzymatic reactions proceeding via the formation of tetrahedral intermediates. Besides, some reports disagreed with the above rule of Jencks, based on the Marcus theory (Marcus, 1965) insisting that the transition state for proton transfer reactions occurs at a value of HAR such that the free energy change for proton transfer is zero. This condition is satisfied when the **pK_a** values of the proton-accepting and proton-donating species are equal (Szawelski, 1981). An illustrative example in distinguishing between concerted and/or stepwise character may be the identification of the mechanism of action of cysteine proteases of the papain C1 family, where a large number of experimental works have contributed a lot in this latter course; however the application of the proton inventory methodology (PI) along with the use of k_{cat}/K_m and k_{cat} vs. pH profiles were shown as decisive and reliable tools in investigating enzymatic mechanisms. In more details and for the hydrolysis of specific substrates by papain, chymopapain and stem bromelain, were estimated the values of the Michaelis-Menten parameters (k_{cat}/K_m, k_{cat}, K_S), the values of other rate constants (k_1, k_{-1}, k_2, k_3) as well as the values of all related **pK_a**s and the corresponding fractionation factors and SIE, from PI studies, and kinetic parameters/rate constant vs. pH profiles (Ishikawa, 2007; Pavlovsky,1999; Theodorou, 2001,2007a). Therefore, by taking into account results like these described above, HAR/PT (heavy atom reorganization/proton transfer) diagrams could be constructed (figure 12); the examples which are given below are referred in the hydrolysis of p-nitroanilide substrates by cysteine proteases of the papain family.

4.2 Particular NMR-spectroscopy methods

4.2.1 Liquid-state NMR spectroscopy: Hydrogen NMR spectroscopy (^{1}H, ^{2}H, and ^{3}H), Heteronuclear NMR spectroscopy (^{13}C, ^{15}N, ^{18}O, and ^{19}F), studies on enzyme dynamics

Both nuclear magnetic resonance (NMR) spectroscopy and X-ray crystallography are the only biophysical methods which can provide high-resolution structures of biological molecules such as proteins and their complexes at atomic resolution. Additional information can also be provided about conformational dynamics and exchange processes of

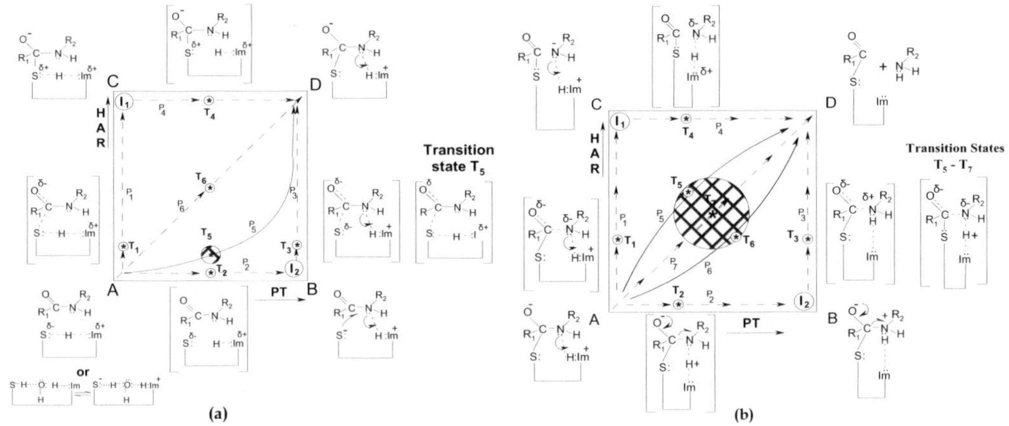

Fig. 12. HAR/PT diagrams where **A** symbolizes the reactants and **D** the products: (a) the boxed diagram represents the most probable transition state $\mathbf{T_5}$, corresponding to a stepwise pathway $\mathbf{P_5}$, (b) the boxed diagram represents the most probable transition states $\mathbf{T_5}$ to $\mathbf{T_7}$, corresponding to the concerted pathways $\mathbf{P_5}$ to $\mathbf{P_7}$.

biomolecules at timescales ranging from picoseconds to seconds, and is very efficient in kinetics of enzymatic reactions (Torchia & Ishima, 2003). NMR results from the absorption of energy by a nucleus changing its spin orientation in a magnetic field. Protons (*^1H*) are the most commonly studied nuclei; because of high natural abundance (99.9885%) and high gyromagnetic ratio; their resonance spectrum is characteristic of the various groups in the molecule. Modern NMR goes far beyond analysis of groups. Two types of NMR interactions through-bond spin-spin and the through-space nuclear Overhauser effects can be used to determine the three-dimensional structure and dynamics of macromolecules in solution (van Holde et al., 2006). Moreover, the deuterium nucleus has a spin of 1, resulting in three energy levels in a magnetic field and a non-zero quadrupole moment, and has found a wide use. Deuterium NMR spectroscopy in solutions yields spectra that are similar to proton NMR spectra except that the deuterium peaks are slightly broader due to quadrupole interactions. Liquid-state deuterium NMR has been used extensively to monitor deuterium labeled species in kinetic and mechanistic studies (van Holde, 2006). For historical and practical reasons, a differentiation between proton and heteronuclear NMR was generally taken into account. However, this distinction is not justified regarding chemical shift and spin coupling, as the basics of NMR spectroscopy are identical for all nuclei. In practice, a differentiation is reasonable for a few important principles i.e. the occurrence of nuclei (Holzgrabe,2008). Nowadays, most successful applications of NMR to biological systems have been typically carried out in aqueous solutions, and have utilized spin $I = 1/2$ nuclei, such as ^{1}H, ^{13}C, ^{15}N and ^{31}P and others, whereas NMR spectroscopy has proved less powerful when applied to nuclei with spin quantum number $\boldsymbol{I >> 1/2}$, i.e. those having a non-spherical charge distribution and an electric quadrupole moment. Unfortunately, for a large number of biologically relevant elements, the only NMR-active isotopes are those with nuclear spins greater than ½ (Ronconi & Sadler 2008). The study of ^{13}C nuclei through NMR spectroscopy is an important technique for determining the number of nonequivalent carbons and to identify the types of carbon atoms that may be present in a compound (Pavia et al., 2009). A complication in using ^{13}C in NMR spectroscopy was the occurrence of ^{13}C-^{1}H coupling involving the many protons normally present in organic compounds; this latter problem was solved by the development of wide band proton decoupling. It is often necessary to prepare compounds enriched in ^{13}C beyond the natural abundance. The ^{17}O is the only NMR-active oxygen isotope (***I* = 5/2**) and its application in NMR has been hindered by several of its intrinsic nuclear properties resulting in low sensitivity and complex spectra; however, ^{17}O NMR spectroscopy in solutions is a useful technique to solve structural problems for small organic molecules. The large quadrupolar interaction of oxygen-containing functional groups can cause highly effective relaxation, which leads to strong broadening of the NMR signals, which can be severe for large molecules. On the other hand, the ^{19}F has many favorable NMR characteristics, including a nuclear spin ***I* = 1/2**, 100% natural abundance, high sensitivity and large chemical shift range (<500 ppm) (Battiste & Newmark, 2006). Endogenous fluorine has a very short T_2 relaxation time and the resulting signal is below the limits of NMR detection in most biological systems of interest (Yu et al., 2005). The ^{15}N Nitrogen nuclei are frequently located at the interaction sites of biomolecules; for example, amide nitrogens in peptides are the key in maintaining the peptide backbone conformation by hydrogen bonding. The side chains of amino acids H, W, and R contain nitrogen atoms which are often located at the active sites of enzymes. To detect interaction sites and to study the interaction mechanism of these biomolecules, the use of nitrogen NMR seems promising (Inomata et al, 2009). The natural abundance of ^{15}N nuclei with a spin quantum number I = 1/2 (which give a sharp resonance signal) is only 0.3%. But recent developments in the instrumentation of NMR spectroscopy have made it possible to observe the resonance of the nuclei with low natural abundance. For such experiments, enrichment of ^{15}N nuclei in the molecules is required and it is performed by chemical syntheses. The study of larger proteins required the development of 2-4D heteronuclear NMR spectroscopy.

As we have already mentioned above, the most basic principle of enzyme catalysis is the ability of enzymes to lower the transition state energy. What it is important in kinetics and thermodynamics in enzyme-catalyzed reactions it has been obtained by monitoring substrate conversion into products; however, much less is known about the kinetics and energetics of conformational changes in the enzyme molecule (Kern et al, 2005). Many enzymatic reactions occur on time scales of microseconds to milliseconds and it has been suggested that dynamics of the enzyme on these time scales is linked to catalysis (Fersht, 1999). Several techniques have been used to detect dynamic processes of enzymes during catalysis, such as fluorescence resonance energy transfer (FRET), atomic force microscopy and stopped flow fluorescence. While those methods report on dynamics of individual sites, or motions of the entire enzyme molecule, NMR spectroscopy of proteins in solution allows detection of motions at a multitude of specific atomic sites simultaneously over a time from picoseconds (Palmer, 1997). These studies suggest that protein motion plays important roles in all aspects of catalysis.

4.2.2 Solid-state NMR spectroscopy

Although progress in protein structure determination has been tremendous over the last years, however large classes of proteins cannot be investigated using liquid state NMR or X-ray crystallography, because either the proteins cannot be crystallized to a sufficient diffraction quality for X-ray diffraction, or they cannot be brought into a sufficiently concentrated solution, or are too large for liquid-state NMR (Böckmann, 2006). Therefore there is a considerable interest in the development of methods for protein structure determination, which do not have these limitations. High-resolution solid-state NMR (SSNMR) is a very promising technique in this respect, and is becoming of increasingly importance in studying enzymes whose active sites in complex with substrates exhibit compression, and where key reactive groups have particularly short non-bonded distances and are expected to show unusual dynamics (McDermott & Polenova, 2007). Chemically detailed information inherent to NMR, along with the opportunity in stabilizing species at lower temperatures or even study catalysis in its native biological environment, makes SSNMR an especially powerful method.

4.3 Neutron scattering and X-ray diffraction methods

4.3.1 Diffraction data measurements, collection refinement

In the X-ray diffraction data of crystals are included critical 3D-structural information of the crystallized molecules. Such a data collection for single crystals refers to the process of measuring diffracted intensities and to their standard deviations (noise) (McDermott & Polenova, 2007). The quality of the diffraction data determines the accuracy of the final model. Although for macromolecular crystallography, there are many factors that compromise the data quality, however the key to obtain the highest possible quality of diffraction data lies in the data collection strategy (the wavelength, attenuation, detector-to-crystal distance, exposure time, start angle, scan range and oscillation angle) (Cianci et al., 2008). Macromolecular crystals diffract X-rays poorly as compared to crystals of small molecules, and usually tend to have a much shorter lifetime in the X-ray beam. Next step in a protein crystallography project after the diffraction data collection is the processing of data in order to extract the relative intensities of the diffracted X-ray beam. The methodology and software used for data acquisition and structure solution allow the experimenter to obtain a preliminary structure solution within minutes at the end of the data-collection session (Dauter, 2006). The extracted intensities are then used for the calculation of an electron density map into which a model of the protein is built.

4.3.2 Small angle X-ray diffraction

Small-angle X-ray scattering (SAXS) is a technique that allows the study of the structure and interactions of biological macromolecules in solution. SAXS can be used to probe proteins, nucleic acids, and their complexes under various conditions, without the need of crystallizing the sample and without molecular weight limitations inherent in other methods such as NMR spectroscopy (Das & Doniach, 2006). This progress has been achieved by improving the brightness of synchrotron radiation x-ray sources combined with a wide availability of new computational tools for interpreting SAXS measurements. The basic principle of SAXS is to scatter X-ray photons elastically off molecules in solution and to record the scattering intensity as a function of the scattering angle (Pollack, 2011a). The parameters most frequently extracted from a SAXS profile for a biomolecule in solution, sufficiently diluted to avoid the effects of interparticle interference, are radius of gyration Rg and forward scattering intensity $I(0)$ which are obtained from the Guinier formula $I(q) \approx I(0)\, exp(-q^2R_g^2/3)$, for small momentum transfer q (Lipfert & Doniach 2007). With the introduction of high-brilliance synchrotron sources, it is now possible to obtain high signal-to-noise SAXS profiles of biomolecule samples with x-ray exposures of milliseconds, or even less, with continuous flow mixing (Pollack, 2011b). The SAXS methodology allows the time resolved characterization of the size and shape of structure ranging from small peptides up to whole viruses by means of beam line setups and appropriate mixers; these structures undergo changes on time scales much faster than one second (Das & Doniach, 2006).

4.4 CD-spectroscopy

4.4.1 Protein folding determination

The rapid characterization of new proteins gets of great importance in the fields of proteomics and structural genomics. Circular Dichroism (CD) relies on the differential absorption of left and right circularly polarized radiation by chromophores which either possess intrinsic chirality or are placed in chiral environments. Proteins possess a number of chromophores which can give rise to CD signals. This spectroscopic technique is widely used in the evaluation of the conformation and stability of proteins under various environmental conditions including temperature, ionic strength, etc. The mechanism of protein folding represents one of the major unsolved problems in molecular biology. Knowledge of protein folding pathways and structural characterization of their states are necessary for a thorough understanding of folding which would have an immediate practical impact, as folding and unfolding participate in the control of a variety of cellular processes (Dobson & Karplus 1999). The task for the experimental scientist is to employ a variety of techniques to gather structural and kinetic data which allow models for folding to be proposed and tested. In view of the rates of the various processes, it is usually necessary to use rapid kinetic methods (stopped or quenched flow) as well as manual mixing methods (dead time typically 10-15 sec) in order to probe as much of the refolding process as possible. Stopped flow methods typically have dead times in the range 1 to 10 msec, and involve dilutions of 11-fold or greater).

4.4.2 Characterization of protein (enzyme) secondary structure and stability upon pH, temperature, denaturizing agents etc

One of the main applications of CD for the study of proteins is the estimation of secondary structure of proteins as their peptide bonds are asymmetric; molecules without symmetry show the phenomenon of circular dichroism. In that case, the chromophores of the polypeptide backbone of proteins are aligned in arrays, and their optical transitions are shifted or split into multiple transitions due to "exciton" interactions resulting different structural elements having characteristic CD spectra as it is shown in figure 13 (Sreerama & Woody, 2004). In addition to the intrinsic CD of the protein backbone, when ligands with chromophores bind to proteins they may develop useful strong extrinsic CD bands; also, the aromatic chromophores of proteins, which have bands in the near ultraviolet region, are often in asymmetric environments and can be used to examine whether mutations change the tertiary structure of proteins (Greenfield, 2006).

4.5 Mass-spectroscopy

4.5.1 Enzyme kinetics: Reaction monitoring, proton transfer

Mass spectrometry has emerged as a valuable tool in biochemistry offering unique insight into biological systems with respect to sensitivity and accuracy. More specifically, mass

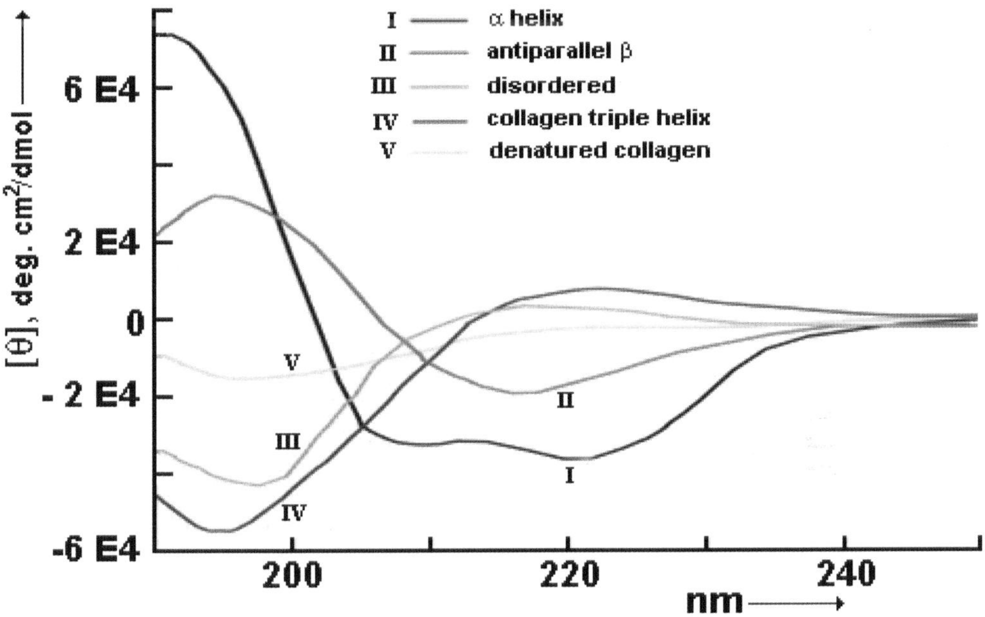

Fig. 13. CD spectra of polypeptides and proteins secondary structures (as modified from Sreerama & Woody, 2004).

spectrometry permits protein sequencing, elucidation of protein folding pathways, characterization of post-translational modifications on peptides and proteins, and detection of covalent and non-covalent protein ligand complexes (Bothner et al, 2000). Recently, the potential of mass spectrometry in studying enzyme catalysis has been widely demonstrated. The development of soft ionization techniques, such as electrospray ionization (ESI) and matrix-assisted laser desorption (MALDI), has made mass spectrometry an excellent complementary technique to conventional spectrophotometric methods for studying enzyme kinetics. Enzyme mechanisms range from simple two-step processes to complex multi-step reactions and they could be elucidated by means of suitable kinetic experimentation. After the initiation of an enzymatic reaction, there is a short period of time during which reaction intermediates are accumulated; in this "pre-steady-state" period the rate constants of individual steps could be measured. With very few exceptions, pre-steady-state kinetic studies require a time resolution in the millisecond range, which can only be achieved by using automated rapid mixing techniques (Johnson, 1995). Typically, the kinetics in these types of rapid mixing experiments are monitored optically, e.g., by UV-visible absorption or by fluorescence spectroscopy; enzyme kineticists use chromogenic substrate analogues and/or radiolabeled substrates which undergo a change upon turnover. Relatively recently, mass spectrometry (MS)-based techniques have shown great promise in the area of chemical and biochemical kinetics as they do not require chromophoric substrates or radioactive labeling. More important developments of MS spectrometry includes its ability to measure pre-steady-state kinetics of "time-resolved" ESIMS by coupling a continuous-flow-mixing capillary directly to an ESI source (Zechel et al,1998).

Moreover, the kinetics of amide H/D exchange can be measured also by NMR and MS spectroscopy; this latter has been emerged as an attractive alternative to NMR method, with significant contributions to the understanding of the role of protein dynamics in enzyme-catalyzed reactions (Kaltashov & Eyles, 2002).

4.5.2 Protein structure and identification

The determination of protein structure, function and interactions is vital in understanding biological processes. Many biophysical methods have been reported for the investigation of protein structure, dynamics and interactions, in the quest to relate protein structure and function. In the post-genomic era, mass spectrometry (MS) has become the cornerstone of proteomics in identifying cellular proteins and characterizing their expression levels, post-translational modifications, network relationships and metabolism products; they have been developed gentle ionizations techniques for mass spectrometry, matrix-assisted laser desorption ionization (MALDI) and electrospray ionization (ESI), which expanded remarkably the impact of mass spectrometry in the protein chemistry. The majority of these techniques remain in the area of primary structure determination; however, nowadays mass spectra can provide important clues about higher-order structure of protein by applying several approaches in using MS to study protein higher order structure involving H/D exchange, radical-mediated protein foot-printing and chemical cross-linking with MS (Chance, 2008).

4.5.3 Protein-protein and protein – ligands interactions

As enzyme structure and function are strongly related, the high resolution determination of the molecular structure of proteins gets of great importance in biochemical research. NMR spectroscopy and X-ray crystallography are two important techniques in obtaining high-resolution structural information; however many protein systems are not amenable to these methods due to their size, conformational flexibility, aggregation propensity, or limited sample amount. Therefore, higher throughput methods are necessary to unravel the relationships between protein structural interactions and cellular function, and in this way mass spectrometry (MS) plays an ever-increasing role in protein structure determination due to its speed, sensitivity, and specificity (Heck & van den Heuvel, 2003). The identification and deconvolution of multi-protein complexes helps in understanding protein function and cell regulation, while it is essential to recognize the individual components of protein complexes and their stoichiometries, as well as the nature of interactions, the kinetics and any resulting conformational changes during complex formation. Many protein interactions are non-covalent ones and they can be investigated with MS if the experimental conditions favor retention of non-covalent association (e.g. electro-spray MS, as well as matrix-assisted laser desorption ionization MS) (Heck & van den Heuvel, 2003). More recent applications of mass spectrometry utilize isotopic labeling of proteins via amide hydrogen/deuterium exchange followed by proteolytic fragmentation of labeled protein and analysis; this latter application of MS can measure rates of amide hydrogen exchange with solvent in defined regions of proteins.

4.6 Inorganic mechanisms as probes in investigating enzymatic mechanisms

Sometimes the elucidation of inorganic mechanisms can be used as a probe in investigating particular enzymatic mechanisms which otherwise they may remain at least not clarified or even unexplored. A good example could be an insight in the mechanism of action of carbonic anhydrase II (EC 4.2.1.1.), a zinc metalloenzyme widespread in nature, which catalyzes the reversible reaction of hydration of CO_2. In living organisms, carbonic anhydrase is involved in various physiological functions including respiration, pH and acid-base regulation, CO_2 and HCO_3^- transport, water and electrolyte balance, and biomineralization; the activity of carbonic anhydrase increases as preceding to the occurrence of the first calcite and quartz crystals formation, in embryos of *Mytilus edulis* L., due to the acceleration of bicarbonate formation. Our example comprises a detailed experimental and theoretical evidence of the effect of carbonic anhydrase II on the dissolution process of carbonate minerals of phosphate ores by dilute acetic acid solutions in the pH range from 2.37 to 6.40. Besides, the elucidation of the mechanism of carbonic anhydrase was based on two relative detailed mechanisms which were reported previously on the selective dissolution of calcite from low-grade phosphate ores. Carbonic anhydrase II was found active at pH values as low as 2.37, even though this enzyme was considered as having a relatively limited pH range of activity at pH 6.0 to 7.8 (Vaimakis & Papamichael, 2002). As a conclusion, two possible mechanisms (figure 14) of action for this enzyme were proposed from pH 2.37 up to 6.40, while the role of carbonic anhydrase in the biomineralization process of marine and other organisms was elucidated.

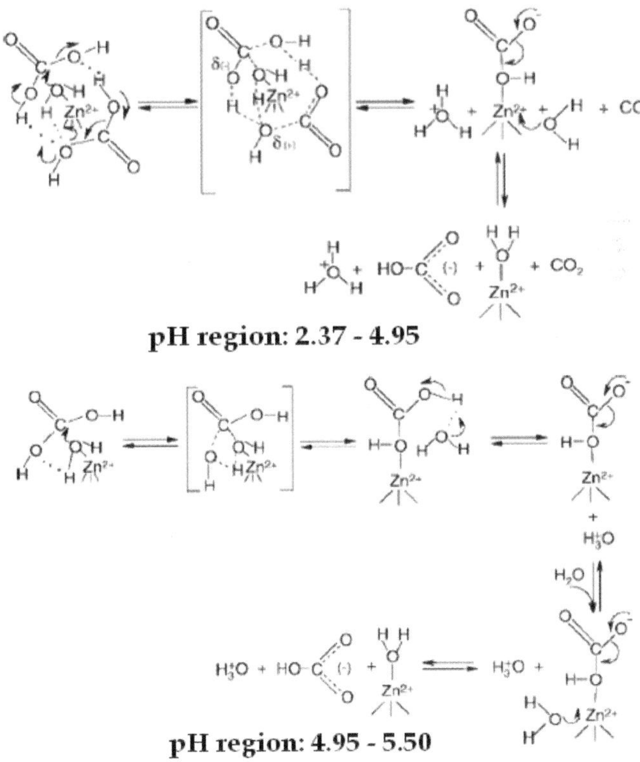

Fig. 14. Two possible mechanisms of action of carbonic anhydrase II (EC 4.2.1.1.), in acid pH-values

5. References

Aloulou, A., Rodriguez, JA. & Frédéric, C. (2006). Exploring the specific features of interfacial enzymology based on lipase studies. *Biochimica et Biophysica Acta(Molecular & cell biology og lipids),* Vol. 1761,Vol.9, pp. 995–1013

Böckmann, A. C. R. (2006). Structural and dynamic studies of proteins by high-resolution solid-state NMR. *Chimie,* Vol 9, No.3-4, pp 381–392

Auld, D. S. (1997). Zinc Catalysis in Metalloproteases. *Structure and Bonding,* Vol. 89, pp. 29-50

Bachovchin, W.W. (2001). Contributions of NMR spectroscopy to the study of hydrogen bonds in serine protease active sites. *Magn. Reson. Chem.,*Vol. 39, No.1,(December 2001), pp. S199–S213

Battiste, J. & Newmark, R.A. (2006). Applications of ^{19}F multidimensional NMR. *Prog. Nucl. Magn. Reson. Spectrosc.,* Vol 48, No.1,(March 2006), pp 1-23, ISSN 00796565

Bieth JG. (1978). Elastases: Structure, function, and pathological role. *Front Matrix Biol,*Vol. 6, pp. 1-82.

Bieth, J.G., Dirrig, S., Jung, M-L., Boudier, C., Papamichael, E.M., Sakarellos, C. & Dimicoli J-L. (1989) "Investigation of the active center of rat pancreatic elastase", *B.B.A.* (Protein Structure and Molecular Enzymology/*Proteins and Proteimics)* 994, pp. 64-74 , ISSN: 0167-4838

Bothner,B., Chavez,R., Wei J., Strupp C., Phung Q., Schneemann,.A. & Siuzdak G. (2000). Monitoring Enzyme Catalysis with Mass Spectrometry. *J. Biol. Chem.,* Vol 275, No.18,(May 2000),pp 13455–13459

Box, M.J. (1971). Bias in nonlinear estimation. *Journal of the Royal Statistical Society Series B,* Vol. 33 ,pp. 171-201

Brocklehurst, K., Malthouse, J.P.G. & Shipton, M. (1979). Evidence that binding to the S_2-subsite of papain may be coupled with catalytically relevant structural change involving the cysteine-25–histidine-159 diad. Kinetics of the reaction of papain with a two-protonic-state reactivity probe containing a hydrophobic side chain. Biochem. J., Vol. 183, No.2, pp. 223-231

Buckle, A. M. &. Fersht, A. R. (1994). *Biochemistry,* Vol. 33, No.7, pp. 1644-1653

Chance, M. (2008). *Mass Spectrometry Analysis for Protein-Protein Interactions and Dynamics,* Wiley-VCH, ISBN 978-0470-2588-66,Weinheim, Germany

Cianci, M., Helliwell, J. R. & Suzuki, A. (2008). The interdependence of wavelength, redundancy and dose in sulfur SAD experiments. *Acta Cryst.* Vol D64, (November 2008),pp 1196–1209

Clarke, D.T. & Jones, G.R. (1999) *Biochemistry,* Vol. 38, No.32, pp.10457-10462

Cleland, W. W. (2000). Low barrier hydrogen bonds in enzymatic catalysis. *Arch. Biochem. Biophys.,* Vol. 382, No.1, pp. 1-5

Cleland, W.W. (1979). Statistical analysis of Enzyme Kinetic Data. *Methods in Enzymol.,* Vol. 63, pp. 103-138

Comish-Bowden A. & Eisenthal, R. (1974). Statistical considerations in the estimation of enzyme kinetic parameters by the direct linear plot and other methods. *Biochemical Journal,* Vol. 139, pp. 721-730

Cornish-Bowden, A. (1995), Analysis of Enzyme Kinetic Data. Oxford University Press, ISBN: 019-854878-8, Oxford

Dall'Acqua, W.& Carter, P (2000) Substrate-assisted catalysis: Molecular basis and biological significance, *Protein Science* , Vol.9, No.1, pp.1-9

Das, R. & Doniach, S. (2006). Structural studies of proteins and nucleic acids in solution using small angle x-ray scattering (SAXS), In Soft Matter: *Scattering, Imaging and Manipulation*, Pecora, R. & Borsali, R., pp 1084-1408, Springer, ISBN 978-1-4020-4464-9,Berlin

Dauter, Z. (2006). Estimation of anomalous signal in diffraction data. *Acta Cryst.* Vol D62, No.8, pp 867–876

Davies, G. & Henrissat, B. (1995). Structures and mechanisms of glycosyl hydrolases. *Structure,* Vol. 3, No.9, pp. 853-859.

De Caro, JD., Boudouard, M., Bonicel, J., Guidoni, A., Densuelle, P. & Rovery, M. (1981). Porcine pancreatic lipase: Completion of the primary structure. *Biochimica et Biophysica Acta,* (Protein Structure and Molecular Enzymology/*Proteins and Proteimics),* Vol. 671, No.2, pp. 129-138

De la Sierra, I-L., Papamichael, E. M., Sakarellos, C., Dimicoli, J-L. & Prangé, T. (1990).Interaction of the Peptide CF_3CO-Leu-Ala-NH-C_6H_4-CF_3 (TFLA) with Porcine Pancreatic Elastase. x-Ray Studies at 1.8 Å. *J. Molecular Recogn,* Vol. 3, No.1, pp. 36-44

Dimicoli, J-L., Papamichael, E.M.& Sakarellos, C. (1987). Dynamics of Elastase peptide complexes. A ^{13}C NMR Study. *Protides of the biological fluids,* Vol. 35, pp 449-452

Dixon, M. M. & Matthews, B. W. (1989). Is γ-Chymotrypsin a tetrapeptide acyl-enzyme adduct of α-Chymotrypsin? *Biochemistry,* Vol. 28, No. 17, pp. 7033-7038

Dobson C.M. & Karplus M., (1999). The fundamentals of protein folding: bringing together theory and experiment. *Curr. Opin. Struct. Biol.,* Vol 9, No.1, (February 1999),pp 92-101

Dune, B.M., Jimenez, M., Parten, B.F., Valler, M.J., Rolph, C.E. & Kay, J. (1986) A systematic series of synthetic chromophoric substrates for aspartic proteinases. *Biochem. J.,* Vol. 237, pp. 899-906

Evmiridis, N.P. & Papamichael, E.M. (1991). Investigation of the error structure of the calibration curve for periodate determination by flow-injection analysis and chemiluminescence detection. *Chemom. Intell. Lab. Systems,*Vol. 12, pp. 39-47

Fersht, A. (1999) *Structure and Mechanism in Protein Science: A Guide to Enzyme Catalysis and Protein Folding,* (1st edition),W.H. Freeman, ISBN-10 0-7167-3268-8, New York]

Fletcher, R. (1965). Function minimization without evaluating derivatives - a review. *Computer Journal,* Vol..8, pp. 33-41

Gosalia, D.N, Salisbury, C.M., Maly, D.J,. Ellman J.A. &. Diamond, S.L.(2005). Profiling serine protease substrate specificity with solution phase fluorogenic peptide microarrays, Proteomics, Vol. 5, pp. 1292–1298

Greenfield., N.J. (2006) Using circular dichroism spectra to estimate protein secondary structure. Nat Protoc., Vol.1, No.6, pp. 2876–2890

Gupton, B.F., Carroll, D.L., Tuhy, P.M., Kam, C.M.& Powers, J.C. (1984). *J. Biol. Chem.,* Vol. 259, No.7, pp. 4279-4287

Heck,A.J.R., & van den Heuvel, R.H.H.(2003). Investigation of intact protein complexes by mass spectrometry. *Mass Spectrometry Reviews,* Vol 23,No.5, (October 2003), pp 368–389

Henrissat, B. & Romeu, A. (1995). Families, superfamilies and subfamilies of glycosyl hydrolases. *Biochem. J.*, Vol. 311,(October 1995), pp 350-351

Henrissat, B. (1991). A classification of glycosyl hydrolases based on amino acid sequence similarities.*Biochem. J.*, Vol. 280,(December, 1991) pp. 309-316

Hill, V. (1913). The Combinations of Haemoglobin with Oxygen and Carbon Monoxide. *Biochemical Journal*, Vol. 7, pp. 471-480

Hiromi, K., Ohnishi, M. & Tanaka, A. (1983). Subsite structure and Ligand binding mechanism of glucoamylase, *Molecular and Cellular Biochemistry*, Vol. 51, No.1, pp. 79-95.

Hogan, M.C. & Woodley, J.M. (2000). Modelling of two enzyme reactions in a linked cofactor recycle system for chiral lactones synthesis. *Chemical Engineering Science*, Vol. 55, No.11, (June 2000), pp 2001–2008

Holzgrabe,U., Wawer I.& Diehl,B. (2008). *NMR Spectroscopy in Pharmaceutical Analysis, Elsevier*, ISBN 978-0-444-53173-5, Amsterdam, The Netherlands

Hunkapiller, M., Forgac, M., & Richards J. (1976). Mechanism of action of serine proteases: tetrahedral intermediate and concerted proton transfer.*Biochemistry*, Vol. 15, No.25, pp. 5581-5588

Inomata, K., Ohno, A., Tochio, H., Isogai, S., Tenno, T., Nakase, I., Takeuchi, T., Futaki, S., Ito, Y., Hiroaki, H. & Shirakawa, M. (2009). High-resolution multi-dimensional NMR spectroscopy of proteins in human cells .*Nature* Vol 458, (March 2009),pp 106-10

Ishikawa, K., Nakatani, H., Katsuya, Y. & Fukazawa, C. (2007). Kinetic and Structural Analysis of Enzyme Sliding on a Substrate: Multiple Attack in β-Amylase. *Biochemistry*, Vol. 46, No.3, pp. 792-798

Jencks, W.P. (1972) General acid-base catalysis of complex reactions in water, *Chemical Reviews*, Vol. 72, No.6, pp. 705-718

Johnson, K. A. (1995). Rapid quench kinetic analysis of polymerases, adenosinetriphosphatases, and enzyme intermediates. *Methods Enzymol.*, Vol. 249, pp 38-61

Kafarov, V. (1976), *Cybernetic Methods in Chemistry & Chemical Engineering*, MIR Publishers, Moscow

Kaltashov,I.A.& Eyles, S.J. (2002) Crossing the phase boundary to study, protein dynamics and function: combination of amide hydrogen exchange in solution and ion fragmentation in the gas phase. *J. Mass. Spectrom.* ,Vol 37, No.6, pp 557–565

Kern, D., Eisenmesser, E.Z. & Wolf-Watz, M. (2005). Enzyme dynamics during catalysis measured by NMR spectroscopy.Methods in Enzymology, Vol 394, pp 507-524

Kidd, R.D., Sears, P., Huang, D.H., Witte, K., Wong, C.H. & Farber, G.K. (1999). *Protein Sci.*, Vol. 8, No.2, pp. 410-417

Kim, M-J., Yamamoto, D., Matsumoto, K., Inoue, M. Ishida, T., Mizuno, H., Sumiya, S. & Kitamura, K., (1992). Crystal structure of papain-E64-c complex. Binding diversity of E64-c to papain S_2 and S_3 subsites. *Biochem. J.*,Vol. 287, No. 3,pp. 797-803

Kirby, A. J. (2001).The lysozyme mechanism sorted after 50 years.*Nature Struct. & Mol. Biol.*, Vol. 8, No.9, pp. 737-739

Knowles, J.R. (1976) Whither enzyme mechanisms. *FEBS Lett.*, Vol. 62, pp. E53-E61, ISSN 0014-5793

Kokkinou, M., Theodorou, L.G & E.M. Papamichael (2011).Aspects on the Catalysis of Lipase from Porcine Pancreas (type VI-s) in aqueous media: development of ion-pairs. *BRAZ. ARCH. BIOL. TECHNOL.*, Accepted for publication , ISSN 1516-8913

Liese, A., Seelbach, K. & Wandrey, C. (2006). *Industrial biotransformations*, Wiley-VCH, ISBN-13 978-3-527-31001-2, Weinheim

Lipfert, J. & Doniach S.(2007). Small-angle X-ray scattering from RNA, proteins, and protein complexes.*Annu. Rev. Biophys. Biomol. Struct.*, Vol 36,(February 2007), pp.307–27

Lymperopoulos, K., Kosmas, M. & Papamichael, E. M. (1998). A Formulation of Different Equations Applied in Enzyme Kinetics". *Journal of Scientific and Industrial Res.*, Vol. 57, special issue, pp. 604-606, ISSN 0022-4456

Mannervik, B. (1982). Regression Analysis, Experimental Error, and Statistical Criteria in the Design and Analysis of Experiments for Discrimination Between Rival Kinetic Models. *Methods in Enzymol.*, Vol. 87, pp. 370-390

Manzettia, S., McCullocha, D.R., Heringtona, A.C. & van der Spoel, D. (2003). Modeling of enzyme-substrate complexes for the metalloproteases MMP-3, ADAM-9 and ADAM-10. *Journal of Computer-Aided Molecular Design*, Vol. 17, pp. 551–565

Marcus, R. A. (1965). On the theory of electron-transfer reaction. VI. Unified treatment for homogeneous and electron reactions. *J. Chem. Phys.* Vol. 43, No.2 67-683

Mazur, A.K., & Nakatani, H. (1993). Multiple Attack Mechanism in the Porcine Pancreatic α-Amylase Hydrolysis of Amylose and Amylopectin, *Archives of Biochemistry and Biophysics*, Vol..306, No.1, pp. 29-38

Mc Carter, J.D. & Withers, S.G. (1994). Mechanisms of enzymatic glycoside hydrolysis. *Current Opinion in Structural Biology*, Vol. 4, No.6, pp. 885-892

McDermott, A. & Polenova T. (2007). Solid state NMR: new tools for insight into enzyme function.*Current Opinion in Structural Biology*, Vol 17,No.5,(October 2007), pp 617–622

Meschede, L., & Limbach, H-H. (1991). Dynamic NMR Study of the Kinetic HH/HD/DD Isotope Effects on the Double Proton Transfer in Cyclic Bis(p-fluorophenyl)formamidine Dimers. *J. Phys. Chem.*, Vol.95, pp. 10267-10280

Michaelis, L. & Menten, M.L., (1913). Die Kinetik der Invertinwirkung. *Biochemisches Zeitschrift*, Vol. 49, pp. 333-369.

Muralikrishnaa, G.& Nirmala, M. (2005). Cereal α-amylases – An overview. *Carbohydrate Polymers*, Vol. 60,No.2, (May 2005), pp. 163–173

NC-IUB (Nomenclature Committee of the International Union of Biochemistry). (1983). Symbolism and terminology in enzyme kinetics. *Biochemical Journal*, Vol. 213, No.3, pp.561-571

Northrop, D.B. (2001). Follow the Protons: A Low-Barrier Hydrogen Bond Unifies the Mechanisms of the Aspartic Proteases. *Acc. Chem. Res.*, Vol. 34, No.10, pp. 790-797

Ohtaki, A., Kondo, S., Shimura, Y., Tonozuka, T., Sakano, b Y., Kamitori, b S. (2001). Role of Phe286 in the recognition mechanism of cyclomaltooligosaccharides (cyclodextrins) by *Thermoactinomyces _ulgaris* R-47 _-amylase 2 (TVAII). X-ray structures of the mutant TVAIIs, F286A and F286Y, and kinetic analyses of the Phe286-replaced mutant TVAIIs. *Carbohydrate Research*, Vol. 334, No.4, pp. 309–313

Ollis, DL., Cheah, E., Cygle,r M., Dijkstra, B., Frolow, F., Franken, SM., Harel, M., Remington, SJ., Silman, I., Schrag, J., Sussman, JL., Verschueren, KHG.& Goldman,

A. (1992). The Alpha/Beta - Hydrolase Fold. *Protein Engineering,design & selectiom* Vol. 5, No.3 pp. 197-211

Palmer, A.G. (1997). Probing molecular motion by NMR.*Curr.Opin.Struct.Biol.*,Vol 7,No.5, (October 1996),pp 732-737

Papamichael, E.M. & Evmiridis, N.P. (1988). Program based on the pattern search method: application to periodate determination using flow injection analysis and chemiluminescence detection. *TRENDS in Anal. Chem.*,Vol. 7, No.10, pp. 366-370

Papamichael, E.M. & Lymperopoulos. (1998) K. Elastase and Cathepsin-G from Human PMN activated by PAF: Relation between their Kinetic Behavior and Pathophysiological Role In *Advances in Biotechnology,* Pandey, A. , pp.221-234, New Delhi, ISBN 81-87198-03-6, India

Papamichael, E.M. & Theodorou, L.G. Experimental and theoretical approaches in investigating enzymatic mechanisms: Applications on the thermo-stable extracellular Protease-A-17N-1 from Bacillus sp., with possible biotechnological interest, in *Current Topics on Bioprocesses in Food Industry Vol III.* (2010). pp. 130-139, Rao, L.V., Pandey, A., Larroche, C., Soccol, C-R. & C-G., pp. 130-139, Dussap, Asiatech Publishers, Inc., ISBN 81-87680-21-0, New Delhi, India

Papamichael, E.M. &. Theodorou, L.G.(2005).Enzyme Kinetics and Modeling of Enzymatic Systems, In *Enzyme Technology* , Pandey, A., Webb, C., Soccol, C.R. & Larroche, C., pp. 37-62, Asiatech Publishers Inc., ISBN 81-87680-12-1 New Delhi

Papamichael, E.M. (1987). Least squares Fitting of Tabular Data to Rational Functions in *BASIC. ANALYST,* Vol. 112, pp. 815-819

Papamichael, E.M., Bieth, J.G., Theodorou, L.G., Lymperopoulos, K.& Valasaki. K. (2009) The elucidation of the mechanism of action of cysteine proteinases of the Papain-C1 family: possible biotechnological applications, In *New Horizons in Biotechnology,* Pandey, A., Larroche,C., Soccol,C.R. &. Dussap,G.C., pp. 104-122, Asiatech Publishers, Inc., ISBN 81-87680-19-9 New Delhi, India

Papamichael, E.M., Evmiridis, N.P. & Potosis, C (2000).Non-parametric Fitting of Nonlinear Equations to Experimental Data without Use of Initial Guessing: A *Basic* Computer Program. *BRAZ. ARCH. BIOL. TECHNOL.*, Vol. 43, No.1,pp. 1-9

Papamichael, E.M., Evmiridis, N.P., Thanasoulias, N. & Stefanou, D. (1995). Design of experiments for a precise estimation of the calibration curve of periodate in its determination by F.I.A. and CL-detection. *Chemom. Intell. Lab. Systems, Vol* 30, pp 227-237

Papamichael, E.M., Koukkou, A-I., Douka, E., Vartholomatos, G., Masavetas, K.A & Drainas, C. (2002). Diagnostic tests on the mode of ligand binding to proteins: application to *Zymomonas mobilis* strains. *Indian Journal of Biotechnology,*Vol 1, pp 386-392

Papamichael, E.M., Roustas, M.K., Bieth, J.G. (1999). Detection of S_1-P_1 and S_3-P_3 interactions between papain and four synthetic substrates. *BRAZ. ARCH. BIOL. TECHNOL.*, Vol. 42, No.3, pp. 277-280, ISSN 1516-8913

Patel, M., Kayani, I. S., Mellor, G.W., Sreedharan, S., Templeton, W., Thomas, E.W., Thomas, M. & Brocklehurst, K. (1992). Variation in the P_2- S_2 stereochemical selectivity towards the enantiomeric N-acetyl-phenylalanylglycine 4-nitroanilides among the cysteine proteinases papain, ficin and actinidin. *Biochem. J.*, Vol. 281, No.2,pp. 553-559.

Pavia, D.L., Lampman, G.M., Kriz, G.S.& Vyvyan, J.R.(2009). *Introduction to Spectroscopy*, (4th edition), Brooks/Cole Cengage Learning, ISBN-13 978-0-495-11478-9, USA

Pavlovsky, A., Ye, Q.-Z., Ortwine, D. F., Humblet, C., Purchase, C., White, A., Roth, B., Johnson, L., Hupe, D., Williams, M., Dhanaraj, V. & Blundell, T. (1999). *Protein Sci.*, Vol. 8, No.7. pp. 1455-1462

Pelmenschikov, V. & Siegbahn, P.E.M. (2002). Catalytic Mechanism of Matrix Metalloproteinases: Two-Layered Piana, S. & Carloni, P. (2000). Conformational flexibility of the catalytic asp dyad in HIV-1 protease: an ab initio study on the free enzyme. *Proteins: Struct., Funct. Genet.*, Vol. 39, No.1, pp. 26-36

Polgár, L. (1989). *Mechanisms of Protease Action*, pp 157-182, CRC Press, Inc., Boca Raton, FL

Pollack, L. (2011a). SAXS Studies of Ion–Nucleic Acid Interactions.*Annual Review of Biophysics* Vol 40,(June 2011),pp 225-242

Pollack, L. (2011b). Time resolved SAXS and RNA folding.*Biopolymers*, Vol.95, No.8, pp543-549

Qian M., Haser R., Buisson G., Duee E. & Payan F. (1994). The active centre of a mammalian α-amylase. Structure of the complex of a pancreatic α-amylase with a carbohydrate inhibitor refined to 2.2A resolution. *Biochemistry*, Vol. 33, No.20, pp. 6284-6294

Rawlings, N. D., & Barrett, A. J. (1993). Evolutionary families of peptidases. *Biochem. J*, Vol.290, (February 1993), pp. 205–218

Rawlings, N.D. & Barret, A.J. (1994). Families of Cysteine Peptidases. *Methods in Enzymology*, Vol. 244, pp. 461-486, ISSN 0076-6879

Rebholz, K.L. & Northrop, D.B. (1991). Slow step after bond-breaking by Porcine Pepsin identified usingsolvent deuterium isotope effects. *Biochem. Bophys. Res. Commun.*, Vol. 176, No.1, pp. 65-69

Ronconi, L.& Sadler, P.J. (2008). Applications of heteronuclear NMR spectroscopy in biological and medicinal inorganic chemistry.*Coordination Chemistry Reviews*, Vol 252, (January 2008),pp 2239–2277

Salleh, A.B., Rahman, R.N.Z.R.A. & Basri, M. (2006). *New Lipases and Proteases, Nova Science Publishers*, Inc. ISBN 1-600221-068-6, New York.

Savageau, MA. (1998). Development of fractal kinetic theory for enzyme-catalysed reactions and implications for the design of biochemical pathways. *Biosystems*, Vol. 47, pp. 9-36

Schechter, I. & Berger, A. (1967). On the size of the active site in protease: I. Papain. *Biochem. Biophys. Res. Commun*,Vol 27, No.2, pp 157-162

Schramm, V.L. (1998). Enzymatic transition state and transition state analog design. *Annu. Rev. Biochem*, Vol. 67,pp. 693-720

Segel I.H, 1975, *Enzyme Kinetics: Behavior and Analysis of Rapid Equilibrium and Steady-State Enzyme Systems*, John Wiley & Sons, ISBN 0-471-77425-1, Canada

Sreerama, N. & Woody, R.W. (2004). Computation and analysis of protein circular dichroism spectra. *Methods Enzymol*, Vol 383, pp 318–351

Stein, R.L., Strimpler, A.M., Hori, H. & Powers, J.C., (1987). Catalysis by Human Leukocyte Elastase: the Proton Inventory as a Mechanistic Probe. *Biochemistry*, Vol. 26, No.5, pp. 1305-1314

Svensson, B. (1994). Protein engineering in the co-amylase family: catalyfic mechanism, substrate specificity, and stability. *Plant Mol Biol*, Vol. 25, No.2, pp. 141-157

Szawelski, R. J., and Wharton, C. W. (1981) Kinetic sovent isotope effects on the deacylation og specific acyl-papains. Proton inventory studies on the papain –catalyzed hydrolyses of specific ester substrates: analysis of possible transition state structures.*Biochem. J,*.Vol. 199, No.3, pp.681-692

Taylor, K.(2004) *Enzyme Kinetics and Mechanisms*, Kluwer AcademicPublishers, New York

Theodorou, L.G., Bieth, J.G. & Papamichael, E.M. (2004). Insight Into Catalytic Mechanism of Papain-Like Cysteine Proteinases: the case of D^{158}. *Applied Biochemistry and Biotechnology-Part A Enzyme Engineering & Biotechnology*, Vol. 118, No. 1-3, pp. 171-175, ISSN 0273-2289

Theodorou, L.G., Bieth, J.G. & Papamichael, E.M. (2007a). The catalytic mode of cysteine proteinases of papain (C1) family. *Bioresource Technology*, Vol. 98, No.10, pp. 1931-1939, ISSN: 0960-8524

Theodorou, L.G., Lymperopoulos, K., Bieth, J.G. & Papamichael, E.M. (2001). Insight into the Catalysis of Hydrolysis of four Newly Synthesized Substrates by Papain: A Proton Inventory Study. *Biochemistry-US,* Vol. 40, pp. 3996-4004

Theodorou, L.G., Perisynakis, A., Valasaki, K., Drainas, C. & Papamichael, E.M. (2007b). Proton Inventories Constitute Reliable Tools in Investigating Enzymatic Mechanisms: Application on a novel Thermo-stable Extracellular Protease from a Halo-Alkalophilic *Bacillus* sp. *(The) J. Biochemistry (Tokyo)*, Vol. 142, No.2, pp. 293-300

Torchia, D.A. & Ishima R. (2003). Molecular structure and dynamics of proteins in solution: Insights derived from high-resolution. NMR approaches. *Pure Appl. Chem.*, Vol 75, No.10,pp 371–1381

Vaimakis, T.C. & Papamichael, E.M. (2002). Dissolution Kinetics of Ores, an invited contribution to *Encyclopedia of Surface & Colloid Science*, Hubbard, A., pp. 1471-1485 Marcel Dekker, ISBN 13- 9780824706333, New York

Van Holde, K.E., Johnson, W.C. & Shing P.(2006). Nuclear Magnetic Resonance Spectroscopy, In: *Principles of Physical Biochemistry*, pp 535-577, Pearson Prentice Hall, ISBN 0-13-046427-9, New Jersey

Van Tilbeurgh, H., Egloff, M.P., Martinez, C., Rugani, N., Verger, R. & Cambillau, C. (1993). Interfacial activation of the lipase procolipase complex by mixed micelles revealed by X-ray crystallography. *Nature,* Vol. 362, No.6423, pp. 814-820

Verger, R. & de Haas, G.H. (1976). Interfacial enzyme kinetics of lipolysis. *Annu. Rev. Biophys. Bioeng*, Vol. 5, pp. 77-117

Wilmouth, R.C., Edman, K., Neutze, R., Wright1, P.A., Clifton, I.J., Schneider, T.R., Schofield, C.J. & Hajdu, J. (2001). X-ray snapshots of serine protease catalysis reveal a tetrahedral intermediate. *Nature structural biology (lett*), Vol. 8, pp. 689-694

Yu, J.X., Kodibagkar, V.D., Cui, W. & Mason, R.P. (2005). 19F: A Versatile Reporter for Non-Invasive Physiology and Pharmacology Using Magnetic Resonance. *Curr. Med. Chem.*, Vol 12, No 7, pp 819-848, ISSN 0929-8673

Zechel, D. J., Konermann, L., Withers, S. G. & Douglas, D. J. (1998). Pre-steady state kinetic analysis of an enzymatic reaction monitored by time-resolved electrospray ionization mass spectrometry. *Biochemistry* ,Vol37,No.21, pp 7664-7669, ISSN 0006-2960

12

Supraventricular Tachycardia Due to Dopamine Infused Through Epidural Catheter Accidentally (A Case Report and Review)

Demet Coskun* and Ahmet Mahli
Department of Anesthesiology and Reanimation
Gazi University Faculty of Medicine
Ankara
Turkey

1. Introduction

Ensuring analgesia both intraoperatively and postoperatively by the administration of local anesthetics or opioid through epidural catheter is a widespread method. On the other hand, after thoracic and major abdominal surgery, optimal perioperative anesthesia and analgesia can be provided through thoracic epidural analgesia and thus, postoperative morbidity and mortality can be decreased specifically by blocking sympathetic nerve fibers (1). In spite of the availability of epidural technique, in cases of the inadvertent administration of nonepidural medications into the epidural space, serious morbidity and mortality can be caused by a direct drug or drug-additive neurotoxic, pH, or osmolality effect (2).

In literature, there are several reports of various substances infused through epidural catheter inadvertently (2-10). However, there have been no reports describing inadvertent administration of dopamine through epidural catheter as in the case we present here. We present, review and discuss this case in the light of literature.

2. Case report

A 54-year-old man who was 1.68 m tall and weighed 70 kg, was admitted to cardiovascular surgery intensive care unit after 3 vessel coronary by-pass surgery. All hemodynamic data were within normal limits with the help of inotropic support. The weaning from the ventilator was uneventful. It is our policy to use thoracal epidural anlgesia for all patients following open heart surgery. The catheter is placed a night before the operation after getting informed consent. The infusion liquid that is administered through the epidural catheter in order to ensure analgesia in the patient in the postoperative period in intensive care unit is prepared as 100 mg of mepedrine in 50 mL of isotonic solution and according to the clinical status of the patient, the infusion speed of the infusion device is adjusted as

*Corresponding Author

0.1-0.3 mg/kg/hour. The patient in question was receiving 0.2 mg/kg/hour of meperidine through thoracal epidural catheter by the help of an infusion device.

After 10 hours following the operation, while there was no instability regarding his hemodynamical status, he suddenly started to complain of severe abdominal pain and dizziness followed by vomiting with intervals of two or three seconds. The evaluation of vomited matter showed no abnormal material. He developed a supraventricular tachycardia (with normal ORS complex and no discernible P waves) that reached up to 180 bpm. His blood pressure was monitored as 200/120 mmHg during the constrained period. His physical findings were evaluated as normal except tachycardia and high blood pressure. He had no abnormal abdominal findings and there was no reason for projectile vomiting. All consultations were done and an emergency abdominal ultrasound was performed. Both of them, besides laboratory findings, revealed no positive answer to what caused all these suddenly developed symptoms.

The constrained period lasted for about 20 minutes until it was recognized that a nursing mistake had been made while transferring the meperidine mixed solution into microperfusion device. Dopamine solution had been placed into perfusion device instead of meperidine solution and the patient had received 5 µg/kg/min of dopamin through epidural catheter for 20 minutes. As soon as it was understood, the infusion was discontinued. The intravenous infusion liquid that contains dopamine is prepared as 200 mg of dopamine in 50 mL of isotonic solution and the infusion speed is adjusted according to the clinical status of the patient. Once the nursing mistake was discovered, the records were studied and it was understood that the patient's complaints had started about 7 minutes after the onset of the infusion of dopamine through epidural catheter.

The patient's complaints started to improve 3 minutes after the discontinuation of the infusion and eventually all the symptoms disappeared. The patient's follow-up was uneventful during his stay in intensive care unit and he was discharged from the hospital in the 5th post-operative day. A long-term follow-up including all laboratory evaluations revealed no abnormal findings. Besides, there were no pathological findings in the neurological examination of the patient during the 6-month-period following the operation.

3. Discussion

Thoracic epidural anesthesia which is followed by postoperative epidural analgesia is increasingly being used for abdominal, major vascular and cardiothoracic surgery. The main merit of thoracic epidural postoperative analgesia is the optimal analgesia which it provides for several days and its minimal side-effects without the need for rescue medication (11). Segmental sympathetic block and analgesia are among the potential mechanisms for thorasic epidural analgesia that may influence mortality and myocardial infarction after coronary artery bypass graft surgery in a favorable way (12). It has been reported that the use of local anesthetics in thoracic epidural analgesia may reduce myocardial oxygen demand by way of decreasing heart rate, inotropy, and systemic vascular resistance (13). It has also been reported that thoracic epidural anesthesia may improve myocardial oxygen supply by dilating stenotic coronary arteries (14). Fewer arrhythmic episodes and postoperative myocardial infarction were reported, and patients could be extubated earlier with the aid of thoracic epidural analgesia. The risk of pulmonary complications is decreased by optimized pain control and early mobilization, and this results in a shortened stay in intensive care units. When combined with early enteral nutrition, thoracal epidural analgesia ensures an earlier return of gastrointestinal function. It has been reported that patients treated with thoracic epidural anesthesia and analgesia have a better health-related quality of life (1). However, apart from all these advantages, in patients who have undergone full anticoagulation for cardiopulmonary bypass, the risk of spinal hematoma associated with central neuraxial analgesia is still unknown (12).

Many comparisons of local anesthetic alone, opioid alone or the combination of both have been made in order to ensure thoracic epidural analgesia (11). In cases where opiates are combined with local anesthetics and given either epidurally or spinally, the opiate action is at receptors mediating pain in the dorsal horn of the spinal cord, whereas the action of the local anesthetic is at the dorsal root ganglion. Thus, the effect of combining the two produces a better quality of analgesia and a less risk of systemic toxicity or any other undesirable side effects than when compared with the use of the same degree of analgesia or anesthesia achieved with a single agent (15,16).

Various substances belonging to different pharmacological classes are used as adjuvant in regional anesthesia as they are known to enhance and prolong analgesia of local anesthetics and opioids. The dose requirements of local anesthetics and opioids may be lowered by use of such substances, and thus the dose-dependent side effects of local anesthetics and opioids (e.g. motor block, nausea) may be reduced. Such drugs may also produce analgesia themselves. The list of adjuvants studied during the review period includes adrenaline, clonidine, ketamine, neostigmine, nondepolarizing muscle relaxants, and nonsteroidal anti-inflammatory drugs (17).

Although continuous infusion is the most popular means of administration, it is generally associated with sensory block regression, notably with local anesthetic alone. The time to first analgesic rescue is increased by addition of opioid. The long-known popularity of infusion is the result of the perception that the cardiovascular and respiratory side-effects of it are less when compared to with bolus alone (11).

The following data were obtained as the result of a review on drug error in anesthetic practice: The rate of administration errors was 14%, only four of which were pre-errors. The most common errors were inadvertent arterial injection, subcutaneous injection due to tissued intravenous catheter and inadvertent intravenous injection when performing epidural and peripheral nerve blocks. The most common contributing factors cited were fault of technique (19%), haste (16%) and error of judgement (14%). In the same study, the most frequently cited factors to minimize the incident were prior experience or training (32%) and skilled assistance (11%) (18).

In another study performed, the main sources of inadvertent administration of nonepidural medications into the epidural space were found to be "syringe swap", "ampoule error", and epidural/intravenous line confusion, and it was reported that in spite of all measures that are currently undertaken, accidents would occur inevitably (2).

A literature review on human medicine identified numerous drugs that were inadvertently injected epidurally, and these included thiopental, methohexital, vecuronium, midazolam with fentanyl, morphine with dextrose, ephedrine, cefazolin, gentamicin, amoxicillin clavulanic acid, potassium chloride, magnesium sulphate, total parenteral nutrition, intralipid infusion, phenol containing ranitidine, ether, and paraldehyde (2). Respiratory depression with remifentanil (3), sensory blockade, muscle spasms, and hypertension with potassium chloride (4), and a significant decrease in blood glucose level with insulin (5) are among the complications which were reported in humans as a result of accidental epidural drug administration. Accidental epidural injections of vecuronium, atracurium, cisatracurium, and rocuronium were reported to have no neurological or cardiovascular side effects or other symptoms of local or systemic toxicity (6-8,10). Again, in a reported case, the inadvertent injection of a mixture of rocuronium and morphine into the caudal epidural space in awake patient showed miosis without any neurological abnormality (9). In our case, on the other hand, dopamine was administered inadevrtently through epidural catheter and following the onset of administration, clinical symptoms such as abdominal pain, dizziness, supraventricular tachycardia, hypertension and vomiting were observed.

In cases of inadvertent epidural injection, some practitioners flush the epidural space with distilled water or saline in order to dilute the concentration of the drug. Some others use epidural or intravenous corticosteroids in order to reduce the inflammatory response (2).These attempts were speculative, however, and because of the upward spread of the drugs, they could potentially worsen the situation (10).

In a related study on animals, it was reported that methylprednisolone sodium succinate as a treatment for acute spinal cord injury is a commonly used but controversial practice (19). Again in other studies on animals, it has been reported that it can be used as a neuroprotective agent as it decreases lipid peroxidation (20) that may contribute to free radical formation after acute spinal cord injury (21). In a study performed by O'Kell ve Ambros (22) on animals, the authors were concerned that secondary to vasoconstriction, acute inflammation and ischemia could occur, and therefore, to minimize these potentially detrimental effects, methylprednisolone sodium succinate was administered. In our case, where dopamine was administered inadvertently through epidural catheter, no pathological findings were observed as a result of the examination performed as soon as the error was discovered and in the following 6-month clinical follow-up period.

The first studies on the spread of analgesic solutions in the epidural space and penetration into the neuraxis were performed by Bromage et al (23). These studies have shown that local anesthetic appeared in the cerebrospinal fluid (CSF) very soon after epidural injection and reached a peak concentration in about 10 to 15 minutes. Plasma venous levels of epidurally administered agents are reached quickly and much sooner than after spinal anesthesia. In another study, it was reported that following lumbar epidural injection of 75 mg lidocaine (3.75 ml of a 2% solution), the drug became detectable in 1 to 2 minutes and it reached a concentration of 0.3 mcg/ml within 5 minutes (24). The rich internal vertebral venous plexus forming four extensive, longitudinal channels in the posterior and anterolateral locations constitutes the ground for rapid absorption from the epidural space. These are thin walled veins without valves. Therefore, the epidural drugs are exposed to a large vascular surface (23).

A large proportion of patients who undergo anesthesia and surgery suffer from nausea and vomiting afterwards. This may be peripheral or central in origin, vomiting may arise either from stimulation of the chemoreceptor trigger zone (CTZ) or by activation of labyrinthine reflexes. Anti-emetic drugs are known to act centrally either at the CTZ by antagonism of dopamine receptors or at the vomiting center by antagonism of muscarinic cholinoceptors or histamine receptors, or both (25). The CTZ is situated in the area postrema near the base of the 4th ventricle and, although it is found within the brain, it is not protected by the blood-brain barrier. The capillary endothelial cells are not bound tightly and therefore, they allow for relatively free passage of large and small molecules into this area. This is an important afferent limb of the vomiting reflex and when this area is stimulated by toxins or drugs in the blood or CSF, vomiting often occurs as a result. Many antiemetics are known to act at this site (26).

In the CTZ, dopaminergic fibres are found, and the stimulation of this area causes nausea and vomiting. Dopaminergic and sympathomimetic receptors have been identified in the coronary, renal, cerebral and mesenteric vessels. Dopamine receptors are also found on the presynaptic membrane of postganglionic sympathetic nerves (27). Dopamine is not only the immediate metabolic precursor of norepinephrine and epinephrine, but also a central neurotransmitter and has important intrinsic pharmacological properties. While specific dopaminergic receptors are found in the central nervous system, injected dopamine does not readily cross the blood-brain barrier and therefore, it usually has no central effects (28). In our case where dopamine was administered through epidural catheter, thus, dopamine had an influence on CTZ not through blood but through CSF, and caused the patient to vomit.

Dopamine stimulates both α- and β-adrenoceptors as well as specific dopamine receptors in renal and mesenteric arteries. In low dosage (2-5 mcg/kg/min), dopamine reduces regional arterial resistance in renal and mesenteric vascular beds by an action on specific dopamine receptors. Besides, dopamine receptors are found in basal ganglia, the substantia nigra, corpus striatum and the limbic system. In basal ganglia, dopamine is antagonistic to acetylcholine. Dopaminergic system connects the limbic cortex, basal ganglia and hypothalamus and it is known to be concerned with behaviour (27).

In cases of overdose, adverse effects are generally attributable to excessive sympathomimetic activity. Nausea, vomiting, tachycardia, anginal pain, arrhythmias, headache, hypertension, and vasoconstriction are among effects that may be encountered during infusion of dopamine. These effects usually disappear quickly when the infusion is slowed or discontinued as the drug has an extremely short half-life in plasma (28). In our case also, symptoms such as abdominal pain, dizziness, tachycardia, hypertension and vomiting disappeared once dopamine administered through epidural was discontinued.

In a previous study, Jensen et al (29) collected related recommendations using reports of drug errors. In that study, one general and five specific strong recommendations were discussed: in order to decrease the number of drug administration errors in anesthesia, systematic countermeasures should be used; prior to the injection of a drug, the label on the drug ampoule or syringe should be read carefully; the legibility and contents of labels on ampoules and syringes should be optimized according to agreed standards; syringes should (almost) always be labeled as convenient; drug drawers and workspaces should be organized formally; before a drug is drawn up or administered, its label should be double-checked with a second person or a device.

According to Abeysekara et al (18), the reasons for drug errors in anesthetic practices include inattention, haste, drug labeling error, communication failure and fatigue. They reported that in order to minimize such events, prior experience and training, rechecking equipment and monitors capable of detecting the incident were necessary.

It is reported that with respect to epidural management, in order to detect the early signs of permanent neurological damage such as epidural hematoma or abscess and immediate life-threatening events such as respiratory and cardiovascular depression, protocols should be strictly followed by trained nurses who should also take records on an hourly basis (11). Consequently, in order to prevent inadvertent injection of drugs, nameplates or labels should be found on syringes for both test doses and drugs, and doctors and nurses should double-check before the administration of drugs (10).

4. Conclusion

The area where a thoracic epidural catheter is placed has a distinctive property as it is close to heart innervation. For this reason, injection of any drug through thoracic epidural bears great importance. The drug injected through epidural directly affects the plexus in that region. If thoracic region is in question, the drug injected through epidural directly affects the sympathetic nerves innervating the heart. The drug then passes on to CSF affecting the spinal cord, and the administered drug then enters the systematic cycle and thus shows its effects.

We believe that drugs given through epidural, specifically thoracic epidural, should be used very carefully, and the name of the drug should be written on the syringe carefully. In order to prevent inadvertent administration of drugs through epidural, as the case is for all catheters used, the epidural catheter should also bear its name clearly.

5. References

[1] Waurick R, Van Aken H. Update in thoracic epidural anaesthesia. Best Pract Res Clin Anaesthesiol 2005; 19: 201-13.
[2] Hew CM, Cyna AM, Simmons SW. Avoiding inadvertent epidural injection of drugs intended for non-epidural use. Anaesth Intensive Care. 2003; 31: 44-9.
[3] Xu X, She S, Yao S, Mok M, Zuo Z. Respiratory depression and difficult ventilation after inadvertent epidural administration of remifentanil (letter). Anesth Analg 2007; 104: 1004.
[4] Tessler MJ, White I, Naugler-Colville M, Biehl DR. Inadvertent epidural administration of potassium chloride. A case report. Can J Anaesth 1988; 35: 631-3.
[5] Kal JL, Vlassak EEW, Bulder ER, Franssen EJF. Inadvertent epidural administration of insulin. Anaesthesia 2007; 62: 621-3.
[6] Kostopanagiotou G, Mylona M, Massoura L, Siafaka I. Accidental epidural injection of vecuronium. Anesth Analg 2000; 91: 1550-1.
[7] Sanchez-Bailen MJ, Roca P, Benlloch R. Accidental administration of atracurium through an epidural catheter. Rev Esp Anestesiol Reanim 2006; 53: 455-6.
[8] Vassilakos D, Tsakiliotis S, Veroniki F, Zachariadou C, Giala M. Inadvertent epidural administration of cisatracurium. Eur J Anaesthesiol 2004; 21: 671-2.

[9] Cesur M, Alici HA, Erdem AF, Boga I. Accidental caudal injection of rocuronium in an awake patients. Anesthesiology 2005; 103: 444-5.

[10] Shin SW, Yoon JU, Baik SW, Lee HJ, Ri HS. Accidental epidural injection of rocuronium. J Anesth 2011; 25:753-5.

[11] McLeod GA, Cumming C. Thoracic epidural anaesthesia and analgesia 2004. Continuing Education in Anaesthesia, Critical Care and Pain 2004; 4: 16-9.

[12] Liu SS, Block BM, Wu CL. Effects of perioperative central neuraxial analgesia on outcome after coronary artery bypass surgery: a meta-analysis. Anesthesiology 2004; 101:153-61.

[13] Gramling-Babb PM, Zile MR, Reeves ST. Preliminary report on high thoracic epidural analgesia: Relationship between its therapeutic effects and myocardial blood flow as assessed by stress thallium distribution. J Cardiothorac Vasc Anesth 2000; 14: 657–61.

[14] Meissner A, Rolf N, Van Aken H: Thoracic epidural anesthesia and the patient with heart disease: Benefits, risks, and controversies. Anesth Analg 1997; 85: 517–28.

[15] Fischer RL, Lubenow TR, Liceaga A, McCarthy RJ, Ivankovich AD. Comparison of continuous epidural infusion of fentanyl-bupivacaine and morphine-bupivacaine in management of postoperative pain. Anesth Analg 1988; 67: 559-63.

[16] Chestnut DH, Owen CL, Bates JN , Ostman LG, Choi WW, Geiger MW. Continuous infusion epidural analgesia during labor: A randomized double-blind comparison of 0.0625% bupivacaine/0.0002% fentanyl versus 0.125% bupivacaine. Anesthesiology 1988; 68: 754-9.

[17] Förster JG, Rosenberg PH. Clinically useful adjuvants in regional anaesthesia. Curr Opin Anaesthesiol 2003; 16: 477-86.

[18] Abeysekera A, Bergman IJ, Kluger MT, Short TG. Drug error in anaesthetic practice: a review of 896 reports from the Australian Incident Monitoring Study database. Anaesthesia. 2005; 60: 220-7.

[19] Jeffery ND, Blakemore WF. Spinal cord injury in small animals 2. Current and future options for therapy. Vet Rec 1999; 145: 183-90.

[20] Braughler JM, Hall ED. Correlation of methylprednisolone levels in cat spinal cord with its effects on (Na+ + K+)-ATPase, lipid peroxidation, and alpha motor neuron function. J Neurosurg 1982; 56: 838-44

[21] Tator CH, Fehlings MG. Review of the secondary injury theory of acute spinal cord trauma with emphasis on vascular mechanisms. J Neurosurg 1991; 75: 15-26.

[22] O'Kell AL, Ambros B. Accidental epidural injection of thiopental in a dog. Can Vet J 2010; 51: 305-7.

[23] Colins VJ. Epidural Anesthesia. In: Principles of Anesthesiology General and Regional Anesthesia. Vincent J. Collins (Ed), 3rd edi. Lea and Febiger, Philadelphia, 1993; pp. 1571-610.

[24] Giasi RM, D'Agostino E, Covino BG. Absorption of lidocaine following subarachnoid and epidural administration. Anesth Analg 1979; 58: 360-3.

[25] Churchill-Davidson HC. Psychotropic Agents and Anti-Emetics. In: A Practice of Anaesthesia. HC Churchill-Davidson (Ed.), 5th edi. Lloyd-Luke (Medical Books) Ltd, London, 1984; pp. 649-59.

[26] Fukuda K. Intravenous Opioid Anesthetics. In: Anesthesia. Ronald D. Miller (Ed.), 6th edi. Elsevier Churchill Livingstone, Philadelphia, 2005; pp. 379-438.

[27] Aitkenhead AR, Smith G. Drugs Affecting The Autonomic Nervous System. In: Textbook of Anaesthesia. Alan R. Aitkenhead, Graham Smith (Eds.), 3rd edi. Churchill Livingstone, Bell and Bain Ltd, Glasgow, 1996; pp.195-210.
[28] Hoffman BB, Lefkowitz RJ. Catecholamines and Sympathomimetic Drugs. In: Goodman and Gilman's The Pharmacological Basis of Therapeutics. Alfred Goodman Gilman, Theodore W. Rall, Alan S. Nies, Palmer Taylor (Edits.), 8th edi, Pergamon Press, Inc 1990; pp. 187-220.
[29] Jensen LS, Merry AF, Webster CS, Weller J, Larsson L. Evidence-based strategies for preventing drug administration errors during anaesthesia. Anaesthesia 2004; 59: 493-504.

13

Aluminium – Non-Essential Activator of Pepsin: Kinetics and Thermodynamics

Vesna Pavelkic[1], Tanja Brdaric[1] and Kristina Gopcevic[2]
[1]*Institute "Kirilo Savic" Belgrade*
[2]*University of Belgrade, School of Medicine*
Serbia

1. Introduction

The stability of proteins and their interactions with other molecules, especially with toxic ones, is a topic of special interest in biochemistry because many cellular processes depend on that. These interactions have immediate consequences for protein stability, as shown by varying the thermodynamic properties of the system. This fact provides an extra variable to study protein unfolding linked to ligand binding (Lumry et al. 1966, Crothers 1971, Schellman 1975, McGhee 1976).

Porcine pepsin A (EC 3.4.23.1), belongs to the aspartic protease family and plays an integral role in the digestion process of vertebrates. As all aspartic proteases pepsin molecule consist of two homologous lobes composed predominantly of β-sheets separated by a hinged substrate-binding cleft. Two active site aspartic residues, Asp32 and Asp215, occupy the cleft to which admittance is restricted by a hinged flexible flap region (Andreeva et al. 1984, Baldwin et al. 1993, Blundell et al. 1990). One of two Asp residues has to be protonated and the other deprotonated, for the protein to be active (Lumry et al. 1966). Due to the catalytic residues, the active pH ranges from 1.0 to 5.0 (Blundell et al. 1990, Sielecki et al. 1990, Brandts & Lin 1990, Shrake & Ross 1992, Celey et al. 2005).

Pepsin undergoes a conformational transition from the native to the denatured state in a narrow pH range. Refolding of an immobilized form of the denatured pepsin was achieved without the prosequence (Kurimoto et al. 2001), but its refolding mechanism is still unsolved. Thermal denaturation of proteins is being studied intensively today. Investigation of denaturation may help to elucidate mechanisms of the reverse process, i.e. protein folding. Complex structures such as proteins, that undergo transitions originated from conformational changes, are suitable to be studied by Differential Scanning Calorimetry (DSC). DSC is primarily used to characterize stability and folding, and to study binding interactions between proteins and small molecules, drugs, and other proteins (Powers et al. 1977). The consequences of protein interactions with other molecules on interactions on protein stability were shown through varying the thermodynamic properties of the system. This fact provides an extra variable to study protein unfolding linked to ligand binding. Various approaches that describe macromolecular unfolding coupled to ligand binding were reported by several authors many years ago (Lumry et al. 1966, Crothers 1971, Schellman 1975, McGhee 1976). More recently, with the application of theory, DSC has been proved to be a very useful tool to estimate very tight binding constants (Brandts & Lin 1990, Shrake & Ross 1992,) as well as to characterize the energetic of binding and unfolding (Celey et al. 2005, Celey et al. 2006).

DSC is used to measure the binding constants from temperature melting points (T_m) shifts small molecule binding to a protein. The binding constant of the ligand can be estimated from the T_m in the presence and absence of ligand, as long as the concentration of ligand in the DSC cell is known. Binding of a ligand to a protein occurs only if there is a release of free energy. Accordingly, the protein–ligand complex is more stable than the free partners are. The extent of stabilization depends upon the magnitude of the binding energy. Comparison of stability of the complex with that of the free partners allows estimation of binding energy.

Through calorimetric studies, Privalov showed that thermal denaturation of porcine pepsin is a complex process that proceeds by two distinct stages occurring at different temperatures. Because pepsin has been well structurally characterized, it represents an appropriate model to study the effects of metal ions on structure, function and kinetic behaviour (Privalov et al. 1981).

Trivalent aluminium ion, Al^{3+}, is a typical metal ion that exist as a hydrated $A1(H_20)_6{}^{3+}$ in acid pH solutions. Acid digestion in the stomach would solubilise most of the ingested aluminium compounds to the monomolecular species Al^{3+} (e.g. hydrated $Al(H_20)_6{}^{3+}$). After absorption, aluminium distributes unequally to all tissues in humans and accumulates in some. About one-half of the total body burdens of aluminium are in the skeleton and about one fourth is in the lungs (from accumulation of inhaled insoluble aluminium compounds). Aluminium has also been found in most soft tissue organs and its levels have been found to increase with ageing of experimental animals. Aluminium compounds have a wide variety of uses, including production of pharmaceuticals and food additives. A variety of complexes may be formed with the ligands present in biological systems and/or in foods.

The complexes between ligands and aluminium have different physicochemical properties, such as solubility in aqueous medium, stability at different pH, electric charge etc. This can greatly influence the toxicokinetic and toxicodynamic profile of aluminium. Although aluminium is toxic to humans, animals and plants, its biochemistry has been little studied and is poorly understood (Gomez et al.1994, Kerr & Ward 1988.). Because of the lack of quantitative information, it is not easy to assess the biological relevance and possible biological role of such interactions.

The Al^{3+} interacts with a large number of proteins, glycoproteins and carbohydrates, but very little is known about the chemistry, binding strength and binding mode of these complexes. The most likely binding sites of $A1(H_20)_6{}^{3+}$ in bio systems are oxygen donors, and especially negatively charged oxygen donors. Carboxylate, phenolate, catecholate and phosphate are the strongest Al^{3+} binders. Biomolecules containing such functions may be involved in the uptake and transport processes of Al^{3+} (Scientific Opinion of the Panel on Food Additives, Flavourings, Processing Aids and Food Contact Materials on a request from European Commission on Safety of aluminium from dietary intake, 2008).

Recently it has been shown that Al^{3+} ions increase pepsin activity (Krejpcio & Wojciak 2002).

Gel electrophoresis is a broad subject encompassing many different techniques and can provide information about the molecular weights and charges of proteins, the subunit structures of proteins and a purity of a particular protein preparation. It is relatively simple to use and it is highly reproducible. The most common use of gel electrophoresis is the qualitative analysis of complex mixtures of proteins. Microanalytical methods are sensitive, linear image analysis system make gel electrophoresis useful for quantitative and preparative purposes as well. The technique provides the highest resolution of all methods available for separating proteins. Polypeptides differing in molecular weights by as little as a few hundreds of Daltons and proteins differing less than 0.1 pH unit in their isoelectric points are routinely resolved in gels.

Sodium dodecyl sulphate-polyacrylamide gel electrophoresis (SDS-PAGE) is the most commonly practiced polyacrilamide gel electrophoresis technique used for proteins. The method provides an easy way to estimate the number of polypeptides in a sample and thus assess the complexity of the sample or the purity of a preparation. SDS-PAGE is particularly useful for monitoring the fractions obtained during chromatographic or other purification procedures. One of the more important features of SDS-PAGE is that it is a simple, reliable method with which is easy to estimate the molecular weights of proteins. SDS-PAGE requires that proteins be denatured to their constituted polypeptide chains, so that it is limited in the information it can provide. In those situations where it is desirable to maintain biological activity, non-denaturing systems must be employed. However, the gel patterns from non-denaturing gels are more difficult to interpret than are those from SDS-PAGE. Non-denaturing systems also give information about the charge isomers of proteins.

The subject of electrophoresis deals with the controlled motion of charged particles in electrical fields. Since proteins are charged molecules, they migrate under the influence of electrical fields. From the point of view of electrophoresis, the two most important physical properties of proteins are their electrophoretic mobility and charge and its isoelectric points. The electrophoretic mobility depends on its charge, size, and shape, and it is very different in gels than in free solution. Pepsin has been studied by electrophoresis since its isolation from different sources (Herriot 1940, Porcellii, 1968, Cunningham 1970, Cann 1962, Varilova 2005).

In our previous studies, the in vitro influence of different concentrations of Al^{3+} ions, physiological and toxic ones, on pepsin activity was investigated. Kinetic studies were undertaken to determine the nature of the enzyme modulation (type and mechanism) by investigated metal ion. The mechanism of Al^{3+} ions on pepsin activity evaluated from kinetic studies and was classified as a case of non-essential activation with partial non-competitive character (Pavelkic et al. 2008). With the application of theory, DSC method has been used as a tool to estimate binding constants (Pavelkic et al. 2011) as well as to characterize the energetic of binding and unfolding.

The present paper summarizes the current knowledge of activating and stabilizing effect of Al^{3+} ions on gastrointestinal fluids, especially on main gastrointestinal enzyme - pepsin. Therefore, there is a lack of information about thermal stability of pepsin in a presence of Al^{3+} ions. As the binding mechanism of Al^{3+} ions on pepsin is not still clear the objective of this study is to investigate the *in vitro* conditions the influence of different concentrations of

Al^{3+} ions, physiological and toxic ones, on pepsin conformational stability during the process of thermal unfolding, with a purpose of better understanding of pepsin/aluminium interaction.

2. The effect of activator on the reaction rate and kinetic parameters – Theory

The mode of activation, essential or non-essential, depends on the values of the equilibrium constants, the rate constants of the limiting velocity steps and substrate concentration. Reversible enzyme activation implies the binding of the enzyme to the activator (A) which affects the rate of an enzyme-catalyzed reaction. A simple scheme to describe the interactions between an enzyme (E), a substrate (S) and the activator (A) is presented below.

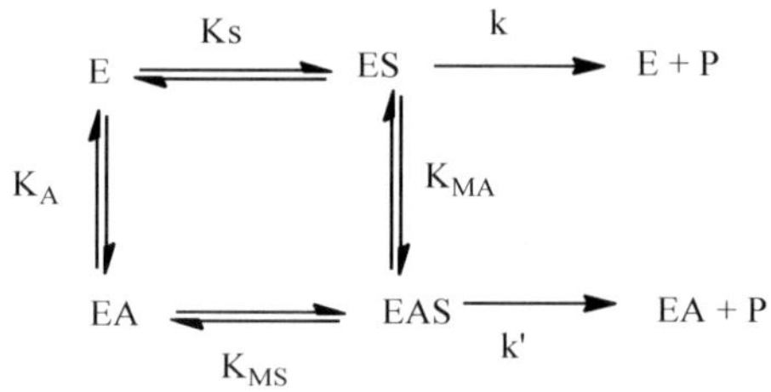

Fig. 1. Reaction scheme representing the mechanism of the enzyme catalyzed reaction and interactions of the enzyme (E) with activator (A) and the substrate (S).

In this model, a molecule of enzyme (E) can bind one molecule of substrate (S) and/or one molecule of activator (A). Equilibrium constants for the dissociation reactions ES ↔ E + S, EAS ↔ EA + S, EA ↔ E + A and EAS ↔ ES + A, are K_S, K_{MS}, K_A and K_{MA} respectively. The rate constants k and k′ are the rate constants for reactions ES → E + P (product) and EAS → EA + P respectively. The reaction scheme is based on the assumption that equilibrium between enzyme, substrate and activator, and their complexes is set up almost immediately and during the time required to measure initial velocity. Also, the higher concentrations of S and A than total enzyme concentration, as well as the velocities of product formation from the enzyme-substrate and enzyme-activator-substrate complexes as a velocity limiting steps in transformation S → P, were assumed. The rate constants k and k′ are related to the parameters V_1 and V_2 through following equations:

$$V_1 = k[E_t] \tag{1}$$

$$V_1 = k'[E_t] \tag{2}$$

Where $[E_t]$ is the total enzyme concentration: $[E_t] = [E] + [ES] + [EA] + [EAS]$.

The equilibrium constants K_S, K_{MS}, K_A and K_{MA} for the dissociation reaction mentioned above are respectively:

$$K_S = \frac{[E][S]}{[ES]} \tag{3}$$

$$K_{MS} = \frac{[EA][S]}{[EAS]} \tag{4}$$

$$K_A = \frac{[E][A]}{[EA]} \tag{5}$$

$$K_{MA} = \frac{[ES][A]}{[EAS]} \tag{6}$$

These equilibrium constants are related by the equation:

$$K_S \cdot K_A = K_{MS} \cdot K_{MA} \tag{7}$$

If activator is not present in the reaction solution, the enzyme follows typical Michaelis-Menten kinetics, with apparent values of V_{max} and K_M (V_1 and K_S in the reaction scheme represented in Figure 1, respectively). When activator is present in saturating concentrations, Michaelis kinetics is still obeyed, but with V_{max} and K_M equal to V_2 and K_{MS}. The analysis of such of system (Figure 1), assuming that equilibrium conditions applied to substrate binding, give the following possibilities: partially competitive activation if k = k', partially non-competitive activation if $K_S = K_{MS}$, $K_A = K_{MA}$ and k< k', or partially mixed case if $K_S \neq K_{MS}$, $K_A \neq K_{MA}$ and k< k' (Dixon 1979, Fontes 2000).

Assuming that equilibrium conditions apply, for the above system (Figure 1) the equation that can be derived takes the form:

$$v = \frac{V_{\max}\frac{[S]}{K_S} + V_{\max}\frac{[A][S]}{K_A K_S}}{1 + \frac{[S]}{K_S} + \frac{[A]}{K_A} + \frac{[A][S]}{K_{MA}K_{MS}}} \tag{8}$$

Or

$$v = \frac{V_{\max}[S]}{K_S \frac{\left(1 + \frac{[A]}{K_{MA}}\right)}{\left(1 + \frac{k'}{k}\frac{[A]}{K_{MA}}\right)} + [S]\frac{\left(1 + \frac{[A]}{K_{MA}}\right)}{\left(1 + \frac{k'}{k}\frac{[A]}{K_{MA}}\right)}} \tag{9}$$

When activator is not present in the system, i.e. [A]=0 M, the above equation attain the form of well known Michaelis-Menten equation. If the activator is present in the system at any concentration, the reaction rate is defined as apparent so the maximal velocity and dissociation constants too:

$$v_{app} = \frac{V_{\max}\frac{\left(1+\frac{k'}{k}\frac{[A]}{K_{MA}}\right)}{\left(1+\frac{[A]}{K_{MA}}\right)}[S]}{K_S\frac{\left(1+\frac{[A]}{K_{MA}}\right)}{\left(1+\frac{k'}{k}\frac{[A]}{K_{MA}}\right)}+[S]} \tag{10}$$

And

$$V_{\max app} = V_{\max}\frac{\left(1+\frac{k'}{k}\frac{[A]}{K_{MA}}\right)}{\left(1+\frac{[A]}{k \cdot K_{MA}}\right)} \tag{11}$$

$$K_{Sapp} = K_S\frac{\left(1+\frac{[A]}{K_{MA}}\right)}{\left(1+\frac{[A]}{k \cdot K_{MA}}\right)} \tag{12}$$

Consequently double reciprocal plots (Lineweaver-Burk) of 1/V = f (1/[S]), will be linear when [A] varied. Secondary plots of the slopes and intercepts of the plots of 1/v =f (1/[S]) against [A] will be hyperbolic.

The linearization of that can be exceeded via plotting double reciprocal plots of the change in slope or intercept (Δ_{slope} or $\Delta_{intercept}$ must be determined by subtracting the values in the presence of activator from that in its absence) will be linear. These give a possibility for easy graphical evaluation of important kinetic constants.

3. The effect of activator on the thermal stability of protein – Theory

Treatment of non-two-state transitions includes both calorimetric and van't Hoff heat changes. Indicating the temperature-dependent parameters heat capacity function can be expressed by the equation:

$$C_p(T) = \left[\frac{K_A(T)\Delta \cdot H_{mA}^{VH}\Delta H_{mA}}{\left(1+K_A(T)\right)^2 RT^2}\right] + \cdots \tag{13}$$

In this case, the equilibrium constant will be:

$$K_A(T) = \exp\left[\frac{-\Delta H_{mA}^{VH}}{RT\left(\frac{1-T}{T_{mA}}\right)}\right] \tag{14}$$

where ΔH_{mA}^{VH} is a van`t Hoff enthalpy for the transition with characteristic T_{mA} .

In order to define the stability of a protein consisting of several structural subunits and assuming that interaction between the units are negligible we estimate the Gibb's energy for a unit from experimental data using the following equation:

$$\Delta G(T) = \Delta H_{mA}^{VH}\left(\frac{1-T}{T_{MA}}\right) \tag{15}$$

To obtain detailed information about thermodynamic properties of pepsin in a strong acid media, DSC profiles were analyzed within the framework of "Non-2-State, with zero ΔC_p model" (that use the Leveberg-Marquardt non-linear least-square method). Non-2-State model involved the next parameters: T_m, H^{cal}, and H^{VH}. The model is applied to transitions with no ΔC_p effects. Before curve fitting, a baseline was subtracted from the experimental data to remove ΔC_p effects and sets C_p to zero at all temperatures (ΔC_p given in Table are evaluated before curve fitting).

The DSC protein stability data contain information on related aspects of protein structure and interactions, and may be used to estimate metal binding affinities in metalloprotein complex.

To estimate the magnitude of Al^{3+} binding affinity to pepsin, we used an expression for equilibrium binding affinity (Brandts et al. 1989, Brandts et al. 1990, Lin et al. 1993) derived from the theory of coupled equilibrium,

$$K_{Al^{3+}}(T_{Al}) = \frac{\exp\left[\frac{-\Delta H_0^{VH}}{R}\left(\frac{1}{T_{Al}} - \frac{1}{T_0}\right) + \frac{\Delta C_p}{R}\left(\ln\frac{T_{Al}}{T_0} + \frac{T_0}{T_{Al}} - 1\right)\right]}{\left[Al^{3+}\right]_{T_{Al}}} \tag{16}$$

Where $K_{Al^{3+}}(T_{Al})$ is the equilibrium binding affinity for formation of the pepsin – Al^{3+} complex at the transition temperature for unfolding Al^{3+}-pepsin, ΔH_0^{VH} is the transition enthalpy for pepsin unfolding, T_0 is the transition temperature for pepsin unfolding, T_{Al} is the transition temperature for pepsin – Al^{3+} complex, and $\left[Al^{3+}\right]_{T_{Al}}$ is the concentration of free metal ion at T_{Al} .

From the shift in T_m, the changes in the apparent stability of the particular units of protein treated with activator (aluminium treated pepsin in investigated model system) relative to the native form $\Delta(\Delta G)$ was evaluated at the transition temperature as a difference between ΔG calculated for native and activator treated protein (Lin et al. 1993, Brewer et al. 2001):

$$\Delta\left(\Delta G\right)=\Delta G_{(\text{activator treated protein})}-\Delta G^{0}_{(\text{native protein})} \qquad (17)$$

Estimation of the average number of ligands bound to the native protein $\overline{X}_N$ can be accomplished in a term of total Gibbs energy of unfolding that is defined by the difference between the Gibbs energies of the denatured and native state, with the assumption that no ligand - binding occurs in the unfolded state (Brewer & Wampler 2001).

Starting from relation

$$\left(\frac{\partial \Delta G^{0}_{tot}}{\partial \ln[A]}\right)_T = RT\left(\frac{\partial \ln(Q-K_0)}{\partial \ln[A]}\right)_T = RT\overline{X_N} \qquad (18)$$

Where,

ΔG^{0}_{tot} is a total Gibbs energy,

Q - partition function of all residual native states which include native ligand free and native ligand bounded protein molecules,

K_0 - the equilibrium constant of unfolding, and

$\overline{X}_N$ - an average number of ligands bound to the native protein,

the average numbers of ligands bound to the native protein could be graphically determined from the slope of G^{0}_{tot} *versus* $\ln[A]$.

Indirect determination of the enthalpy of unfolding assumes the knowledge of the equilibrium as a function of temperature. Starting from spectroscopic data spectroscopic signal for 100% denaturated (random coil) sample and 100% native protein was determined. The temperature range where protein transitions from native to denatured form was covered. Fraction of native protein as a function of temperature and the fraction of unfolded protein as a function of temperature f_N and f_D respectively, were defined in terms of measured absorbance $A(T)$ as:

$$f_D = \frac{A(T)-A_N(T)}{A_D(T)-A_N(T)} \text{ and } f_N = 1-f_D \qquad (19)$$

N and D refer to the native and unfolded state respectively.

Determined fraction of native and unfolded protein could be used for further determination of enthalpy of unfolding using the relation:

$$\ln\left(K_{eq}\right)=\left(\frac{-\Delta H^{VH}_{unf}}{RT}\right)+\frac{\Delta S}{R} \qquad (20)$$

Previous equation give possibility for simple graphical determination equilibrium constant. The plot ln (K_{eq}) *vs.* *1/T* describes a straight line with slope equal to $\Delta H^{VH}_{unf} / R$.

The application of gel electrophoresis to the measurement of dissociation constants of protein-ligand complexes has been studied previously (Yen HC et al. 1993). The dissociation constant in the gel (K_d^{gel}) is defined by following equations:

$$K_d = \frac{[P][L]}{[PL]} \tag{21}$$

$$R_S = \frac{r}{R_0} = \frac{[P]}{[P]+[PL]} \tag{22}$$

$$\frac{1}{R_f} = 1 + \frac{[L]}{K_d} \tag{23}$$

$$[L]R_f = K_d - K_d R_f \tag{24}$$

Where $[L]$ is ligand concentration, $[P]$ is concentration of sample protein, R_0 and r protein electrophoretic mobility in the absence and the presence of ligand. Obtained dissociation constant K_d is apparent dissociation constant in gel, and may be different from dissociation constant in solution.

4. Materials and methods

Pepsin, lyophilized powder, was purchased from Sigma–Aldrich, and used without further purification. Hemoglobin from bovine blood was purchased from Sigma–Aldrich and was used as substrate. PAGE-reagents were purchased fromSigma–Aldrich. Other chemicals aluminum chloride ($AlCl_3 \cdot 6H_2O$), hydrochloric (HCl), trichloroacetic acid (TCA) were obtained from MERCK. All used chemicals are of reagent grade and were prepared prior to use.

4.1 Enzyme assay

The Worthington method based on enzyme-catalyzed measured rate of hydrolysis of denatured hemoglobin (Hb) substrate was used for evaluation of enzyme activity in the absence (control) and presence of Al^{3+} ions (Anson 1938). Pepsin activity was determined in an incubation medium containing 1mL of pepsin solution (20 mg/mL in 0.01M HCl, pH2) and 5 mL of haemoglobin solution (2% solution of hemoglobin in 0.01M HCl). The working solutions were incubated for 10 min at 37°C. The reaction was stopped by addition of 10 mL 5% TCA. The absorbance of clear filtrates recorded at 280 nm, and activities were calculated by the equation:

$$U_{units/mg} = \frac{\left(A_{280nm(filtrate)} - A_{280nm(blank)}\right)\cdot 1000}{10\,\text{min}\cdot mg_{\text{enzyme in reaction mixture}}} \tag{25}$$

Kinetic analysis was carried out by following the initial velocity of the enzymatic reaction in the absence and presence of Al^{3+} in concentration range from $1.7 \cdot 10^{-6}$ to $8.7 \cdot 10^{-3}$ M, and increasing concentrations of hemoglobin from $2.5 \cdot 10^{-2}$ to $4 \cdot 10^{-3}$ M. All the assays were performed at pH 2. The data analyzed by the software package Origin 6.1 and the results were recalculated using EZ FIT program (Perrela 1988).

4.2 Native PAGE electrophoresis

Native electrophoresis of pepsin and hemoglobin on 10% polyacrylamide gel carried out at 48 °C during 90 min, according to the Laemmli procedure, at pH 8.3 (Laemly 1970). Water solutions of all samples of enzyme (pepsin dissolved in water to final concentration of 2 mg/mL) were titrated with HCl to pH 2 and incubated at 37 °C , with addition of different concentrations of Al^{3+} ion (1, 5 and 10 mM). The samples were diluted with sample buffer in ratio 1:1 (v/v) and applied on gel in volume of 20 μL. Visualization was performed with Commassie Brilliant Blue G-250 dye. The gels scanned and processed using Corel Draw 11.0 software package. Quantification of electrophoretic mobility of the molecule is carried out via R_S value, where it is defined by:

$$R_S = \frac{\text{Distance of protein migration}}{\text{Distance of tracing dye migration}} \tag{26}$$

4.3 Differential scanning calorimetry

DSC measurements were carried out on a MicroCall "MC-2" Differential Scanning Calorimeter (MicroCall Inc., Northampton, MA) with cell volumes 1.14 mL, at heating rates 1.5 °C/min. DSC scans were obtained in the temperature range from 10 to 100 °C. For all the measurements the protein concentrations were 0.03 mM, pH were set at 2. Degassing during the calorimetric measurements was prevented by additional constant pressure of 1 atm over the liquids in the cells. At first, the solvent was placed in both the sample and reference compartments. A DSC curve corresponding to solvent *vs.* solvent run was used as an instrumental baseline. The calorimetric data were corrected for the calorimetric baseline (by subtracting solvent – solvent scan). The data were converted to molar excess heat capacity by using the protein concentration (0.03 mM pepsin) and cell volume of 1.14 mL and than corrected for the difference in heat capacity between the initial and the final state by using linear baseline. The calorimetric reversibility of thermally induced transition was checked by reheating the protein solution in the calorimetric cell after cooling from the first run.

5. Results and discussion

5.1 The effect of Al^{3+} ions on the reaction rate and kinetic parameters of pepsin

The influence of Al^{3+} ions on porcine pepsin activity were examined in a wide range of Al^{3+} ions concentration included physiological and toxic ones, *in vitro* conditions, and at pH 2. All investigated concentration of Al^{3+} ions cause increase of pepsin activity. The increasing concentrations of metal ions induced increase of enzymatic activity. The observed effects are presented at Figure 2, and it is indicative that increase of pepsin activity follows in a dose dependent manner the concentrations of bounded aluminium. The obtained results are in agreement with previously reported (Krejpcio 2002) stimulatory effect of Al^{3+} ions on porcine pepsin activity. The authors reported that applying concentration of $1.1 \cdot 10^{-3}$ M Al^{3+} ions induce the activation of 191%, while we obtained 135.8% activation of pepsin activity, in applied concentration of Al^{3+} ions of $8.7 \cdot 10^{-3}$ M. The observed disagreements could be explained by differences in experimental conditions (different pH, enzyme/substrate ratio).

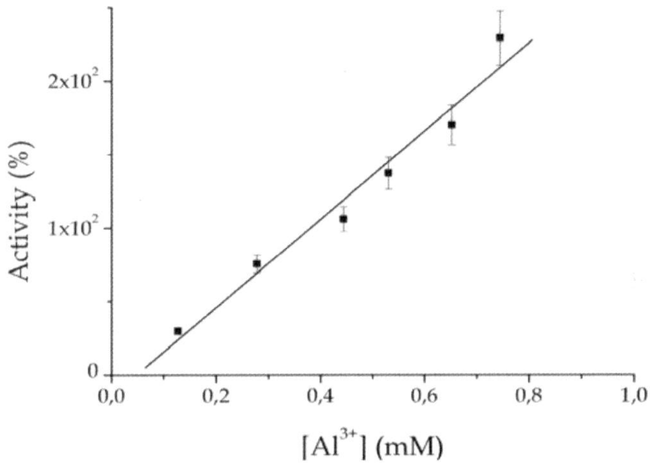

Fig. 2. The *in vitro* effects of Al^{3+} ions on pepsin activity; the effects were investigated in concentration range from $1.7 \cdot 10^{-6}$ to $8.7 \cdot 10^{-3}$ M of Al^{3+} ions. The increasing concentrations of Al^{3+} ions induced increase of enzymatic activity. Values are expressed as the percent of increased activity related to the control, which considered as 100%. Aluminum was found to stimulate the enzyme activity in dose-dependent manner. Investigated concentrations of Al^{3+} ions, induce the increase of pepsin activity from 30.7% to 135.8% ($p < 0.01$), in comparison with corresponding control. The degree of activation is expressed as % of increased activity considering the pepsin activity in the absence of aluminum as 100%. Data are expressed as a mean of at least three independent experiments performed in triplicate. Data from Pavelkic et al. (2008) are modified.

Initial reaction rates were determined by monitoring the change in absorbance at 280 nm due to formed reaction products in a Beckman UV 5260 UV-VIS spectrophotometer, in cells of path length 1cm, thermostatically controlled at 37 ± 0.1 °C. A typical kinetic experiment consisted of numerous steady – state rates at different combinations of substrate and activator concentrations was performed and presented at Figure 3.

The results obtained from Lineweaver-Burk plots, are used for calculation of kinetic constants. The secondary plots of the slopes and intersects *vs.* activator concentrations are not linear (data not shown), but the reciprocal of the change in slope and intercept (Δ_{slope} and $\Delta_{intercept}$) that are determined by subtracting the values in the presence of activator from that in its absence, are linear. The intercepts of a plot $1/\Delta_{slope}$ and $1/\Delta_{intercept}$ *vs.* $1/[Al^{3+}]$ on $1/\Delta$ axis, and intercepts of both plots on $1/[Al^{3+}]$ axis are used for calculating equilibrium constants K_{MS} and K_{MA} for dissociation of formed binary enzyme-activator (Al^{3+}) and ternary enzyme activator- substrate complexes (Figure 4). The calculated values for constants are (0.904 ± 0.083) mM and (8.56 ± 0.51) mM, respectively.

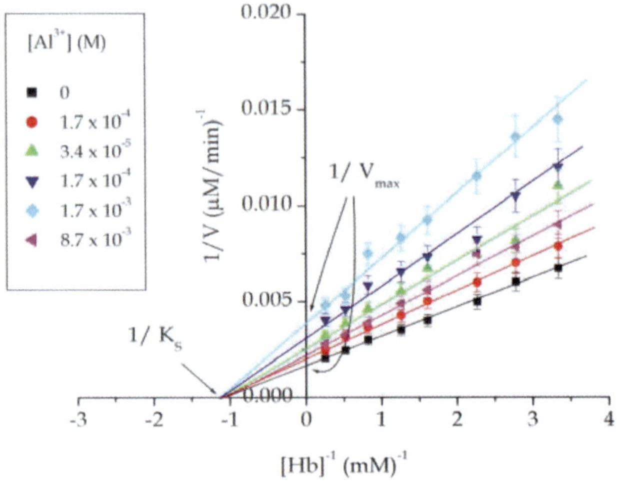

Fig. 3. Double reciprocal Lineweaver – Burk plot of influence of Al^{3+} ions on reaction kinetics of pepsin at pH2; Increase of reaction velocity in a presence of activator (inset: various concentration of Al^{3+} ions) is proportional to increased activator concentration. Increasing of aluminium concentrations increased V_{max} values, without significant change in the value of apparent enzyme affinity for substrate K_S. Graphically determined apparent enzyme affinity for substrate, K_S, in the presence of 1.7 μM activator is (0.907 ± 0.083) mM L^{-1}, while in the presence of maximal activator concentration (8.7 mM) K_S is (0.917 ± 0.073) mM L^{-1}. V_{max} is changed in a concentration depending manner. Without presence of activator maximal reaction rates changes from (254 ± 7) μM min^{-1}, to (599 ± 17) μM min^{-1} at maximal activator concentration. Data from Pavelkic et al. (2008) are modified.

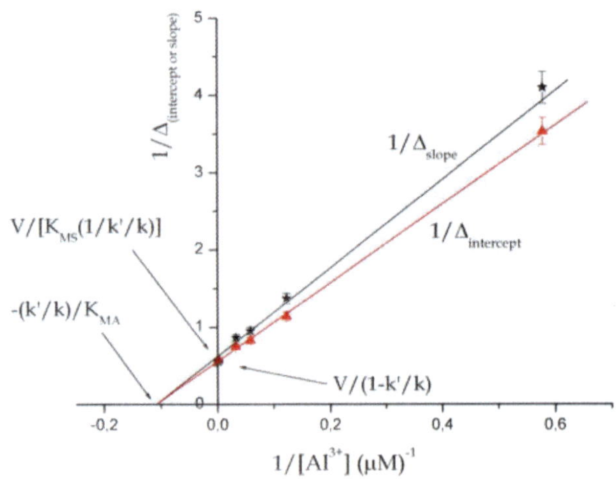

Fig. 4. The reciprocal of the change in slope and intercept (Δ_{slope} and $\Delta_{intercept}$) against reciprocal of activator concentration, where Δ is defined as slope or intercept in the absence of activator, Al^{3+} ions, minus that in its presence. Data from Pavelkic et al. (2008) are modified.

Simple geometrical considerations illustrated in Figure 5 show that kinetic data could be used for graphical determination of the activator concentration that gives a reaction rate equal to the half of saturation concentration of activator (A_{50}), as well as the dissociation constant K_A for enzyme-activator complex. If the abscissa variable is $1/[A]$, then the intercept is $- 1/ [A_{50}]$, where $[A_{50}]$ is activator concentration that gives a rate equal to the half that at a saturating concentration of activator.

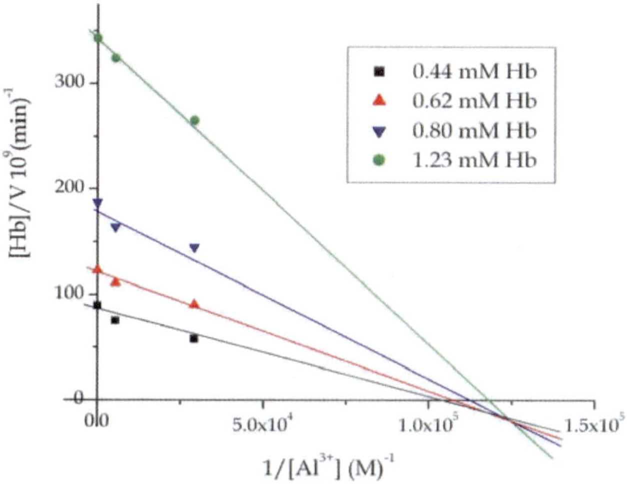

Fig. 5. Activation effects of different aluminium concentrations on pepsin. The intercepts on the abscissa of the plot [Hb]/V *vs.* reciprocal of aluminium concentrations represents the values of A_{50}. The obtained kinetic data were used for determination of dissociation constant K_A for pepsin-aluminium (EA) complex. The calculated values of A_{50} and K_A were (8.05 ± 0.48) μM and (8.82 ± 0.90) μM, respectively. Data from Pavelkic et al. (2008) are modified.

5.2 The influence of Al^{3+} ions on electrophoretic mobility of pepsin

Native PAGE profiles of untreated and aluminium treated pepsin solutions at pH 2 were studied to verify the conformational changes of pepsin induced by Al^{3+} ions that resulting in activation effect. Electrophoretic mobility in the presence of Al^{3+} ions (from 1 to 10 mM) inducing the highest activation (producing around the 100% activation or more upon the enzyme assay data) and in the absence of activator were compared. The electrophoregrams of pepsin samples in absence or in the presence of different concentrations of Al^{3+} ion are presented in Figure 6 and Figure 7, respectively.

The presence of Al^{3+} cause the decrease of pepsin electrophoretic mobility at all investigated concentrations. The degree of decrease is proportional to Al^{3+} concentrations, which the one has been exposed. In the absence of Al^{3+} ion, the electrophoretic mobility of pepsin under the physiological conditions the obtained Rs value for pepsin is 0.47 while in the presence of 1, 5 and 10 mM Al^{3+} ions the obtained Rs values were 0.46, 0.44 and 0.42, respectively.

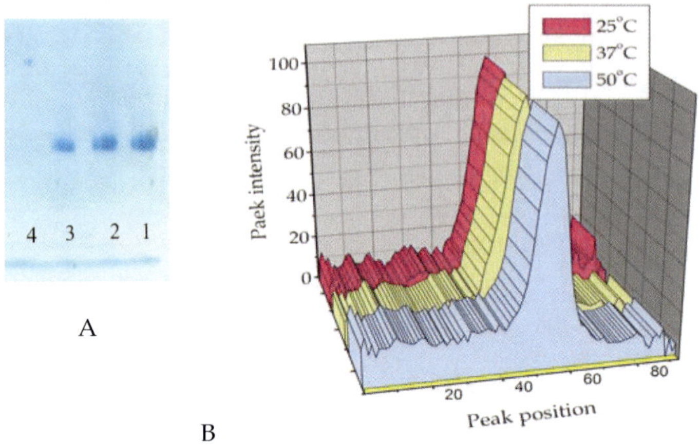

Fig. 6. A - Native PAGE electrophoregram of pepsin without Al^{3+} ions at pH 2. B – Visualization of quantified electrophoretic mobility of pepsin molecule treated at different temperatures.

Native PAGE electrophoresis of pepsin on 10% polyacrylamide gel carried out at 4°C during 90 min, according to the Laemmli procedure, at pH 8.3. Water solutions of all samples of enzyme (pepsin dissolved in water to final concentration of 2 mg/mL) were titrated with HCl to pH 2 and incubated at 25°C, 37°C, 50°C and 70°C (band 1 to 4 respectively). Visualization was performed with Commassie Brilliant Blue G-250 dye. B - The gels were scanned and processed using Corel Draw 11.0 software package.

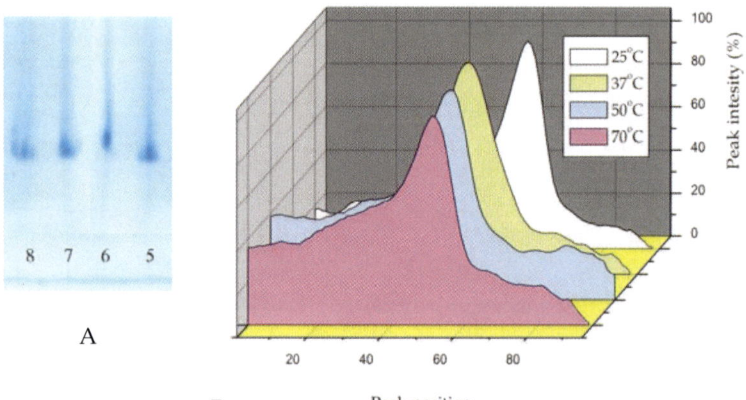

Fig. 7. A - Native PAGE electrophoregram of pepsin in a presence of 5 mM Al^{3+} ions at pH 2. B – Scanned and processed gel of pepsin samples with addition 5 mM Al^{3+}, previously incubated at 25°C, 37°C, 50°C and 70°C (band 5 to 8 respectively).

Quantification of electrophoretic mobility of the molecule is carried out via R_S value, where it is defined as:

R_S = distance of protein migration / distance of tracing dye migration.

In all cases increasing the temperature causes the decrease in electrophoretic mobility of pepsin. The cause of decrease in electrophoretic mobility can be explained by thermally induced conformational changes in pepsin molecule. The pepsin bend is absent in samples treated at 70°C, in the absence of Al^{+3} ion as well as in the presence of all investigated Al^{+3} concentrations, except 5 mM Al^{+3}. This result is in agreement with previously reported data that temperatures of 70°C and higher induce unfolding of an enzyme (Sepulveda et al. 1975). The degree of pepsin electrophoretic mobility decrease depends on Al^{3+} concentration that the one has been exposed. The difference between Rs values obtained at 25 °C and 50 °C in absence of Al^{3+} ion is 0.02, while in the presence of 10 mM Al^{3+} it is 0.05. If the influence of Al^{3+} ion concentration on pepsin mobility at defined temperature we discuss it could be seen that increase in concentration of Al^{3+} decelerate the migration of pepsin samples on concentration dependent manner. Rs values of pepsin at 37°C in the absence of Al^{3+} is 0.47, while Rs values are 0.46, 0.44 and 0,42 in the presence 1 mM, 5 mM and 10 mM of Al^{3+} respectively (data not shown). The same trend has been obtained for the other tested temperatures, except for 70°C. The slow down in pepsin migration can be explained by conformational changes caused by Al^{3+} binding to enzyme.

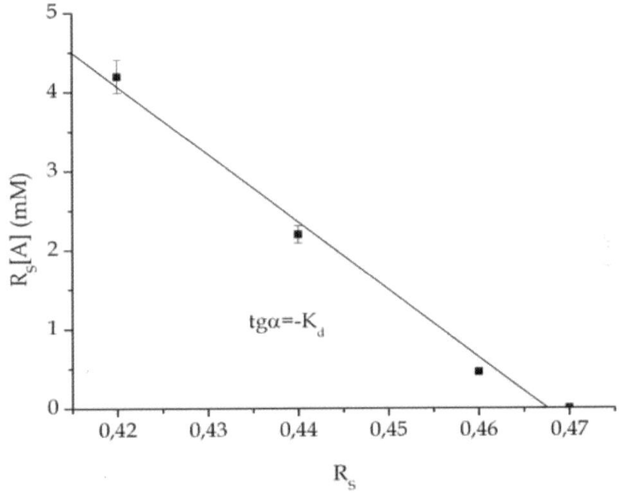

Fig. 8. Graphical determination of dissociation constant from obtained R_s values from electrophoregrams of pepsin in a presence different concentration of Al^{3+} ions. Calculated value of (0.856 ± 0.007) mM is in a good agreement with those determined via kinetic experiments.

5.3 Thermal stability of pepsin in a presence of Al^{3+} ions followed by differential scanning calorimetry

Calorimetric enthalpy for the complete transition was estimated from the total peak area, and also the enthalpy from the temperature dependence of the equilibrium according to the van't Hoff equation, as well as the enthalpy for the each stage of pepsin unfolding. The van't

Hoff enthalpy, ΔH^{VH}, was determined for each scan by subtracting the baseline to remove the heat capacity effect and then curve fitting to a non-two state model (Table 1).

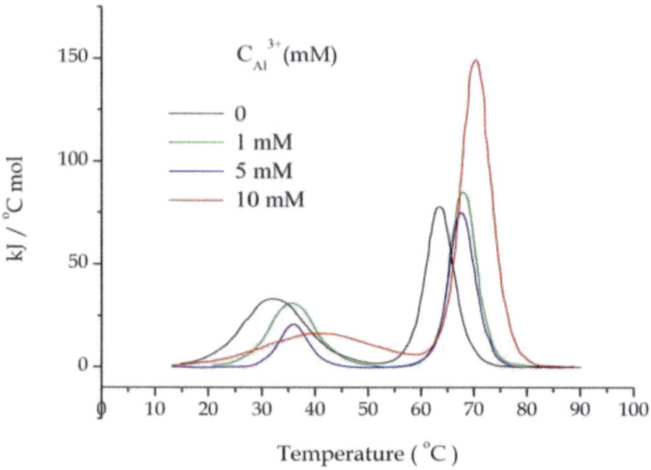

Fig. 9. Thermograms of pepsin with addition different concentrations of Al^{3+} at different concentrations, at pH 2.

A presence of aluminium affects the position of the first peak, and changes its shape. Compared with the DSC profile of pepsin for all Al^{3+} concentrations (1, 5, 10 mM) the first peak becomes more broadened and asymmetric. Van't Hoff enthalpies calculated for the first transition temperature are more than twice larger than calorimetric enthalpies observed for the same transition temperatures. For these transitions calorimetric and van't Hoff enthalpies are calculated and are presented in Table 1.

C_{Al+3} (mM)	peak	T_m (K)	ΔH^{cal} (kJ/mol)	ΔH^{VH} (kJ/mol)	$\Delta(\Delta G^0)$ (kJ/mol)	$K_{L(Tm)}$ (M^{-1})
0	1	304.5 ± 0.2	535 ± 21	196 ± 8	0	-
	2	336.9 ± 0.2	556 ± 12	531± 17	0	-
1	1	308.6 ± 0.2	138 ± 12	389± 42	7.94±0.76	$1.05 \cdot 10^3$
	2	340.9 ± 0.2	769 ± 21	568 ± 8	-0.52±0.05	$9.26 \cdot 10^8$
5	1	309.2 ± 0.2	171 ± 4	422 ± 8	9.32±0.91	$7.30 \cdot 10^2$
	2	342.5 ± 0.2	518 ± 35	627± 42	3.74±0.04	$5.71 \cdot 10^8$
10	1	315.6 ± 0.2	159 ± 21	529± 44	8.78±0.88	$6.76 \cdot 10^5$
	2	343.5 ± 0.2	481 ± 17	567± 21	0.23±0.01	$1.43 \cdot 10^6$

Table 1. Thermodynamic parameters of pepsin unfolding in a presence of Al^{3+}. Standard Gibb's energy was calculated at 25°C; K_L is equilibrium-binding affinity; Reported values are the means of minimum three independent replicates.

In contrast to ΔH^{cal} of value 535 kJ/mol calculated for the first transition temperature for intact pepsin, in a presence of Al^{3+} for each applied concentrations values are reduced of approximately 138 to 170 kJ/mol. For the second transition temperature, calorimetric enthalpies are very close to each other. At the same time, calculated values for van't Hoff enthalpies, for both transition temperatures, are close to each other. With the exceptions of the first transition temperature for the aluminium non-treated pepsin, all other examined cases have a ΔH^{VH} that is smaller than ΔH^{cal}. At the first transition temperature, the ratio $n = \Delta H^{cal}/\Delta H^{VH}$ ranges from 0.35 for pepsin treated with 1 mM Al^{3+} to 2.72 for native pepsin. At the second transition temperature, those ratios vary from 0.83 for pepsin treated with 5 mM Al^{3+} to 1.35 for native form of pepsin.

The fact that the ratio is larger than unity for some cases suggests that multiple transitions occur within a single peak and that the transitions are coupled less then 100%. Each lobe of pepsin is composed of two almost identical sub-domains (Andreeva 1989, Brandts 1990, Blundel 1990) forming a part of the binding cleft, and the structural feature might well contribute to the transitions causes deviation from two-state behaviour for most forms. At low temperature, there were essentially no unbound aluminium ions (all excess Al^{3+} was dialysed before DSC experiments). Depending on concentrations of bound Al^{3+} the shifts in T_m values ranges of about 4 to 11 degrees for the first transition, and for the second transition T_m values for all aluminium concentrations are shifted from 4 to about 7 degrees. From the shift in T_m values the changes in apparent stability of the treated pepsin relative to the native form was evaluated from the equation:

$$\Delta\left(\Delta G\right) = \Delta G_{Al^{3+}} - \Delta G^{0}_{(native)} \quad (27)$$

Where $\Delta G^{0}_{(native)}$ is zero at T_m, while $\Delta G_{Al^{3+}}$ was obtained from Gibbs-Helmholtz equation. The obtained values of $\Delta\left(\Delta G\right)$, the Gibbs free energy of aluminium binding, are listed in Table 1. As the process of pepsin unfolding is complex process, and proceeds in two different stages, the free energy of unfolding was calculated at both temperatures of transition. Compared to the temperatures where native pepsin unfolds, and to calculated free energies for the both transition temperatures, aluminium binding causes stabilisation of the pepsin structure for all applied concentrations.

Binding of Al^{3+} at the first part of pepsin molecule causes structural changes and during the melting process, intermolecular interactions are present probably because of partially denaturised initially part of the protein. At the second transition temperature in a presence of various Al^{3+} concentrations at pH 2, the observed values of van't Hoff and calorimetric enthalpies are very close to each other. Unfolding of the second part of the molecule in presence of Al^{3+} take place as a two state process, at which the second part of molecule behave as a single domain.

The DSC curve profiles suggest two kinds of binding sites for Al^{3+} on pepsin. At each transition midpoints, T_{m_1} and T_{m_2}, and from ligand-induced shifts and calorimetric parameters for reversible transitions, an equilibrium binding affinity K_L were calculated (Table 1).

The average number of ligands bound per molecule of native pepsin, as estimated from DSC data, was $\overline{X}_{NI}$ =1.35 for the first transition temperature, and $\overline{X}_{NII}$ =3.58 for the second transition temperature. The obtained values for average number of bound ligands per molecule of pepsin for both transition temperatures are in agreement with calculated binding constants (Table 1).

UV melting experiments, as indirect mode for following thermal unfolding parameters, were conducted in the absence and presence of Al^{3+} ions to assess the impact of bound Al^{3+} ions on the thermal stability of pepsin. The resulting melting profiles of pepsin at 280 nm, pH 2 without and in a presence of 5 mM Al^{3+} ions are presented on Figure 10. Both melting curves showed typical sigmoid behaviour. Addition of 5 mM solution of Al^{3+} produces biphasic denaturation of pepsin at pH 2. Spectroscopic signals for thermal denaturation of pepsin in a presence of Al^{3+} ions at pH 2 are presented at Figure 10.

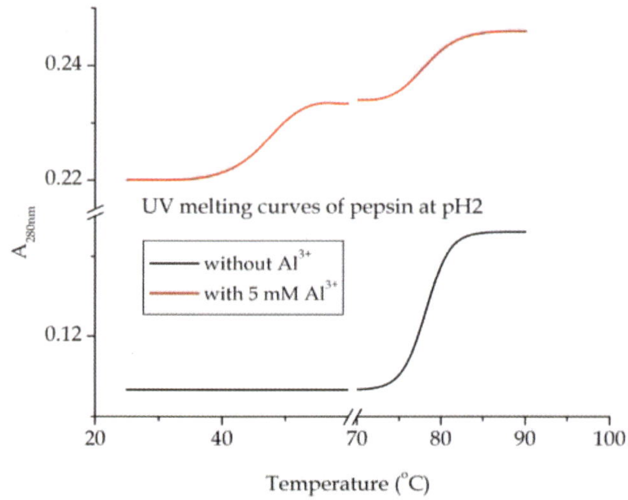

Fig. 10. UV absorbance measurements were carried out on Beckman UV 5260 UV-VIS spectrophotometer with an electro thermal temperature control cell unit. The temperature control was performed with digital voltmeter with thermocouples. A quartz cell with 1 cm path length was used for all the absorbance studies. Absorbance was measured directly as a temperature function. Thermal unfolding of pepsin was monitored by recording absorbance at 280 nm in temperature interval from 20 °C to 90 °C with heating rate of 1 °C/min and samples were allowed to equilibrate for one minute at each temperature setting, while the reference cell, containing just a solvent, was monitored at room temperature. The resulting increase of the absorbance of the sample solution recorded over the temperature range. Pepsin concentration was 0.3 mg / $ml_{solution}$.

The calculated values of van't Hoff enthalpy from spectroscopic data of unfolding of pepsin and corresponding values of temperatue midpoints for thermally induced conformational transitions of pepsin at pH 2 and in a presence of 5 mM Al^{3+} ions were calculated and presented in Table 2.

	λ = 280 nm
T_{m1} (K)	320.5
$\Delta H^{UV}{}_{unf1}$ (kcal/K mol)	97
T_{m2} (K)	352.1
$\Delta H^{UV}{}_{unf2}$ (kcal/K mol)	140

Table 2. Thermodynamic characteristics of pepsin denaturation at pH 2 in a presence of 10 mM Al^{3+} ions, obtained by UV spectroscopy.

6. Conclusion

Results of our study showed that aluminium cause increase pepsin activity. The obtained activation of pepsin is probably a consequence of conformational changes of enzyme molecule induced by bounded aluminium. As it were previously reported in analogy to the other aspartic proteases, bounded aluminium ions could causes significant conformational changes and induce increase in beta structure content (Flaten et al. 1992, Bittar et al. 1992, Clauberg et al. 1993).

The kinetic data implies that activation of pepsin is a non-essential partial non-competitive type. That suggests that bound aluminium do not influence on substrate binding sites on pepsin, but causes conformational changes that increase the rate of substrate converting to the reaction products. The results are consistent with a partial activation system presented in scheme in Figure1. Calculated dissociation constants from kinetic and indirect UV melting assay data are in good agreement to each other.

The present thermodynamic analyses show that DSC method is useful to measure the binding constants from *Tm* shifts. The stabilization effect of Al^{3+} binding on pepsin molecule, as well as an average number of ligands bound to the native protein, equilibrium binding affinity K_L were also calculated. The obtained values for binding affinity for site I are lower than on site II, which is in agreement with obtained values for average number of bound ligand. In addition, it can be assumed that the site II has a higher affinity for Al^{3+}than site I.

7. Acknowledgment

This study was supported by Ministry of Science of Republic of Serbia, Project No. 172015.

8. References

Andreeva, N.S.; Zdanov, A.S.; Fedorov, A.A.; Gushchina, A.E.; Shutskever, N.E.; (1984) X-ray analysis of pepsin. VI. Atomic structure of the enzyme at 2-angstrom resolution. *Mol Biol*, Vol. 18, pp. 313–322.

Anson, M. (1938) The estimation of pepsin, trypsin, papain and cathepsin with hemoglobin, *J Gen Physiol*, Vol. 22, pp. 79–89.

Baldwin, E.T.; Bhat, T.N.; Gulnik, S.; Hosur, M.V.; Sowder, R.C.; Cachau, R.E.; Collins, J.; Silva, A.M.; Erickson, J.W. (1993) Crystal structures of native and inhibited forms of human cathepsin D: Implications for lysosomal targeting and drug design. *Proc Nat Acad Sci USA* Vol.90, pp. 6796–6800.

Bittar, E.E.; Xiang, Z.; Huang, Y.P.; (1992) Citrate as an aluminium chelator and positive effector of the sodium efflux in single bamacle muscle fibers, *Biochim Biophys Acta,* Vol. 1108, pp. 210-214.

Blundell, T.L.; Jenkin, J.; Sewell, B.T.; Pearl, L.H.; Cooper, J.B.; Tickle, I.J.; Veerapandian, B.; Wood, S.P. (1990) X-ray analyses of aspartic proteinases. The three-dimensional structure at 2.1 A resolution of endothiapepsin. *J Mol Biol*, Vol. 211, pp. 919–941.

Brandts, J. F.; Hu, C. Q.; & Lin, L.-N. (1989) A simple model for proteins with interacting domains. Application to scanning calorimetry data, *Biochemistry* 28, 8588–8596.

Brandts, J.F.; Lin L.-N., (1990) Study of strong to ultratight protein interaction using differential scanning calorimetry, *Biochemistry,* Vol. 29, pp. 6927–6940.

Brewer, J. M., and Wampler, J. E. (2001) A differential scanning calorimetric study of the effects of metal ions, substrate/product, substrate analogues and chaotropic anions on the thermal denaturation of yeast enolase 1, *Int. J. Biol. Macromol.* Vol. 28, pp. 213-218.

Cann, J.R. (1962) Electrophoretic Demonstration of Specific Enzyme-Substrate Complex between Pepsin and Serum albumin. II. Inhibiition of complex formation by acetyl-L-tryptophan and fatty acids, *The Journal of Biological Chemistry,* Vol. 237, No. 3, pp. 707-711.

Celey, M.S.; Dassie, S.A.; Freire, E.; Bianconi, M.L.; Fidelio, G.D. (2005) Ligand induced thermostability in proteins: Thermodynamic analysis of ANS-albumin interaction. *Biochim. Biophys. Acta,* Vol. 1750, pp. 122-133.

Celey, M.S.; Dassie, S.A.; Gonzales, M.; Bianconi, M.L.; Fidelio, G.D. (2006) Differential scanning calorimetry as a tool to estimate binding parameters in multiligand binding proteins. *Anal Biochem,* Vol. 350, pp. 277-284.

Chu, Y.H., Chen, J.K., & Whitesides, G.M. (1993) Affinity Electrophoresis Multisectional Polyacrylamide Slab Gels Is a Useful and Convenien Technique for Measuring Binding Constants of Aryl Sulfonamides to Bovine Carbonic Anhydrase B, *Analytical Chemistry,* Vol. 65, pp. 1314-1322.

Clauberg, M.; Joshi, J.G. (1993) Regulation of serine protease activity by aluminium: Implications for Alzheimer disease, *Proc Nat Acad Sci,* Vol. 90, pp. 1009-1012.

Crothers, D.M. (1971) Statistical thermodynamics of nucleic acid melting transitions with coupled binding equilibria, *Biopolymers* Vol. 10, pp. 2147-2160.

Cunningham, L.; Rasch, E.M.; Lewis, A.L. & Heitsch, R. (1970) Discontinuous electrophoresis of pepsin and pepsinogen in thin sheets of polyacrylamide gel, *The Journal of Histochemistry and Cytochemistry,* Vol. 18, No. 12, pp. 853-861., http://jhc.sagepub.org/content/18/12/853

Dixon, M. & Webb, E.C., (1979) Enzymes, 3rd ed. London: Longmans; pp. 227-272.

Flaten, T.P.; Garruto, R.M. (1992) Polinuclear ions in aluminium toxicity, *J Theoret Biol*, Vol. 152, pp. 129-132.

Fontes, R.; Ribeiro, J.M. & Sillero, A., (2000) Inhibition and activation of enzymes. Effect of a modifier on the reaction rate on kinetic parameters, *Acta Biochimica Polonica,* Vol. 47, No. 1, pp. 233-357.

Gomez, M.; Domingo, J.L.; Del Castillo, D.; Llobet, J.M.; Corbella, J. (1994) Comparative aluminium mobilizing actions of several chelators in aluminium-loaded ureamic rats. *Hum Exp Toxicol*; Vol. 13, pp. 135–139.

Herriott, R. M.; Desreux, V. & Northrop J. H. (1940) Electrophoresis of Pepsin, *J Gen Physiol.*; Vol. 23, No.4, pp. 439–447.

Kerr, D.N.S.; Ward, M.K. Aluminium intoxication: History of its clinical recognition and management. In: Sigel H, Sigel A, editors. Metal ions in biological systems: Aluminium and its role in biology. New York: Marcel Dekker; 1988. p 217–258.

Krejpcio, Z.; Wojciak, R.W. (2002) The influence of Al^{3+} ions on pepsin and trypsin activity in vitro. *Pol J Environ stud*; Vol. 11, pp. 251–254.

Kurimoto, E.; Harada, T.; Akiyama, A.; Sakai, T., & Kato, K. (2001) In vitro refolding of porcine pepsin immobilized on agarose beads. *J. Biochem. (Tokyo)*.130, pp. 295–297.

Laemmli. (1970) Cleavage of structural proteins during the assembly of the head of bacteriophage. Nature, Vol. 227, pp. 680-685.

Lin, L.-N., Mason, A. B., Woodworth, R. C., and Brandts, J. F. (1993) Calorimetric studies of the N-terminal half-molecule of transferrin and mutant forms modified near the Fe(3+)-binding site. *Biochem. J*, Vol. 293, pp. 517–522

Lumry, R.; Biltonen, R.; Brandts, J.F. (1966) Validity of the "two-state" hypothesis for conformational transitions of proteins, *Biopolymers*, Vol. 4, pp. 917–944.

McGhee, J.D. (1976) Theoretical calculations of the helix–coil transition of DNA in the presence of large, cooperatively binding ligands, *Biopolymers*, Vol. 15, pp. 1345–1375.

Pavelkic, V. M.; Beljanski, M. V.; Antic, K. M.; Babic, M. M.; Brdaric, T. P.; & Gopcevic, K. R. (2011) Thermal Stability of Porcine Pepsin Influenced by Al(III) Ion: DSC Study, *Russian Journal of Physical Chemistry A*, Vol. 85, No. 13, pp. 2245–2250, ISSN 0036-0244.

Pavelkic, V.M.; Gopcevic, K.R.; Krstic, D.Z.; Ilic, M.A.; (2008) The influence of Al^{3+} ions on porcine pepsin activity in vitro, *Journal of enzyme inhibition and medicinal chemistry*, Vol. 23, No. 6, pp. 1002-1010.

Perrela, W.F.; (1988), A Practical Curve Fitting microcomputer program for the analysis of kinetic data on IBM-PC compatible computers, *Anal Biochem*, Vol. 174, pp. 437–447.

Porcelli, G. (1968) Molecular properties of pepsin as studied by gel filtration, *Experientia*, Vol. 15, No. 211, pp. 707-711.

Powers, J.C.; Harley, A.D. & Myers, D.V. (1977) Subsite specificity of porcine pepsin. *Adv. Exp. Med. Biol.*, Vol. 95, pp. 141-157.

Privalov, P.L.; Mateo, P.L.; Khechinashvili, N.N. (1981) Comparative thermodynamic study of pepsinogen and pepsin structure. *J. Mol.Biol.*, Vol. 152, pp. 445-464.

Schellman, J.A. (1975) Macromolecular binding, *Biopolymers*, Vol. 14, pp. 999–1018.

Sepulveda, P.; Marciniszyn, J.; Lui, D.; Tang, J. (1975) Primary structure of porcine pepsin. III. Amino acid sequence of a cyanogens bromide fragment, CB2A, and the complete structure of porcine pepsin, *J Biol Chem*; Vol. 250, pp. 5082–5088.

Shrake, A.; Ross, P.D. (1992) Origin and consequences of ligand-induced multiphasic thermal protein denaturation, *Biopolymers*, Vol. 32, pp. 925–940.

Sielecki, A.R.; Fedorov, A.A.; Boodho, A.; Andreeva, A.; James, M.N.G. (1990) Molecular and crystal structures of monoclinic porcine pepsin refined at 1.8A resolutions. *J Mol Biol*; Vol. 214, pp. 43–170.

14

Peptides and Peptidomimetics in Medicinal Chemistry

Paolo Ruzza
Institute of Biomolecular Chemistry of C.N.R.
Italy

1. Introduction

Peptides show great pharmaceutical potential as active drugs and diagnostics in several clinical areas such as endocrinology, urology, obstetrics, oncology, etc. and as functional excipients in drug delivery systems to overcome tissue and cellular membrane barriers (Nestor, 2009). From a pharmaceutical point of view, peptides are situated somewhere between classical organic drug substances and high molecular weight biopharmaceuticals.

The importance of peptides to life is evident from the most primitive organism to man. In man, a myriad of roles is filled by peptides spanning hormonal, neuromodulatory, mucosal defense, et al.

Despite the obvious importance of peptides to homeostasis in man, there are few peptides resulting from medicinal chemistry that are commercialized pharmaceutical products in the USA and Europe. The shortcomings of peptides as pharmaceutical products have been long known: typically short duration of action, lack of receptor subtype selectivity, lack of oral bioavailability. However medicinal chemistry offers solutions to the first two limitations and oral bioavailability issues have been addressed by novel routes of administration (e.g. intranasal, inhalation) and injectable depot formulations (Nestor, 2009).

2. Peptide design considerations

The physical and chemical properties of peptides and proteins are determined by the nature of the constituent amino acid side chains and by the polyamide peptide backbone itself.

The structures of the 20 primary amino acids are given in Figure 1. Amino acids are divided into hydrophobic and hydrophilic residues. The first group includes those with aliphatic side chains (Ala, Val, Ile, Leu, Met) and those with aromatic side chains (Phe, Tyr, Trp). The hydrophilic group includes amino acids with neutral, polar side chains (Ser, Thr, Asn, Gln), those with acidic (Asp and Glu) or with basic side chains as Lys, Arg and His.

Two amino acids, Cys and Pro, have special properties that set them apart. Cys containing a thiol group that can be oxidatively couple to another Cys residue to form a disulfide bond that stabilizes secondary and/or tertiary structure or to hold two different peptide chains together. On the other hand, free thiols are present in some protein, where they serve as ligand for metal chelation, as nucleophiles in proteolitic enzymes, or as carboxyl activators in acyl transferases. Pro is a cyclic residue that has specific conformational effects on the peptide or protein backbone. Indeed, cyclic structure locks Pro φ backbone dihedral angle at approximately -75°. Additionally, several residues can undergo post-traslational modification to yield new amino-acids.

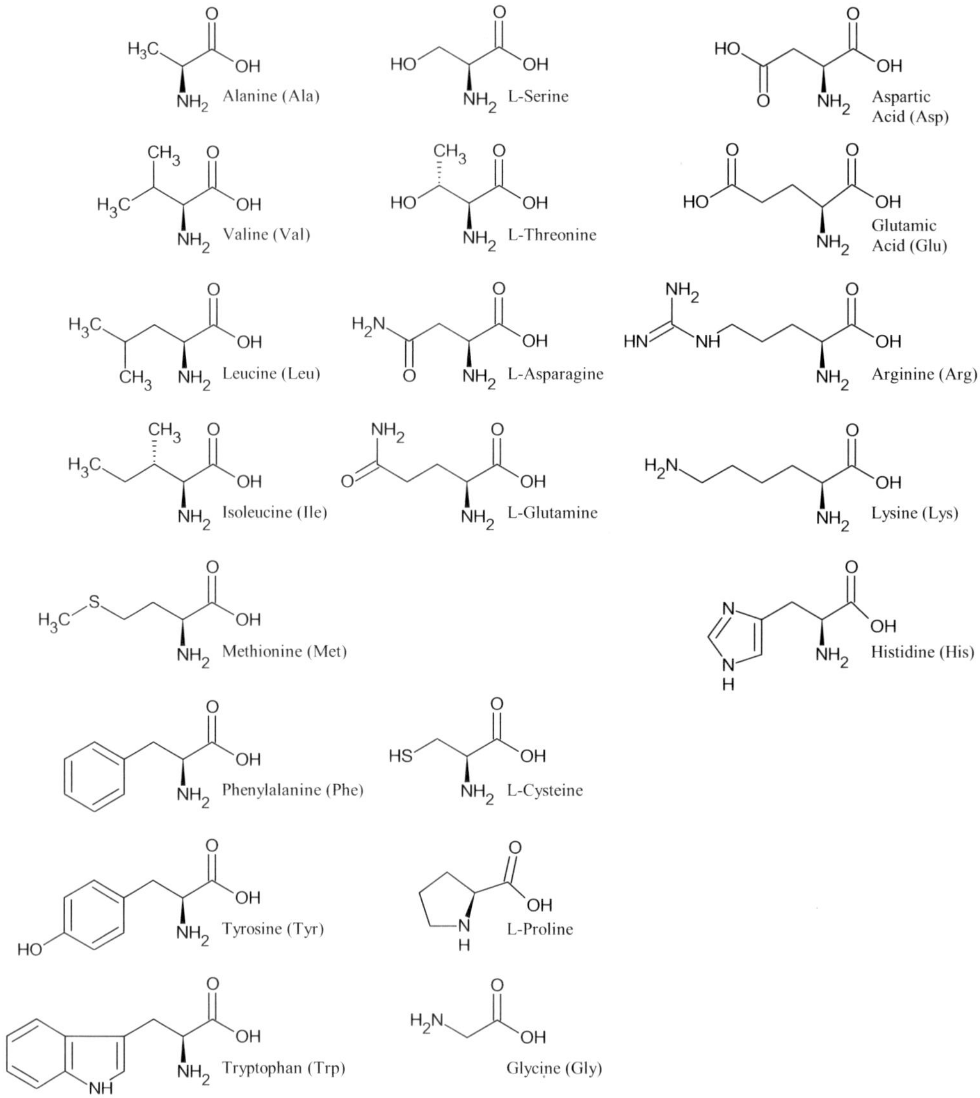

Fig. 1. L-Amino acid structures.

Small peptides typically show high conformational flexibility due to the multiple conformations that are energetically possible for each residue. The conformation of the peptide backbone can be described by three torsional angles (Figure 2): φ, which is the angle defined by C(O)−N−Cα−C(O); ψ, which is defined by N−Cα−C(O)−N; and ω, which is defined by Cα−C(O)−N−Cα. The ω angle for the peptide bond is generally trans (ω = 180°) except for the Xaa-Pro bond, which can be cis (ω = 0°) or trans. Pioneering work of Ramachandran et al. (1965) resulted in the so-called Ramachandran plots which restrict the allowed values for the torsional angles φ and ψ to most amino acids. The conformational space accessible to the L-amino acids is about one third of the total structural space. Nevertheless the remaining degrees of freedom still make a prediction of structure extremely difficult. There are only few examples reported in the literature where short to medium sized peptides (<30-50 residues) adopt a stable structures in aqueous solution (Grauer & Köning, 2009). In most cases they exist in numerous dynamically interconverting conformations.

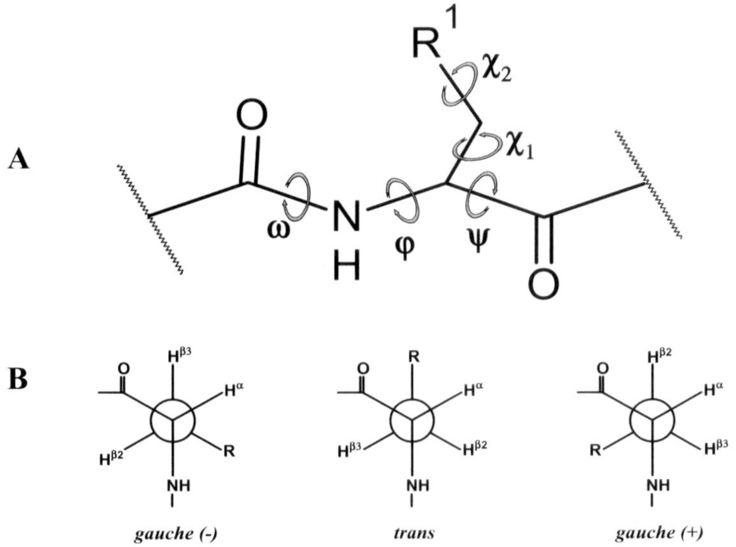

Fig. 2. (**A**) Backbone and side chain torsional angles; (**B**) Newman projection of three staggered rotamers in L-amino acids.

An equally critical area for the design of bioactive peptides, though much less explored, is that of the three-dimensional structures of the side chain moieties. This is described by the side chain χ torsional angle (χ_1 is defined by the N-Cα-Cβ-Cγ) (Figure 2). It can assume three low energy staggered conformations (rotamers): *gauche*(+); *gauche*(-); and *trans*. The energy differences between these conformations is not high, but the orientation of the side chain group of an L-amino acid residue relative to the peptide backbone is dramatically different: for *gauche*(-) χ_1, the side chain points toward the N-terminus of the peptide chain; for *trans*, the side chain points toward the C-terminus; and for *gauche*(+), the side chain points over the peptide backbone (Hruby et al., 1997). The consequences for both the surface that is created by the peptide ligand and its complimentarity for a receptor/acceptor are critical for successful recruitment of the target from small peptides as confirmed by structure-activity relationship studies (Hruby et al., 1997).

The most important technique for structural determination of biomolecules is the x-ray diffraction analysis on single crystal, even if it is questionable whether the solid state conformation determined by X-ray analysis are identical to those occurring in solution or during the interactions with the biological target (Kessler, 1982; Wuthrich et al, 1991). Over the last decade, NMR spectroscopy has emerged as an important tool for structural determination of biomolecule in solution. The increase in magnet technology and in the speed and data storage capacity of modern PCs allowed the development of multi-dimensional NMR methods which permit to solve in detail the resonance assignment of biomolecules and to determine proton-proton distances at the base of NMR structures determination.

In addition to these powerful techniques, also fluorescence and circular dichroism (CD) studies provide useful information about the peptide conformation in solution and its capability to interact with target molecules (Ruzza, 2001; Siligardi, 2011).

2.1 Methodologies for design peptides

Conformational considerations in peptide synthesis remain one of the greatest challenges in the design of biologically active peptides. Peptides will usually be an ensemble of conformation states in solution. If biological activity involves only one discrete conformer, this conformational ensemble represents a dilution of the biologically active species.

This problem is more acute for peptides designed to mimic a portion of a protein structure, where the intramolecular interactions characteristic of the protein structure are lost (Figure 3). A strategy for reducing the number of the accessible conformations and rendering the selectivity of synthetic peptides more stringent than that afford by the sequence could take advantage by the introduction of local or global constraints into peptide sequences.

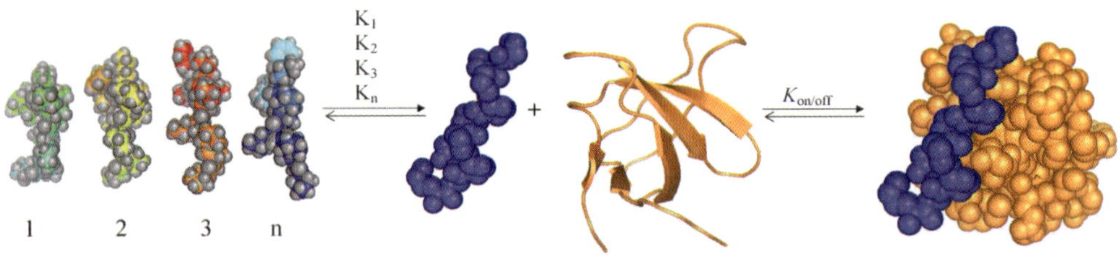

Fig. 3. Binding equilibrium involving a conformational manifold of the proline-rich peptide. The association process consists of the redistribution of the conformational ensemble from the binding-incompetent to the binding-competent (PPII) species, and then of the interaction of the latter with the SH3 domain (adapted from Ruzza et al., 2006).

2.1.1 Global restrictions

The simplest way to introduce a conformational constraint into a peptide sequence is by cyclization (Figure 4). This typically increases the *in vivo* stability of the cyclic peptides compared to their linear analogs. Cyclization can be obtained by connecting the N- with the C-terminus (head-to-tail) portion of the peptide sequence, or the couple of either the N- or the C-terminus with one of the side chains (backbone-to-side chain), or the couple of side chains not involved in specific interactions with other (side chain-to-side chain).

The most common side chain-to-side chain cyclization is the oxidation of two Cys residues with the formation of a disulfide bond. Alternatively, the formation of amide bonds between the side chains of Lys and Asp/Glu can occur. One limiting factor of side chain-to-side chain cyclization is that a limited section of the polypeptide is constrained. To overcome this problem several covalent bridges may be incorporated into one sequence (Grauer & Köning, 2009).

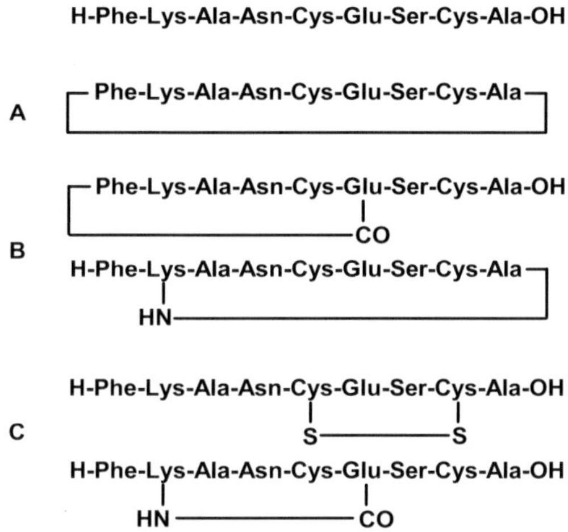

Fig. 4. Examples of peptide cyclization: (**A**) head-to-tail, (**B**) backbone-to-side chain, and (**C**) side chain-to-side chain.

2.1.2 Local restrictions

The simplest local constraints that can be placed on a given residue involve the substitution of a methyl group for an hydrogen adjacent to a rotable bond (Figure 5). One substitution which have been extensively investigated in the last years involve the α-hydrogen yielding Cα-tetrasubstituted α-amino acids (Toniolo, 2001, and reference therein). For example, replacing the α-hydrogen on alanine with a methyl group gives α-aminoisobutyric acid (Aib). This residue was found in peptide sequences from a fungal source. The steric bulk of the methyl group reduced the rotational freedom of the two peptide backbone angles φ and ψ. In the case of Aib, the allowable φ and ψ backbone angles in peptides are restricted to values near –57°, -47° and +57°, +47° (Karle, 1996).

The introduction of an alkyl group either at the β-position or on aromatic ring of naturally occurring amino acids rigidifies the conformational flexibility of the side chain. Three of natural amino acids show β-disubstitutions: Val (two methyl groups), Ile (a methyl and an ethyl) and Thr (a methyl and a hydroxyl). Additionally, β-substitution leads to a second asymmetric center in the amino acid structure. These modifications do not greatly perturb the backbone, allowing the peptide backbone and the side chain some degree of flexibility, which often is crucial for the activity of peptide mimetic. Another advantage of these modifications is that the extra alkyl groups can enhance the lipophility of peptide, and therefore can help it to overcome membrane barrier (Hruby et al., 1997; and references therein).

Surely, the introduction of a covalent bond between the aromatic ring of an α-amino acid residue and the peptide backbone has proven to be a useful further conformation restriction. For example, 1,2,3,4-tetrahydroisoquinoline carboxylic acid (Tic) is a cyclic constrained analog of phenylalanine (Figure 5), in which a methylene bridge is placed between the α-nitrogen, and 2′-carbon of the aromatic ring (Kazmierski & Hruby, 1988).

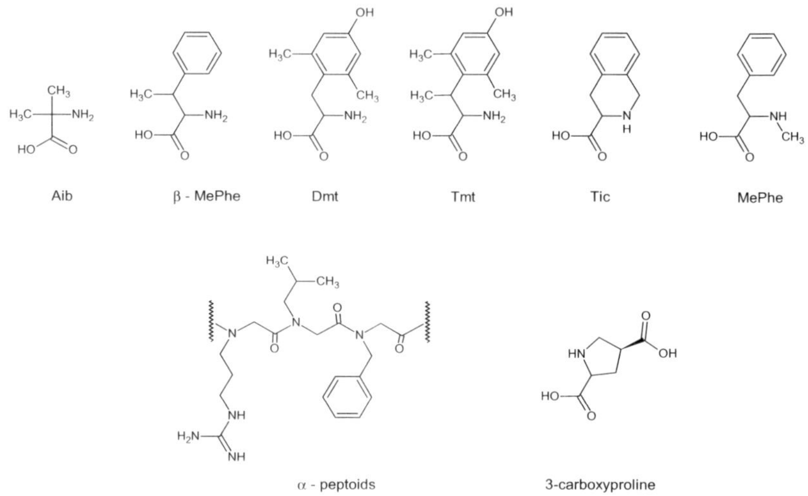

Fig. 5. Structures of some local constraints.

N-alkylated residue, and in particular N-methylation is an important modification of the peptide bond that influence the conformational freedom of the peptide backbone. The steric constraints introduced by the N-alkyl group have also effect on the side chain freedom of the neighboring amino acids. Additionally, the number of inter- and intra-molecular hydrogen bonds decreases due to the removal of the backbone NH groups, destabilizing both α-helix and β-sheet conformations. Finally, the attached carbonyl group shows an increased basicity and decreased polarity.

Oligomers of N-substituted glycines, where the side chain is attached to the amine nitrogen instead of the α-carbon, are called α-peptoids (Figure 5) (Zuckermann & Kodadek, 2009). The conformational change in the N-substituted glycines makes the α-carbon achiral so that peptoids are less restricted in their spatial conformation. Neither peptoids can form intramolecular hydrogen bonds through backbone–backbone interactions, because of the lack of amide protons that help peptides stabilize both α-helical structures and β-sheet conformations. However, the same backbone structure renders the peptoids highly resistant to proteases.

A further investigated group of local constraints are derivatives of the natural amino acids proline. Proline analogs displaying the characteristics of other amino acids are referred to as proline-amino acid chimeras, and have been used to study the spatial requirements for receptor affinity and biological activity of both natural amino acids and peptides. For example, β-substituted-prolines such as 3-carboxyproline, 3-phenylproline, and 3-di-methylproline combine amino acid side chain functionality with proline's conformational rigidity. In these cases, replacement of the natural amino acids in peptides by proline-amino acid chimeras provided better understanding of the bioactive conformations of peptides binding to receptors (Quancard et al., 2004; and references therein).

2.1.3 Backbone modification

The backbone of a peptide can be modified in various ways by isosteric or isoeletronic substitution (Cudic & Stawikowski, 2007; and reference therein). Figure 6 summarizes the most important ways to modify the peptide backbone.

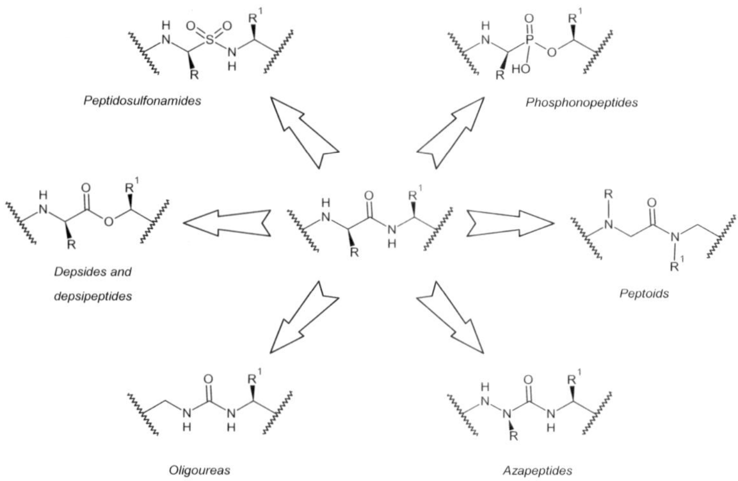

Fig. 6. Most important peptide bond surrogates (adapted from Cudic & Stawikowski, 2007).

Various peptidomimetics containing pseudopeptides or peptide bond surrogates, in which peptide bonds have been replaced with other chemical groups, are designed and synthesized with the aim to obtain peptide analogs with improved pharmacological properties. This is mainly because such approaches create an amide bond surrogate with defined three dimensional structures and with significant differences in polarity, hydrogen bonding capability and acid-base character. Also important, the structural and stereochemical integrities of the adjacent pair of α-carbon atoms in these pseudopeptides are unchanged. The psi-bracket (ψ[ ]) nomenclature, introduced by A. Spatola (1983), is used for this type of modification. The introduction of such modifications to the peptide sequence is expected to completely prevent protease cleavage of amide bond and significantly improve the peptides metabolic stability. However, such modifications may also have some negative effects on peptides biophysical and biochemical properties, in particular their conformation, flexibility and hydrophobicity. Therefore, the choice of an amide bond surrogate is a compromise between positive effects on pharmacokinetics and bioavailability and potential negative effects on activity and specificity (Cudic & Stawikowski, 2007). The ability of the surrogate to mimic the steric, electronic and solvation properties of the amide bond is certainly the most important characteristic in determining the potency of pseudopeptide analogs. From the synthetic point of view, the methods for assembly of peptidosulfonamides, phosphonopeptides, oligoureas, depsides, depsipeptides, peptoids and azapeptides are parallel those for standard solid-phase peptide synthesis, although different reagents and different coupling and protecting strategies need to be employed.

2.2 Methodologies for peptide synthesis

Methods for synthesizing peptides are divided into two classes: solution or liquid phase (classical) and solid phase (SPPS). The classical methods have evolved since the beginning of the last century, and they are described amply in several books and reviews (Goodman et al., 2004; Bodansky, 1993). The SPPS was conceived and elaborated by R.B. Merrifield beginning in 1959, and it has also been covered compressively (Merrifield, 2006; Chan and White, 2000).

Solution synthesis retains value in large-scale manufacturing and for specialized laboratory application. However, the need to optimize reaction condition and purification procedures for the different intermediate renders this method time-consuming and laboratory-intensive. Consequently, most workers, now requiring peptides for their research, opt for the more accessible SPPS approach.

The concept of the SPPS can be illustrated in Figure 7 where the C-terminal protected amino acid is attached to an insoluble polymeric support via a labile linker. Subsequently, the anchored peptide is extended by a series of deprotection/coupling cycles, which are required to proceed with high yields and fidelities. The reactions are driven to completion by the use of excess soluble reagents, which can be removed by simple filtration and washing without losses. Once peptide has been accomplished, it is necessary to release protected residues and to cleave the crude peptide from the solid support. These two operations can be performed simultaneously or in separate step, according to the successive destine of the peptide. Finally, the synthetic peptide must undergo purification step and characterization to verify the desired structure.

The two major chemistries for SPPS involve the use of either base labile α-amino protecting group (Fmoc) or acid labile α-amino protecting group (Boc). Each method involves different side chain protecting group, and consequent cleavage/deprotection methods and resins (Table 1).

Peptide purification and peptide quality evaluation is performed by HPLC. Most crude peptides are purified by reversed phase HPLC to achieve the desired purity. The combination of cation or anion exchange HPLC purification followed by RP-HPLC provides a powerful technique to purify a crude peptide with inferior quality. Mass spectra by MALDI or ESI-TOF and mono- and bi-dimensional NMR are the standard analytical procedure to assess peptide identity.

Recently, convergent synthesis strategies for the generation of highly complex branched peptides or scaffolded peptides and proteins have been developed. Such ligation reactions include the formation of thiazolidines or oximes from mutually reactive precursors, as well as native chemical ligation through reaction of a peptide thioester with an N-terminal cysteine in aqueous buffers, or the generation of [1,2,3]-triazoles through 1,3-dipolar cycloadditions of alkynes to azides, which belongs to a group of reactions referred to as click chemistry, which proceed at room temperature in the presence of copper(I) as a catalyst.

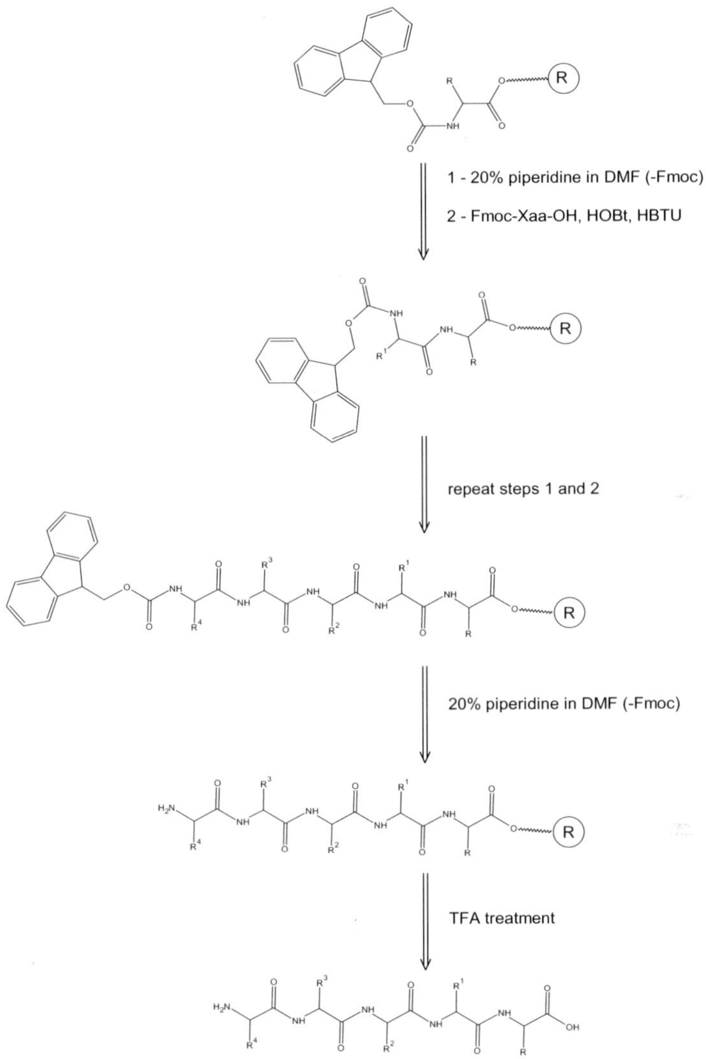

Fig. 7. Fmoc solid-phase peptide synthesis procedure.

Topic	Fmoc chemistry	Boc chemistry
Side chain protection	Acid sensitive	Strong acid sensitive (HF)
N$^{\alpha}$-deprotection	20% piperidine in DMF	50% TFA in DCM
Final cleavage	TFA in SPPS vessel	HF (special equipment)
Automation	Yes	Yes
Synthetic steps	Deblock, wash, couple, wash	Deblock, neutralization, wash, couple, wash
Resin	Acid or super-acid sensitive	Merrifield type

Table 1. Comparison of Fmoc- and Boc-SPPS.

3. Peptides and molecular recognition

In the post-genomic era, the importance of protein-protein interactions is becoming even more apparent. Proteins continuously interact each other to govern signaling pathways within and between cells. Biological signaling requires that protein complexes are formed and activated at the right time and in the right place, and that their formation is both reversible and transient. The strength and duration of a signal may be critical for the effects of hormones, cytokines and growth factors, and a large number of specific protein interaction domains are known which mediate this machinery (Pawson, 2004).

Although it is possible to derive some general principles of protein-protein recognition from experimentally determined structures, recent structural studies on protein complexes formed during signal transduction illustrate the remarkable diversity of interactions, both in term of interfacial size and nature. There are two broad classes of complexes: "domain-domain," in which both components comprise pre-folded structural units, and "domain-peptide," in which one component is a short motif that is unstructured in the absence of its binding partner.

Structure-based drug design seeks to identify and modulate such interactions. This optimization process requires knowledge about interaction geometries and approximate affinity contributions of attractive interactions that can be gleaned from crystal structure and associated affinity data.

3.1 Peptide-receptor ligands in cancer imaging

Since the first histological evidence of the high expression of somatostatin receptors in pituitary adenomas (Reubi, 1984), many other human cancers were found to overexpress peptide receptors in vitro (Table 2). Based on these results, peptide receptor ligands labeled with different probes (radionuclides, magnetic and optical probes) have been started to be developed for the in vivo targeting and imaging of tumors.

Receptor	Tumor type
Somatostatin (hSSTR1 – hSSTR5)	Neuroendocrine, non-Hodgkin's lymphoma, melanoma, breast, pancreatic, gastric, colon, prostate, lung, SCLC, MTC
Cholecystokinin (CCK-A and CCK-B)	MTC, SCLC, pancreatic, astrocytoma, ovarian
Vasoactive Intestinal Peptide (VPAC1 and VPAC2)	SCLC, colon, gastric, breast, pancreatic, prostate, urinary bladder, lymphoma, meningioma
Neurotensin (NTR1 – NTR3)	SCLC, colon, exocrine pancreatic, prostate
Bombesin (BRS-1 – BRS-4)	SCLC, glioblastoma, colorectal, gastric, prostate, ovarian, breast
$\alpha_v\beta_3$ Integrin	Melanoma, neuroblastoma, breast
α-MSH (MC1R – MC5R)	Melanoma
Neuropeptide Y (Y1 – Y6)	Neuroblastoma, glioblastoma, breast
Substance P	SCLC, MTC, glioblastoma, astrocytoma, breast

Table 2. Peptide receptors overexpressed in tumors (adapted from Ruzza & Calderan, 2011).

The distribution and significance of the different peptide receptors as well as the properties and characteristics of their ligands have been discussed in manifold reviews (Bolzati, 2010; Lee, 2010; and references therein).

Development of labeled peptide probes relied on isolation of naturally occurring peptides (Table 3), screening of synthetic or phage libraries, and structure-based rational design. Generally, peptide-based probes are designed starting from naturally occurring peptide hormones, which, excepting the indispensable amino acids involved in biological activity, are modified to prolong their half-lives in vivo.

Peptide	Sequence
Somatostatin (14)	H-Ala-Gly-c(Cys-Lys-Asn-Phe-Phe-Trp-Lys-Thr-Phe-Thr-Ser-Cys)-OH
Somatostatin (28)	H-Ser-Ala-Asn-Ser-Asn-Pro-Ala-Met-Ala-Pro-Arg-Glu-Arg-Lys-Ala-Gly-c(Cys-Lys-Asn-Phe-Phe-Trp-Lys-Thr-Phe-Thr-Ser-Cys)-OH
Chlocystokinin	H-Lys-Ala-Pro-Ser-Gly-Arg-Met-Ser-Ile-Val-Lys-Asn-Leu-Gln-Asn-Leu-Asp-Pro-Ser-His-Arg-Ile-Ser-Asp-Arg-Asp-Tyr(SO_3H)-Met-Gly-Trp-Met-Asp-Phe-NH_2
Gastrin	Pyr-Leu-Gly-Pro-Gln-Gly-Pro-Pro-His-Leu-Val-Ala-Asp-Pro-Ser-Lys-Lys-Gln-Gly-Pro-Trp-Leu-Glu-Glu-Glu-Glu-Glu-Ala-Tyr-Gly-Trp-Met-Asp-Phe-NH_2
CCK8	H-Asp-Tyr(SO_3H)-Met-Gly-Trp-Met-Asp-Phe-NH_2
Minigastrin	H-Leu-Glu-Glu-Glu-Glu-Glu-Ala-Tyr-Gly-Trp-Met-Asp-Phe-NH_2
Vasoactive Intestinal Peptide (VIP)	H-His-Ser-Asp-Ala-Val-Phe-Thr-Asp-Asn-Tyr-Thr-Arg-Leu-Arg-Lys-Gln-Met-Ala-Val-Lys-Lys-Tyr-Leu-Asn-Ser-Ile-Leu-Asn-NH_2
Neurotensin	Pyr-Leu-Tyr-Glu-Asn-Lys-Pro-Arg-Arg-Pro-Tyr-Ile-Leu-OH
Bombesin	Pyr-Gln-Arg-Leu-Gly-Asn-Gln-Trp-Ala-Val-Gly-His-Leu-Met-NH_2
Gastrin Releasing Peptide	H-Val-Pro-Leu-Pro-Ala-Gly-Gly-Gly-Thr-Val-Leu-Thr-Lys-Met-Tyr-Pro-Arg-Gly-Asn-His-Trp-Ala-Val-Gly-His-Leu-Met-NH_2
Neuromedin B	H-Gly-Asn-Leu-Trp-Ala-Thr-Gly-His-Phe-Met-NH_2
RGD	$_c$[Arg-Gly-Asp-D-Phe-Lys]
α-MSH	Ac-Ser-Tyr-Ser-Met-Glu-His-Phe-Arg-Trp-Gly-Lys-Pro-Val-NH_2
β-MSH	H-Ala-Glu-Lys-Lys-Asp-Glu-Gly-Pro-Tyr-Arg-Met-Glu-His-Phe-Arg-Trp-Gly-Ser-Pro-Pro-Lys-Asp-OH
γ-MSH	H-Tyr-Val-Met-Gly-His-Phe-Arg-Trp-Asp-Arg-Phe-NH_2
ACTH	H-Ser-Tyr-Ser-Met-Glu-His-Phe-Arg-Trp-Gly-Lys-Pro-Val-Gly-Lys-Lys-Arg-Arg-Pro-Val-Lys-Val-Tyr-Pro-Asn-Gly-Ala-Glu-Asp-Glu-Ser-Ala-Glu-Ala-Phe-Pro-Leu-Glu-Phe-OH
GLP-1	H-His-Asp-Glu-Phe-Glu-Arg-His-Ala-Glu-Gly-Thr-Phe-Thr-Ser-Asp-Val-Ser-Ser-Tyr-Leu-Glu-Gly-Gln-Ala-Ala-Lys-Glu-Phe-Ile-Ala-Trp-Leu-Val-Lys-Gly-Arg-NH_2
Neuro Peptide Y	H-Tyr-Pro-Ser-Lys-Pro-Asp-Asn-Pro-Gly-Glu-Asp-Ala-Pro-Ala-Glu-Asp-Met-Ala-Arg-Tyr-Tyr-Ser-Ala-Leu-Arg-His-Tyr-Ile-Asn-Leu-Ile-Thr-Arg-Gln-Arg-Tyr-NH_2
Calcitonin	H-$_c$(Cys-Gly-Asn-Leu-Ser-Thr-Cys)-Met-Leu-Gly-Thr-Tyr-Thr-Gln-Asp-Phe-Asn-Lys-Phe-His-Thr-Phe-Pro-Gln-Thr-Ala-Ile-Gly-Val-Gly-Ala-Pro-NH_2

Table 3. Peptide receptor ligand sequences.

A linker is usually introduced between the imaging probe and the ligand, with the aim to preclude or minimize unwanted interferences between these two moieties. Linkers may act as a pharmacokinetic modifier and have a profound impact on the biodistribution of the whole molecule (Rufini, 2006; Schottelius, 2004). The most popular linkers are short amino acid sequences (i.e., dimer o trimer of β-Ala, Gly or N^{ε}-amino hexanoic acid) or low molecular weight polyethylene glycole (PEG) or hydrocarbon chains. Lipophilic molecules are cleared from the body by the hepatobiliary route, whereas hydrophilic probes are mainly cleared via the renal system.

Natural occurring peptide-ligands are usually recognized by more than one receptor subtype. A great debate is ongoing about the opportunity to increase the ligand-specificity towards receptor subtypes expressed on tumor cells. Several studies demonstrated that there are significant variations in the expression profile of subtype peptide receptors also between the primary tumor and its metastases or even within the same tumor (Reubi, 2002; Reubi, 2003) and so, an increase of receptor subtypes selectivity might be counterproductive in the development of imaging molecules. On the other hand, subtype-selective ligands are useful tools for functional imaging purposes as well as to study the changes in receptor expression and response to therapeutic interventions.

Until recently the use of receptor-antagonists has not been considered for in vivo targeting of tumors overexpressing G-protein coupled receptors and this due to the low capability of antagonist to internalize into tumor cells. Indeed, the cell internalization of imaging probes has been regarded for a long time as a fundamental prerequisite of labeled peptides, providing high contrast imaging. Recently, interesting results have been obtained with two somatostatin antagonists towards SST2 and SST3 receptor subtypes, which showed high tumor accumulation and retention, resulting in matchless imaging properties (Ginj, 2006). The benefit of the use of antagonist peptide ligands has a considerable impact on those systems, in which the binding of agonist-ligand either stimulates tumor growth or exerts unwanted pharmacological action.

Many authors have demonstrated that different peptide receptors are co-expressed on tumors in a heterogeneous manner, e.g., breast cancer (expressing concomitantly GRP- and NPY-receptors), gastrointestinal stromal tumor (GRP, CCK-B, and VPAC2 receptors), gastroenteropancreatic neuroendocrine tumors (GLP-1, CCK, and VPAC1 receptors), and the prostate cancer (prostate-specific membrane antigen or PSMA, and integrin or GRP receptors) (Ruzza & Calderan, 2011). These suggest that targeting more than one receptor class simultaneously would greatly enhance the sensitivity of tumor detection. In addition, some peptide receptors (e.g., αvβ3 integrin) are characterized by a low ligand internalization capacity, which improves in the presence of multimer ligands (Liu, 2010).

These aspects (co-expression on tumors and low internalization capacity) stimulate the development of multivalent and/or multireceptor ligands able to bind either to multiple homo (multivalent) or to hetero (multireceptor) receptors present on the surface of the tumor cell. The presence of more ligands induces a number of peculiar biological characteristics to the targeting molecules that are not present in the monovalent ligand. Polyvalent interactions are generally much stronger than the corresponding monovalent and offer the basis for mechanisms of agonizing or antagonizing biological activities that are fundamentally different from those available in monovalent system. Multivalent interactions may become particularly attractive and biologically relevant when the ligand-receptor binding is weak or the receptor density is low.

Linkers and/or scaffolds structure is important because it must present ligands simultaneously to their cognate receptors with minimal entropic penalty. The development of suitable linkers and/or scaffold structures, permitting the correct simultaneous presentation of ligands to their receptors, as well as the choice of opportune ligands for multivalency and/or multireceptor approaches may provide both new targets and strategies for designing new imaging agents.

3.2 Peptides in protein-protein interactions: The SH3 domain

From the huge array of "domain-peptide" complex class, a super-family of small domains is represented by the SH3 domains that it is identified in more than 350 different proteins in organisms ranging from yeasts to humans, showing a completely conserved structure.

The SH3 domain is a 60-amino acids non-catalytic protein domain identified in the sequence similarity region between the Src and Abl families of non-receptor tyrosine kinases (Mayer, 1988). This domain is structured on five β-strands arranged into two sheets packed at right angle. The first sheet is formed by strands A, E and the first half of B, while the second is formed by β-strands C, D, and the second half of B. The βA-strand is connected to the βB-strand by the long RT loop, which contain the ALY(F)DY(F) motif. The loops connecting strands βB and βC and strands βC and βD are called N-Src and Distal loop, respectively. The βC strand contains the WW dipeptide motif. After the βD strand, the polypeptide chain adopts a 3_{10} helix containing the PxxY motif that connects βD and βE strands (Marchiani, 2009; and references therein).

Crystal and solution structures of SH3 domain-ligand complexes reveal that the SH3 region involved in the interaction with the proline-rich peptide is a surface patch formed by the side chains of a few well-conserved residues: 1) one of the two aromatic residues in the ALY(F)DY(F) motif; 2) the first tryptophan of the WW dipeptide; 3) the PxxY motif. These residues are aligned to form a surface patch, quite hydrophobic, in which the aromatic side chains are stacked against each other (Figure 8).

The majority of SH3 domains recognize proline-rich peptides that adopt a left-handed poly-proline type II (PPII) helix containing two XP dipeptides, separated by a scaffolding residue (often a proline), forming the XPxXP core element (Feng, 1994). A basic residue, Lys or more frequently an Arg, is present either at the N-terminal or at the C-terminal to the XPxXP motif, permitting to classify Pro-rich ligands into two distinct groups named classes I and II, respectively.

The capability to recognize Lys or Arg residue into the binding motif is a selectivity mechanism found in SH3-ligands. For example, the Crk SH3 domain is selective for class II peptide-ligands containing a Lys residue (Knudsen, 1995). High resolution crystal structures of this domain bound to proline-rich peptides containing either lysine or arginine residue shown that while the lysine side-chain is in a extended configuration and the ε-amino group makes strong hydrogen bonds with three acidic residues (Asp147, Glu149 and Asp150), the arginine side chain does not adopt a low energy extended configuration and is involved in only two hydrogen-bonding interactions with proteins (Wu, 1995).

Structural analysis of either class I or class II peptides – SH3 complexes showed that these two ligand classes bind to SH3 domains in opposite orientations at the same binding site. The fact that ligands can bind either N-to-C or C-to-N orientations is a consequence of the two-fold rotational pseudo-symmetry possessed by the left-handed PPII helix (Siligardi &

Drake, 1995). This apparent ambiguity is resolved by the observation that important determinant for the binding to the two XP pockets is the surface presented by the alkylated amide nitrogen of the proline residue, and the carbonyl, the α-carbon and the side-chain of the preceding residue (Fernandez-Ballester, 2004).

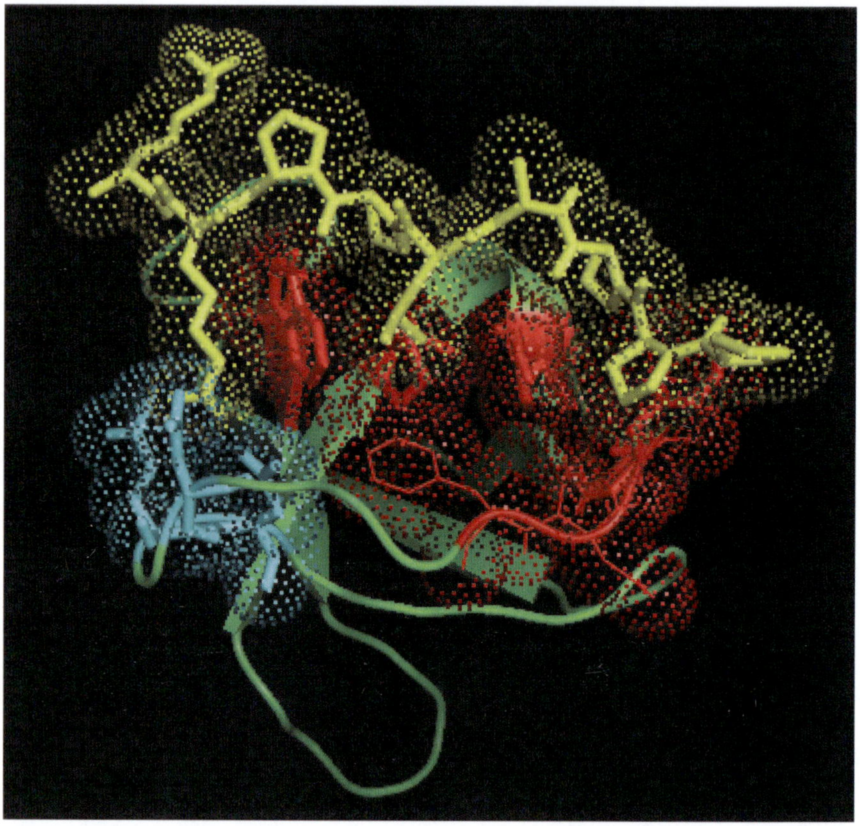

Fig. 8. The interactions occurring between the N-terminal SH3 domain of c-Crk and a lysine-containing proline-rich peptide are shown (PDB file 1CKA). The the ligand-peptide is highlighted in yellow. The aromatic surface patch is depicted in red, while the anionic side chain of the Asp and Glu residues involved in the interaction with the Lys residue in cyan. The Figure was drawn using the program PYMOL (K.L. DeLano, www.pymol.org).

Studies on the SH3 Fyn tyrosine kinase domain revealed that the Trp residue in the binding pocket can adopt two different orientations, determining the type of ligand able to bind to the domain. The motion of this residue is closely related to the presence of specific residues located in a key position; e.g. the residue numbering 132 of Fyn. When the conserved Trp residue can move, upon ligand binding, the structural conformation of the ligand fixes the conserved Trp either to SH3 class I or class II orientations. Unlike, when the motion of conserved Trp is hindered, the SH3 domain invariably presents the conserved Trp residue in a SH3 class II orientation, either in free or ligand-bound state (Fernandez-Ballester, 2004).

A recent finding demonstrated as some SH3 domains recognized not only the XPxXP sequences but that also other contacts are involved in the recruitment (Li, 2005), which may be classified into three arbitrary categories: (1) interactions that involve the XPxXP-motif docking surface of the SH3 domain to a peptide that does not conform to a classic XPxXP consensus; (2) interactions that do not involve the XPxXP-motif docking surface of the SH3 domain and (3) complex interactions, which may or may not involve residues contributing to the PxxP docking surface, but differ strongly from typical SH3 target peptide recognition.

4. Conclusion

The focus of medicinal chemistry is on the design of molecules that can manipulate disease-related biological targets for beneficial effects with low toxicity. As we have seen, peptides show great potential as both active drugs and diagnostics. The discovery and development of peptide-based drugs have both rational and empirical aspects. Random screening procedures can be used to identify ligands for known functional domains of target proteins, which can be followed by successive structural and computational analysis.

The principal medicinal chemistry challenges for a peptide chemist are to design molecules characterized by a sufficient duration of action, sufficient receptor specificity, and a both stable and appropriate formulation. Recently, studies of self-organizing peptides (amyloids) yielded important information for the development of long-acting peptides. Peptide constraint has been used both to prevent proteolysis and to bias binding toward particular receptor subtypes. The latter activity appears still to be evolving into a rational design approach but still requires attention to an appropriate strategy for successful commercial development.

Many of these issues are reminiscent of the "rocky road" which other biotecnology drugs, e.g., monoclonal antibodies, had to take before they became a commercial success. However, the development of peptides into tools for diagnostic purposes and drugs, based on their specificity of target recognition and their versatility of mechanisms, offers enormous promise. While peptides as drugs is a concept that still involves considerable challenge, encouragement may be gleaned from the words of Arthur C. Clarke (1917 – 2008) "...we do not have all the answers, but we have plenty of questions certainly worth thinking about; and when the technology is finally sufficiently advanced it is indistinguishable from magic".

5. Acknowledgment

I am very grateful to B. Biondi for the helpful discussions.

6. References

Bodansky, M. (1993) Principles of Peptide Synthesis. Springer-Verlag.

Bolzati, C., Refosco, F., Marchiani, A. & Ruzza, P. (2010) Tc-99m-Radiolabelled Peptides for Tumour Imaging: Present and Future *Curr. Med. Chem.*, Vol. 17, No. 24, pp. 2656-2683.

Chan, W.C. & White, P.D. (2000) Fmoc Solid Phase Peptide Synthesis: A Practical Approach. Oxford University Press.

Cudic, P. & Stawikowski, M. (2007) Pseudopeptide synthesis via Fmoc solid-phase synthetic methodology *Mini-Rev. Org. Chem.*, Vol. 4, No. 4, pp. 268-280.

Feng, S.B., Chen, J.K., Yu, H.T., Simon, J.A. & Schreiber, S.L. (1994) 2 Binding Orientations for Peptides to the Src Sh3 Domain - Development of a General-Model for Sh3-Ligand Interactions *Science*, Vol. 266, No. 5188, pp. 1241-1247.

Fernandez-Ballester, G., Blanes-Mira, C. & Serrano, L. (2004) The tryptophan switch: Changing ligand-binding specificity from type I to type II in SH3 domains *J. Mol. Biol.*, Vol. 335, No. 2, pp. 619-629.

Ginj, M., Zhang, H.W., Waser, B., Cescato, R., Wild, D., Wang, X.J., Erchegyi, J., Rivier, J., Macke, H.R. & Reubi, J.C. (2006) Radiolabeled somatostatin receptor antagonists are preferable to agonists for in vivo peptide receptor targeting of tumors *Proc. Natl. Acad. Sci. U. S. A.*, Vol. 103, No. 44, pp. 16436-16441.

Goodman, M., Toniolo, C., Moroder, L. & Felix, A. (2004) Houben-Weyl Methods in Organic Chemistry. Synthesis of Peptides and Peptidomimetics, Vol. E22a, E22b, E22c, E22d, E22e., Thieme, Stuttgart, New York.

Grauer, A. & Koenig, B. (2009) Peptidomimetics - A versatile route to biologically active compounds *Eur. J. Org. Chem.*, No. 30, pp. 5099-5111.

Hruby, V.J., Li, G.G., HaskellLuevano, C. & Shenderovich, M. (1997) Design of peptides, proteins, and peptidomimetics in chi space *Biopolymers*, Vol. 43, No. 3, pp. 219-266.

Karle, I.L. (1996) Flexibility in peptide molecules and restraints imposed by hydrogen bonds, the AiB residue, and core inserts *Biopolymers*, Vol. 40, No. 1, pp. 157-180.

Kazmierski, W. & Hruby, V.J. (1988) A New Approach to Receptor Ligand Design - Synthesis and Conformation of a New Class of Potent and Highly Selective Mu-Opioid Antagonists Utilizing Tetrahydroisoquinoline Carboxylic-Acid *Tetrahedron*, Vol. 44, No. 3, pp. 697-710.

Kessler, H. (1982) Conformation and Biological Activity of Cyclic Peptides *Angew. Chem. Int. Ed. Engl.*, Vol. 21, No. 7, pp. 512-523.

Knudsen, B.S., Zheng, J., Feller, S.M., Mayer, J.P., Burrell, S.K., Cowburn, D. & Hanafusa, H. (1995) Affinity and Specificity Requirements for the First Src Homology-3 Domain of the Crk Proteins *Embo J.*, Vol. 14, No. 10, pp. 2191-2198.

Lee, S., Xie, J. & Chen, X.Y. (2010) Peptides and Peptide Hormones for Molecular Imaging and Disease Diagnosis *Chem. Rev.*, Vol. 110, No. 5, pp. 3087-3111.

Li, S.S.C. (2005) Specificity and versatility of SH3 and other proline-recognition domains: structural basis and implications for cellular signal transduction *Biochem. J.*, Vol. 390, pp. 641-653.

Marchiani, A., Antolini, N., Calderan, A. & Ruzza, P. (2009) Atypical SH3 domain binding motifs: features and properties *Curr. Top. Pept. Protein Res.*, Vol. 10, pp. 45-56.

Mayer, B.J., Hamaguchi, M. & Hanafusa, H. (1988) A novel viral oncogene with structural similarity to phospholipase C *Nature*, Vol. 332, No. 6161, pp. 272-275.

Merrifield, R.B. (2006) Solid-Phase Peptide Synthesis. In: *Advances in Enzymology and Related Areas of Molecular Biology*, John Wiley & Sons, Inc., pp. 221-296.

Nestor, J.J., Jr. (2009) The medicinal chemistry of peptides *Curr. Med. Chem.*, Vol. 16, No. 33, pp. 4399-4418.

Pawson, T. (2004) Protein interactions in signaling and cell polarity *Faseb J.*, Vol. 18, No. 8, pp. C220.

Quancard, J., Labonne, A.l., Jacquot, Y., Chassaing, G.r., Lavielle, S. & Karoyan, P. (2004) Asymmetric synthesis of 3-substituted proline chimeras bearing polar side chains of proteinogenic amino acids. J. Org. Chem., Vol. 69, No. 23, pp. 7940-7948.

Ramachandran, G.N., Ramakrishnan, C. & Sasisekharan, V. (1963) Stereochemistry of polypeptide chain configurations *J. Mol. Biol.*, Vol. 7, No. 4, pp. 95-99.

Reubi, J.C. & Landolt, A.M. (1984) High density of somatostatin receptors in pituitary tumors from acromegalic patients. *J. Clin. Endocrinol. Metab*, Vol. 59, pp. 1148-1151.

Reubi, J.C. (2003) Peptide receptors as molecular targets for cancer diagnosis and therapy *Endocr. Rev.*, Vol. 24, No. 4, pp. 389-427.

Reubi, J.C., Gugger, M. & Waser, B. (2002) Co-expressed peptide receptors in breast cancer as a molecular basis for in vivo multireceptor tumour targeting *Eur. J. Nucl. Med. Mol. Imaging*, Vol. 29, No. 7, pp. 855-862.

Rufini, V., Calcagni, M.L. & Baum, R.P. (2006) Imaging of neuroendocrine tumors *Semin. Nucl. Med.*, Vol. 36, No. 3, pp. 228-247.

Ruzza, P. & Calderan, A. (2011) Radiolabeled peptide-receptor ligands in tumor imaging *Expert Opin. Med. Diagn.*, Vol. 5, No. 5, pp. 411-424.

Ruzza, P., Donella-Deana, A., Calderan, A., Brunati, A., Massimino, M.L., Elardo, S., Mattiazzo, A., Pinna, L.A. & Borin, G. (2001) Antennapedia/HS1 chimeric phosphotyrosyl peptide: Conformational properties, binding capability to c-Fgr SH2 domain and cell permeability *Biopolymers*, Vol. 60, No. 4, pp. 290-306.

Ruzza, P., Siligardi, G., Donella-Deana, A., Calderan, A., Hussain, R., Rubini, C., Cesaro, L., Osler, A., Guiotto, A., Pinna, L.A. & Borin, G. (2006) 4-Fluoroproline derivative peptides: effect on PPII conformation and SH3 affinity *J. Pept. Sci.*, Vol. 12, No. 7, pp. 462-471.

Schottelius, M., Poethko, T., Herz, M., Reubi, J.C., Kessler, H., Schwaiger, M. & Wester, H.J. (2004) First F-18-labeled tracer suitable for routine clinical imaging of sst receptor-expressing tumors using positron emission tomography *Clin. Cancer Res.*, Vol. 10, No. 11, pp. 3593-3606.

Siligardi, G. & Drake, A.F. (1995) The Importance of Extended Conformations and, in Particular, the P-Ii Conformation for the Molecular Recognition of Peptides *Biopolymers*, Vol. 37, No. 4, pp. 281-292.

Siligardi, G., Ruzza, P., Hussain, R., Cesaro, L., Brunati, A., Pinna, L. & Donella-Deana, A. (2011) The SH3 domain of HS1 protein recognizes lysine-rich polyproline motifs *Amino Acids*, published on-line.

Spatola, A. (1983) In: *Peptides and Proteins*, Weinstein, B., Ed.; Marcel Dekker Inc.: New York, Vol. 3, pp. 267-357.

Toniolo, C., Crisma, M., Formaggio, F. & Peggion, C. (2001) Control of peptide conformation by the Thorpe-Ingold effect (C^{α}-tetrasubstitution) *Biopolymers*, Vol. 60, No. 6, pp. 396-419.

Wu, X.D., Knudsen, B., Feller, S.M., Zheng, J., Sali, A., Cowburn, D., Hanafusa, H. & Kuriyan, J. (1995) Structural Basis for the Specific Interaction of Lysine- Containing Proline-Rich Peptides with the N-Terminal Sh3 Domain of C-Crk *Structure*, Vol. 3, No. 2, pp. 215-226.

Wuthrich, K., Vonfreyberg, B., Weber, C., Wider, G., Traber, R., Widmer, H. & Braun, W. (1991) Receptor-Induced Conformation Change of the Immunosuppressant Cyclosporine-A *Science*, Vol. 254, No. 5034, pp. 953-954.

Zuckermann, R.N. & Kodadek, T. (2009) Peptoids as potential therapeutics *Curr. Opin. Mol. Ther.*, Vol. 11, No. 3, pp. 299-307.

15

Carbonic Anhydrase Inhibitors and Activators: Small Organic Molecules as Drugs and Prodrugs

Murat Şentürk[1], Hüseyin Çavdar[2], Oktay Talaz[3] and Claudiu T. Supuran[4]
[1]*Ağrı İbrahim Çeçen University*
[2]*Dumlupınar University*
[3]*Karamanoğlu Mehmetbey University*
[4]*University of Florence*
[1,2,3]*Turkey*
[4]*Italy*

1. Introduction

This chapter concerns influences of inhibitors and activators on carbonic anhydrase isoenzymes of various living systems. Carbonic anhydrase (EC 4.2.1.1., CA) is a pH regulatory/metabolic enzyme in all life kingdoms, found in organisms all over the phylogenetic tree (Supuran, 2008a,b,c) catalyzing the hydration of carbon dioxide to bicarbonate and the corresponding dehydration of bicarbonate in acidic medium with regeneration of CO_2 (Sly and Hu, 1995). 16 isozymes have been described up to now in mammals, the most active ones as catalysts for carbon dioxide hydration being CA II and CA IX (Sly and Hu, 1995; Ozensoy et al., 2004; Bayram et al., 2008; Senturk et al., 2009; Hilvo et al, 2008). The sixteen isozymes differ in their subcellular localization, catalytic activity and susceptibility to different classes of inhibitors. Some of them are cytosolic (CA I, CA II, CA III, CA VII and CA XIII), others are membrane bound (CA IV, CA IX, CA XII and CA XIV), two are mitochondrial (CA VA and CA VB), and one is secreted in saliva (CA VI). It has been reported that CA XV isoform is not expressed in humans or in other primates, but it is abundant in rodents and other vertebrates (Table 1.) (Nair et al., 1994; Parkkila et al., 1996; Pastorekava et al., 2004; Bayram et al., 2008; Innocenti et al., 2008a,b; Senturk et al., 2009; Ekinci et al., 2011). CAs are produced in a variety of tissues where they participate in several important biological processes such as acid-base balance, respiration, carbon dioxide and ion transport, bone resorption, ureagenesis, gluconeogenesis, lipogenesis and body fluid generation (Supuran, 2008a,b,c). CA isozymes involved in these processes are important therapeutic targets with the potential to be inhibited / activated for the treatment of a range of disorders such as edema, glaucoma, obesity, cancer, epilepsy and osteoporosis (Innocenti et al., 2008b; Ekinci et al., 2007; Ekinci et al., 2011).

Isozyme	Catalytic activity (CO_2 hydration)	Affinity for sulfonamides	Sub-cellular localization
CA I	Low (10%of thatof CAII)	Medium	Cytosol
CA II	High	Very high	Cytosol
CA III	Very low (0.3%of thatof CAII)	Very low	Cytosol
CA IV	High	High	Membrane-bound
CA VA	Moderate-high[a]	High	Mitochondria
CA VB	Moderate	High	Mitochondria
CA VI	Moderate	Medium-High	Secreted into saliva/milk
CA VII	High	Very high	Cytosol
CARP VIII	Acatalytic	*	Cytosol
CA IX	High	High	Membrane-bound
CARP X	Acatalytic	*	Cytosol
CARP XI	Acatalytic	*	Cytosol
CA XII	Medium-Low	Very high	Membrane-bound
CA XIII	LOW	High	Unknown
CA XIV	Moderate	High	Membrane-bound

[a]Moderate at pH 7.4, high at pH 8.2 or higher.
[b]CA XIII has not been isolated as a protein but has been identified from an expressed sequence tag (EST) derived from a mouse mammary gland cDNA library.
*The native CARP isozymes do not contain Zn (II), so that their affinity for the sulfonamide inhibitors has not been measured. By site-directed mutagenesis it is possible to modify these proteins and transform them in enzymes with CA-like activity which probably are inhibited by sulfonamides, but no studies on this subject are available presently.

Table 1. Higher vertebrate α-CA isozymes, their Relative CO_2 hydrase activity, affinity for sulfonamide inhibitors, and sub-cellular localization

In addition to the physiological reaction, the reversible hydration of CO_2 to bicarbonate (reaction 1, Scheme 1), CAs catalyze a variety of other reactions, such as: the hydration of cyanate to carbamic acid, or of cyanamide to urea (reactions 2 and 3); the aldehyde hydration to gem-diols (reaction 4); the hydrolysis of carboxylic, or sulfonic (reactions 5, 6), as well as other less investigated hydrolytic processes, such as those described by equations 7-10 in Scheme 1 (Supuran et al., 1997; Supuran and Scozzafava, 2000b; Guerri et al., 2000). It should be mentioned that the previously reported phosphatase activity of CA III was recently proved to be an artefact (Kim et al., 2000). It is unclear at this moment whether CA catalyzed reactions other than the CO_2 hydration has physiological significance.

2. Carbonic anhydrase inhibitors

As will be discussed shortly, many of these isozymes are important targets for the design of inhibitors with clinical applications. CA inhibition with sulfanilamide (**1**) discovered by Mann and Keilin (Krebs, 1948) was the beginning of a great scientific adventure that led to important drugs, such as the antihypertensives of benzothiadiazine and high-ceiling diuretics type (Supuran 1994), the sulfonamides with CA inhibitory properties mainly used as antiglaucoma agents (Krebs, 1948; Supuran, 1994; Mansoor et al., 2000), some antithyroid drugs (Krebs, 1948), the hypoglycemic sulphonamides (Maren et al., 1983) and, ultimately,

$$O{=}C{=}O + H_2O \longleftrightarrow HCO_3^- + H^+ \quad (1)$$

$$O{=}C{=}NH + H_2O \longleftrightarrow NH_2COOH \quad (2)$$

$$HN{=}C{=}NH + H_2O \longleftrightarrow NH_2CONH_2 \quad (3)$$

$$RCHO + H_2O \longleftrightarrow RCH(OH)_2 \quad (4)$$

$$RCOOAr + H_2O \longleftrightarrow RCOOH + ArOH \quad (5)$$

$$RSO_3Ar + H_2O \longleftrightarrow RSO_3H + ArOH \quad (6)$$

$$ArF + H_2O \longleftrightarrow HF + ArOH \quad (7)$$

(Ar = 2,4-dinitrophenyl)

$$PhCH_2OCOCl + H_2O \longleftrightarrow PhCH_2OH + CO_2 + HCl \quad (8)$$

$$RSO_2Cl + H_2O \longleftrightarrow RSO_3H + HCl \quad (9)$$

(R = Me; Ph)

$$ArOPO_3H_2 + H_2O \longleftrightarrow ArOH + H_3PO_4 \quad (10)$$

Scheme 1. Reactions (1-10) catalyzed by α-CAs.

some novel types of anticancer agents (Supuran and Scozzafava, 2000). The report of Krebs (1948) that mainly the unsubstituted aromatic sulfonamides of type $ArSO_2NH_2$ act as strong CAIs, and that the potency of such compounds is drastically reduced by N-substitution of the sulfonamide moiety, constituted the beginning of extensive structure-activity correlations, which led to some valuable drugs during a short period of time. Among the active structures found by Krebs were also the azodyes **2** (prontosil red) and **3**, derived from sulfanilamide (Maren, 1976; Krebs, 1948; Supuran et al., 2003). The early stages of CAIs development have thouroughly been reviewed by Maren (Maren, 1976; Maren, 1967) whereas literature till 1993 was reviewed by Supuran (Supuran and Scozzafava, 2000; Supuran et al., 2003) and more incompletely (up to 1996) by Mansoor et al. (2000). Thus, in this review we will concentrate on the recent developments in this field that led to important advances in the design of topically acting antiglaucoma sulfonamides, isozyme-specific inhibitors, inhibitors with modified sulfonamide moieties, antitumor sulfonamides, as well as diagnostic tools and biosensors based on this class of pharmacological agents (Supuran et al., 2003).

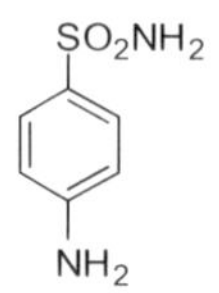

1

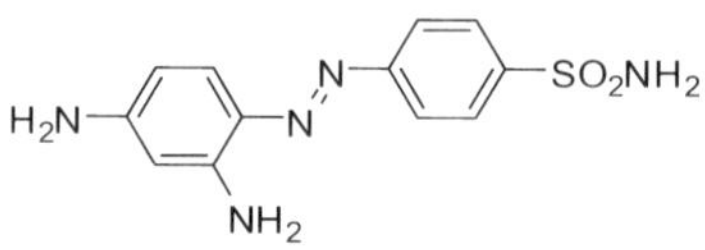

2

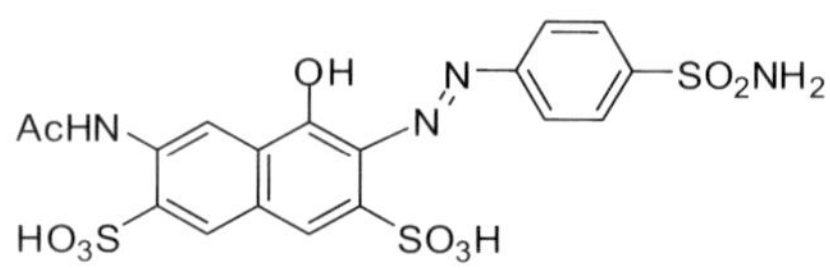

3

CAs are inhibited by four main mechanisms: (*i*) coordination of the inhibitor to the Zn(II) ion by replacing the zinc-bound water/hydroxide ion and leading to a tetrahedral geometry of Zn(II) (e.g., the sulfonamides, Fig. 1A) (Supuran 2008a; Alterio et al., 2009). (*ii*) Addition of the inhibitor to the metal coordination sphere, when the Zn(II) ion is in a trigonal bipyramidal geometry (e.g., the thiocyanate adduct, Fig. 1B) (Supuran 2008a; Alterio et al., 2009). (*iii*) Anchoring of the inhibitor to the Zn(II)-bound solvent molecule, i.e., a water or hydroxide ion (e.g. phenol, Fig. 1C) (Nair et al., 1994) (*iv*) Occlusion of the CA active site entrance, with coumarins (Maresca et al., 2009; Maresca et al., 2010) lacosamide (Temperini et al., 2010) and fullerenes (Innocenti et al., 2010) binding in this way, as shown schematically in Fig. 1D for a hydrolyzed coumarin derivative (Maresca et al., 2009). All these binding modes have been demonstrated by means of X-ray crystallography of enzyme-inhibitor adducts (Nair et al., 1994; Supuran, 2008a; Maresca et al., 2009; Durdagi et al., 2011). It should be noted that passing from sulfonamides and their bioisosteres (sulfamates, sulfamides, etc.) to inhibitors occluding the entrance of the active site, the role of the Zn(II) ion is constantly diminishing in its interaction with the inhibitor molecule (Nair et al., 1994; Supuran, 2008a; Maresca et al., 2009; Durdagi et al., 2011). This phenomenon has important consequences for the drug design of CA inhibitors (CAIs), because the bottom of the active site cavity is very much conserved in the 16 CA isozymes described so far in mammals, whereas the regions with the highest variation in amino acid sequence, therefore the highest degree of structural diversity, are just those at the entrance of the active site (Supuran and Scozzafava, 2007b; Supuran, 2008a; Alterio et al., 2009). Indeed, phenols, (Ekinci et al., 2010; Durdagi et al., 2011) but also coumarins (Maresca et al., 2009; Maresca et al., 2010) and other types of non-zinc binder inhibitors (Alterio et al., 2009; Ekinci et al.,

2011) were recently shown to lead to isozyme-selective CAIs, a goal difficult to achieve with the classical sulfonamide/sulfamate inhibitors (Supuran, 2008a; Zu and Sly, 1990).

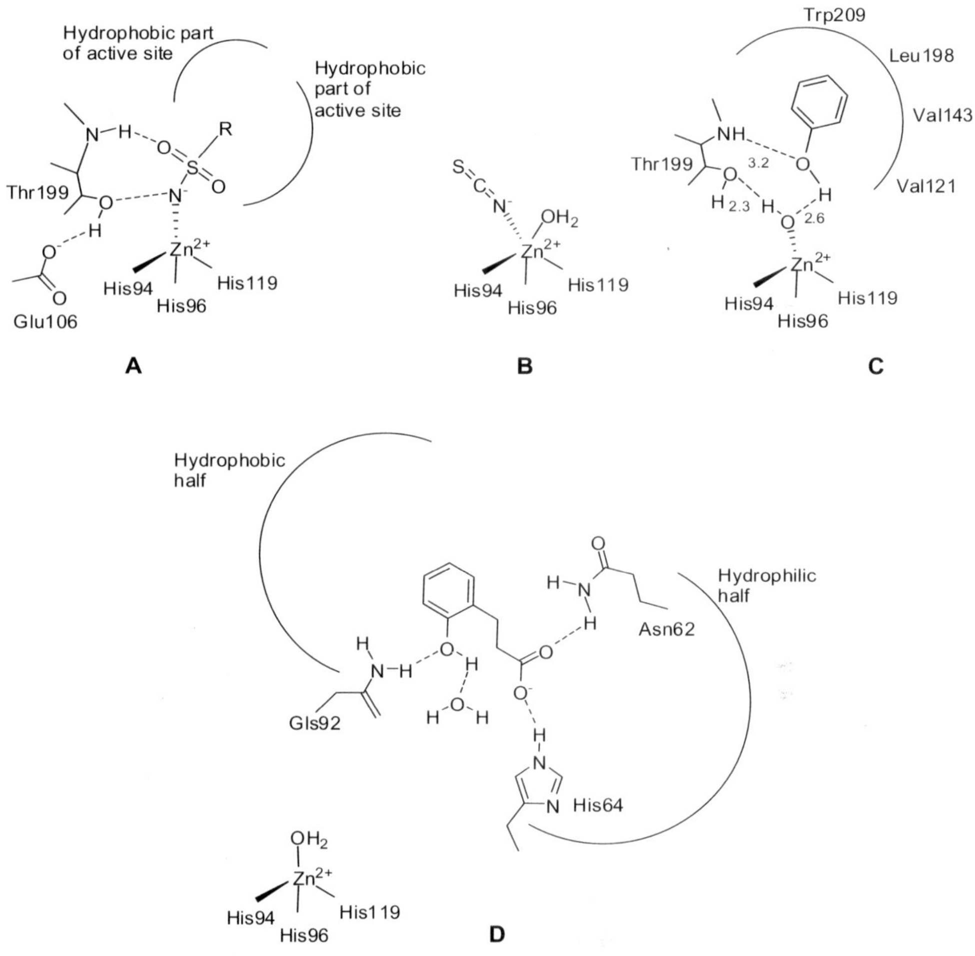

Fig. 1. Schematic representation for the three main CA inhibition mechanisms: (**A**) Sulfonamides (and their isosteres, sulfamate, and sulfamide) substitute the fourth zinc ligand and bind in tetrahedral geometry of the metal ion (Alterio et al., 2009); (**B**) Inorganic anion inhibitors (thiocyanate as an example) add to the metal ion coordination sphere leading to trigonal bipyramidal adducts (Alterio et al., 2009); (**C**) Phenols anchor to the Zn(II) coordinated water molecule/hydroxide ion (Nair et al., 1994); (**D**) Coumarins (hydrolyzed in situ to 2-hydroxycinnamic acids) occlude the entrance of the active site cavity, interacting both with hydrophilic and hydrophobic amino acid residues. The inhibitor does not interact at all with the catalytically crucial Zn(II) ion which is coordinated by three His residues and a water molecule (Maresca et al., 2009; Maresca et al., 2010).

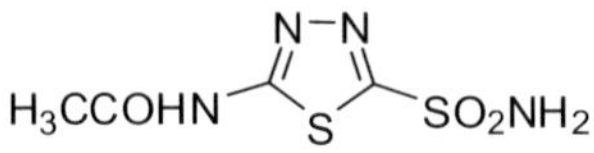
4

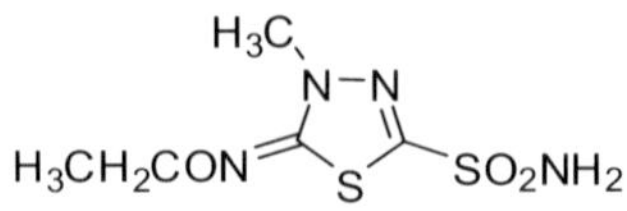
5

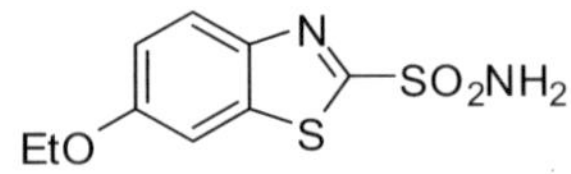
6

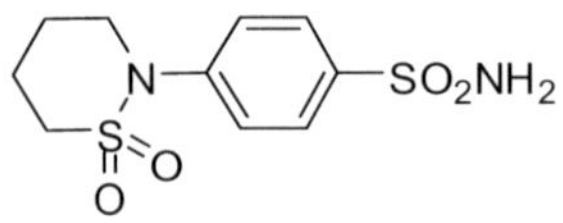
7

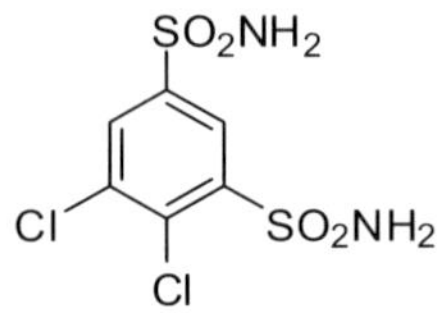
8

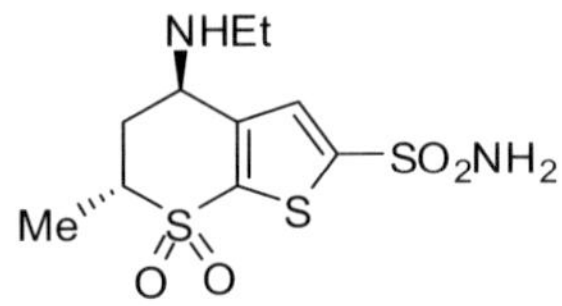
9

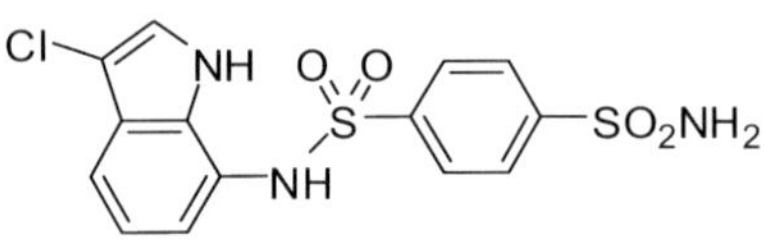
10

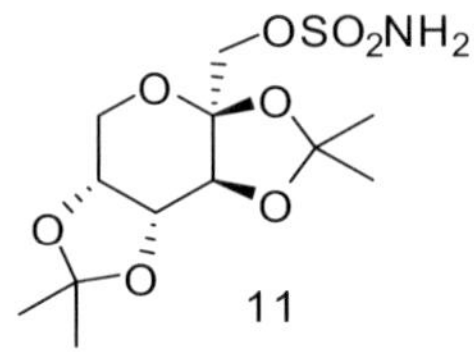
11

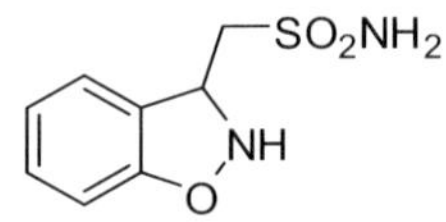
12

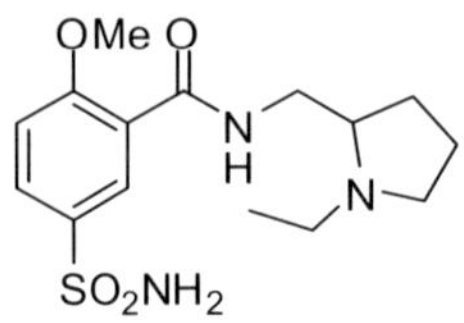
13

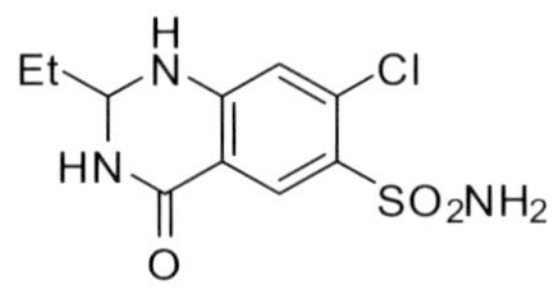
14

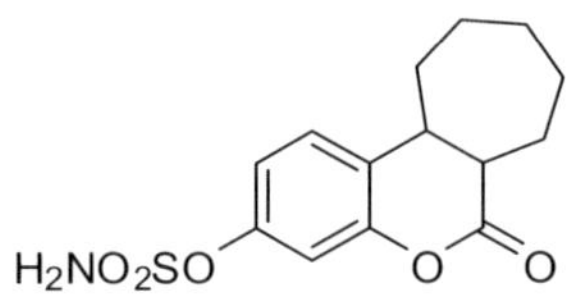
15

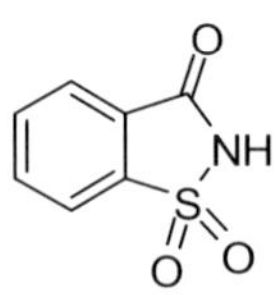
16

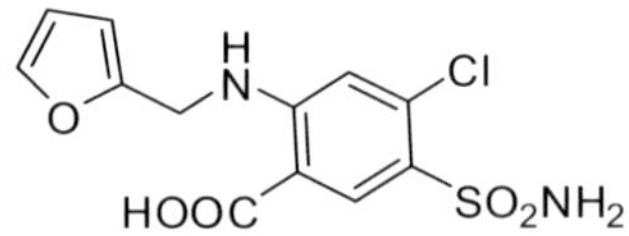
17

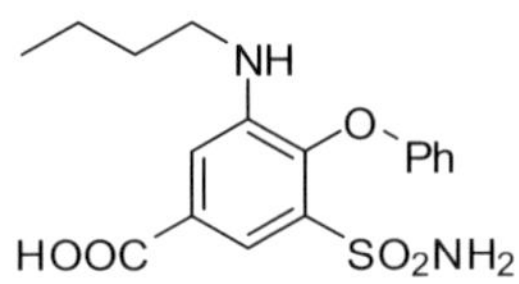
18

Fig. 2. CAIs include the classical inhibitors acetazolamide (**4**), methazolamide, (**5**) ethoxzolamide (**6**), sulthiame (**7**) and dichlorophenamide (**8**). CAIs also include more recent drugs/investigational agents such as dorzolamide (**9**), indisulam (**10**), topiramate (**11**), zonisamide (**12**), sulpiride (**13**), COUMATE (**15**), saccharin (**16**). Many of these compounds were initially developed years ago during the search for diuretics, among which the thiazides, compounds, as well as derivative **14** are stil widely clinically used (Supuran, 2008a). However, some of these enzyme inhibitors could also be used for the systemic treatment of glaucoma (see below), and more recently, newer derivatives have been discovered that have the potential as topical antiglaucoma agents, as well as antitumour, anti-obesity or anti-infective drugs (Supuran, 2008a,b,c).

3. Carbonic anhydrase activators

Carbonic anhydrase (CA, EC 4.2.1.1) inhibition with sulfonamides, discovered by Mann and Keilin (1940), and its activation by different classes of compounds, reported by Leiner (1940), although simultaneous, had completely different consequences for research of these enzymes and their modulators of activity. Whereas CA inhibitors (CAIs) were extensively studied, leading to a detailed understanding of the catalytic and inhibition mechanisms and also to several valuable drugs ((Supuran and Scozzafava, 2001), CA activators (CAAs) constituted a controversial issue immediately after they were first described (Kiese, 1941). Thus, activation of crude human red cell enzyme (a mixture of isozymes CA I and CA II) by different compounds, such as histamine, amino acids, and some purine derivatives, has been reported and retracted several times by the above mentioned and other authors (van Goor, 1948; Supuran and Scozzafava, 2000), without arriving at a clear-cut answer regarding the mere existence of such a class of CA activity modulators. This topic, then, received little attention from the scientific community for at least two reasons: (i) the statement by Clark and Perrin (1951) that activators of CA do not exist and (ii) the idea that the reported activation is not a phenomenon per se but an artifact generally due to restoration of CA activity possibly lost in the presence of adventitious metal ions or other impurities (or due to enzyme adsorption at interfaces, or even due to enzyme denaturation followed by renaturation in the presence of activators) (Maren, 1967) Leiner (1940), the researcher whose role in discovering this important class of modulators of CA activity should be completely revaluated, observed among others that the activation was readily detected when working with highly purified enzyme preparations, and this may explain the large discrepancies between the different early studies describing this phenomenon. Only recently Supuran's group reported the X-ray crystallographic structures of adducts of the human isozyme hCA II with different activators, proving undoubtedly the existence of this class of modulators of enzyme activity as well as elucidating their mechanism of action at the molecular level (Maren, 1967; Briganti et al., 1997; Briganti et al., 1998; Scozzafava and Supuran, 2002). The very recent report (Briganti et al., 1998) that some CAAs (such as phenylalanine and imidazole) administered to experimental animals may produce an important pharmacological enhancement of synaptic efficacy, spatial learning, and memory proves that this class of relatively unexplored enzyme modulators may have pharmacological applications in conditions in which learning and memory are impaired, such as for example Alzheimer's disease or aging. One must also mention that it was previously reported that the levels of CA are significantly diminished in the brain of patients affected by Alzheimer's disease (Sun and Alkon, 2001), and these facts strongly support the involvement of different CA isozymes in cognitive functions (Briganti et al., 1997; Briganti et al., 1998; Sun and Alkon, 2001; Meier-Roge et al., 1984; Scozzafava and Supuran, 2002).

The binding of CA activators (CAAs) to various isozymes, such as CA I, II and IV, was studied by kinetic and X-ray crystallographic techniques (the last techniques were applied only for the cytosolic isozymes I and II) (Ilies et al., 2002; Scozzafava and Supuran 2002a,b;

Temperini et al., 2007), which showed the activator to intervene in the rate-determining step of the catalytic cycle, that is, the shuttling of protons between the active site and the reaction medium, a process which in most CA isoforms is assisted by a histidine residue (His64, CA I numbering) placed in the middle of the active site cavity (Scozzafava and Supuran 2002a,b; Temperini et al., 2007). CAAs, there is the possibility of alternative proton transfer pathways, involving a protonatable moiety of the activator bound within the enzyme active site, which explains the enhanced overall catalytic efficiency, reflected in the augmentation of k_{cat}, without any effect on K_M, for all isoforms investigated up to now in detail (i.e., CA I, II, IV, VA, VII, XIII, and XIV) (Ilies et al., 2002; Scozzafava and Supuran 2002a,b; Temperini et al., 2007). X-Ray crystallography of adducts of human CA (hCA) II with histamine (**19**) (Birganti et al., 1997), L- and D-phenylalanine (**20**) (Temperini et al., 2005), and L- and D-histidine (**21**) (Temperini et al., 2006a), as well as the adduct of hCA I with L-His (**21**) (Temperini et al., 2006b), allowed a better understanding of the CA activation phenomenon at the molecular level, bringing also new insights into problems of ligand recognition by an enzyme active site, since it has been observed that enantiomers such as L-/D-His and L-/D-Phe bind in a very different manner to hCA II, interacting with different amino acid residues from the activator binding site. In addition, the interaction between the two best studied isozymes, that is, hCA I and II, with the same activator, L-His, was also very different, with the activator binding deep within the active site cavity in the case of hCA I, and toward the external of the cavity for hCA II. These studies are helpful for the design of better CAAs or for obtaining compounds with selectivity for an isozyme, and less affinity for another one which is not desirable to be activated (or inhibited) (Scozzafava and Supuran 2002a,b; Temperini et al., 2005a,b; Temperini et al., 2007).

L-Adrenaline (**22**), one of the neurotransmitter catecholamines released by the sympathetic nervous system and adrenal medulla in response to a range of stresses in order to regulate the host physiological functions, is involved in regulation of blood pressure, vasoconstriction, cardiac stimulation, relaxation of the smooth muscles (such as the bronchial ones) as well as in several metabolic processes (Hoffman, and Lefkowitz, 1996). As a consequence, 4 has a variety of clinical uses, such as among others for relieving respiratory distress in asthma, in treating hypersensitivity reactions due to various allergens, cardiac arrest, or as a topical hemostatic agent, etc . (Hoffman, and Lefkowitz, 1996; Rawas-Qalaji, et al., 2006).

The activating effects of adrenaline (**22**) on CA II (of bovine origin, bCA II) were first investigated by this group (Supuran and Puscas, 1994), being shown that the compound is a weaker CAA, as compared to histamine, aromatic/heterocyclic amino acids or other structurally related amines investigated in the same study. Temperini et al. (2007) decided to investigate in more detail its interaction with various physiologically relevant CA isozymes,1-5 such as CA I, II, IV, VA, VII, and XIV (all of them present among others in the brain).1 Temperini et al. (2007) reported kinetic investigations regarding the activation of the above-mentioned isoforms with L-adrenline (**22**), as well as an X-ray crystallographic study of the hCA II–4 adduct. Same study work may bring a better understanding of the CA activation processes, potentially useful for the design of pharmacological agents, whereas from the chemical point of view, it reveals a completely new interaction between the activator and the enzyme, which explains at the molecular level the lower efficacy of adrenaline as a CA II activator (Temperini et al., 2007).

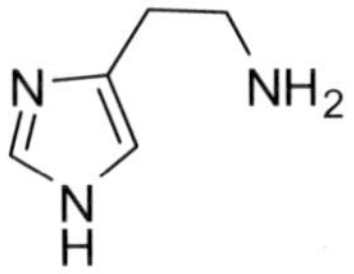

19

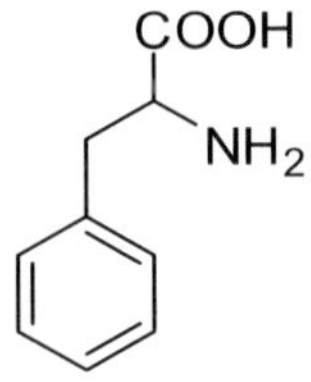

20

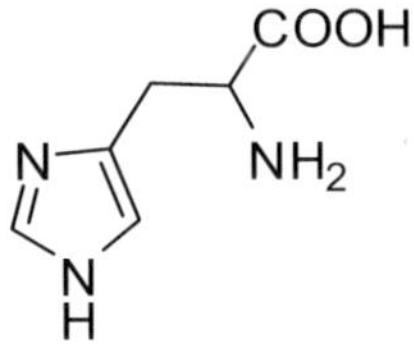

21

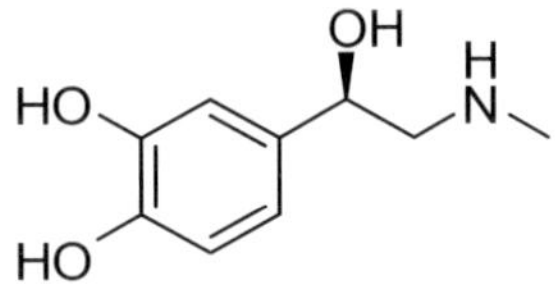

22

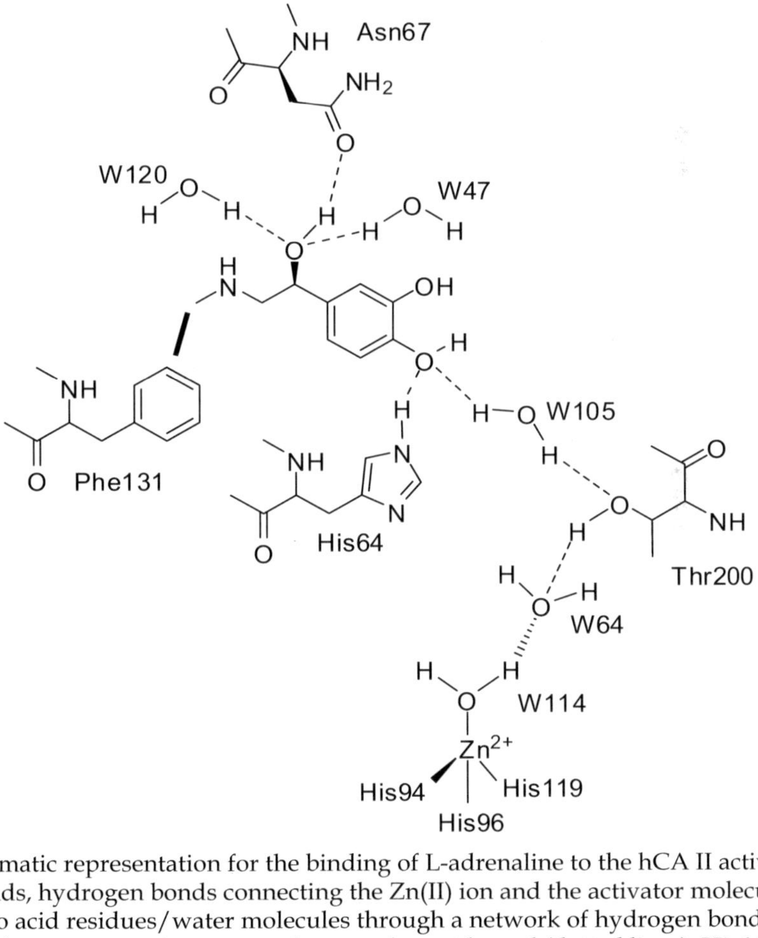

Fig. 3. Schematic representation for the binding of L-adrenaline to the hCA II active site. The Zn(II) ligands, hydrogen bonds connecting the Zn(II) ion and the activator molecule with other amino acid residues/water molecules through a network of hydrogen bonds, stabilizing the enzyme-activator complex, are also evidenced (dotted lines). His64 is shown only in the 'in' conformation, the only one making a hydrogen bond with the activator molecule. The 'out' conformation of His64 does not interact with the activator. The methylamino group of 4 does not participate in any polar interaction, being rather close to the phenyl ring of Phe131 (bold line) (Temperini et al., 2007).

Temperini et al. (2007) studied may also shed new light in the recognition processes by metalloenzymes of ligands which do not directly interact with the metal ion, phenomena far less investigated up to now, since the majority of ligands interacting with metalloenzymes usually directly coordinate the metal ion(s) from the enzyme active site.

The X-ray crystal structure of the CA II L-adrenaline adduct revealed the reason why this compound is a weaker activator as compared to histamine (**19**) and related biogenic amines/amino acids. Thus, in contrast to other activators investigated earlier, L-adrenaline (**22**) plugs the entrance of the active site cavity, obstructing it almost completely. In this conformation, it is unable to facilitate the shuttling of protons between the active site and the environment, also because the pKas of its protonatable moieties are in the range of 8.6–11.34. On the contrary, histamine bound to the enzyme active site adopts a conformation that allows its imidazolic moiety (with a pKa around 7) to easily participate in proton shuttling, similarly with residue His64, the natural proton shuttle amino acid in the CA II active site. These findings explain thus that both the steric requirements (orientation in which the activator binds within the active site) and electronic factors (pKa of the proton shuttle moiety) are important for a compound to act as an effective CA activator, and may shed new light in the recognition processes by metalloenzymes of ligands which do not directly interact with the metal ion (Temperini et al., 2007).

4. References

Alterio, V.; Hilvo, M.; Di Fiore, A.; Supuran, C.T.; Pan, P.; Parkkila, S.; Scaloni, A.; Pastorek, J.; Pastorekova, S.; Pedone, C.; Scozzafava, A.; Monti, S.M. & De Simone, G. (2009). Crystal structure of the extracellular catalytic domain of the tumor-associated human carbonic anhydrase IX. *Proceedings of the National Academy of Sciences of the United States of America*, 106, 16233-16238.

Bayram, E.; Senturk, M.; Kufrevioglu, O.I. & Supuran, C.T. (2008). In vitro inhibition of salicylic acid derivatives on human cytosolic carbonic anhydrase isozymes I and II. *Bioorganic and Medicinal Chemistry*, 16, 9101-9105.

Briganti, F.; Iaconi, V.; Mangani, S.; Orioli, P.; Scozzafava, A.; Vernaglione, G. & Supuran, C.T. (1998). A ternary complex of carbonic anhydrase: X-ray crystallographic structure of the adduct of human carbonic anhydrase II with the activator phenylalanine and the inhibitor azide. *Inorganica Chimica Acta*, 275-276, 295-300.

Briganti, F.; Mangani, S.; Orioli, P.; Scozzafava, A.; Vernaglione, G. & Supuran, C.T. (1997). Carbonic anhydrase activators: X-ray crystallographic and spectroscopic investigations for the interaction of isozymes I and II with histamine. *Biochemistry*, 36, 10384-10392.

Clark, A.M. & Perrin, D.D. (1951). A reinvestigation of the question of activators of carbonic anhydrase. *Biochemical Journal*, 48, 495-503.

Durdagi, S.; Senturk, M.; Ekinci, D.; Balaydin, H.T.; Goksu, S.; Kufrevioglu, O.I.; Innocenti, A.; Scozzafava, A. & Supuran, C.T. (2011). Kinetic and docking studies of phenol-based inhibitors of carbonic anhydrase isoforms I, II, IX and XII evidence a new binding mode within the enzyme active site. *Bioorganic & Medicinal Chemistry*, 19, 1381-1389.

Ekinci, D.; Beydemir, S. & Kufrevioglu, O.I. (2007). In vitro inhibitory effects of some heavy metals on human erythrocyte carbonic anhydrases. *Journal of Enzyme Inhibition and Medicinal Chemistry*, 22, 745-750.

Ekinci, D.; Cavdar, H.; Talaz, O.; Senturk, M. & Supuran, C.T. (2010). NO-releasing esters show carbonic anhydrase inhibitory action against human isoforms I and II. *Bioorganic & Medicinal Chemistry*, 18, 3559-3563.

Ekinci, D.; Ceyhun, S.B.; Senturk, M.; Erdem, D.; Kufrevioglu, O.I. & Supuran, C.T. (2011). Characterization and anions inhibition studies of an α-carbonic anhydrase from the teleost fish Dicentrarchus labrax. *Bioorganic & Medicinal Chemistry*, 19, 744-748.

Guerri, A.; Briganti, F.; Scozzafava, A.; Supuran, C.T. & Mangani, S. (2000). Mechanism of cyanamide hydration catalyzed by carbonic anhydrase II suggested by cryogenic X-ray diffraction. *Biochemistry*, 39, 12391-12397.

Hilvo, M.; Baranauskiene, L.; Salzano, A.M.; Scaloni, A.; Matulis, D.; Innocenti, A.; Scozzafava, A.; Monti, S.M.; Di Fiore, A.; De Simone, G.; Lindfors, M.; Janis, J.; Valjakka, J.; Pastorekova, S.; Pastorek, J.; Kulomaa, M.S.; Nordlund, H.R.; Supuran, C.T. & Parkkila, S. (2008). Biochemical Characterization of CA IX, One of the Most Active Carbonic Anhydrase Isozymes. *Journal of Biological Chemistry*, 283, 27799-27809.

Hoffman, B.B.; Lefkowitz, R.J. (1996). Catecholamines, sympathomimetic drugs, and adrenergic receptor antagonists. In Goodman's the pharmacological basis of therapeutics; Hardman, J.G.; Limbird, L.E.; Molinoff, P.B.; Ruddon, R.W.; Goodman Gilman, A., Eds., 9th ed.; McGraw-Hill: New York, pp 199-237.

Ilies, M.; Banciu, M.D.; Ilies, M.A.; Scozzafava, A.; Caproiu, M.T. & Supuran, C.T. (2002). Carbonic anhydrase activators: Design of high affinity isozymes I, II, and IV activators, incorporating Tri-/Tetrasubstituted-pyridinium-azole moieties. *Journal of Medicinal Chemistry*, 45, 504-510.

Innocenti, A.; Hilvo, M.; Scozzafava, A.; Parkkila, S. & Supuran, C.T. (2008a). Carbonic anhydrase inhibitors: Inhibition of the new membrane-associated isoform XV with phenols *Bioorganic & Medicinal Chemistry Letters*, 18, 3593-3596.

Innocenti, A.; Vullo, D.; Scozzafava, A. & Supuran, C.T. (2008b). Carbonic anhydrase inhibitors. Interactions of phenols with the 12 catalytically active mammalian isoforms (CA I-XIV). *Bioorganic & Medicinal Chemistry Letters*, 18, 1583-1587.

Innocenti, A.; Durdagi, S.; Doostdar, N.; Strom, T.A.; Barron, A.R. & Supuran, C.T. (2010) Nanoscale enzyme inhibitors: fullerenes inhibit carbonic anhydrase by occluding the active site entrance. *Bioorganic & Medicinal Chemistry*, 18, 2822-2828.

Kiese, M. (1941). Die Aktivierung der Kohlensaureanhydrase. *Naturwissenschaften*, 29, 116-117.

Kim, G.; Selengut, J. & Levine, R.L. (2000). Carbonic anhydrase III: The phosphatase activity is extrinsic. *Archives of Biochemistry and Biophysics*, 377, 334-340.

Krebs, H.A. (1948). Inhibition of carbonic anhydrase by sulfonamides. *Biochemical Journal*, 43, 525-528.

Leiner, M. (1940). Das Ferment Kohlensaureanhydrase im Tierkorper. *Naturwissenschaften*, 28, 316-317.

Mann, T. & Keilin, D. (1940). Sulphanilamide as a specific inhibitor of carbonic anhydrase. *Nature*, 146, 164-165.

Mansoor, U.F.; Zhang, Y.R. & Blackburn, G.M. (2000). The design of newcarbonic anhydrase inhibitors. In: Chegwidden, W.R.; Edwards, Y.; Carter, N. Editors. The carbonic anhydrases-New horizons. Basel: Birkhauser Verlag, pp 437–460.

Maren, T.H. (1967). Carbonic anhydrase: Chemistry, physiology and inhibition. *Physiological Reviews*, 47, 595-781.

Maren, T.H. (1967). Carbonic anhydrase: Chemistry, physiology and inhibition. *Physiological Reviews*, 47, 595-781.

Maren, T.H. (1976). Relations between structure and biological activity of sulfonamides. *Annual Review of Pharmacology and Toxicology*, 16, 309-327.

Maren, T.H.; Jankowska, L.; Sanyal, G. & Edelhauser, H.F. (1983). The transcorneal permeability of sulphonamide carbonic anhydrase innhibitors and their effect on aqueous humor secretion. *Experimental Eye Research*, 36, 457-480.

Maresca, A.; Temperini, C.; Vu, H.; Pham, N.B.; Poulsen, S.A.; Scozzafava, A.; Quinn, R.J. & Supuran, C.T. (2009). Non-zinc mediated inhibition of carbonic anhydrases: coumarins are a new class of suicide inhibitors. *Journal of the American Chemical Society*, 131, 3057-3062.

Maresca, A.; Temperini, C.; Pochet, L.; Masereel, B.; Scozzafava, A. & Supuran, C.T. (2010). Deciphering the mechanism of carbonic anhydrase inhibition with coumarins and thiocoumarins. *Journal of Medicinal Chemistry*, 53, 335-344.

Meier-Ruge, W.; Iwangoff, P. & Reichlmeier, K. (1984). Neurochemical enzyme changes in Alzheimer's and Pick's disease. *Archives of Gerontology and Geriatrics*, 3, 161-165.

Nair, S.K.; Ludwig, P.A. & Christianson, D.W. (1994). Two-site binding of phenol in the active site of human carbonic anhydrase II: structural implications for substrate association. *Journal of the American Chemical Society*, 116, 3659-3660.

Ozensoy, O.; Arslan, O. & Sinan, O.S. (2004). A new method for the purification of carbonic anhydrase isozymes by affinity chromatography. *Biochemistry (Moscow)*, 69, 216-219.

Parkkila, S. & Parkkila, A.K. (1996). Carbonic anhydrase in the alimentary tract. Roles of the different isozymes and salivary factors in the maintenance of optimal conditions in the gastrointestinal canal. *Scandinavian Journal of Gastroenterology*, 31, 305-317.

Pastorekova, S.; Parkkila, S.; Pastorek, J. & Supuran, C.T. (2004). Carbonic anhydrases: current state of the art, therapeutic applications and future prospects. *Journal of Enzyme Inhibition and Medicinal Chemistry*, 19, 199-229.

Rawas-Qalaji, M.M.; Simons, F.E.R.; Simons, K.J.J. (2006). *Allergy Clin. Immunol*. 117, 398.

Scozzafava, A. & Supuran, C.T. (2002a). Carbonic Anhydrase Activators: High Affinity Isozymes I, II, and IV Activators, Incorporating a β-Alanyl-histidine Scaffold. *Journal of Medicinal Chemistry*, 45, 284-291.

Scozzafava, A. & Supuran, C.T. (2002b). Carbonic Anhydrase Activators: Human Isozyme II is Strongly Activated by Oligopeptides Incorporating the Carboxyterminal Sequence of the Bicarbonate Anion Exchanger AE1. *Bioorganic & Medicinal Chemistry Letters*, 12, 1177-1180.

Senturk, M.; Talaz, O.; Ekinci, D.; Cavdar, H. & Kufrevioglu, O.I. (2009). In vitro inhibition of human erythrocyte glutathione reductase by some new organic nitrates. *Bioorganic & Medicinal Chemistry Letters*, 19, 3661-3663.

Sly, W.S. & Hu, P.Y. (1995). Human carbonic anhydrases and carbonic anhydrase deficiencies. *Annual Review of Biochemistry* 64, 375-401.

Sun, M.K. & Alkon, D.L. (2001). Pharmacological enhancement of synaptic efficacy, spatial learning and memory through carbonic anhydrase activation in rats. *Journal of Pharmacology and Experimental Therapeutics*, 297, 961-967.

Supuran, C.T. & Puscas, I. (1994). Carbonic anhydrase activators. In carbonic anhydrase and modulation of physiologic and pathologic processes in the organism; Puscas, I., Ed.; *Helicon Press: Timisoara*, pp 113-145.

Supuran, C.T. (2008a). Carbonic anhydrases: novel therapeutic applications for inhibitors and activators. *Nature Reviews Drug Discovery*, 7, 168-181.

Supuran, C.T. (2008b). Carbonic anhydrases-an overview. *Current Pharmaceutical Design*, 14, 603-614.

Supuran, C.T. (2008c). Diuretics: From Classical Carbonic Anhydrase Inhibitors to Novel Applications of the Sulfonamides. *Current Pharmaceutical Design*, 14, 641-648.

Supuran, C.T. & Scozzafava, A. (2000a). Activation of carbonic anhydrase isozymes. In The Carbonic Anhydrases - New Horizons; Chegwidden, W.R.; Carter, N.; Edwards, Y.; Eds.; Birkhauser Verlag: Basel, Switzerland, pp 197-219.

Supuran, C.T. & Scozzafava, A. (2000b). Carbonic anhydrase inhibitors and their therapeutic potential. *Expert Opinion on Therapeutic Patents*, 10, 575-600.

Supuran, C.T. & Scozzafava, A. (2001). Carbonic anhydrase inhibitors. *Current Medicinal Chemistry*, 1, 61-97.

Supuran, C.T. (1994). Carbonic anhydrase inhibitors. In: Puscas, I. (Ed). Carbonic anhydrase and modulation of physiologic and pathologic processes in the organism. Timisoara (Romania): Helicon, pp 29-111.

Supuran, C.T.; Scozzafava, A. & Casini, A. (2003). Carbonic anhydrase inhibitors. *Medicinal Research Reviews*, 23, 146-189.

Supuran, C.T.; Conroy, C.W. & Maren, T.H. (1997). Is cyanate a carbonic anhydrase substrate? *Proteins: Structure, Function and Genetics*, 27, 272-278.

Temperini, C.; Innocenti, A.; Scozzafava, A.; Mastrolorenzo, A. & Supuran, C.T. (2007). Carbonic anhydrase activators: L-Adrenaline plugs the active site entrance of isozyme II, activating better isoforms I, IV, VA, VII, and XIV. *Bioorganic & Medicinal Chemistry Letters*, 17, 628-635.

Temperini, C.; Innocenti, A.; Scozzafava, A.; Parkkila, S. & Supuran, C.T. (2010). The Coumarin-binding site in carbonic anhydrase accommodates structurally diverse inhibitors: The antiepileptic lacosamide as an example and lead molecule for novel classes of carbonic anhydrase inhibitors. *Journal of Medicinal Chemistry*, 53, 850-854.

van Goor, H. (1948). Carbonic anhydrase: its properties, distribution and significance for carbon dioxide transport. *Enzymologia*, 13, 73-164.

Zhu, X.L. & Sly, W.S. (1990). Carbonic anhydrase IV from human lung. Purification, characterization, and comparison with membrane carbonic anhydrase from human kidney. Journal of Biological Chemistry, 265, 8795-8801.

16

Stochastic Simulation for Biochemical Reaction Networks in Infectious Disease

Shailza Singh and Sonali Shinde
National Centre for Cell Science NCCS Complex, Ganeskhind, Pune University Campus, Pune India

1. Introduction

Modern computational science is converging on complex problems in the general field of systems biology. There is now a credible possibility of modeling drug delivery vesicles (liposomes) and their properties with qualitative and quantitative insight coming from atomistic calculations. Understanding the formation of vesicles from phospholipids bilayers and their fluidity and permeability properties is the basis of a large number of applications in the domain of drug delivery, in particular release of the active species according to the pH or ionic concentration changes. Prediction of structural changes (phase transition in particular) of membranes by modification of one or several constituents or addition of external molecular species may have potential therapeutic applications. Understanding the basic principles of biomembranes (lipid bilayers) governing and mediating various biologically relevant processes on the microscopic level is one of the great challenges in biology (Singh 2011). Molecular dynamic (MD) simulations are well suited for detailed analysis of the interactions between lipid bilayers and various small molecules, including water, chemicals, co-enzymes, peptides, oligonucleotides and proteins, as evidenced by the extensive body of published literature. Density Functional Theory (DFT) methods and recent theoretical studies of the properties of phospholipid molecules, consistent QM/MM and MM methodologies as well as their counterparts as function of time, Born-Oppenheimer dynamics (BOMD) and molecular dynamics (MD) are applied to understand and predict the properties of liposomes in water, in particular, fluidity, and their evolution in the presence of ions and biological agents. This has subsequently been achieved through the Dipalmitoylphosphatidylcholine (DPPC) bilayer systems and its partitioning with an ether lipid drug. Hence, membrane-lipid therapy plays a dominant role in molecular medicine.

1.1 Cellular model of lipid membranes and drug partitioning

The model of the DPPC bilayer was used for simulation of the phospholipid environment around the drug. The lipid parameters were taken from the literature (Lipka et al., 1984). The partial atomic charges were calculated at DFT/B3LYP/6- 31G** level using Gaussian 09 package. Also, the partitioning of large molecular systems was done by following ONIOM (Our-own-N-layered integrated molecular orbital and molecular mechanics) method, whereby the whole system is partitioned into onion-skin-like layers, using QM/MM. The total energy can be obtained from following:

$$E= E[Low, real] + E[Med, int] + E[High, inner]-E[Low,int]-E[Med, inner] = E6+E5+E4-E3-E2$$

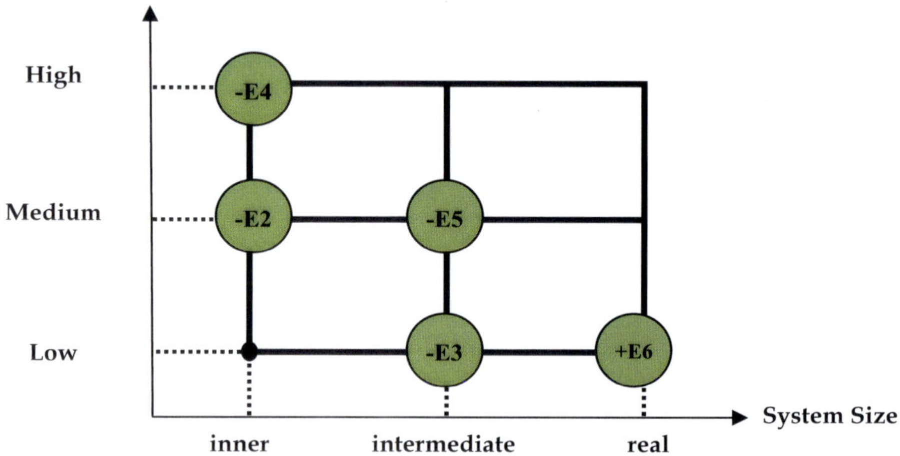

where real denotes the entire system, which is treated at low level, while int denotes the part of the system partitioned to be the intermediate layers for which the energy is calculated at both medium and high levels. Here inner denotes the inner layer of the system partitioning, whose energy is calculated at both high and medium levels.

Chemical potential profile, μ(z), of solute across a lipid bilayer and adjacent water phase is obtained by inserting the solute numerous times into randomly selected positions in the system obtained by MD simulation and calculating the interaction energy, E(z), between the inserted solute and all the molecules in the system. From $\langle \exp(-E(z)/RT) \rangle_t$, where $\langle \ldots \rangle_t$ denotes the thermal average over insertions of solute with randomly chosen orientations into configurations of the system at depth z unperturbed by the solute, the excess chemical potential, μ(z), and thereby the free energy of transfer, ΔG(z), from bulk water to the bilayer interior at the depth z are obtained: $\Delta G(z) = \mu(z) - \mu(\text{water})$

$$= -RT\ln \langle e^{-E(z)/RT} \rangle / \langle e^{-E(\text{water})/RT} \rangle$$

This simulation may enable us to understand the thermodynamic interactions between the lipid and drug molecules, the role of electrostatics in such adducts, and the permeability of drug (Fig. 1A & 1B). Degree of penetration into the membrane interior obtained from computer simulations may also be useful in estimating the extent to which a drug or prodrug that is unstable in a given solution or biological fluid might be protected when bound to a lipid bilayer membrane (Fig.1B&C). Multi-scale modeling and simulation revealed that the interactions between the drug and membrane are both electrostatic and hydrophobic. Increasing the chain length and lipophilicity may strengthen the binding interactions and overcome the problem of drug resistance.

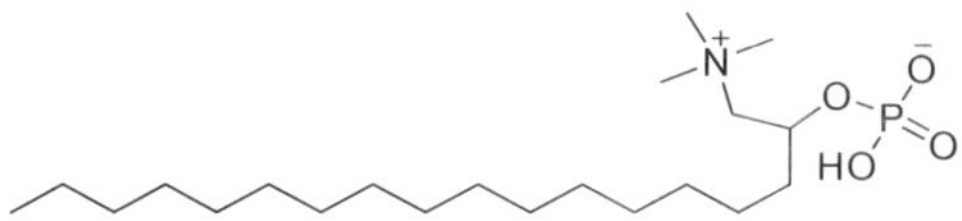

1-(triimethylamino)octadecan-2-yl monohydrogen phosphate

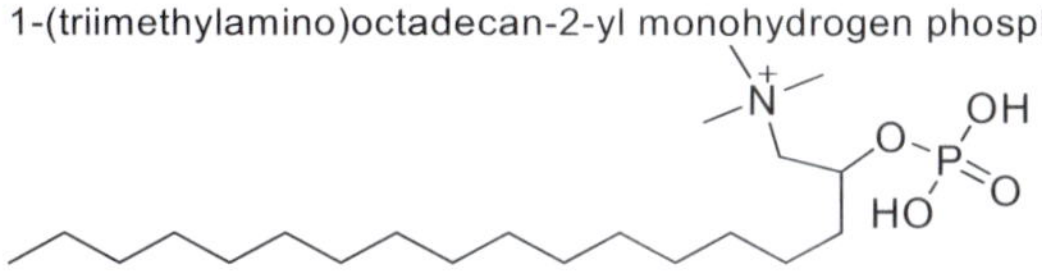

1-(triimethylamino)octadecan-2-yl dihydrogen phosphate

Fig. 1. A) Neutral and charged states of miltefosine

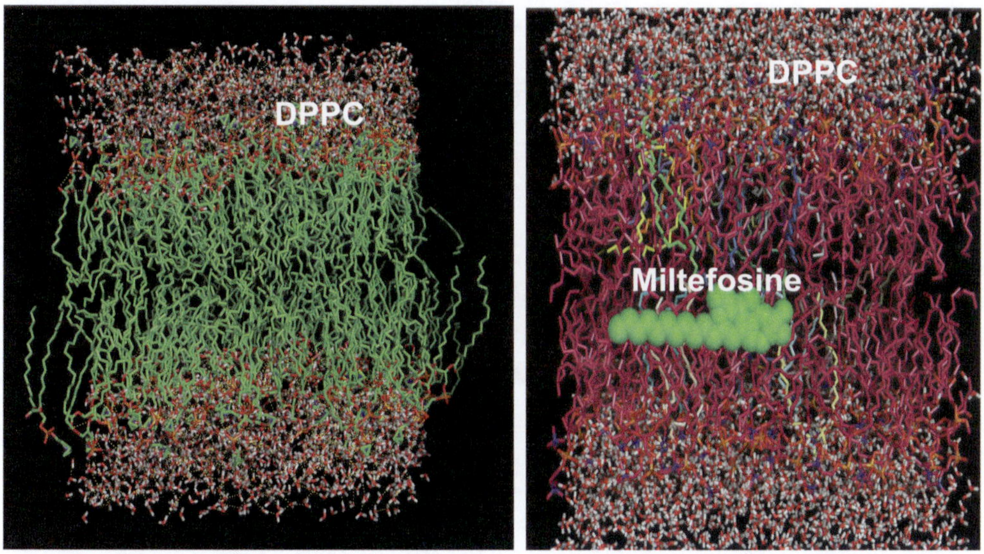

B C

Fig. 1. B) Model representing DPPC bilayer system, C) Miltefosine with the lipid bilayer system.

2. Membrane permeability, lipid metabolism and multi-drug resistance in *Leishmania major*

Membrane impermeability is the major contributing factor to multidrug resistance in clinical isolates of *Leishmania major* (Perez Victoria et al., 2006). Reductionism which dominated biological research for over a century has provided a wealth of information about individual cellular components and their functions. Understanding the structure and the dynamics of the complex intercellular web of interactions that contribute to the structure and function of a living cell is a key challenge for biology in the 21st century.

The recent developments in genome sequencing (complete for *L. major, L. braziliensis*, and *L. infantum*) and lipidomic tools conceive a powerful platform for the study of lipid metabolism in Leishmania. Lipid concentration changes in biological systems reflect regulation at multiple spatial and dynamic scales, e.g., biochemical reactions in the cells, intercellular lipid trafficking, changes in cell membrane composition, systemic lipid metabolism or lipid oxidation [Niemela et al., 2009]. Excluding the transport reactions, the percentage of intracellular reactions participating in lipid metabolism in *L.major* was the greatest, when compared to reactions across other metabolic subsystems [Chavali et al., 2008]. In order to address the intricacies of lipid regulation, it is quite obligatory to analyze the lipid metabolic mechanisms (Fig.2).

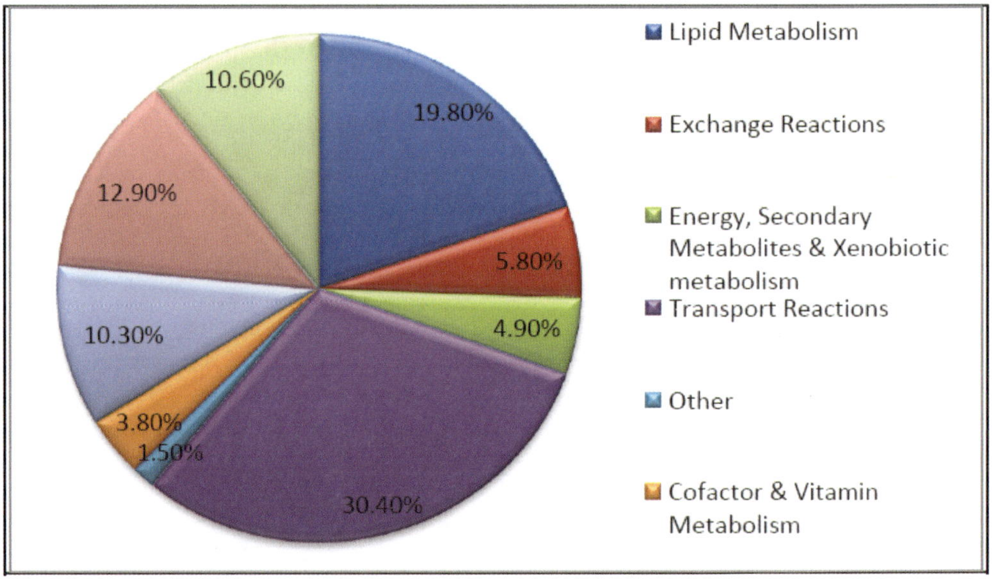

Fig. 2. Distribution of Metabolic Pathways according to the Cellular Processes. Neglecting the Transport Reactions, the Lipid Metabolism shows the highest no. of intracellular reactions signifying the abundance of the lipid biochemical networks.

The *L.major* pathogen is decoded at the interactome level, and the study is converged into the Lipid Metabolic Pathway, to serve the purpose of targeting the probable ligand via Liposomal Drug Delivery. Lipids play an active role in a variety of dynamic processes involving the membranes that compartmentalize the cell. To achieve this, cell must regulate the mechanical properties of the membrane and it can do so partly by controlling its lipid composition. The underlying biophysical question is to understand the variability and chemical diversity of membrane lipid composition, the mechanical properties of the membrane and the associated protein functions. Lipid metabolism is essential to the development, multiplication, virulence and differentiation of Leishmania species in the host, thus making the pathways for synthesis of parasite lipids good targets for development of new anti-leishmanial drugs [Zufferey and Mamoun, 2005; Zhang K. et al., 2003; Zufferey et al., 2003; Haughan et al.,1995]. Thereby, the diversity between Leishmania and mammals in lipid composition could be exploited towards selective chemotherapy. Lipids being a crucial entity of the pathogen cell surface are given extensive importance and moreover due to the liposomal drug delivery system, targeting the lipids organized in the membrane of the pathogen would be an added advantage for the smooth release of the encapsulated drug.

The cell surface of Leishmania spp. has been shown to play a role in host-pathogen interactions and in the ability of the pathogen to evade the host-immune system. LPGs are essential for adhesion of the parasite to the midgut of the insect and therefore are important for transmission of the parasite to the human host. The basic LPG structure in all Leishmania species consists of several domains like the GPI anchor, with an 1-O-alkyl-2-lyso-phosphatidyl inositol lipid joined to a heptasaccharide glycan core, a long phosphoglycan (PG) domain composed of (Gal β1-4manα1-PO4)n repeat units (n=15-30), and a small neutral oligosaccharide cap [Bergter and Vermelho, 2010]. In different Leishmania species the phosphoglycan repeat units contain additional substitutions that mediate key roles in stage-specific adhesion. Deletion of LPG in *L.major* indicates that the glycosylated structures are involved in resistance to oxidative stress and the human immune system [Oppenheimer et al., 2011]. Henceforth, it is evident that lipids are essential cell constituents and therefore must be constantly synthesized to allow multiplication of the parasite. This suggests that the pathways leading to their synthesis are essential for parasite proliferation and pathogenesis and thus offers a reasonable target for rational design of novel antileishmanial drugs. Gal*f* plays an important role in host specific cell recognition, parasitic growth and pathogenesis. Since Gal*f* is not present in humans, the Galf biosynthetic pathway is an attractive target for the development of novel anti-parasitic drugs. In this pathway, UDP-galactopyranose mutase (UGM) catalyzes the conversion of UDP-galactopyranose to form UPD-Galf, which serves as a precursor for all the Galf found on the cell surface. Deletion of UGM gene may lead to the identification of specific inhibitors of this enzyme. [Oppenheimer et al., 2011]

Interactome Network Building is a crucial step for advancing towards Mathematical modeling, using the Systems Biology Markup Language. Metabolic network reconstruction has become an indispensable tool for studying the systems biology of metabolism. The focus is laid onto reviewing the mathematical foundations for analyzing chemical reactions, and describing how these systems of coupled chemical reactions can provide insight into the behavior of complex regulatory mechanisms. This is accomplished using the simulation mechanisms based on the certain defined kinetic laws such as Convenience Kinetics, Generalized Mass Action Kinetics and the Hill-Hinze equation. A saturable rate law "Convenience Kinetics" - a generalised form of Michaelis-Menten kinetics, covers all possible stoichiometries, describes enzyme regulation by activators and inhibitors, and can be derived from a rapid-equilibrium random-order enzyme mechanism. Convenience kinetics is used to translate a biochemical network – manually into a dynamical model with rational biological properties. It implements enzyme saturation and regulation by activators and inhibitors, covers all possible reaction stoichiometries, and can be specified by a small number of parameters. Their mathematical forms make it especially suitable for parameter assessment and optimisation. To ensure thermodynamic correctness, it is written in terms of thermodynamically independent parameters [Liebermeister and Klipp, 2006]. Moreover, the classes of generalized kinetic expressions of GMA also ensure consistency with the extended thermodynamic conditions [Horn and Jackson, 2004].

Simulation can provide the ultimate detail concerning individual particle motions as a function of time [Karplus and McCammon, 2002]. Thus, they can be used to address specific questions about the properties of a model system, often more easily than experiments on the actual system. These techniques are carried out upon treating a biological process as a system of equations, represented by their rate constants and other parameters and simulating their interactions through numerical techniques. The numerical simulations capture the effects of genes and their expression level through the time-course of evolution at molecular concentration. Thus, it is a biochemical characterization of the enzymatic network using the systems biology approach by interconnecting mathematical, biological, and physical sciences with the aim to capture the behavioural sciences of the enzymes, in the temporal and spatial scales, eventually leading to the discrete stochastic kinetic simulation. The integration of genomic and physiological information is now increasingly important with the emergence of "systems biology", which attempts to simultaneously study the expression patterns and activity of all genes, together with proteomic and metabolomic data [Cavalieri and Filippo, 2005]. When combined with a specific method of analysis like flux balance analysis (FBA), constraint-based models can be used to generate quantitative predictions (e.g., growth rate of an organism) and yield testable hypotheses for future experimental investigations [Roberts et al., 2009; Lee et al., 2006]. This permits an iterative process of model development, hypothesis generation and testing, and further model development and refinement [Reed et al., 2006]. Hence, looking at the disease as "perturbation of networks" can provide such a framework which may offer insights from systems biology into the practicalities of personalized, preventive, predictive and participative (P4) medicine [Antonio del Sol et al., 2010]. Using this approach, a base is formulated for the appropriate selection of an inhibitor, taking into account the dynamics of the enzyme kinetics.

2.1 Lipophosphoglycan & GIPL structure

The parasite surface is the primary interface of Leishmania with the host, and is comprised largely of three abundant classes of glycosylphosphatidylinositol (GPI)-anchored molecules: lipophosphoglycan (LPG), a smaller heterogeneous group of glycoinositolphospholipids (GIPLs), and proteins such as gp63, gp46, PSA-2, and proteophosphoglycans (PPGs) [G.F. Spath, 2000]. This LPG is held together with a phosphoinositide membrane anchor, and has a tripartite structure consisting of a lipid domain, a neutral hexasaccharide, and a phosphorylated galactose-mannose, with a termination in a neutral cap [G.F. Spath, 2000] (Fig.3). LPG is in abundance in the cell membrane and is extended from the cell surface. In the mammalian host, LPG confers resistance to complement-mediated lysis, oxidative stress, and inhibits phagolysosomal fusion. In Leishmania major, the core of the abundant surface lipophosphoglycan (LPG) is structurally related to that of the smaller glycosylinositolphospholipids (GIPLs) in containing galactosylfuranose (Galf) residues in a Gal0-2Galf (β3)Man motif [Zhang et al., 2004]. However, deletion of the putative Galf - transferase (Galf T) LPG1 affected Galf incorporation in LPG but not GIPLs [G.F. Spath, 2000]. Thus, LPG and LPG1 satisfy the requirements for virulence factors genes as set forth by the modern "Molecular Koch's postulates", establishing LPG itself as a Leishmania virulence factor [Falkow S, 1988].

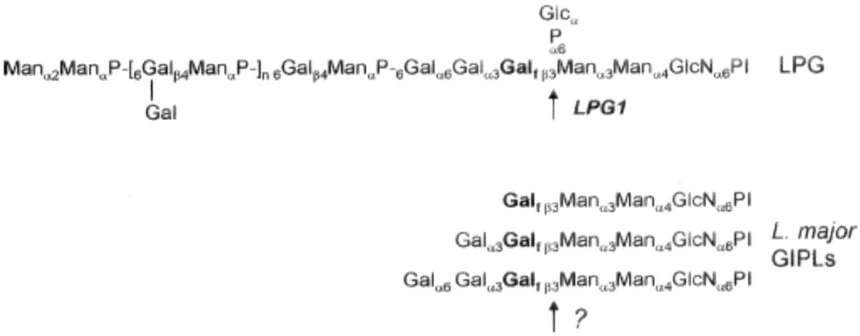

Fig. 3. Structure of GIPLs and LPGs in *L. major*.

2.2 Stochastic simulation

The study of metabolic networks is of high relevance, because of their implications for the basic understanding of living cells and organisms and for medical applications, especially with respect to discovering drug targets [Pavlopoulos et al., 2008]. Defining a system by the dynamic state of its metabolome relies on the effective integration of omics data because the metabolic state of the system is largely derived from the global expression of its genome and proteome [Davidov et al., 2003]. Recent advances enable the production of metabolic network models reconstructed from genome sequences, as well as experimental measurements of much of the metabolome [Douglas B. Kell, 2006]. The network-based representation and analysis of biological systems contributes to a greater understanding of their structures and functions at different levels of complexity. These techniques can also be used to identify potential novel therapeutic targets based on the characterisation of vulnerable or highly influential network components [Azuaje et al., 2010]. Recently developed computational tools enable rational and graphical composition of genetic circuits for standard parts, and subsequent simulation for testing the predicted functions *in silico* [Marchisio and Stelling, 2009]. Model construction typically involves the translation of prior knowledge into a list of reactants and reactions [Aldridge et al., 2006]. These models require information about the kinetics of each of the reactions participating in the network, such as the kinetic laws describing the dynamics of the reactions with their respective parameters. Thereafter, kinetic equations are mapped to the reaction model through either stochastic or deterministic approaches, and at times a hybrid model may be adopted. Several modelling approaches are derived from assuming different simplistic kinetic mechanisms: Convenience rate law, mass-action, Michaelis-Menten, power-law, LinLog [Sergio Grimbs, 2009]. There are several modes of modeling these metabolic networks: Structural modeling, Flux balance Analysis and Metabolic control Analysis. Thus, using the concept of mathematical modeling and applying the science of systems biology, the simulation of metabolic pathway is carried out based on certain kinetic laws and their parameters.

Once a target is identified, whole cell screening assays can be designed, using synthetic biology strategies [Weber and Fusseneger, 2009]. Temporal information from computer simulations are validated by those done on simplified versions of yeast cell cycle and have shown to be in good agreement with experiment [Tyson et al., 2001]. The conversion of a reconstruction into a mathematical format facilitates a myriad of computational biological studies, including evaluation of network content, hypothesis testing and generation, analysis of phenotypic characteristics and metabolic engineering [Thiele and Bernhard , 2010].

2.3 Enzymes unique to *L.major* and absent in *H.sapiens*

It was noted that these distinctive enzymes listed below restricted only to *L.major* catalyzed reactions are involved in some of the metabolic pathways (Table 1).

Sr. No.	Enzymes	Metabolic Pathways
1	side-chain/ phosphoglycan β-1,3 galactosyltransferase 7	LPG,GIPL,GPI Biosynthetic Pathway
2	side-chain/ phosphoglycan β-1,3 galactosyltransferase 6	
3	side-chain/ phosphoglycan β-1,3 galactosyltransferase 5	
4	side-chain/ phosphoglycan β-1,3 galactosyltransferase 4	
5	side-chain/ phosphoglycan β-1,3 galactosyltransferase 3	
6	side-chain/ phosphoglycan β-1,3 galactosyltransferase 2	
7	side-chain/ phosphoglycan β-1,3 galactosyltransferase 1	
8	side-chain/ phosphoglycan β-1,3 galactosyltransferase related protein 6	
9	side-chain/ phosphoglycan β-1,3 galactosyltransferase related protein 5	
10	side-chain/ phosphoglycan β-1,3 galactosyltransferase related protein 4	
11	side-chain/ phosphoglycan β-1,3 galactosyltransferase related protein 3	
12	side-chain/ phosphoglycan β-1,3 galactosyltransferase related protein 2	
13	side-chain/ phosphoglycan β-1,3 galactosyltransferase related protein 1	
14	phosphoglycan β-1,2 arabinosyltransferase	
15	side- chain β-1,2 arabinosyltransferase	
16	mannosyltransferase (GPI14)	
17	GIPL galf transferase	
18	β- galactofuranosyltransferase like protein (LPG1)	
19	galactofuranosyltransferase like protein lpg1 - like protein	
20	β- galactofuranosyltransferase	
21	GPI 18/ PIG V	
22	GPI 10/ GPI anchor biosynthetic protein	
23	gpi transamidase complex	
24	Sterol C-24 reductase,putative	Ergosterol Biosynthesis
25	C-5 sterol desaturase,putative	
26	Sterol 24-C methyltransferase	
27	Δ6 desaturase	Fatty Acid Elongation
28	Δ4 desaturase	
29	Δ6 elongase	
30	Δ5 elongase	
31	Δ5 desaturase	
32	Δ12 desaturase	
33	stearic acid desaturase	
34	enoyl-[-ACP] reductase, putative	
35	fatty acid elongase	Fatty Acid Biosynthesis
36	β- ketoacyl ACP synthase	
37	cardiolipin synthase, putative	Ester Biosynthesis

Table 1. Enzymes restricted to *L.major* and the respective Metabolic Pathways belonging to Lipid and Fatty Acid Biochemical Network.

Thus, of the overall 20 metabolic pathways involved in Lipid and Fatty Acid Metabolism, there are 13 such pathways which are exclusively restricted to *L.major*, of which only 7 pathways had the enzymes and reactions unique to *L.major*. From the Table 1 it is found that the maximum number of the genes and the resultant gene products (enzymes), distinctive to the *L.major* are specifically engaged in the LPG and GIPL Biosynthesis Pathway followed by the fatty acid metabolism.

2.4 Gene Regulatory Network (GRN) and lipid metabolism

The prior mentioned metabolic pathways (Fig.4) are taken into account to form an interacting regulatory network of genes in order to lay an emphasis upon the clustering of the genes into metabolic pathways of related functions.

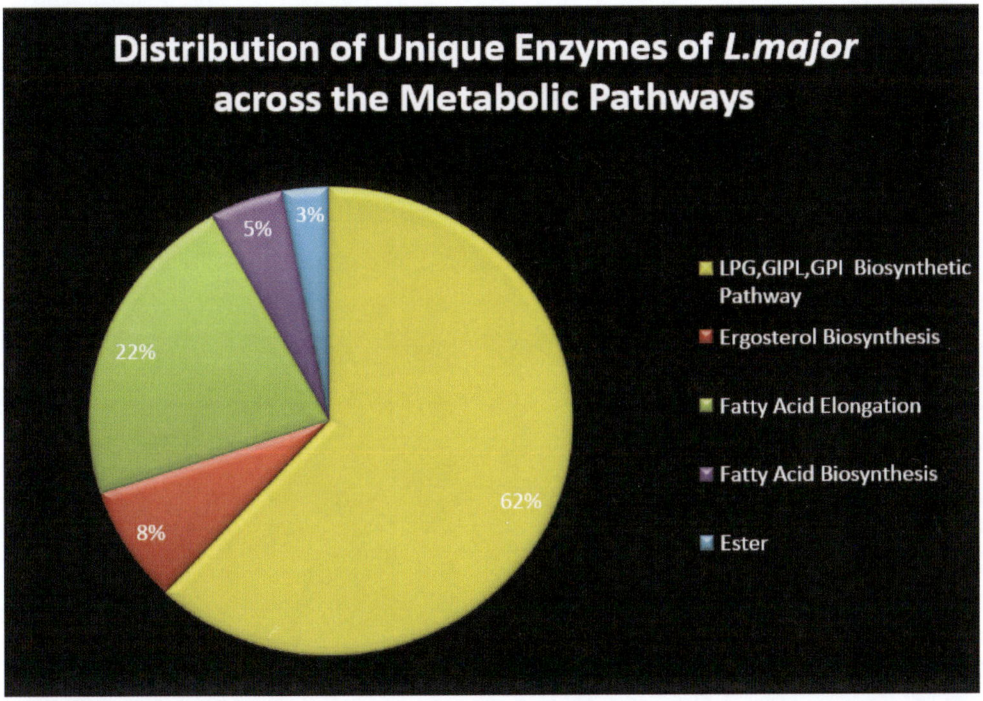

Fig. 4. Pie chart showing the abundance of unique enzymes present in LPG, GPI anchor and GIPL biosynthetic pathway.

A gene regulatory network (GRN) aims to capture the dependencies between these molecular entities and is often modeled as a network composed of nodes which represents genes, proteins and/or metabolites) and edges representing molecular interactions such as protein-DNA and protein-protein interactions or rather indirect relationships between genes. Network model architectures can be distinguished by the type of model: stochastic or deterministic, static or dynamic and the type of relationships between the variables (directed or undirected; linear or non-linear function or relation table). Although many undirected network representations exist, the focus of this chapter is on directed networks.

From this network it is clearly visible, that LPG Biosynthetic Pathway, GIPL Biosynthesis Pathway, GPI anchor Biosynthesis Pathway, and Dolichyl-diphosphooligosaccharide biosynthesis Pathway are inter-connected through one or more genes involved commonly in the regulation of the proteins which act as enzymes catalyzing the reactions in these pathways (Fig.5).

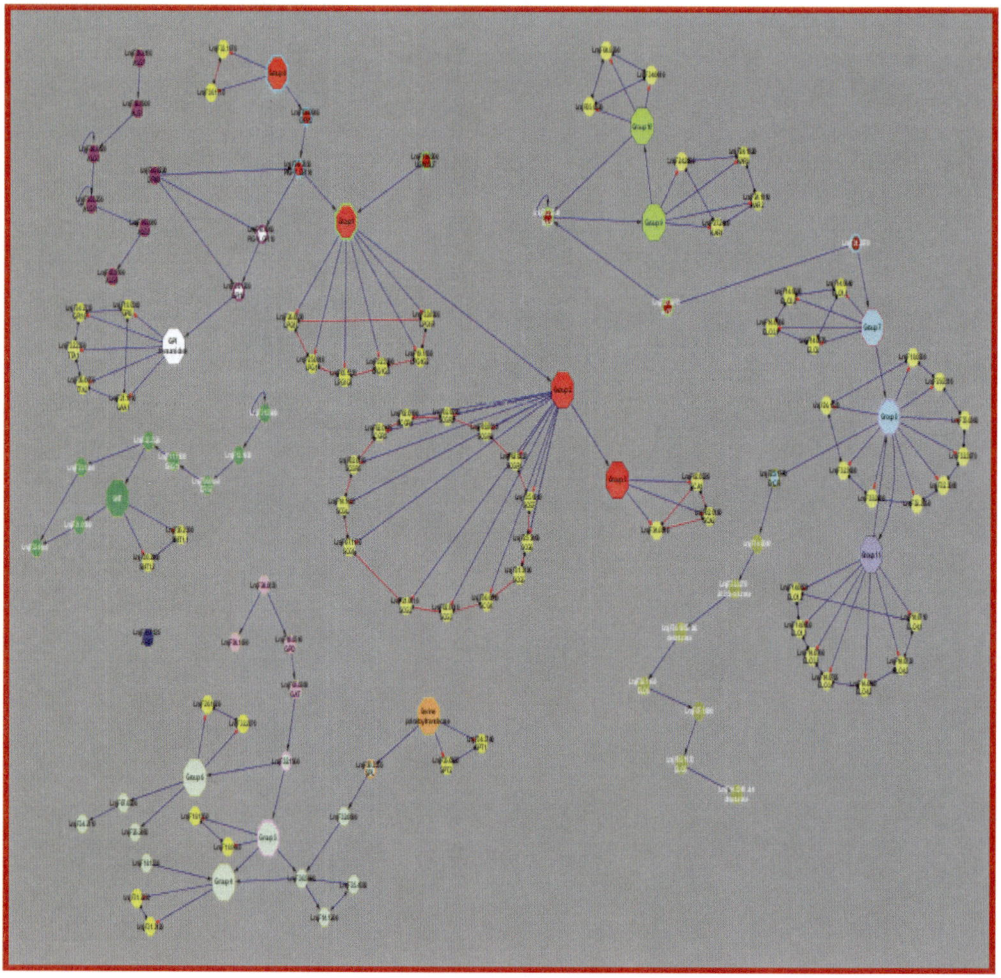

Fig. 5. Gene Regulatory Network constructed using Cytoscape for visualizing the inter-connection of the Lipid Metabolic Pathways restricted to *L.major* *.

*Legend overleaf

LEGEND:

- Lipophosphoglycan Pathway
- LPG + GIPL Biosynthesis Pathway
- LPG + GIPL + GPI- anchor Biosynthesis Pathway

GPI- anchor Biosynthesis Pathway
GPI - anchor + GIPL Biosynthesis Pathway
Dolichyl-diphosphooligosaccharide Biosynthesis
Ergosterol Biosynthesis
Sphingolipid Metabolism
Ester Phospholipid Biosynthesis
Sphingolipid Metabolism + Ester Phospholipid Biosynthesis
Glycerolipid biosynthesis- initial steps
Ester Phospholipid Biosynthesis + Glycerolipid biosynthesis - initial st
Ether Phospholipid Biosynthesis
Fatty acid Biosynthesis Initiation
Fatty acid biosynthesis-- elongase pathway
Very Long Chain Fatty Acid Biosynthesis
Fatty Acid Elongation – Unsaturated
Fatty Acid Elongation - Saturated
F.A. elongase + F.A. initiation
F.A. elongation saturated + F.A. initiation
F.A. elongase + V.L.C. F.A. Biosynthesis
F.A. elongase + F.A. elongation saturated
Group of genes involved in single reaction

Similarly, the pathways Fatty Acid Elongation (Saturated and Unsaturated), Fatty acid biosynthesis Initiation, Very Light Chain Fatty Acid Biosynthesis and Fatty acid biosynthesis-elongase pathway; and the pathways Ester phospholipid biosynthesis, Sphingolipid Metabolism and Glycerolipid biosynthesis- initial steps are respectively inter-related through common intervention of the genes. But, the pathways Ergosterol Biosynthesis and Ether Phospholipid Biosynthesis are the only ones that are not related with any of the other Metabolic Reactions, and are self-contained.

Hence, the gene regulatory network gives an entire overview about the reacting species in the same dimension. The reactions and pathways that are inter-connected and have common enzymes and compounds taking part in the same reactions can further be investigated. Also, it gives an outline and a general idea related to the cluster of genes taking part in the reactions.

From the Cytoscape Regulatory Network of the Lipid Metabolism Pathway, it is found that the maximum number of the genes and the resultant gene products (enzymes), distinctive to the *L.major*, ae specifically clustered in the LPG and GIPL Biosynthesis Pathway, followed by the fatty acid metabolism.

Thereby, from the Cytoscape network and Fig 6, it is established that majority of the enzymes in a large number are present only in the LPG, GIPL and GPI anchor bioynthesis pathways, thus giving a wide scope for the enzymatic studies to be undertaken. Consequently, the Lipophosphoglycan Pathway in conjunction with the GIPL and GPI anchor biosynthesis is of paramount importance.

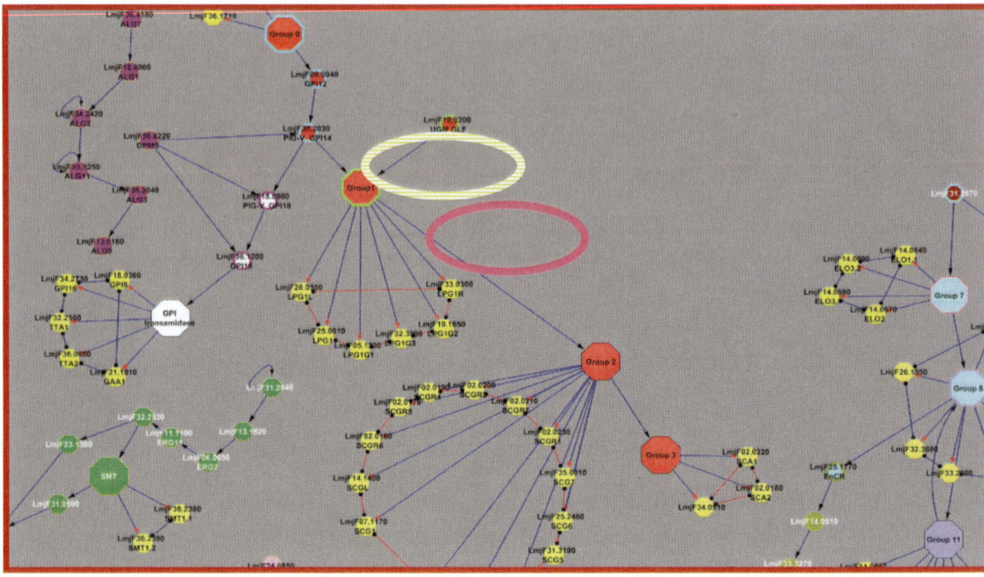

Fig. 6. Enlarged portion of the Gene Regulatory Network focusing on the large number of genes involved in LPG, GIPl and GPI anchor biosynthesis pathway [Pathways marked by red octagon]. Thus it can be concluded that the gene GPI 14 [marked by off-white] can play a crucial role in the pathway since it is at a junction leading to the other 2 pathways- GIPL and GPI. Also, the cluster of genes assembled into Group1 [marked by pink] is at a vital cross-road leading to GIPL and LPG Biosynthetic Pathway.

2.5 Compartmentalization

The sub-cellular localization of the target enzymes plays a very significant role in order to introduce an inhibitor in a cellular system. Hence, the location of the enzymes involved in LPG Biosynthetic Pathway is determined and the presence of the transmembrane domains is also checked (Table 2).

Cellular overview was created using this data to simplify the complexity and for elaborative interpretation of the data. The compartments included are Nucleus, Golgi apparatus, Endoplasmic Reticulum, and the Cell Membrane. The fluxes and the choke-point reactions are also marked to indicate the critical reactions in the pathway (Fig.7).

Sub-cellular Localization of enzymes involved in the LPG Metabolic Pathway					
Sr. No.	Enzymes	TMHMM domains	Sub-cellular Localization	Signal Peptide	Signal Anchor
1	phosphatidylinositol-N-acetylglucos-aminyltransferase subunit c, putative	7	integral to Cell membrane	-	-
2	n-acetylglucosaminyl-phosphatidyl inositol biosynthetic protein,putative	-	cytoplasm	-	-
3	N-acetyl-D-glucosaminyl-phosphatidylinositol deacetylase	1	integral to cell membrane	Present	-
4	***mannosyl transferase,putative***	8	integral to ER	-	-

Sub-cellular Localization of enzymes involved in the LPG Metabolic Pathway					
Sr. No.	Enzymes	TMHMM domains	Sub-cellular Localization	Signal Peptide	Signal Anchor
			membrane		
5	***beta galactofuranosyl transferase***	1	integral to cell membrane	-	Present
6	***GIPL galf transferase, putative***	1	integral to cell membrane	Present	-
7	***beta-galactofuranosyltransferase-like protein***	1	integral to cell membrane	-	Present
8	galactofuranosyltransferase lpg1-like protein	1	integral to cell membrane	-	Present
9	***GIPL galf transferase, putative***	1	integral to cell membrane	-	Present
10	***GIPL galf transferase, putative***	-	cytoplasm	-	-
11	***phosphoglycan beta 1,3 galactosyltransferase 4, scβGalT***	1	Golgi Membrane	Present	-
12	***phosphoglycan beta 1,3 galactosyltransferase 3, scβGalT***	1	Golgi Membrane	-	-
13	***phosphoglycan beta 1,3 galactosyltransferase 2, scβGalT***	1	Golgi Membrane	-	-
14	***phosphoglycan beta 1,3 galactosyltransferase 1, scβGalT***	1	Golgi Membrane	-	-
15	***side chain β1,3 galactosyltransferase-like protein***	1	Golgi Membrane	-	-
16	***side chain β1,3 galactosyltransferase-related protein 6***	1	Golgi Membrane	-	-
17	***side chain β1,3 galactosyltransferase-related protein 5***	1	Golgi Membrane	-	-
18	***side chain β1,3 galactosyltransferase-related protein 4***	1	Golgi Membrane	-	-
19	***side chain β1,3 galactosyltransferase-related protein 3***	1	Golgi Membrane	-	Present
20	***side chain β1,3 galactosyltransferase-related protein 2***	1	Golgi Membrane	-	-
21	***side chain β1,3 galactosyltransferase-related protein 1***	1	Golgi Membrane	-	-
22	***phosphoglycan beta 1,3 galactosyltransferase 7, scβGalT***	1	Golgi Membrane	-	-
23	***phosphoglycan beta 1,3 galactosyltransferase 6, scβGalT***	1	Golgi Membrane	-	-
24	***phosphoglycan beta 1,3 galactosyltransferase 5, scβGalT***	1	Golgi Membrane	-	-
25	***phosphoglycan beta 1,2 arabinosyltransferase, scβAraT-2***	1	Golgi Lumen	-	-
26	***phosphoglycan beta 1,2 arabinosyltransferase, scβAraT***	1	Golgi Lumen	-	-
27	***phosphoglycan beta 1,2 arabinosyltransferase***	1	Golgi Lumen	-	-

Table 2. Sub-cellular Localization of the Enzymes, through Literature Survey, GeneDB and UniProtKB. The enzyme names marked in bold and italicized are the ones that are present exclusively in the *L.major* pathogen.

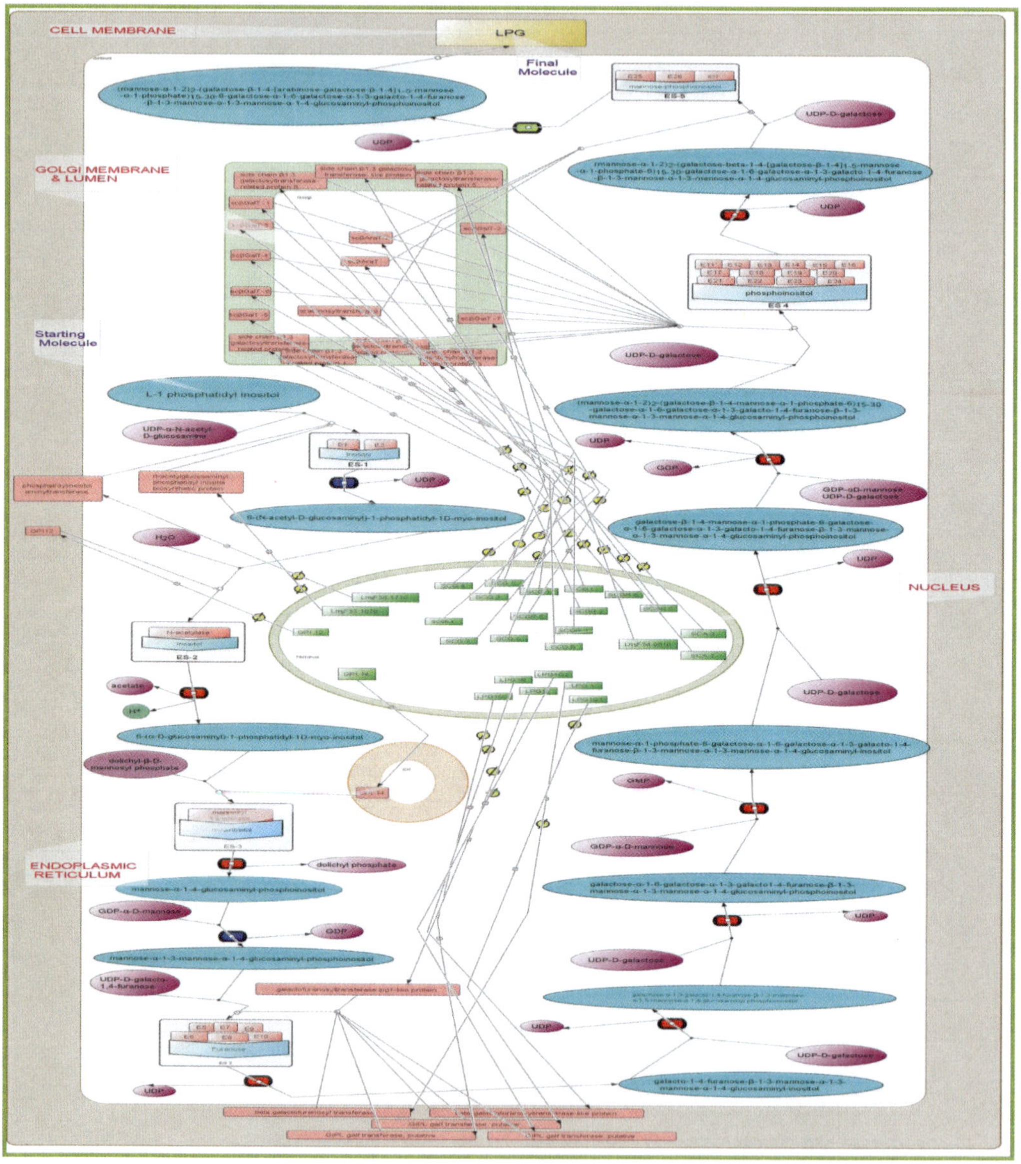

Fig. 7. Cellular Overview of the LPG Biosynthetic Pathway with respect to the Sub-cellular Localization, constructed using Cell Designer. The enzymes, for which the literature data was also not available, were considered to be within the cytosol.*

* Legend overleaf

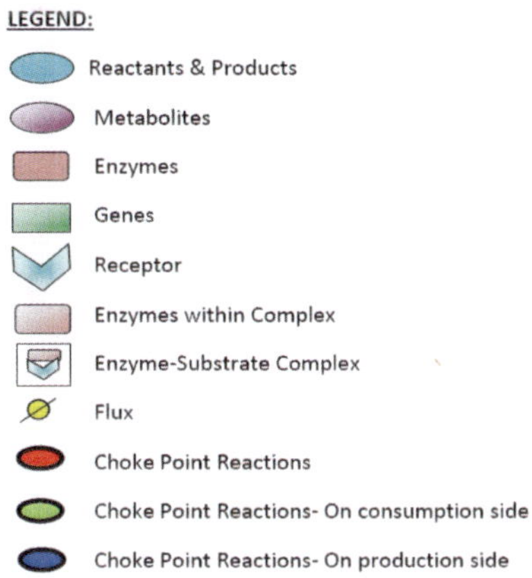

2.6 Biochemical modeling

Since it's established that the **Lipophosphoglycan Biosynthetic Pathway** posed a vital role in the Leishmania Parasite, and is a significant Pathway for identifying the drug targets, it is reconstructed in Cell Designer for generating a Mathematical Model of the same (Fig.8).

The genes coding for the enzymatic proteins, substrates, products, Enzyme-substrate complex, and the metabolites - all the entities are taken into account during the rebuilding of the pathway.

From this reconstruction, an outline of the change in the fluxes through the pathway is created. The fact file of all the contributing moieties is described in Table 3 and Table 4.

LPG Biosynthesis Reaction Summary		
Sr. No.	Species	Figures
1	Enzymes	27
2	Genes	27
3	Metabolites	27
	Consumed	13
	Produced	14
4	Compounds (Reactants & Products)	14
5	Enzyme-Substrate Complexes	6
6	Total no of Reactions	13
	Enzyme Catalyzed Reactions	6
	Non- Enzyme Catalyzed Reactions	7

Table 3. Summary of the LPG Biosynthesis Reaction.

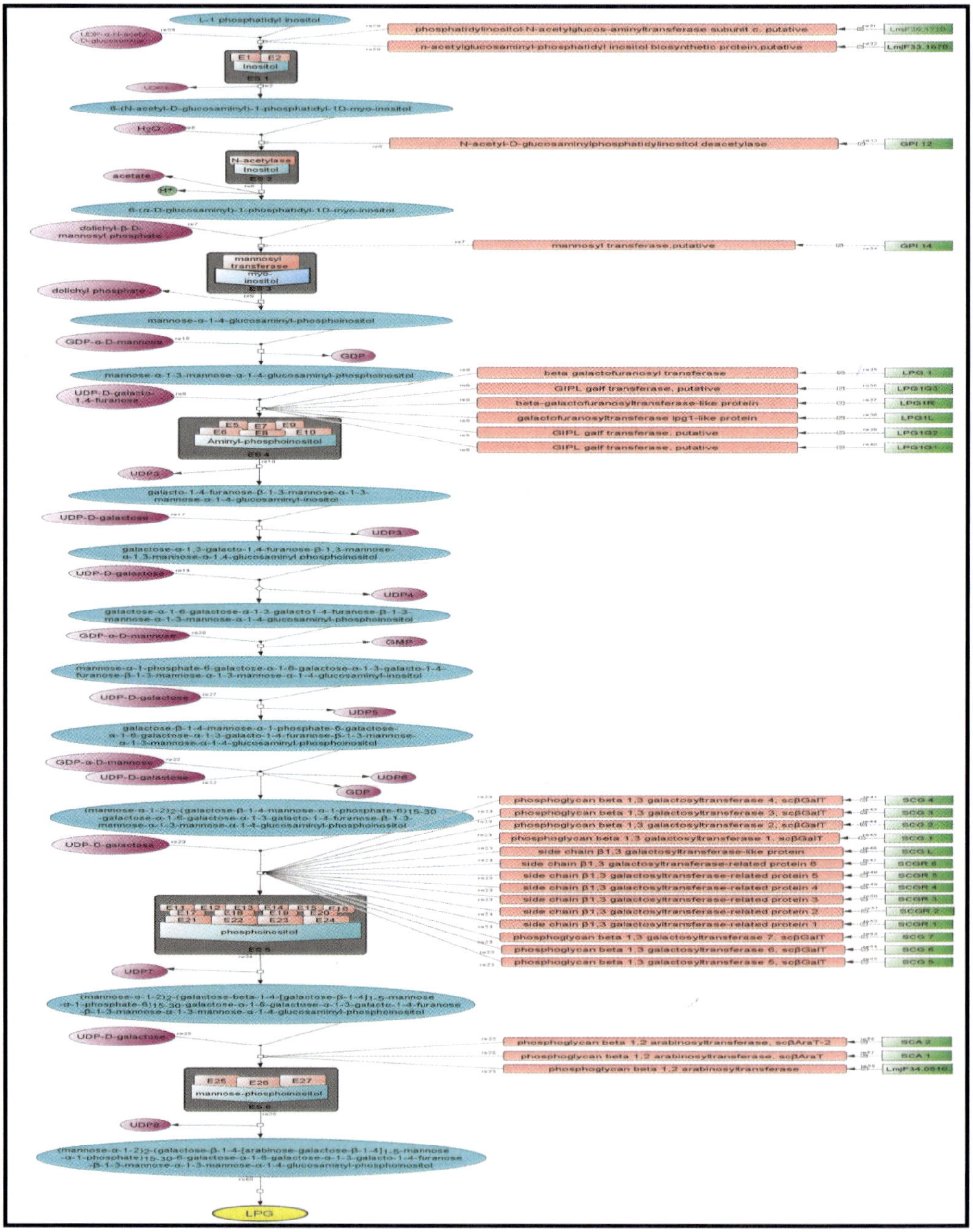

Fig. 8. Mathematical modeling of LPG Biosynthetic Pathway using Cell Designer.

Breakdown of Reactions		
1	Total no of Irreversible Reactions	67
	Enzyme Catalyzed Reactions	54
	Non- Enzyme Catalyzed Reactions	13
2	Transport Reactions	51
	Gene Reactions	27
	Non-gene reactions	24
3	Non- Transport Reactions	16

Table 4. Analysis of the individual reactions occurring in the LPG Biosynthesis Pathway.

Translating a known metabolic network into a dynamic model requires rate laws for all chemical reactions. The mathematical expressions depend on the underlying enzymatic mechanism; they can become quite involved and may contain a large number of parameters. Rate laws and enzyme parameters are still unknown for most enzymes. Convenience kinetics is used to translate a biochemical network – manually into a dynamical model with plausible biological properties. It implements enzyme saturation and regulation by activators and inhibitors, covers all possible reaction stoichiometries, and can be specified by a small number of parameters. Its mathematical form makes it especially suitable for parameter estimation and optimization. In general, the convenience kinetics applies to arbitrary reaction stoichiometries and captures biologically relevant behavior such as saturation, activation, inhibition with a small number of free parameters. It represents a simple molecular reaction mechanism in which substrates bind rapidly and in random order to the enzyme.

2.6.1 Convenience mass action kinetics

For the enzyme catalyzed reaction, i.e. from substrate to the ES-complex formation, the convenience rate law is taken into account. Rate laws and enzyme parameters are still unknown for most enzymes. For reactions with two or more catalysts, one individual rate law is generated for each catalyst. The total rate law for this particular reaction is given as the sum of the individual rates of all participating catalysts. The equation used here for convenience kinetics is:

$$\frac{E}{defult} \times \frac{kcat\_re \times \dfrac{\dfrac{R}{default}}{kcm\_re\_R} \times \dfrac{\dfrac{M}{default}}{kmc\_re\_M}}{1 + \dfrac{\dfrac{R}{default}}{kcm\_re\_R} \times 1 + \dfrac{\dfrac{M}{default}}{kmc\_re\_M}}$$

where, E is the Enzyme concentration, kcat_re is the catalysis constant, R is the Reactant concentration, M is the Metabolite constant, kmc_re_R and kmc_re_M are the reactant and metabolite Michelis constants respectively, default indicates the default initial quantity value defined by us. For reactions with more than 1 enzyme (catalysts), the equation is summed up for each value of the enzymes.

In general, the convenience kinetics applies to arbitrary reaction stoichiometries and captures biologically relevant behavior such as saturation, activation, inhibition with a small number of free parameters. It represents a simple molecular reaction mechanism in which substrates bind rapidly and in random order to the enzyme.

2.6.2 Generalized mass action

For non-enzyme catalyzed reaction, i.e. from the ES to the product formation, generalised mass-action kinetics is used. Mass action kinetics has numerous analytical properties that are of inherent interest from a dynamical systems perspective. These kinetic laws fail to describe enzyme saturation at high substrate concentrations, which is a common and relevant phenomenon.

$$\text{kass\_re} \times \frac{\text{ES} - \text{Co,plex}}{\text{default}}$$

where, kass_re is the association constant, ES-complex is the concentration of the ES-complex, default is the initial quantity value defined by us.

2.6.3 Hill-Hinze equation

SBMLsqueezer offers the general Hill equation as a kinetic law for the formation of gene products:

$$V_{re2} = \text{v max\_re2} \cdot \frac{[R1]^{hic\_re2\_s2}}{[R1]^{hic\_re2\_2} + \text{ksp\_re2\_s2}^{hic\_re2\_s2}}$$

Since it is assumed that the transition from a gene to protein as "a known transition omitted", and ignored the RNA, the Hill equation is modified by the SBML Squeezer as per the reaction"s convenience and the equation is given as: Vmax_re where, vmax is the maximum velocity attained. Now, according to Quassi Steady State rule, d/dt [mRNA] =0 , i.e. for the intermediate compound, and moreover the concentration of the mRNA reaches steady state very quickly, compared to protein concentration, it is considered that [mRNA] concentration is always considered at steady state.

2.7 Numerical simulations

On the basis of these kinetic laws, the numerical simulations are carried out with certain default values of the parameters and the initial quantities. By means of the numerical simulations, certain graphs are obtained which display the interactions of the molecules with each other and the effect of minute variations in the kinetic parameters. The graphs also generate visualization for the fluxes. For each of the enzyme catalyzed reactions the simulation process is carried out separately for reducing the complications in interpretation of the graphs generated.

In each of the graphs, it is postulated that there was a constant decrease in the concentration of the substrate, while the product had a steady increase in the concentration, with the ES complex initially forming up but then gradually decreasing with time when the product formation began each time. Therefore, on an overall basis, from the above generated graphs, it is concluded that as and when the downstream reaction is considered, there is a potential fall in the flux, though not in the reaction 1, indicating that the flux increased from reaction 1 to reaction 2. Moreover, there is a consistent drop in the concentration of the ES complex as well, which signified that the product is gradually being formed. The concentration of gene G1 almost remain unchanged during this process as the transcription does not change the state of the gene. The principal result of this work is laid onto the idea that it shows a simply identifiable class of kinetic expressions, including the familiar detailed balanced kinetics as a proper subclass, which ensures consistency with the extended thermodynamic conditions. The rate laws applied provided a very good fit to the data. With the network model it is identified which steps have strong effect on other parts of the network using sensitivity analysis, and those steps that do indeed have high levels of control are then chosen further for kinetic analysis. This helped to further postulate that GPI 14 (encoding for mannosyltransferase) and Galf (encoding for Galf transferase) could be examined further since they showed a strong effect on the rest of the network model (Fig.9 A,B,C,D,E and F). The most important feature for building a bottom-up biochemical network model is that the relation between the concentration of the effectors and the rate be accurate. The objective is to learn more about how cells work via the means of computational models and not all about the mechanisms of catalysis, except when they are found themselves of importance to cellular function. The concept of "gene function" becomes synonym with the kinetics of its protein product embedded in the cellular biochemical network.

The network-based representation and analysis of biological systems contributes to a greater understanding of their structures and functions at different levels of complexity. By defining the properties of a system as a whole, the approach aids in improvising decision making in the therapeutic drug development, which has a limitation otherwise, to be predicted from the parts. The goal of modeling in systems biology is to provide a background for hypothesis formulation and prediction based on *in silico* simulation of parasite biology across the multiple distance and time scales. The metabolic reconstruction of biochemical pathway serves as a tool for clarifying inconsistencies between data sources, and provides a platform for data integration and hypothesis generation for further scientific research in infectious disease. By means of the Cell Designer, utilizing its SBML language platform, we articulate a succinct representation of the biochemical properties adopted by a biological system and the underlying metabolic networks, and consequently translate them into systems compatible to stochastic simulations. Ensuing such model construction, and subsequent simulations we introduce a time component in the interaction reactions to determine certain physiochemical conditions of the biological system. Simulations aid in transforming the static data into the dynamic sphere of physiological timescales, by revealing insights into the flexibility of energy metabolism. These simulated models of

A

First Reaction :

Simulation graphs of Reaction 1

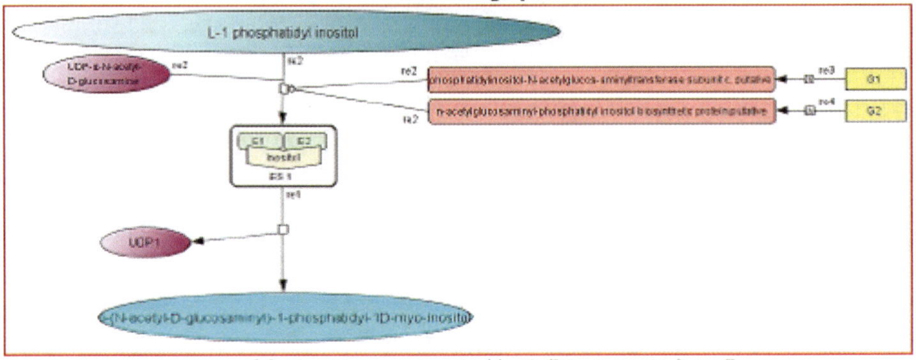

(a) Reaction represented by Cell Designer indiviually

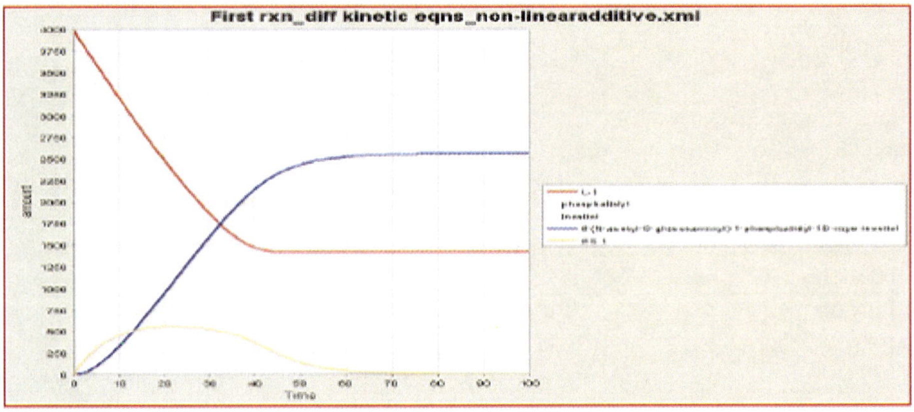

(b) Substrate, ES and Product Formation.

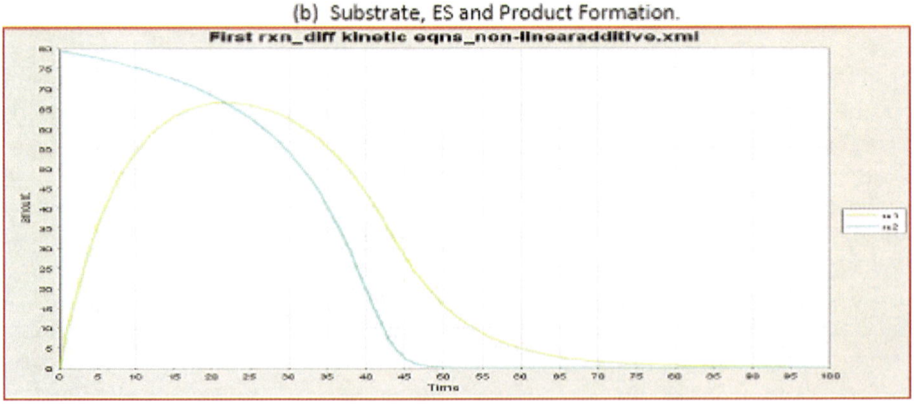

(c) Fluxes of the sub- reaction 1 and sub- reaction 2.

B

Second Reaction:

Simulation graphs of Reaction 2

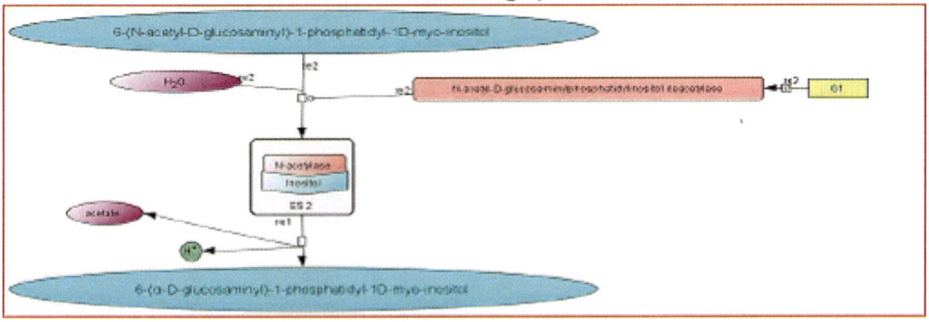

(a) Reaction represented by Cell Designer indiviually

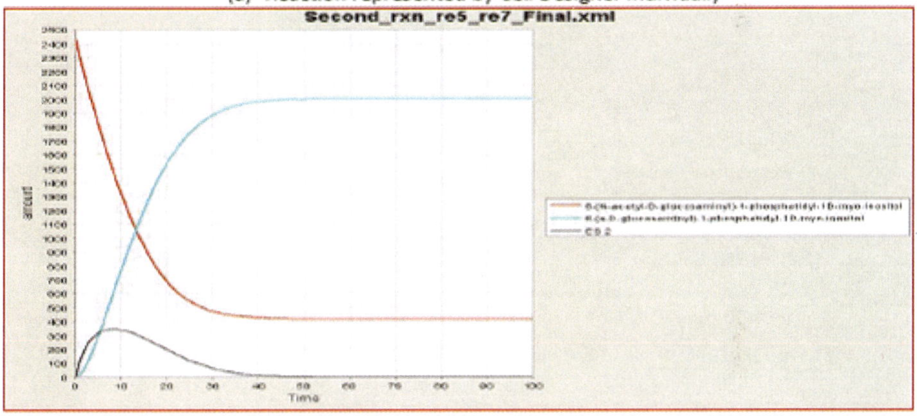

(b) Substrate, ES and Product Formation

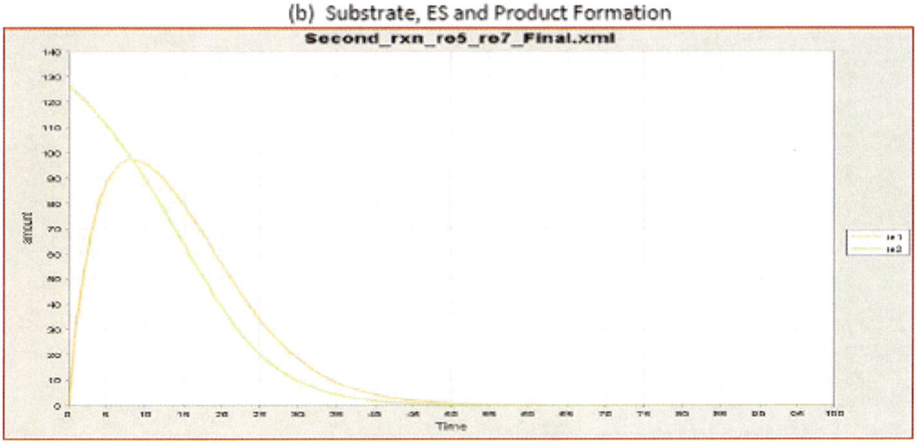

(c) Fluxes of reaction sub-1 and sub-reaction 2.

C

<u>**Third Reaction:**</u>

Simulation graphs of Reaction 3

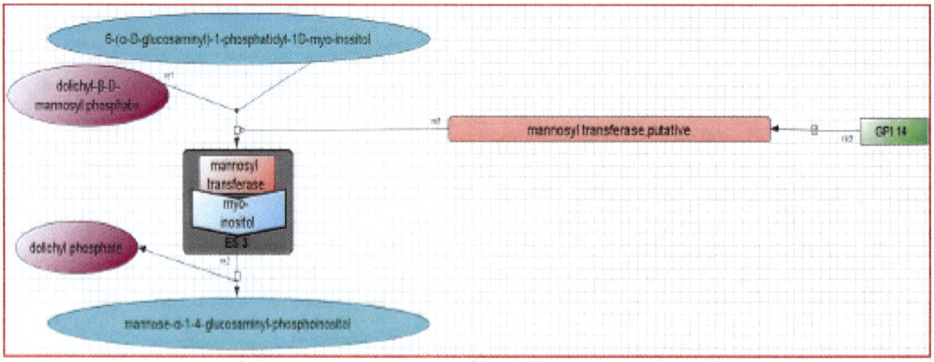

(a) Reaction represented by Cell Designer indiviually

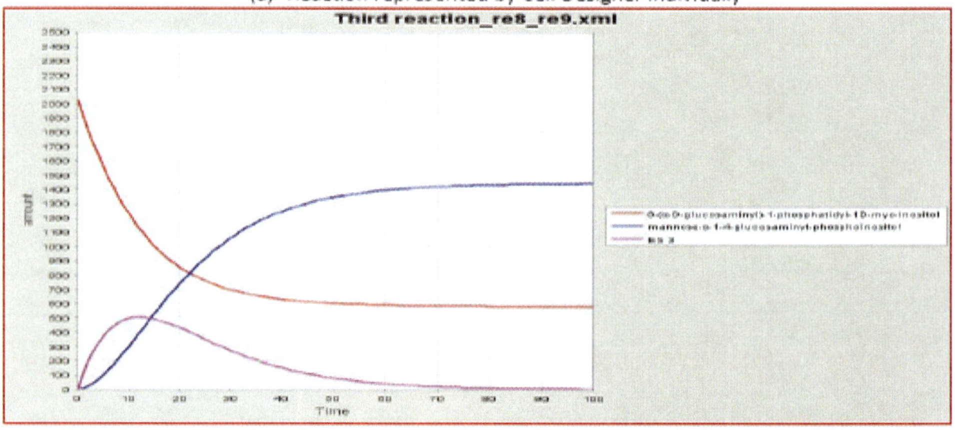

(b) Substrate, ES and Product Formation : the Graph shows a steady formation of the product

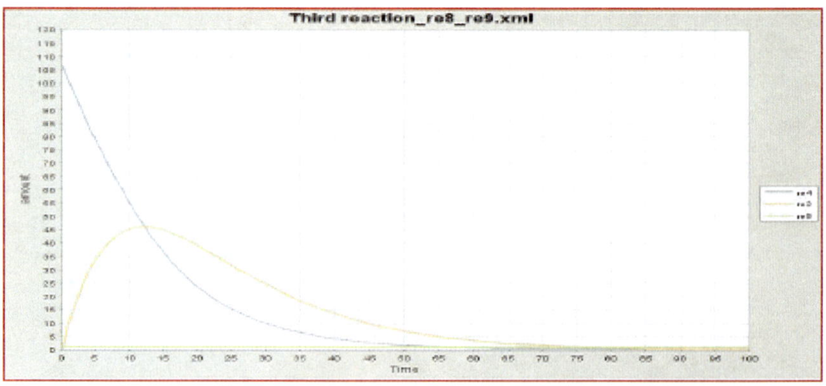

(c) Fluxes of sub- reaction 1,sub-reaction 2 and sub-reaction 3

D

Fourth reaction:

Simulation graphs of Reaction 4

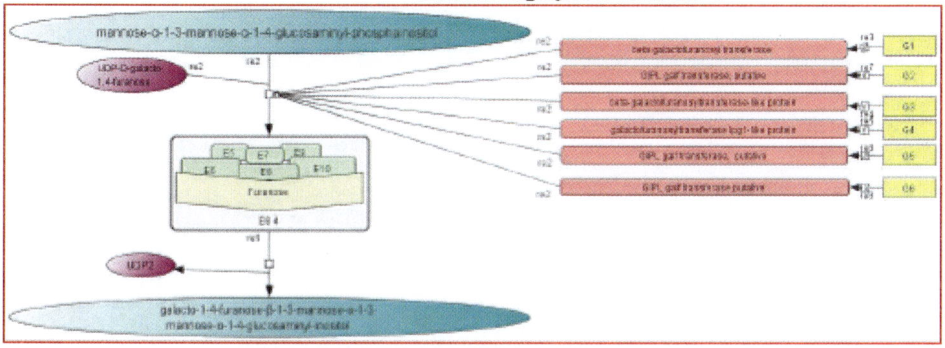

(a) Reaction represented by Cell Designer indiviually

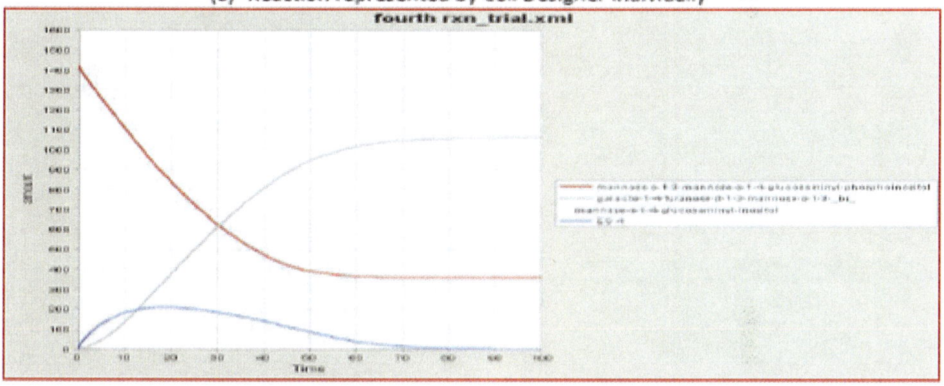

(b) Substrate, ES and Product Formation

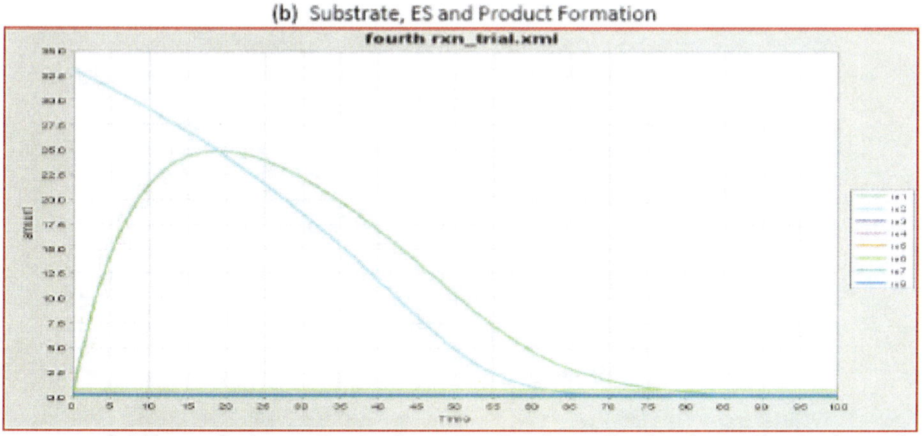

(c) Fluxes of sub- reaction 1,sub-reaction 2, sub-reaction 3, sub- reaction 4,sub-reaction 5, sub- reaction 6,sub-reaction 7, and sub- reaction 8.

E

Fifth Reaction:

Simulation graphs of Reaction 5

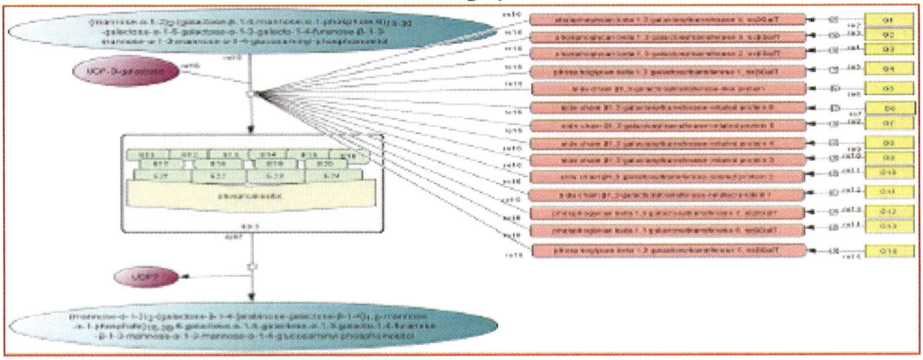

(a) Reaction represented by Cell Designer indiviually

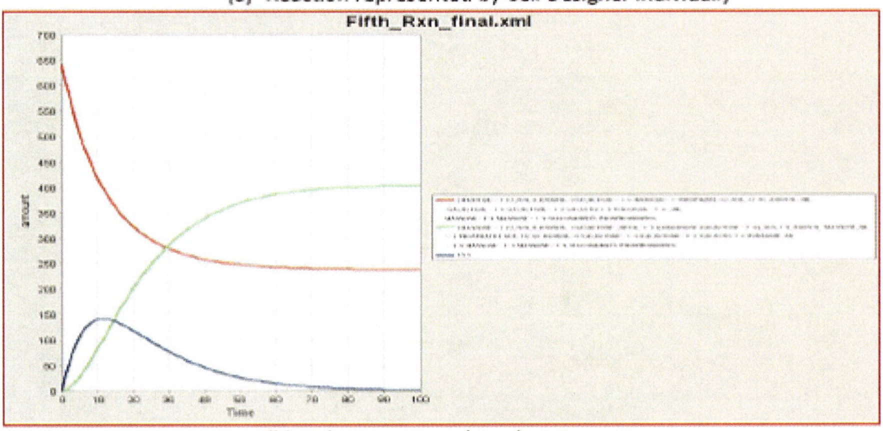

(b) Substrate, ES and Product Formation

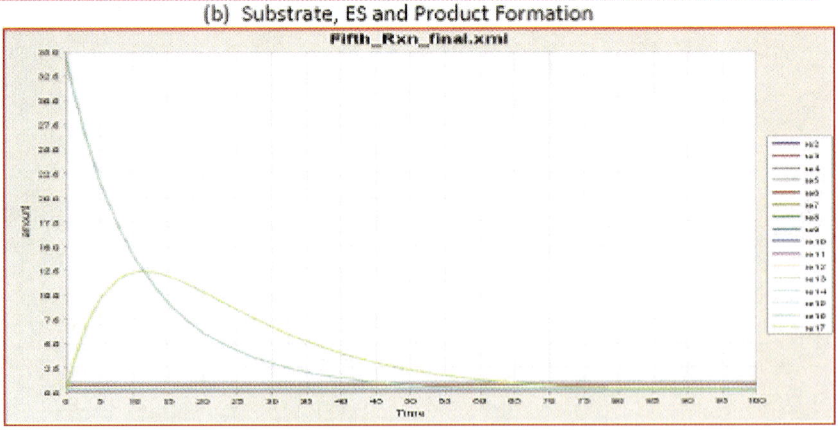

(c) Fluxes of sub- reaction 1 to sub-reaction -17

F

<u>Sixth Reaction:</u>

Simulation graphs of Reaction 6

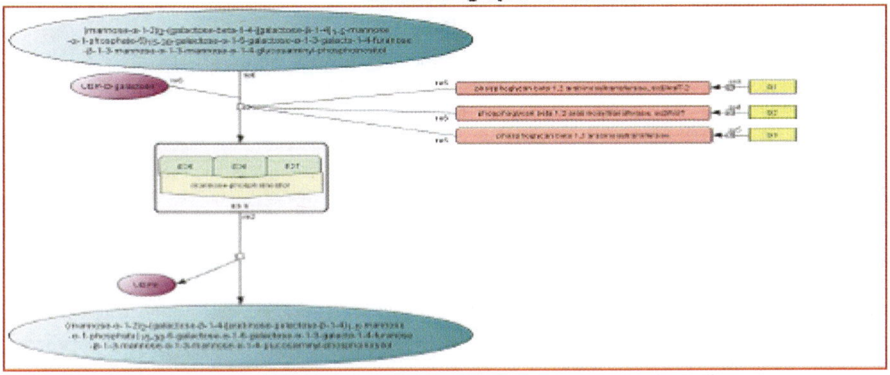

(a) Reaction represented by Cell Designer indiviually

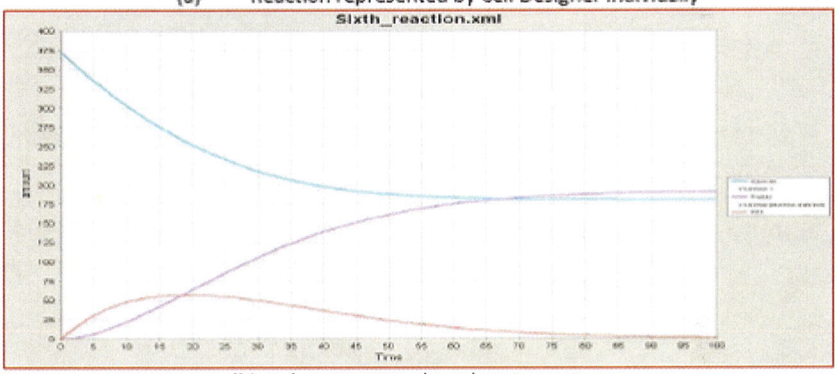

(b) Substrate, ES and Product Formation

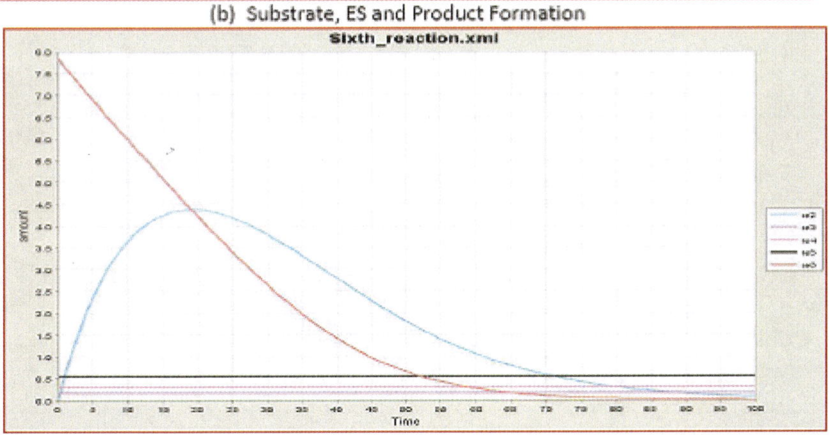

(c) Fluxes of sub-reaction 2, sub-reaction 3, sub- reaction 4,sub-reaction 5 and sub- reaction 6.

Fig. 9. Fluxes across six set of reactions in LPG biosynthetic pathway of *L. major* predicted through discrete stochastic simulation event.

biochemical reaction pathways are quite enthralling since their mathematics provides a means to amalgamate prior knowledge with postulated data and the underlying physical principles, through the graphical visualizations. Thus, we say graphical approaches simplify the process of transforming a network diagram into a set of linked equations. [Aldridge et al., 2006] Thereby, the prediction of potential novel targets can aid in the identification of revolutionary approach for controlling the level of specific, therapeutically relevant genes or proteins. We can test the efficacy of drug targets in the presence of enzyme inhibitors, through the metabolic reconstructions. These techniques can also be used to identify potential novel therapeutic targets based on the characterization of vulnerable or highly influential network components. [Azuaje et al., 2010] To summarize in a nutshell, the *in vivo* and *in silico* understanding of the "Omics" field and the subsequent assimilation of genome, proteome, metabolome and interactome sciences in cellular and multicellular systems is essential for drug discovery.

3. References

Aldridge et al., 2006, Physicochemical modeling of cell signaling pathways, Nature Cell Biology, 8:1195-1203.

Antonio del Sol et al., 2010, Diseases as network perturbations, Current Opinion in Biotechnology, 21:566-571.

Azuaje et al., 2010, Identification of potential targets in biological signaling systems through network perturbation analysis, Biosystems, 100:55-64.

Bergter and Vermelho, 2010. Structures of Glycolipids Found in Trypanosomatids: Contribution to Parasite Functions, The Open Parasitology Journal, 2010, 4:84-97.

Cavalieri and Filippo, 2005, Bioinformatic methods for integrating whole-genome expression results into cellular networks, DrugDiscoveryToday, 10:727-734.

Chavali et al., 2008. Systems analysis of metabolism in the pathogenic trypanosomatid Leishmania major, Molecular Systems Biology, 4:1-19.

Davidov et al., 2003. Advancing drug discovery through systems biology, Drug Discovery Today, 8:175-183.

Douglas B. Kell, 2006. Systems biology, metabolic modeling and metabolomics in drug discovery and development, Drug discovery Today, 11:1085-1092.

Falkow S, 1988, Molecular Koch's postulates applied to microbial pathogenicity, Rev Infect Dis, 10:S274-S276.

Funahashi et al., 2003, Cell Designer: a process diagram editor for gene regulatory and biochemical network, Biosilico, 1: 159-162.

Haughan et al., 1995, Effects of an azasterol inhibitor of sterol 24-transmethylation on sterol biosynthesis and growth of Leishmania donovani promastigotes, Biochem J 308: 31–38.

G.F. Spath, 2000. Lipophosphoglycan is a virulence factor distinct from related glycoconjugates in the protozoan parasite Leishmania major, PNAS, 97:9258–9263.

Horn and Jackson 2004. General mass Action Kinetics. Archive for rational Mechanics and Analysis 47:81-116.

Karplus and McCammon, 2002. Molecular dynamics simulations of biomolecules, Nature structural Biology, 9:646-788.

Lipka, G., Chowdhry, B.Z. and Sturtevant, J.M. 1984 A comparison of the phase transition properties of 1,2-diacylphosphatidylcholines and 1,2-diacylphosphatidylethanolamines in water and deuterium oxide. *J. Phys. Chem.*, 88, pp 5401–5406.

Lee et al., 2006. Flux balance analysis in the era of metabolomics, Brief Bioinform, 7:140-150.

Liebermeister and Klipp. 2006. Bringing metabolic networks to life: convenience rate law and thermodynamic constraints, Theoretical Biology and Medical Modelling, 3:1186- 1192.

Marchisio and Stelling, 2009. Computational design tools for synthetic biology,Current Opinion in biotechnology, 20:479-485.

Niemela et al., 2009. Bioinformatics and Computational method for lipidomics, Journal of Chromatography B, 877:2855-2862.

Oppenheimer et al., 2011. Isolation and characterization of functional Leishmania major virulence factor UDP-galactopyranose mutase, Biochemical and Biophysical Research Communications, 407:552-556.

Perez Victoria,F.J., Sanchez-Canete,M., Seifert,K., Croft, S.L., Sundar,S., Castanys,S., and Gamarro, F. 2006 Mechanisms of experimental resistance of *Leishmania* to miltefosine: Implications for clinical use. Drug Resistance Updates 9, 26–39.

Reed et al., 2006. Towards multidimensional genome annotation, Nat Rev Genet, 7:130-141.

Roberts et al., 2009, Proteomic and network analysis characterize stage-specific metabolism in *Trypanosoma cruzi* ,BMC Systems Biology, 3: 1- 15.

Sergio Grimbs, 2009. Towards structure and dynamics of metabolic networks, Institutional Repository of the University of Potsdam.

Singh 2011 Membrane permeability in Biological Systems: A Systems Biology Perspective. Journal of Computer Science and Systems Biology 4:027-032.

Thiele and Bernhard, 2010, A protocol for generating a high-quality genome-scale metabolic reconstruction,Nature Protocols, 5:93-121.

Tyson et al., 2001, Network dynamics and cell physiology, Nat.Rev.Mol.Cell.Biol. 2:908-916.

Weber and Fusseneger, 2009, The impact of synthetic biology on drug discovery, Drug discovery Today, 14:956-963.

Zhang and Beverley, 2010, Phospholipid and sphingolipid metabolism in Leishmania, Molecular & Biochemical Parasitology, 170:55–64.

Zhang et al., 2004, The LPG1 gene family of *Leishmania major*, Molecular & Biochemical Parasitology, 136:11–23.

Zhang K. et al., 2003, Sphingolipids are essential for differentiation but not growth in Leishmania, EMBO J 22: 6016–6026.

Zufferey and Mamoun 2005. The initial step of glycerolipid metabolism in Leishmania major promastigotes involves a single glycerol-3-phosphate acyltransferase enzyme important for the synthesis of triacylglycerol but not essential for virulence, Molecular Microbiology, 56:800–810.

Zufferey et al. 2003. Ether phospholipids and glycosylinositolphospholipids are not required for amastigote virulence or for inhibition of macrophage activation by Leishmania major, J Biol Chem 278: 44708–44718.

17

Molecular Modeling and Simulation of Membrane Transport Proteins

Andreas Jurik, Freya Klepsch and Barbara Zdrazil
University of Vienna, Department of Medicinal Chemistry
Pharmacoinformatics Research Group
Austria

1. Introduction

Membranes fulfill the essential need of all living species to separate different compartments. On the other hand, in a cell the homeostatic environment can only be maintained by the cellular membrane acting as a selective 'filter', which allows the cell to continuously communicate with other cells. Mechanisms which facilitate the translocation of materials across the membrane regulate the entrance and disposal of ions, amino acids, nutrients, and signaling molecules.

This selective transport across cellular membranes is carried out by two broad classes of specialized proteins, which are associated with or embedded in those lipid bilayers: channels and transmembrane transporters. They work by different mechanisms: Whereas channels catalyze the passage of ions (or water and gas in the case of the aquaporin channel) (Agre, 2006) across the membrane through a watery pore spanning the membrane-embedded protein, transporters are working via a cycle of conformational changes that expose substrate-binding sites alternately to the two sides of the membrane (Theobald & Miller, 2010).

If we regard the force that drives the transport process there is also a huge difference in the way ion channels and transporters act. Channels assist a downhill movement along a concentration gradient (passive diffusion), whereas in transporters it is usually directed against a concentration gradient of the substrate. Thus, in order to comply with their business, transporters are dependent on another source of the cellular energy. Secondary active transporters rely on ionic gradients. In the case of primary active transporters ATP is the driving force (Wang et al., 2010).

A comprehensive list of all annotated transport proteins is freely available online on the TCDB website (http://www.tcdb.org). This Transporter Classification Database uses an International Union of Biochemistry and Molecular Biology (IUBMB) approved system of nomenclature for transport protein classification. The TC system is analogous to the Enzyme Commission (EC) system for classification of enzymes, except that it incorporates both functional and phylogenetic information (Saier et al., 2006; Saier et al., 2009).

According to the TCDB system Membrane Transport proteins can be classified as follows (List of families and subfamilies of the TC system):

1. Pores and channels
   a. Helical channels
   b. Strand porins
   c. Pore-forming toxins
   d. Non-ribosomally synthesized channels
   e. Holins
2. Electrochemical-potential-driven transporters
   a. Transporters or carriers (uniporters, symporters and antiporters)
   b. Non-ribosomally synthesized transporters
3. Primary active transporters
   a. P-P-bond-hydrolysis-driven transporters
   b. Decarboxylation-driven transporters
   c. Methyl-transfer-driven transporters
   d. Oxidoreduction-driven transporters
   e. Light-driven transporters
4. Group translocators
5. Transmembrane electron carriers
6. Accessory factors involved in transport
7. Incompletely characterized transport systems

Our special interest focuses on transmembrane transport proteins ('transporters'). Excellent manuscripts on membrane channels have been provided by other groups (Gumbart et al., 2005; Schmidt et al., 2006).

To date more than 400 membrane proteins have been annotated in the human genome. Two major superfamilies - which are also intensively investigated in our group - are the **ATP- binding cassette transporters** (ABC, e.g. P-glycoprotein), and the **solute carrier superfamily** (SLC). They will be discussed into more detail in section 3 of this chapter.

1.1 Transporters as pharmacological targets

Transport proteins are playing important roles in the whole drug discovery and development process. They regulate absorption, distribution, and excretion of drugs and therefore influence drug disposition, therapeutic efficacy and adverse drug reactions in the human body. This has to be taken into account in pharmacological studies (Giacomini et al., 2010).

It is estimated that transporters account for about 50% of drug targets. However, their modes of (selective) transport are only poorly understood. This is due to difficulties in membrane protein purification, expression, and crystallization (Caffrey, 2003), which is still in its childhood. As a consequence there exists a striking disproportion between the number of entries of resolved structures of soluble proteins and membrane proteins in the protein databank (PDB, http://www.pdb.org/). To date, only about 2% (1462 by Sept 2011) of the structures are from transmembrane proteins (75594 structures in total). Out of these there are only 302 unique structures (proteins of same type but from different species are included) (Irvine). Moreover, a significant number of the membrane protein structures determined are at relatively low resolutions (Lindahl & Sansom, 2008).

However, there are tremendous efforts as to ameliorate the methods in order to obtain atomic resolution structures of membrane protein molecules (Newby et al., 2009). Thus, for the past two decades, the number of available structures of membrane proteins has been climbing the exponential foot of the growth curve, since it is doubling every three years (Theobald & Miller, 2010).

For a medicinal chemist, the availability of a growing number of structures, paves the way for further *in silico* studies. Some are very promising in a way that they can be used as templates in order to build up a homology model of the membrane protein of interest. Those models, which may further be applied for Molecular Dynamics (MD) Simulation and Docking Studies, give us the opportunity to gather new insights into the molecular structure and function of the protein under investigation and the behaviour of certain ligands in the binding site.

As translocation always involves a dynamic process, which cannot easily be studied by mere experimental techniques, above all, the application of long-term MD simulations should be implemented into the whole process of drug discovery and development. Due to significant increase in computational power and improvements in parallelization techniques, nowadays simulations of membrane transport proteins may stretch up to microseconds - that is, to physiologically relevant time scales. In this review we are describing the theory and methodology related to computational techniques used in the modeling of transporters and we will outline the recent developments in the field of ABC transporters and neurotransmitter transporters.

2. Methods

2.1 Homology modeling

2.1.1 Basic concepts

Despite the enormous increase of published structural data for proteins, the particular availability for a protein of interest can vary from the sheer presence of the amino acid sequence to a multitude of high-resolution X-ray structures. Fortunately, Mother Nature was not too generous in providing unique structural folds for functionally related proteins, as the structural arrangement within a family of homologous proteins is much higher conserved than the respective amino acid sequences (Lesk & Chothia, 1980). Thus, in many cases the combination of a primary sequence on the one hand and one or more reasonably well-resolved homologue structures on the other hand can result in homology models surprisingly well representing the molecular reality, paving the way to successful comparative modeling studies. The process of predicting the 3D structure of a protein can be achieved by four main steps: fold assignment, target-template sequence alignment, building and evaluation of the models (Cavasotto, 2011).

2.1.2 Assignment of the basic fold and sequence alignment

The first step towards a good model is the identification and careful selection of structurally related template proteins. Although generally a high percentage of global sequence identity is a good indicator for the model quality to be expected, it must be kept in mind that the identity in the area of interest, i.e. the binding site(s), can differ significantly from overall values. One should strive to put the main focus during template selection on facilitating a maximum of accuracy in modeling those vital regions.

Maybe the best source for structural templates is the Protein Data Bank (Berman et al., 2000). As mentioned earlier, it offers the coordinates of structurally resolved proteins, including large amounts of surplus information like primary sequence, experimental settings or co-bound ligands and ions. Search tools like BLAST and FASTA (Altschul et al., 1997; Pearson, 1990) usually do reasonably well in identifying the correct fold of a protein. The second, even trickier step is the subsequent alignment step of target and template sequence, as it is possible with T-Coffee or CLUSTAL W (Notredame et al., 2000; Thompson et al., 1994). Conserved residues and regions of experimentally determined proximity need to be aligned as accurately as possible. Multiple alignments of sequences belonging to the same gene family can significantly enhance the performance of the search for conserved residues or even regions, but thorough literature search and manual adjustment of the alignment are inevitable in order to achieve best results.

A good example for the importance of taking a comprehensive look at the research subject is the meanwhile annual GPCR Dock competition (Kufareva et al., 2011), where prior to the release of newly resolved G-Protein Coupled Receptors (GPCR) 3D structures, modeling groups get the chance to submit their best efforts of predicting the correct receptor and ligand conformation. It turned out, that advanced modeling tools and human intervention contributed about equally to the success of the individual approaches.

2.1.3 Building and refinement of the models

Once it is assumed that the alignment meets all available experimental data, it can be started to calculate coordinates for the target residues. Although automated homology modeling methods exist, the yielded models tend to lack accuracy, especially in cases of low sequence identity (Dalton & Jackson, 2007).

Usually, the crude model is built by aligning the basic backbone framework, the so-called structurally conserved regions (SCRs). Conserved secondary structural elements like α-helices or β-sheets are inherited, being responsible for the general shape of the model. Several homology modeling approaches also try to include information about known ligands into the binding site construction in order to meet its particular geometry (Evers & Klebe, 2004; Sherman et al., 2006).

Subsequently, assignment of the side chain conformations needs to be done according to steric and energetic constraints. Identical residues usually can be considered to be oriented similarly, likewise highly similar amino acids. For non related residues, rotamer libraries can provide initial geometrical guesses (Schrauber et al., 1993), although other effects like packing energies may lead to significant deviations. Up to 30% of side chain conformations in X-ray structures do not correspond to usual rotamers, yet adopting energetically allowed conformations. Naturally, selecting the most probable side chain orientation solely according to statistical criteria is problematic, so methods including structural features of the local environment have been developed (Deane & Blundell, 2001). Still, some cases require manual adjustment, for instance the incorporation of known disulfide bridges, specific internal hydrogen bonds or ion binding pockets.

The major challenge in comparative modeling is the treatment of structurally variable regions (SVRs). Especially flexible loop regions lacking a structural template are difficult to predict, since the calculation time increases nearly exponentially with the degrees of freedom added by every flexible residue. There are several strategies to meet this issue. Knowledge-based strategies try to find structural guesses by automated database search for related sequence sections in other proteins, possibly not even close to being genetically similar. From a computational point of view, conformational searches by *ab initio* calculation of the desired region are more costly, but recent approaches yielded reasonably good results for a loop length up to 17 residues (Mehler et al., 2002; Zhao et al., 2011). For significantly longer loops, in case that the problematic region is remote from the actual binding site(s) and not considered being directly linked to the binding process, it can be viable to leave it up to the standard modeling software how to build the respective flexible region, and hope for subsequent MD simulations to find a near-to-native conformation (Amaro & Li, 2010).

The model building process bears numerous sources of unfavorable steric strain energies, calling for an appropriate minimization procedure. As one can imagine, this step has to be carefully balanced in order to overcome steric clashes without compromising tediously elaborated side chain orientations or, even worse, entire conserved regions. Instead of global optimization attempts good minimization protocols start with local treatment of clashes with initially fixed backbone atoms. Thus, solvent molecules, ions and hydrogen atoms possibly responsible for large initial forces can adopt energetically more favorable positions. Gradually, initial tethering forces are reduced, avoiding artificial distortions (Höltje et al., 2008). This can be facilitated by molecular mechanics calculations using different force fields like CHARMM (Brooks et al., 1983), OPLS (Jorgensen & Rives, 1988) or AMBER (Weiner et al., 1984). In contrast to force fields for small molecules, they have to handle huge systems, therefore being usually somehow simplified regarding the treatment of long-distance non-bonding interactions or non-polar hydrogen atoms, called united-atom models.

Energy minimized models may be further optimized by molecular dynamics (MD) simulations, as reported in-depth in section 2.3.

2.1.4 Model evaluation

Predictions including as many degrees of freedom as homology models desperately need reliable tools to estimate their quality, as the accuracy of a 3D model is responsible for the amount of information that can be gained by it (Marti-Renom et al., 2000). Several evaluation programs exist; many of them are available online on server-basis. The SWISS-MODEL (Arnold et al., 2006) (http://swissmodel.expasy.org) and the SAVES server (http://nihserver.mbi.ucla.edu/SAVES), for instance, offer a variety of local and global quality estimation tools (Benkert et al., 2011; Hutchinson & Thornton, 1996; Zhou & Zhou, 2002). It is important to look at both, as they are not necessarily mutually related.

A comprehensive stereochemistry check can be carried out using the Procheck suite (Laskowski et al., 1993), searching for geometrically unusual residues in a given protein structure by comparison with stereochemical parameters of high-quality benchmark structures. Likewise, the What_Check module of the WHATIF package and the VADAR web server do a similar job (Vriend, 1990; Willard et al., 2003). The features examined include the planarity of aromatic ring system and peptide bonds, bond lengths and basic checks like C_{α}-chirality.

Once the yielded quality statistics are acceptable within the limitations of the possible, a model can be considered ready for the further use in, for instance, docking studies.

2.2 Molecular docking

Molecular Docking is a versatile tool in structure based drug design. This technique is able to predict possible orientations of one molecule to another. In this section we will focus on protein-ligand docking, describing the interaction of a small molecule in a binding pocket of the protein of interest.

In principle molecular docking is comprised of three consecutive steps: i) the definition of the binding site, ii) the placement of the ligand inside the defined site, and iii) the ensuing evaluation of this placement, called scoring.

2.2.1 Binding site identification

The right determination of the binding site of the ligand is essential for the subsequent docking process. If the active site is not known there are several algorithms that are able to detect potential binding pockets (extensively reviewed in (Henrich et al., 2010)). These programs scan the protein surface for cavities that fulfill certain geometrical constraints, which mark them as possible ligand binding sites. While the program LIGSITE uses a grid for the surface scan (Hendlich et al., 1997), the PASS algorithm utilizes layers of spheres that should describe buried cavities (Stouten & Brady, 2000).

In order to consider also physico-chemical criteria in binding site detection the surface of the protein can be scanned with fragments of ligands with subsequent calculation of their complementarity. Another approach to get an idea about potential active sites can be achieved by comparing the query protein with homologues, as proteins with related function share similar binding sites. For this purpose the program CAVBASE (Kuhn et al., 2007), which relies on the LIGSITE algorithm, has been developed.

As soon as the binding site is known, it has to be characterized in order to get information about specific binding possibilities through non-covalent interactions. To detect these hot spots atom probes, ligand fragments or whole small molecules are positioned inside the binding pocket. The program GRID is able to detect interactions and solvation effects by calculating the interaction energy between grid points of the binding pocket and certain atom probes (Reynolds et al., 1989). On the other hand, the multiple copy simultaneous search (MCSS) method places thousands of probe copies inside the pocket. After energy minimization those probes cluster at certain local minima defining the hot spots (Caflisch et al., 1993).

2.2.2 Search algorithms

The role of the search algorithm is the correct placement of the ligand in the binding pocket. Ideally it should therefore consider all possible degrees of freedom, which leads to higher accuracy. However, due to limitations regarding computer power, this is penalized in favor of higher speed by reducing the number of the degrees of freedom (Sousa et al., 2006).

Although in protein-protein docking the rigid-body approximation is still applied (Kuntz et al., 1982), in protein-ligand docking the small molecule is treated flexible.

Approaches that try to explore all degrees of freedom of the ligand systematically comprise conformational search methods, fragmentation methods or database methods. By applying conformational search methods, every rotatable bond of the ligand is rotated in fixed increments. As this can easily lead to a combinatorial explosion, this technique can only be applied for small or rigid ligands. More prevalently used are the so-called fragmentation methods that place fragments of the ligand in the binding pocket, which are subsequently fused. Depending on the fragmentation and placing of the ligand *place and join* and *incremental approaches* can be distinguished. Popular docking programs utilizing this type of search algorithms include LUDI (Bohm, 1992), FlexX (Rarey et al., 1996), DOCK (Ewing et al., 2001), ADAM (Mizutani et al., 1994) or Hammerhead (Welch et al., 1996).

A computationally efficient way to search for possible orientations forms the database method. For this protocol a conformational library of the ligand is prepared which is docked rigidly into the binding site.

Besides systematic search algorithms there are programs that prefer stochastic principles for binding mode prediction. At this the flexibility of the ligand is provided by random conformational changes that are either kept or rejected on basis of a direct evaluation of the conformation. Among others genetic algorithms present a convenient tool for this purpose. With this optimizing procedure a random population of possible ligand poses is generated, where the characteristics (degrees of freedom) of each are stored in its genetic code (chromosome). By applying genetic operations, like cross-over or mutation, new poses are generated and subsequently scored. Depending on this fitness score the pose is either rejected or it replaces the least fit member of the population. This procedure is conducted over thousands of cycles which ends up in highly optimized ligand orientations. This protocol is included in the popular docking programs GOLD (Jones et al., 1995; Verdonk et al., 2003) and AUTODOCK (Goodsell et al., 1996; Goodsell & Olson, 1990; Olson et al., 1998).

Another possibility to consider ligand flexibility is presented by molecular dynamics simulation of the ligand in the binding pocket. However, this is mainly used in combination with other search algorithms (Kitchen et al., 2004).

In the last years not only the flexibility of the ligand but also protein movements due to ligand binding gained more and more importance (B-Rao et al., 2009; Cozzini et al., 2008). Although it is known that some proteins undergo large structural changes, even domain rearrangements, upon ligand binding, by now it is not possible to cover that in reasonable time and effort. However, since docking a ligand into the right conformation of the binding site is extremely important for the quality of the resulting orientations, efficient workarounds have been developed. Soft docking is one possibility to account small movements of the protein side chains during docking (Jiang & Kim, 1991). For this technique soft potentials are applied on certain side chain atoms in the binding pocket, which therefore tolerate overlap with ligand atoms. The merit of this technique is the easy implementation, as only scoring parameters have to be adapted. On the other hand only small changes can be considered and there might be a bias towards the starting structure.

With the help of rotamer libraries, movements of side chains are included in the search algorithm (Leach, 1994). Depending on the size of the library this method calls on moderate computational power and is able to adapt to certain ligand conformations. Nevertheless, as the backbone is kept rigid large structural movements cannot be covered.

Docking into multiple protein structures (MPS) is therefore highly appreciated as they allow flexibility of the protein during the docking process. Different protein conformations (X-ray structures or taken from MD simulations) are selected and multiple docking runs are performed. As this approach is extremely costly, the more efficient method of ensemble docking should be used preferentially. Therefore an average receptor grid is generated and used for docking (Knegtel et al., 1997).

A hybrid technique that is commonly used to encounter protein flexibility is the induced fit docking protocol of the Schrödinger Suite (Sherman et al., 2006). This method turns major attention on the ligand-induced conformational changes of the protein residues surrounding the binding site. Therefore, the ligand is docked into the rigid binding pocket, amino acid residues that are within a certain radius of the resulting poses are removed and rebuilt using the Schrödinger homology modeling program Prime. After energy minimization of the complex the ligand is redocked into the modified binding pocket.

2.2.3 Scoring functions

The application of a scoring function is important to assess the quality of ligand orientations in the binding pocket that resulted from docking experiments. Basically there are three areas of use for scoring functions. In order to understand the interaction between a defined molecule and the target protein the scoring function needs to be able to identify the true pose among the plethora of orientations, generated by the search algorithm. For lead optimization in particular a scoring function should correctly determine the affinity between the ligand and the protein. However, for virtual screening of large compound databases scoring should provide correct ranking. As there are still limitations regarding computer power, the right balance between accuracy and speed has to be chosen, which is strongly dependent on the field of application (reviewed in (Huang et al., 2010)).

Force field based scoring functions use terms that describe the free energy of binding for evaluating binding poses. In that regard bond stretching, angle bending and dihedral angle forces for the ligand, but also non-bonded VDW and electrostatic interactions with the protein are calculated (Huang et al., 2006). Furthermore the accuracy of these methods depends on their treatment of the solvent. More accurate techniques, like thermodynamic integration or free energy pertubation, treat water molecules explicitly. As these are the most expensive affinity prediction methods, more simplified and computationally less expensive versions are linear interaction energy (LIE) models, where two additional empirical parameters can be used to reduce the number of simulations needed. On the other hand, MM/PBSA and MM/GBSA methods gain speed by using implicit solvent models.

However all of these methods are still not applicable for virtual screening as they are computationally too expensive.

Empirical scoring functions are therefore a fast alternative. They assess the quality of binding by a number of weighted terms that are derived by fitting data of complexes to known affinities (Bohm, 1994; Bohm, 1998). Numerous commonly used scoring functions belong to this group, including ChemScore (Eldridge et al., 1997) and X-Score (Wang et al., 2002). Nevertheless, a disadvantage of this method would be the dependence on the training set, as complexes with binding affinity are essential.

Thus, knowledge-based scoring functions may be preferred in this regard. These scoring functions make use of the statistical occurrence of protein-ligand interactions of complex databases. In contrast to empirical functions they do not aim at reproducing binding-affinities, but experimentally determined structures, wherefore a much larger training set can be used (Tanaka & Scheraga, 1976). Representatives of this group of scoring functions are among others ITScore (Huang & Zou, 2006; Huang & Zou, 2006) and DrugScore (Gohlke et al., 2000). A further development of the ITScore by Zou et al. ITScore/SE managed to include solvation and entropic effects into the scoring function (Huang & Zou, 2008), which lead to a strong increase in scoring accuracy.

As the choice of the scoring function strongly depends on the research query, the combination of several functions, so-called consensus scoring, has been suggested (Charifson et al., 1999).

2.3 Molecular dynamics

It is obvious that the mechanism of action by which certain nutrients or drugs are translocated by a transporter implicates the protein to be flexible. In order to be able to allow for a sufficient comprehension of the dynamics of the transport protein, we can not only rely on experimental techniques. In addition, biomolecular simulations can provide a detailed description of particles in motion as a function of time. Thus, they are an important tool for understanding the physical basis of the structure and function of proteins, and biological macromolecules in general. However, experimental validation should always serve to test the accuracy of the calculated results and also to provide a basis for improving the methodology (Karplus & McCammon, 2002).

It is almost 35 years ago, since for the first time McCommon, Gelin and Karplus have studied the dynamics of the pancreatic trypsin inhibitor by solving the equations of motion for the atoms with an empirical potential energy function (McCammon et al., 1977). In this very beginning of Molecular Dynamics simulations, the calculations were still restricted to the picosecond timescale. However, according to Moore's Law computer power is doubling approximately every two years (Moore, 1965). Thus, MD simulations of biomolecules now are able to stretch up to microseconds. For the study of biological relevant phenomena like enzyme catalysis or even protein folding, MD has become a standard tool - always complementary to experimental techniques.

2.3.1 Theory, fields of application, strengths and limitations of MD simulations

By integrating the Newtonian Equations of Motion, Molecular Dynamics simulations are able to describe the behavior of particles in a certain system within the observed period of time. The interaction of the atoms is described by the potential energy function of the given force field [e.g. Amber (Cornell et al., 1995), CHARMM (Brooks et al., 1983), GROMOS (Scott et al., 1999), OPLS (Jorgensen & Rives, 1988)]. Nowadays, there is an ongoing effort to ameliorate these parameters in a need for models being as less artificial as possible.

The field of application of biomolecular simulations is manifold. It reaches from validation and optimization of previously built homology models, refinement of crystal structures, to the prediction of protein-ligand, and protein-protein interactions, to the study of functional properties of biological systems at the atomic level (e.g. protein-folding, destabilization or structural change of a protein upon mutation), to even *de novo* design of proteins (Park et al., 2005).

Despite obvious drawbacks of classical MD simulations, which include limitations in time scales that can be studied but also certain inaccuracies of the force field, for instance with respect to polarization effects, the ability of bringing molecular structures alive also allows the researcher to sample the conformational space. This is especially interesting in ligand-docking applications. On one hand, various extracted snapshots from a previously MD-equilibrated protein-ligand complex may serve in order to perform an ensemble docking which is said to outperform docking into only one sample structure (Knegtel et al., 1997). Secondly, MD may also be used in order to refine certain poses and study the ligand-protein interactions on a molecular basis as a function of time.

2.3.2 Simulations in a membrane

The setup of a simulation system, which includes a protein embedded into a lipid bilayer requires additional efforts in comparison to a system with a soluble protein. There are different choices the researcher has to make regarding to the nature of the phospholipid bilayer used, the temperature at which the simulations should be performed (this also depends on the nature of the bilayer), the force field, the water model (e.g. SPC, SPC/E, TIP3P, TIP4P, TIP5P; this also depends on the choice of the force field), and many more.

One of the most challenging parts is the correct parameterization of the ligands. According to the force field that has been selected there are diverging approaches, ranging from a pure manual assignment of partial charges and force constants, to the use of scientific software like Gaussian (www.gaussian.com), to an automated procedure by taking advantage of platforms such as the Automated Topology Builder and Repository (Malde et al., 2011). However, it has to be stated clearly that a manual inspection and refinement of suchlike obtained topologies will always be needed.

Membrane proteins should be placed in a bilayer which is as similar as possible to its native environment. There is a diverse spectrum of phosphlipid bilayers available – differing mainly in the charges of their polar head groups, lengths and saturation of their acyl chains. If lipids play key roles in the proteins function, different combinations of lipids will probably better represent the *in vivo* conditions. It should always be kept in mind that in order to simulate the membrane in a liquid-crystalline state the temperature of the simulation needs to be above the melting temperature of the chosen lipids (phase-transition temperature).

The protocols for setting up MD simulations of membrane proteins are manifold. In any case, however, one needs a pre-equilibrated bilayer, which can be retrieved from different groups around the world (e.g. Peter Tieleman, Scott Feller, Helmut Heller, Mikko Karttunen) or an individual bilayer may be generated and equilibrated with regard to the respective size and nature of the protein to be studied.

When it comes to the insertion of the respective protein into the pre-equilibrated bilayer, again no standard protocol has been established up to now. In any case, it is of utmost importance to obtain a system with a tightly packed bilayer around the protein, so that the consecutive equilibration time for the membrane can be kept quite short. Protocols like inflategro (Kandt et al., July 2009; Kandt et al., 2007) or g_membed (Wolf et al., 2010) seem most suitable. Whereas, inflategro inflates the lipid bilayer, insert the protein and then deflate the lipid bilayer again, g_membed does it the other way around. It grows a protein into an already hydrated and equilibrated lipid bilayer during a short MD simulation. A special case of insertion procedure certainly is the use of coarse-grained simulations. Here the lipids are able to self-assemble around the protein. However, as this type of simulations use a very simplified description of interactions, for a lot of investigations the relevant information might not be captured.

An idea of a general protocol for the set up of a MD simulation can be found here:

1. Choose a force field for which you have parameters for the protein and lipids.
2. Insert the protein into the membrane.
3. Solvate the system and add ions to neutralize excess charges and adjust the final ion concentration
4. Energy minimize.
5. Let the membrane adjust to the protein. Typically run MD for ~5-10ns with restraints on all protein heavy atoms.
6. Equilibrate without restraints (gradually release the protein).
7. Run production MD.
8. Analysis.

As seen from this overview, after the insertion of the membrane protein it is inevitable to properly equilibrate the lipid bilayer again. This is done by restraining the protein (plus eventually existing ligands conserved water molecules, ions, and cofactors) during a MD run where the membrane is able to adjust to the protein. Subsequently, the whole system has to undergo an extensive equilibration procedure. The end point of the equilibration phase and simultaneous starting point for the MD production run can be determined mainly by evaluation of system parameters (e.g. total energy, temperature) and parameters concerning the protein (e.g. backbone root mean square deviation). A production run for membrane proteins typically resides somewhere in between 50 ns and hundreds of nanoseconds.

2.3.3 Enhanced sampling techniques

As already mentioned in chapter 2.3.1, classical MD simulations are confronted with their limitations in time scales. The limiting factor is the maximum timestep that can be used for the integration, determined by the fastest motion in the system (e.g. bond vibrations).

Thus, it is not able to study 'slow' biological processes without taking advantage of enhanced sampling techniques. This includes of course always a method, which works at the expense of fidelity.

As outlined in an excellent review of Christen and van Gunsteren (Christen & van Gunsteren, 2008) we have to distinguish three different types of search and sampling enhancement techniques: deformation or smoothening of the potential energy surface (e.g. Coarse-graining the model by reducation of the number of interaction sites), scaling of system parameters (e.g. simulated temperature annealing), and multi-copy searching and sampling (e.g. replica-exchange algorithm).

If we want to study membrane proteins and especially their interactions with ligands sampling along transition pathways will be needed. Such pathways are often characterized by high-energy barriers separating meta-stable states along the ligand/substrate transition. Here, methods like pulling or steered MD (SMD) and targeted MD (TMD) may be used in order to drive the sampling to a specific direction. In the SMD approach external forces are applied on certain atoms in order to accelerate processes that are otherwise too slow to model (Isralewitz et al., 2001). Subsequently, the potential of mean force required to induce the transition can be used to estimate free energy barriers. This method is well established and has been used in many applications (Isralewitz et al., 2001; Lu & Schulten, 1999).

In the TMD method, the reaction coordinate is defined by a single mass-weighted root mean-square 'target distance' between a known initial structure and a fixed final (target) structure. By gradually reducing the constrained target distance to zero, the system is driven from the reactant to product state without explicitly defining the reaction pathway (Schlitter et al., 1994).

3. Recent developments in transporter research – Examples

3.1 ABC Transporters and multidrug resistance

ABC (ATP binding cassette) transporters are ubiquitous proteins that are expressed by prokaryotic and eukaryotic organisms. About 50 human ABC transporters are known, which are divided into seven different subfamilies, designated A-G.

Depending on ABC subfamily substrates include among others drugs, lipids, bile salts, peptides, ions and amino acids. Additionally some ABC proteins are known for transporting a broad variety of chemically diverse molecules, which are therefore referred as multidrug transporters. Besides their physiologically important protecting function of exporting xenotoxins, these efflux pumps affect pharmacokinetic profiles of many drugs. Furthermore the acquisition of multidrug resistance (MDR) can often be traced back to elevated expression of multidrug transporters in the affected cells.

The three ABC transporters mostly associated with MDR are P-glycoprotein (P-gp, ABCB1), multidrug resistance protein 1 (MRP1, ABCC1) and breast cancer resistance protein (BCRP, ABCG2).

P-gp is encoded by the *mdr1* gene and is expressed in epithelial cells of the blood brain barrier, liver, kidney and intestine, where it is located at the apical side of the membrane (Szakacs et al., 2008) (Fig. 1).

The cells of the blood brain barrier (BBB) are closely linked by tight junctions, which practically prevent hydrophilic molecules to diffuse between the cells into the central nervous system (CNS). However, as hydrophobic substances might diffuse through the membrane, it is the role of P-gp to keep those out as well (Neuhaus & Noe, 2009). The protecting function of P-gp at the BBB has been observed with *mdr1* knock-out mice and the dog breed collie, which naturally lacks functional P-gp because of a mutated *mdr1* gene. Collies are extremely susceptible to neurotoxic drugs and thus show dramatic adverse reactions after treatment with the antiparasitic drug ivermectin (Mealey et al., 2001).

This detoxifying role of P-gp can be observed at other barriers as well (e.g. the fetal-maternal barrier), but also in faster clearance of administered drugs as it exports substrates form the hepatocytes into the bile, and from the intestinal epithelium into the intestinal lumen (Schinkel & Jonker, 2003).

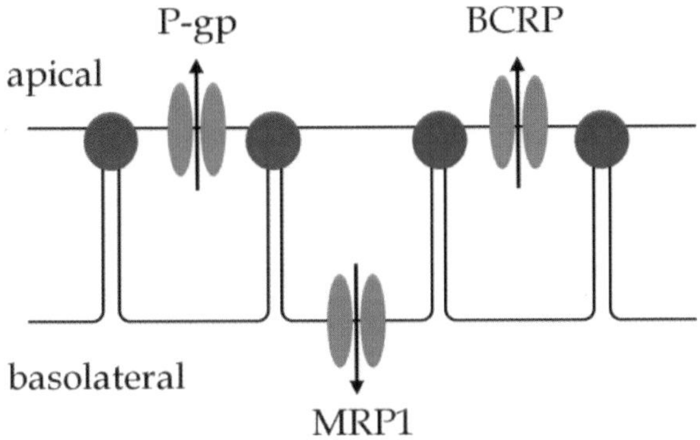

Fig. 1. Localization of the three most important multidrug-transporters.

However, in drug research P-gp poses a large problem, since it highly influences pharmacokinetic properties of drugs. Because of the efflux behavior in the intestinal epithelium the oral bioavailability of drugs is hindered. There are a number of compounds that are able to modulate P-gp activity, which results in modified P-gp concentrations in the target tissue. As a consequence this can lead to adverse drug-drug interactions, when therapeutics are administered at the same time. Furthermore, elevated expression of P-gp, (as it is the case in cancer cells), is one major reason for the acquisition of MDR. One way to overcome these negative effects associated with P-gp activity would be the development of P-gp inhibitors that should restore sensitivity to therapeutics. Already 30 years ago, the reversal of resistance against the vinca alkaloids vincristine and vinblastine by the calcium-channel blocker verapamil was identified (Tsuruo et al., 1981). However, since then no inhibitor reached the market so far. This can be explained by its important physiological functions, rendering them rather antitargets than targets (Ecker & Chiba, 2009).

Another ABC transporter that is highly associated with MDR belongs to the ABCC subfamily. MRP1/ABCC1 is located at the basolateral membrane of epithelial cells of the lung, kidney and the intestine (Fig. 1).

Although the substrate specificity of MRP1 shows some overlap with P-gp especially in terms of hydrophobic substances, MRP1 preferably binds to anionic substances in contrast to the positive charged substrates of P-gp (Borst & Elferink, 2002). Furthermore MRP1 is known for the export of hydrophilic substances as glutathione (GSH) conjugates. Therefore it is not only responsible for preventing xenotoxins entering the cell, but MRP1 also effluxes toxic metabolic compounds, which is highly important for faster clearance.

The role of MRP1 in the acquisition of MDR has particular impact on non-small cell lung carcinoma, a very aggressive cancer type, where high concentrations of MRP1 could be detected in the cancer cells.

The development of MRP1 specific inhibitors faces immense problems as MRP1 substrates and inhibitors show anionic properties, which lack good cell penetration properties (Schinkel & Jonker, 2003).

In 1998 Doyle et al. identified another ABC transporter that conferred resistance to the anthracenedione mitoxantrone, which is a poor substrate for P-gp and MRP1 (Doyle et al., 1998). BCRP belongs to the G or white subfamily of ABC transporters and received the name BCRP because of its isolation from a breast cancer cell line.

As P-gp, BCRP is located at the apical membrane of epithelial cells in the intestine, kidney and placenta (Schinkel & Jonker, 2003) (Fig. 1). Regarding substrate profiles, BCRP shows some overlap with P-gp and MRP1 but does not confer resistance to taxols, cis-platin and verapamil, or vinca alkaloids and anthracyclines. On the other hand, BCRP is known for transporting positively and negatively charged drugs (Sharom, 2008).

A specific inhibitor of BCRP is the tremorgenic mycotoxin fumitremorgin C (FTC). FTC blocked mitoxantrone transport by BCRP without affecting P-gp or MRP1-mediated drug resistance (Rabindran et al., 2000). However, due to neurotoxic effects *in vivo* application is still not possible.

3.1.1 Structure of ABC transporters

The minimal functional unit of an ABC transporter consists of two (pseudo)-symmetric halves that comprise a transmembrane (TM) and a nucleotide binding domain (NBD) (Fig. 2). In the case of P-gp and most other eukaryotic ABC transporters, these subdomains are fused to one polypeptide chain. On the contrary BCRP is a so-called half-transporter (Fig. 2). Half-transporters express each protein half separately and thus need to homo-dimerize to yield functional full transporters.

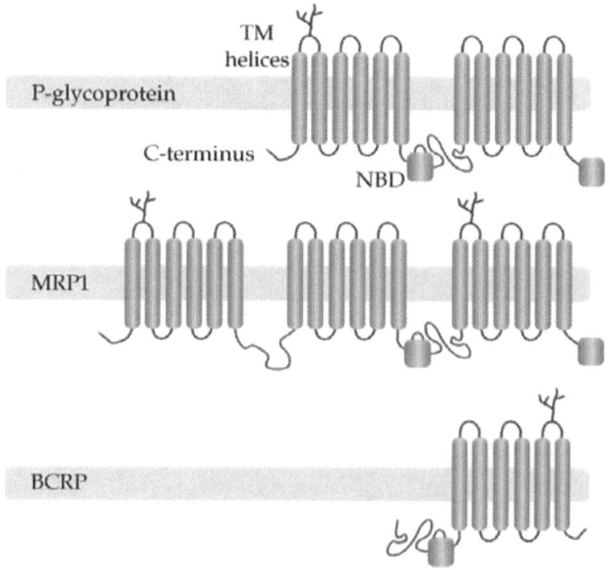

Fig. 2. Topology of the three most relevant multidrug transporters.

The NBDs are responsible for the binding and hydrolysis of ATP, which is needed for the active transport of substrates. On each NBD sequence the characteristic ABC domain consisting of the Walker A and B region, as well as the "signature" or C motif, can be found (Fig. 3). One ATP molecule is supposed to be sandwiched between the Walker A and B of one NBD and the C motif of the other NBD (Fig. 3). As they are highly conserved, the NBDs show large sequence identity among ABC transporters.

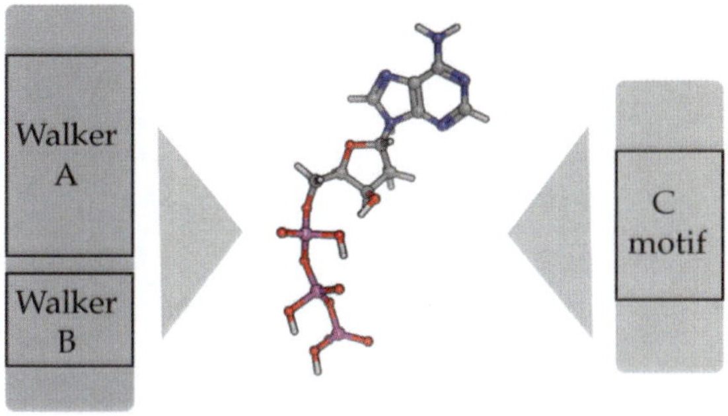

Fig. 3. Position of one ATP molecule in one nucleotide binding domain.

However, substrate binding and transport occurs at the TMDs. Each TMD consists of six TM helices, although this number varies between ABC transporters. The TMDs are much less conserved which leads to a large diversity in substrate profiles among ABC transporters.

During drug transport P-gp and its homologues undergo large conformational changes, converting an open-inward drug-binding state into an open-outward drug-releasing state (Rosenberg et al., 2001). This assumption was confirmed by cryo-electron microscopy and biochemical experiments, where P-gp was trapped in different states of the catalytic cycle (using the non-hydrolysable ATP analog AMP-PNP and ADP-Vi). The detailed mechanism of the energy driven drug transport, rendering the high-affinity into a low-affinity binding site, is currently hypothesized in two different ways and has been extensively reviewed in (Seeger & van Veen, 2009).

3.1.2 Homology modeling of P-gp

As already described in the introduction of this chapter, entries in the protein data bank (PDB) raise exponentially, but the structure determination of membrane proteins is still problematic and only relatively few structures have been resolved up to now. Thus, homology modeling is essential for performing docking or MD studies on most of the ABC transporters.

In 2001 the publication of X-ray structures of *E. coli* MsbA (PDB code: 1JSQ, resolution: 4.5Å), a lipid A transporter, raised a lot of interest in the ABC-transporter community (Chang & Roth, 2001).

The lipid flippase MsbA is an ABC protein that is responsible for the transport for lipid A and lipopolysaccharide (LPS). A non-functional MsbA leads to accumulation of lipopolysaccharide and phospholipids in the inner membrane of gram-negative bacteria.

According to the X-ray structure published in 2001 the association of the two TMDs was interpreted as a chamber that provides alternating access for potential ligands during the catalytic cycle. The theory of MsbA switching between different conformations was confirmed by the subsequent publications of the X-ray structures of Vibrio cholerae MsbA in 2003 (PDB code: 1PF4, resolution: 3.80Å) (Chang, 2003) and of Salmonella typhimurium MsbA in complex with ADP·Vi (PDB code: 1Z2R, resolution: 4.20Å) (Reyes & Chang, 2005). The former presents the apo protein in a closed state, while the latter captures the Protein/ADP·Vi complex in the posthydrolytic state.

At this time these structures were the only source for structure-based design on MsbA and its homologues. Numerous ABCB1 homology models were generated relying on these MsbA templates (Pleban et al., 2005; Seigneuret & Garnier-Suillerot, 2003; Shilling et al., 2003; Stenham et al., 2003; Vandevuer et al., 2006).

However, with the publication of the X-ray structure of the *Staphylococcus aureus* transporter Sav1866, an MsbA homologue (Dawson & Locher, 2006), the previous MsbA and two additional EmrE structures had to be retracted (Chang et al., 2006). According to Chang, an error in the *in-house* software that should process the crystallographic data resulted in a sign change and therefore to a momentous misinterpretation of the data (Matthews, 2007). This incident became the center of numerous discussions, often referred to as the "pentaretraction" (Davis et al., 2008; Penders et al., 2007). In contrast to the retracted MsbA models, the architecture of Sav1866 shows a helix arrangement that is analogous to domain swapping in other enzymes. Thus, TM helices of one TMD are in close contact with the opposite NBD via so-called coupling helices.

One year later, in 2007, Ward et al. published the corrected MsbA structures (Ward et al., 2007), which are in agreement with the SAV1866 architecture.

As SAV1866 (PDB code: 2HYD, resolution: 3.00Å) is one of the best resolved ABC exporters it has been often used as template for further modeling studies. In addition, this structure also fulfills most of the structural restraints that were obtained by cross-linking studies. However SAV1866 was crystallized in the nucleotide-bound conformation, which represents the ligand-releasing state of the protein. Thus the suitability of this template for docking studies can be questioned. In this respect Stockner et al. generated a data-driven homology model on the basis of SAV1866 that should represent the ligand-binding state of the protein by applying structural restraints in TM helices 6 and 12 obtained by cross-linking data on the model (Stockner et al., 2009).

The corrected MsbA coordinates cover different catalytic states, including a nucleotide-free ligand-binding conformation. Unfortunately these structures are resolved at resolutions far from being suitable for docking experiments, with some templates only represented by Cα atoms. Models on basis of the MsbA structures were therefore mainly used for exploring the conformational changes during the catalytic cycle.

With the publication of murine P-gp in March 2009 the first X-ray structure of a eukaryotic ABC exporter was available (Aller et al., 2009) (PDB code: 3G5U, resolution: 3.8Å). Two additionally published structures that include co-crystallized enantiomeric cyclic peptide inhibitors (CPPIs; QZ59-RRR and QZ59-SSS) highlight the binding-competence of these conformations and thus their great value for further docking studies. Furthermore the high sequence identity of 87% with human P-gp highly facilitates the modeling process.

3.1.3 Docking and MD studies

The definition of a binding site is an essential preparation step for docking studies. Regarding P-gp and other ABC transporters, we face the problem that hardly any binding sites for known P-gp ligands have been identified unambiguously. So far, it has been assumed that there is a large binding cavity in the transmembrane region (Loo & Clarke, 1999), which comprises distinct active sites. Furthermore, cysteine-scanning mutagenesis studies showed that the protein is able to bind at least two different molecules simultaneously (Loo et al., 2003). By using biochemical techniques a more detailed characterization of concrete binding sites for distinct substrates was possible (extensively reviewed in (Crowley et al., 2010; Loo & Clarke, 2008; Seeger & van Veen, 2009)). This led to the characterization of the interaction regions of Rhodamine 123 and Hoechst 33342, named R- and the H- site (Loo & Clarke, 2002; Qu & Sharom, 2002), together with a regulatory site, which binds prazosin/progesterone (Shapiro et al., 1999). Furthermore, the release of the P-gp/CPPI-complexes presented another step forward in elucidating drug/P-gp interactions.

Since the co-crystallized enantiomers showed distinct binding patterns, this information raised the assumption of stereoselectivity of P-gp in its ligand binding quality (Aller et al., 2009). Stereoselectivity has also been shown for flupentixol (Dey et al., 1999) and propafenone derivatives (Jabeen et al., 2011). On the other hand there are also ample reports on equal activity of enantiomeres. Thus, as for niguldipine and verapamil both enantiomers showed equivalent activities (Hollt et al., 1992; Luurtsema et al., 2003), the distomers with respect to cardiovascular activity were used for clinical studies.

As the resolution of the hitherto available templates used for constructing protein homology models is quite low, only very few docking studies have been conducted so far. Shortly after the publication of mouse P-gp, Pajeva et al. docked quinazolinones into a homology model of human P-gp based on the murine homologue, which is in complex with the cyclopeptide SSS-QZ59 (Pajeva et al., 2009). The binding site they used was defined by the co-crystallized ligands and was extended by 14Å. The results suggested interaction with TM helices 5, 6 and 11 and were further confirmed by a pharmacophore model.

Becker et al. performed docking studies of the P-glycoprotein modulators colchicine, rhodamine B, verapamil and vinblastine into a homology model based on the nucleotide-free corrected MsbA structure (Becker et al., 2009). The resultant poses predicted that all ligands were able to interact with residues that were experimentally identified as important for ligand binding, strongly involving TM helices 5, 6, 7, 11 and 12. However, none of the drugs was able to contact every identified residue, which favors the hypothesis of distinct interactions sites forming one binding cavity.

Recently Dolghih et al. published a docking approach that was able to discriminate between known P-gp binders and non-binding metabolites (Dolghih et al., 2011). In this study there was a major interest in considering the high flexibility of P-gp. Therefore the induced fit protocol of the Schrödinger Suite was applied (Sherman et al., 2006). However, the discrimination between binders and non-binders can be more efficiently performed on basis of physicochemical properties than different binding mechanisms.

In our group, docking into a homology model based on mouse P-gp was used for explaining the stereoselective P-gp modulating activity of tricyclic benzopyranooxazines (Jabeen et al.,

2011). Besides from activity differences, compounds with 4aS,10bR configuration showed a clear logP-activity correlation (r^2=0.96), which was not the case for the 4aR,10bS series. This characteristic could be partly explained by the received binding hypotheses. The analysis of the docking poses by agglomerative hierarchical clustering resulted in distinct clusters for the different diastereomers. Therefore it has been hypothesized, that activity differences of the diastereomers is due to their different binding modes in the P-gp binding cavity. In addition, molecules with 4aR,10bS chirality were found close to the entry path of the protein, wherefore activity is primarily affected by the molecules' partition coefficient. On the other hand compounds of the 4aS,10bR series also showed docking poses at an active site in the binding pocket of P-gp, thus suggesting that the activity is dependent on multiple factors.

Furthermore, we were able to propose reliable binding hypotheses of propafenone analogs in P-gp by applying a knowledge driven docking protocol (Klepsch et al., 2011). Based on our extensive data from SAR studies on propafenones (Ecker et al., 2008; Pleban et al., 2005), we selected a small set of compounds for docking into a homology model based on mouse P-gp. As propafenone analogs show a clear SAR we assumed a similar binding mode of the docked propafenone derivatives. In that sense the resultant docking poses were clustered according the RMSD of their common scaffold. The clusters were prioritized according a combination of SAR data and protein-ligand interaction fingerprint information. With this protocol a high number of docking poses could be reduced to two reliable binding modes. Key interactions formed by these two clusters were formed with amino acids of TM helices 5, 6, 7 and 12 which were shown previously to be involved in ligand binding (Loo & Clarke, 2008; Seeger & van Veen, 2009).

In contrast to the compounds investigated above steroidal compounds are assumed to bind to the NBD rather than the TMDs. Several docking studies could show ATP-like binding of flavonoids, flavones and chalcones at the ATP-binding site, which is extensively reviewed in (Klepsch et al., 2010).

Regarding P-gp's high flexibility MD simulation represents a convenient technique to consider structural changes of the protein. Unfortunately, a number of MD studies were conducted relying on homology models based on the retracted MsbA X-ray structures (Campbell et al., 2003; Omote & Al-Shawi, 2006; Vandevuer et al., 2006) and are therefore partly no longer valid.

By now MD methods were mainly used for functional investigations of the protein. In order to determine the mechanisms of ATP hydrolysis numerous studies were conducted on isolated NBDs (Campbell & Sansom, 2005; Jones & George, 2007; Jones & George, 2009; Newstead et al., 2009; Wen & Tajkhorshid, 2008), as this comprises the sequence motives essential for ATP-binding. However, recently also studies considering the behaviour of the whole protein upon ATP hydrolysis were published (Becker et al., 2010; Gyimesi et al., 2011; Oliveira et al., 2011). All of those studies relied on the SAV1866 crystal structure, which represents the ligand-releasing and therefore open-outward state of the protein.

While Oliveira et al. (Oliveira et al., 2011) were able to show that replacing both ATP molecules in the NBDs by ADP structural changes in the protein occurred, Gyimesi et al. (Gyimesi et al., 2011) observed structural rearrangements already by exchanging one ATP molecule. This could be of great relevance for heterodimeric ABC proteins like P-gp, where an asymmetric ATP hydrolysis might be possible. In addition movements in TM helices 3 and 6 could be identified, which is in agreement with MD studies conducted by Becker et al. (Becker et al., 2010). Both groups observed closure of the TM domains after ATP hydrolysis.

The investigation of the drug-binding open-inside conformation of P-gp by MD simulation still faces numerous problems, due to instability of the mouse P-gp structure. In that sense the validity of this model is somewhat doubted (Gyimesi et al., 2011; Loo et al., 2010).

3.2 Neurotransmitter transporters

3.2.1 Biological background of the SLC-6 family

The concerted release and reuptake of transmitter substances is a basic principle of proper signal transduction in the nerve cells. In order to terminate a synaptic signal after neural firing, transporter proteins have to remove about 10^5-fold of basal concentrations (Chen et al., 2004; Gouaux, 2009). The transporters practically have to act as selective molecular vacuum cleaners to deal with such huge loads of neurotransmitters in order to re-establish pre-signaling conditions within milliseconds. A major ion gradient serves as driving force and patron for the protein class: the Neurotransmitter:Sodium Symporters (NSS).

Synonymously called the solute carrier 6 family (SLC-6), NSS members include the sodium- and chloride-dependent transporters for GABA, dopamine, serotonin, norepinephrine and glycine, but also just sodium-dependent transporters of amino acids. Thus, the protein family is of particular medical importance, as many CNS diseases like depression, anxiety or epilepsy can be targeted by inhibiting transporters (Iversen, 1971).

They share a basic scaffold consisting of 12 transmembrane regions (TMs), segments 1-5 and 6-10 forming two pseudosymmetric domains housing the substrate and ion binding sites in partially unwound regions half-way across the membrane (Kanner & Zomot, 2008).

The crystal structure of LeuT, a bacterial orthologue of the eukaryotic NSS members, became available in an occluded state conformation in 2005 and in the open to out orientation in 2008 (Singh et al., 2008; Yamashita et al., 2005), thus revealing first detailed insights into the binding site topology. Furthermore, very recently a double mutant stabilized in an inward-open conformation was published (Krishnamurthy & Gouaux, 2012). These crystallographic snapshots fortify the so-called alternating access model for neurotransmitter membrane transport (Jardetzky, 1966). Various attempts have been made to clarify the exact molecular transport mechanism (Forrest et al., 2008; Shi et al., 2008), yet many questions remain unanswered. Concerning the quaternary structure, it is generally assumed that neurotransmitter:sodium symporters form constitutive oligomers (Forrest et al., 2008; Sitte et al., 2004). Despite a comparably poor average overall sequence identity between eu- and prokaryotic SLC-6 members of slightly above 20%, these structures paved the way to comparative modeling studies. Predominantly the monoamine transporters DAT, NET and SERT, but also GAT, have been modeled and studied extensively. For a comprehensive summary of the state of knowledge about the SLC-6 family, the reader is referred to the recent review by Kristensen et al. (Kristensen et al., 2011).

3.2.2 Examples of studies on the hSERT

As mentioned earlier, especially when dealing with low template-target sequence identity, a very careful sequence alignment including all possible experimental knowledge is crucial for the construction of reliable homology models. For the main members of the SLC-6 family a lot of effort has been put into this work, resulting in the comprehensive alignment of NSS sequences with the LeuT published by Beuming et al. in 2006 (Beuming et al., 2006). Since then, some new structural insights into the protein class have been gained leading to slightly altered regions, but still the alignments can be considered a good starting point for experiments with NSS models. In the case of the hSERT, the recent work of Sarker et al. (Sarker et al., 2010) provides a good example for the cumulative value of combining molecular modeling methods with mutagenesis experiments in order to verify *in silico* elaborated hypotheses. For investigating the binding mode of tricyclic antidepressants (TCAs) in the serotonin transporter, comparative modeling marked the starting point for subsequent studies. Using the Beuming alignment, homology models of hSERT were built based on the previously mentioned high-resolution open-to-out structure of the LeuT published in 2008 (PDB code 3F3A). Subsequent docking studies of imipramine resulted in three pose clusters of potential binding modes, showing interactions to previously reported key residues (Andersen et al., 2009; Chen & Rudnick, 2000; White et al., 2006). A diagnostic Y95F mutation, a candidate residue for hydrogen bonding with the imipramine diaminopropyl moiety, significantly decreased imipramine affinity without affecting serotonin binding, ruling out one cluster. Further uptake and docking assays demonstrated that carbamazepine, structurally a truncated and slightly more rigid derivative of imipramine, was able to bind mutually non-exclusive with the substrate serotonin, whereas binding of its large-tailed relative is mutually exclusive. This led to the following conclusions: a) the tricyclic ring system of TCAs binds in an outer vestibule, and b) the basic side chain of imipramine points into the actual substrate binding site.

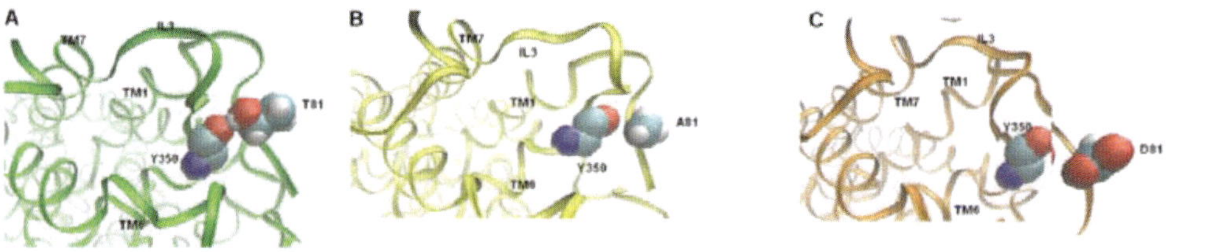

Fig. 4. Molecular dynamics simulations of SERTThr-81 mutants reveal models favoring inward facing states. A, snapshot of wild type SERT after 16 ns of MD simulation. The Thr81 side chain forms a stable H-bond with the backbone carbonyl of Tyr350 in IL3. B, snapshot of SERTT81A after 6 ns of MD simulation; the H-bond is not formed between Ala81 and Tyr350 during the course of the simulation. C, snapshot of SERTT81D after 6 ns of MD simulation; no H-bond is formed between Asp81 and Tyr350 during the course of the simulation. (taken from (Sucic et al., 2010)).

As an example for a more functional study on the SERT, the work of Sucic et al. (Sucic et al., 2010) can be mentioned. As it was analogously reported for the DAT (Guptaroy et al., 2009), the important role of a highly conserved phosphorylation site at the N-terminus of the transporter in mediating the action of amphetamines was studied. Amphetamines are said to induce substrate efflux, but the way they do so is not well understood. Sucic et al. reported that mutating the highly conserved N-terminal residue T81 (a candidate site for phosphorylation by protein kinase C), to alanine or aspartate leads to subsequent fail of the transporter to support amphetamine-induced efflux. As it was also confirmed by molecular dynamics simulations of the wild type transporter, the *in silico* mutated $SERT^{T81A}$ and $SERT^{T81D}$, the data suggested that by phosphorylation or *in silico* mutation of T81 the conformational equilibrium of the serotonin transport cycle alters towards the inward facing conformation. As seen in the MD studies, this happens due to a loss of a hydrogen bond network of T81 with Y350 in IL3 by these mutations. Furthermore, an increased distance between the C terminus (i.e. the most distal point of TM12) and the N terminus after *in silico* mutation was observed. This example nicely indicates how functional MD studies might aid in elucidating biological relevant phenomena.

3.2.3 Studies on hGAT models

The four Na^+- and Cl^--dependent GABA transporters, GAT-1-3 and BGT-1 (SLC6A1, A16, A11, A12), provide a similar percentage of sequence identity to the LeuT. The subtype showing the highest quantity in the CNS is GAT-1. It is also the best-investigated, and the only one currently targeted by a marketed drug, the second-line antiepileptic tiagabine (Gabitril®). Accordingly, systematic synthesis studies in order to discover even more selective compounds have been performed mainly on GAT-1. Nevertheless, other subtypes should not be ignored, as they may be the key to a less side-effect afflicted antiepileptic therapy, as tiagabine efficacy as anticonvulsant is limited, and its use was connected to several adverse effects like sedation, agitation, or even seizure induction. Neuronal GABA reuptake, mainly done by GAT-1, leads to subsequent recycling of the transmitter substance. On the contrary, astroglial uptake of GABA leads to degradation, suggesting subtypes predominantly present in glia cells being an interesting target for enhancing overall GABA levels. For example, the lipophilic GABA analog EF-1502, characterized by GAT1 and GAT2 (BGT-1) selectivity, showed synergistic anticonvulsant activity, when administered with tiagabine (Schousboe et al., 2004), although BGT1 levels in the CNS are about 1000-fold lower, and even a recent study with BGT-1 knockout mice did not show any change in seizure susceptibility (Lehre et al., 2011).

In the search for potent selective non-GAT-1 inhibitors, GABA mimetic moieties (like R-nipecotic acid in tiagabine, β-alanine or THPO [4,5,6,7-Tetrahydroisoxazolo(4,5-c)pyridin-3-ol]) were systematically combined with large aromatic side chains, both in order to increase the affinity and to make the compounds blood-brain barrier permeable (Andersen et al., 1993; Andersen et al., 1999; Clausen et al., 2005; Knutsen et al., 1999; Kragler et al., 2008). Unfortunately, up to now no truly selective tools for the evaluation of non-GAT-1 inhibition are available, although the GAT-1/BGT-1 inhibitor EF1502 and SNAP-5114, showing a certain GAT-2/GAT-3 selectivity, mark a good starting point (Madsen et al., 2010). Thus, further insights into the molecular basis of ligand binding are sought by the aid of *in silico* methods.

GAT-1 has been subject of several comparative modeling studies. Initial studies predominantly aimed at clarifying the GABA binding mode in the occluded transporter state, which is quite well documented so far (Pallo et al., 2007; Wein & Wanner, 2009). Though, compounds with large aromatic tails cannot be accommodated in the occluded-state active site, as the entrance to the binding pocket is barred by the two extracellular gate residues R69 and D451, as well as the F294 side chain, forming the binding site "roof". In order to study tiagabine-like ligands, constructing open-to-out models seemed inevitable, as it was done by Skovstrup et al. (Skovstrup et al., 2010). Structures of both states were modeled and refined exhaustively, as described in section 2.1. The combined use of docking and molecular dynamics simulation was chosen to investigate binding of GABA, its analogue (R)-nipecotic acid and the high active (R)-enantiomer of tiagabine. The results for GABA binding were in line with the earlier mentioned experiments. In case of tiagabine, MD simulations helped to distinguish between the *cis-* and *trans-* conformer, both being possible states due to the protonated state of tiagabine at physiological pH. During the MD, the *trans-* conformer immediately stirred away to the extracellular space, whereas the other one remained stable in the binding site. Summing up, GABA and (R)-tiagabine turned out having two different binding modes, sharing the orientation of the carboxy group towards one of the co-transported sodium ions as a common feature.

For the other GAT subtypes, things are a bit more complicated. Looking at the residues corresponding to LeuT substrate binding site, just a few candidate residues differ significantly, being somehow unlikely to be fully responsible for subtype selective binding. So far, molecular modeling studies have been performed, but highly similar binding sites and the lack of selective ligand data limited their explanatory power (Pallo et al., 2009). Thus, a huge field of activity remains to be explored on the way to fully understand the differences between the GABA subtypes, *in silico* methods being a valuable tool for stepwise adding pieces of information to the big puzzle.

4. Concluding remarks

Membrane transport proteins are responsible for one of the most important processes in living cells: directed transport across barriers. They comprise about 30% of known proteomes and constitute about 50% of pharmacological targets. Although, due to difficulties in expression, purification and crystallization, only about 2% of the high resolution crystal structures in the Protein Data Bank (PDB) are transporters. Thus, computational methods have been utilized extensively to provide significant new insights into protein structure and function. Above all, molecular modeling and molecular dynamics (MD) simulations may deliver atomic level details to reveal the molecular basis of e.g. drug-transporter interactions. As shown on basis of recent research examples, *in silico* methods in many cases can provide additional information to biological experiments, either underpinning pharmacological results or they may even lead to new insight, not being biologically accessible.

5. Acknowledgments

The authors gratefully appreciate financial support provided by the Austrian Science Fund (FWF), grant SFB3502 and SFB3506.

6. References

Agre, P. (2006). The Aquaporin Water Channels. *Proc Am Thorac Soc*, Vol.3, No.1, pp. 5-13

Aller, S.G., Yu, J., Ward, A., Weng, Y., Chittaboina, S., Zhuo, R., Harrell, P.M., Trinh, Y.T., Zhang, Q., Urbatsch, I.L. & Chang, G. (2009). Structure of P-glycoprotein reveals a molecular basis for poly-specific drug binding. *Science*, Vol.323, No.5922, pp. 1718-22

Altschul, S.F., Madden, T.L., Schaffer, A.A., Zhang, J., Zhang, Z., Miller, W. & Lipman, D.J. (1997). Gapped BLAST and PSI-BLAST: a new generation of protein database search programs. *Nucleic Acids Res*, Vol.25, No.17, pp. 3389-402

Amaro, R.E. & Li, W.W. (2010). Emerging methods for ensemble-based virtual screening. *Curr Top Med Chem*, Vol.10, No.1, pp. 3-13

Andersen, J., Taboureau, O., Hansen, K.B., Olsen, L., Egebjerg, J., Stromgaard, K. & Kristensen, A.S. (2009). Location of the antidepressant binding site in the serotonin transporter: importance of Ser-438 in recognition of citalopram and tricyclic antidepressants. *J Biol Chem*, Vol.284, No.15, pp. 10276-84

Andersen, K.E., Braestrup, C., Gronwald, F.C., Jorgensen, A.S., Nielsen, E.B., Sonnewald, U., Sorensen, P.O., Suzdak, P.D. & Knutsen, L.J. (1993). The synthesis of novel GABA uptake inhibitors. 1. Elucidation of the structure-activity studies leading to the choice of (R)-1-[4,4-bis(3-methyl-2-thienyl)-3-butenyl]-3-piperidinecarboxylic acid (tiagabine) as an anticonvulsant drug candidate. *J Med Chem*, Vol.36, No.12, pp. 1716-25

Andersen, K.E., Sorensen, J.L., Huusfeldt, P.O., Knutsen, L.J., Lau, J., Lundt, B.F., Petersen, H., Suzdak, P.D. & Swedberg, M.D. (1999). Synthesis of novel GABA uptake inhibitors. 4. Bioisosteric transformation and successive optimization of known GABA uptake inhibitors leading to a series of potent anticonvulsant drug candidates. *J Med Chem*, Vol.42, No.21, pp. 4281-91

Arnold, K., Bordoli, L., Kopp, J. & Schwede, T. (2006). The SWISS-MODEL workspace: a web-based environment for protein structure homology modelling. *Bioinformatics*, Vol.22, No.2, pp. 195-201

B-Rao, C., Subramanian, J. & Sharma, S.D. (2009). Managing protein flexibility in docking and its applications. *Drug Discov Today*, Vol.14, No.7-8, pp. 394-400

Becker, J.P., Depret, G., Van Bambeke, F., Tulkens, P.M. & Prevost, M. (2009). Molecular models of human P-glycoprotein in two different catalytic states. *BMC Struct Biol*, Vol.9, 3

Becker, J.P., Van Bambeke, F., Tulkens, P.M. & Prevost, M. (2010). Dynamics and structural changes induced by ATP binding in SAV1866, a bacterial ABC exporter. *Journal of Physical Chemistry B*, Vol.114, No.48, pp. 15948-57

Benkert, P., Biasini, M. & Schwede, T. (2011). Toward the estimation of the absolute quality of individual protein structure models. *Bioinformatics*, Vol.27, No.3, pp. 343-50

Berman, H.M., Westbrook, J., Feng, Z., Gilliland, G., Bhat, T.N., Weissig, H., Shindyalov, I.N. & Bourne, P.E. (2000). The Protein Data Bank. *Nucleic Acids Res*, Vol.28, No.1, pp. 235-42

Beuming, T., Shi, L., Javitch, J.A. & Weinstein, H. (2006). A comprehensive structure-based alignment of prokaryotic and eukaryotic neurotransmitter/Na+ symporters (NSS) aids in the use of the LeuT structure to probe NSS structure and function. *Mol Pharmacol*, Vol.70, No.5, pp. 1630-42

Bohm, H.J. (1992). LUDI: rule-based automatic design of new substituents for enzyme inhibitor leads. *J Comput Aided Mol Des*, Vol.6, No.6, pp. 593-606

Bohm, H.J. (1994). The development of a simple empirical scoring function to estimate the binding constant for a protein-ligand complex of known three-dimensional structure. *J Comput Aided Mol Des*, Vol.8, No.3, pp. 243-56

Bohm, H.J. (1998). Prediction of binding constants of protein ligands: a fast method for the prioritization of hits obtained from de novo design or 3D database search programs. *J Comput Aided Mol Des*, Vol.12, No.4, pp. 309-23

Borst, P. & Elferink, R.O. (2002). Mammalian ABC transporters in health and disease. *Annu Rev Biochem*, Vol.71, 537-92

Brooks, B.R., Bruccoleri, R.E., Olafson, B.D., States, D.J., Swaminathan, S. & Karplus, M. (1983). Charmm - a Program for Macromolecular Energy, Minimization, and Dynamics Calculations. *Journal of Computational Chemistry*, Vol.4, No.2, pp. 187-217

Brooks, B.R., Bruccoleri, R.E., Olafson, B.D., States, D.J., Swaminathan, S. & Karplus, M. (1983). CHARMM: A program for macromolecular energy, minimization, and dynamics calculations. *Journal of Computational Chemistry*, Vol.4, No.2, pp. 187-217

Caffrey, M. (2003). Membrane protein crystallization. *J Struct Biol*, Vol.142, No.1, pp. 108-132

Caflisch, A., Miranker, A. & Karplus, M. (1993). Multiple copy simultaneous search and construction of ligands in binding sites: application to inhibitors of HIV-1 aspartic proteinase. *J Med Chem*, Vol.36, No.15, pp. 2142-67

Campbell, J.D., Biggin, P.C., Baaden, M. & Sansom, M.S. (2003). Extending the structure of an ABC transporter to atomic resolution: modeling and simulation studies of MsbA. *Biochemistry*, Vol.42, No.13, pp. 3666-73

Campbell, J.D. & Sansom, M.S. (2005). Nucleotide binding to the homodimeric MJ0796 protein: a computational study of a prokaryotic ABC transporter NBD dimer. *FEBS Lett*, Vol.579, No.19, pp. 4193-9

Cavasotto, C.N. (2011). Homology models in docking and high-throughput docking. *Curr Top Med Chem*, Vol.11, No.12, pp. 1528-34

Chang, G. (2003). Structure of MsbA from Vibrio cholera: a multidrug resistance ABC transporter homolog in a closed conformation. *J Mol Biol*, Vol.330, No.2, pp. 419-30

Chang, G. & Roth, C.B. (2001). Structure of MsbA from E. coli: a homolog of the multidrug resistance ATP binding cassette (ABC) transporters. *Science*, Vol.293, No.5536, pp. 1793-800

Chang, G., Roth, C.B., Reyes, C.L., Pornillos, O., Chen, Y.J. & Chen, A.P. (2006). Retraction. *Science*, Vol.314, No.5807, pp. 1875

Charifson, P.S., Corkery, J.J., Murcko, M.A. & Walters, W.P. (1999). Consensus scoring: A method for obtaining improved hit rates from docking databases of three-dimensional structures into proteins. *J Med Chem*, Vol.42, No.25, pp. 5100-9

Chen, J.G. & Rudnick, G. (2000). Permeation and gating residues in serotonin transporter. *Proc Natl Acad Sci U S A*, Vol.97, No.3, pp. 1044-9

Chen, N.H., Reith, M.E. & Quick, M.W. (2004). Synaptic uptake and beyond: the sodium- and chloride-dependent neurotransmitter transporter family SLC6. *Pflugers Arch*, Vol.447, No.5, pp. 519-31

Christen, M. & van Gunsteren, W.F. (2008). On searching in, sampling of, and dynamically moving through conformational space of biomolecular systems: A review. *Journal of Computational Chemistry*, Vol.29, No.2, pp. 157-166

Clausen, R.P., Moltzen, E.K., Perregaard, J., Lenz, S.M., Sanchez, C., Falch, E., Frolund, B., Bolvig, T., Sarup, A., Larsson, O.M., Schousboe, A. & Krogsgaard-Larsen, P. (2005). Selective inhibitors of GABA uptake: synthesis and molecular pharmacology of 4-N-methylamino-4,5,6,7-tetrahydrobenzo[d]isoxazol-3-ol analogues. *Bioorg Med Chem*, Vol.13, No.3, pp. 895-908

Cornell, W.D., Cieplak, P., Bayly, C.I., Gould, I.R., Merz, K.M., Ferguson, D.M., Spellmeyer, D.C., Fox, T., Caldwell, J.W. & Kollman, P.A. (1995). A Second Generation Force Field for the Simulation of Proteins, Nucleic Acids, and Organic Molecules. *Journal of the American Chemical Society*, Vol.117, No.19, pp. 5179-5197

Cozzini, P., Kellogg, G.E., Spyrakis, F., Abraham, D.J., Costantino, G., Emerson, A., Fanelli, F., Gohlke, H., Kuhn, L.A., Morris, G.M., Orozco, M., Pertinhez, T.A., Rizzi, M. & Sotriffer, C.A. (2008). Target flexibility: an emerging consideration in drug discovery and design. *J Med Chem*, Vol.51, No.20, pp. 6237-55

Crowley, E., O'Mara, M.L., Kerr, I.D. & Callaghan, R. (2010). Transmembrane helix 12 plays a pivotal role in coupling energy provision and drug binding in ABCB1. *FEBS J*, Vol.277, No.19, pp. 3974-85

Dalton, J.A. & Jackson, R.M. (2007). An evaluation of automated homology modelling methods at low target template sequence similarity. *Bioinformatics*, Vol.23, No.15, pp. 1901-8

Davis, A.M., St-Gallay, S.A. & Kleywegt, G.J. (2008). Limitations and lessons in the use of X-ray structural information in drug design. *Drug Discov Today*, Vol.13, No.19-20, pp. 831-41

Dawson, R.J. & Locher, K.P. (2006). Structure of a bacterial multidrug ABC transporter. *Nature*, Vol.443, No.7108, pp. 180-5

Deane, C.M. & Blundell, T.L. (2001). CODA: a combined algorithm for predicting the structurally variable regions of protein models. *Protein Sci*, Vol.10, No.3, pp. 599-612

Dey, S., Hafkemeyer, P., Pastan, I. & Gottesman, M.M. (1999). A single amino acid residue contributes to distinct mechanisms of inhibition of the human multidrug transporter by stereoisomers of the dopamine receptor antagonist flupentixol. *Biochemistry*, Vol.38, No.20, pp. 6630-9

Dolghih, E., Bryant, C., Renslo, A.R. & Jacobson, M.P. (2011). Predicting binding to p-glycoprotein by flexible receptor docking. *PLoS Comput Biol*, Vol.7, No.6, pp. e1002083

Doyle, L.A., Yang, W., Abruzzo, L.V., Krogmann, T., Gao, Y., Rishi, A.K. & Ross, D.D. (1998). A multidrug resistance transporter from human MCF-7 breast cancer cells. *Proc Natl Acad Sci U S A*, Vol.95, No.26, pp. 15665-70

Ecker, G.F. & Chiba, P. (2009). ABC Transporters - From Targets to Antitargets? Transporters as Drug Carriers. G. F. Ecker and P. Chiba. Weinheim, Wiley-VCH. 1: 349-362

Ecker, G.F., Stockner, T. & Chiba, P. (2008). Computational models for prediction of interactions with ABC-transporters. *Drug Discov Today*, Vol.13, No.7-8, pp. 311-7

Eldridge, M.D., Murray, C.W., Auton, T.R., Paolini, G.V. & Mee, R.P. (1997). Empirical scoring functions: I. The development of a fast empirical scoring function to estimate the binding affinity of ligands in receptor complexes. *J Comput Aided Mol Des*, Vol.11, No.5, pp. 425-45

Evers, A. & Klebe, G. (2004). Successful virtual screening for a submicromolar antagonist of the neurokinin-1 receptor based on a ligand-supported homology model. *J Med Chem*, Vol.47, No.22, pp. 5381-92

Ewing, T.J., Makino, S., Skillman, A.G. & Kuntz, I.D. (2001). DOCK 4.0: search strategies for automated molecular docking of flexible molecule databases. *J Comput Aided Mol Des*, Vol.15, No.5, pp. 411-28

Forrest, L.R., Zhang, Y.W., Jacobs, M.T., Gesmonde, J., Xie, L., Honig, B.H. & Rudnick, G. (2008). Mechanism for alternating access in neurotransmitter transporters. *Proc Natl Acad Sci U S A*, Vol.105, No.30, pp. 10338-43

Giacomini, K.M., Huang, S.M., Tweedie, D.J., Benet, L.Z., Brouwer, K.L., Chu, X., Dahlin, A., Evers, R., Fischer, V., Hillgren, K.M., Hoffmaster, K.A., Ishikawa, T., Keppler, D., Kim, R.B., Lee, C.A., Niemi, M., Polli, J.W., Sugiyama, Y., Swaan, P.W., Ware, J.A., Wright, S.H., Yee, S.W., Zamek-Gliszczynski, M.J. & Zhang, L. (2010). Membrane transporters in drug development. *Nat Rev Drug Discov*, Vol.9, No.3, pp. 215-36

Gohlke, H., Hendlich, M. & Klebe, G. (2000). Knowledge-based scoring function to predict protein-ligand interactions. *J Mol Biol*, Vol.295, No.2, pp. 337-56

Goodsell, D.S., Morris, G.M. & Olson, A.J. (1996). Automated docking of flexible ligands: Applications of AutoDock. *Journal of Molecular Recognition*, Vol.9, No.1, pp. 1-5

Goodsell, D.S. & Olson, A.J. (1990). Automated docking of substrates to proteins by simulated annealing. *Proteins*, Vol.8, No.3, pp. 195-202

Gouaux, E. (2009). Review. The molecular logic of sodium-coupled neurotransmitter transporters. *Philos Trans R Soc Lond B Biol Sci*, Vol.364, No.1514, pp. 149-54

Gumbart, J., Wang, Y., Aksimentiev, A., Tajkhorshid, E. & Schulten, K. (2005). Molecular dynamics simulations of proteins in lipid bilayers. *Curr Opin Struct Biol*, Vol.15, No.4, pp. 423-431

Guptaroy, B., Zhang, M., Bowton, E., Binda, F., Shi, L., Weinstein, H., Galli, A., Javitch, J.A., Neubig, R.R. & Gnegy, M.E. (2009). A juxtamembrane mutation in the N terminus of the dopamine transporter induces preference for an inward-facing conformation. *Mol Pharmacol*, Vol.75, No.3, pp. 514-24

Gyimesi, G., Ramachandran, S., Kota, P., Dokholyan, N.V., Sarkadi, B. & Hegedus, T. (2011). ATP hydrolysis at one of the two sites in ABC transporters initiates transport related conformational transitions. *Biochim Biophys Acta*, Vol.

Hendlich, M., Rippmann, F. & Barnickel, G. (1997). LIGSITE: automatic and efficient detection of potential small molecule-binding sites in proteins. *Journal of Molecular Graphics & Modelling*, Vol.15, No.6, pp. 359-63, 389

Henrich, S., Salo-Ahen, O.M., Huang, B., Rippmann, F.F., Cruciani, G. & Wade, R.C. (2010). Computational approaches to identifying and characterizing protein binding sites for ligand design. *J Mol Recognit*, Vol.23, No.2, pp. 209-19

Hollt, V., Kouba, M., Dietel, M. & Vogt, G. (1992). Stereoisomers of calcium antagonists which differ markedly in their potencies as calcium blockers are equally effective in modulating drug transport by P-glycoprotein. *Biochem Pharmacol*, Vol.43, No.12, pp. 2601-8

Höltje, H.D., Sippl, W., Rognan, D. & Folkers, G. (2008). Molecular Modeling. Basic Principles and Applications. Weinheim, Germany, Wiley-VCH Verlag GmbH & CoKGaA

Huang, N., Kalyanaraman, C., Irwin, J.J. & Jacobson, M.P. (2006). Physics-based scoring of protein-ligand complexes: enrichment of known inhibitors in large-scale virtual screening. *J Chem Inf Model*, Vol.46, No.1, pp. 243-53

Huang, S.Y., Grinter, S.Z. & Zou, X. (2010). Scoring functions and their evaluation methods for protein-ligand docking: recent advances and future directions. *Phys Chem Chem Phys*, Vol.12, No.40, pp. 12899-908

Huang, S.Y. & Zou, X. (2006). An iterative knowledge-based scoring function to predict protein-ligand interactions: I. Derivation of interaction potentials. *J Comput Chem*, Vol.27, No.15, pp. 1866-75

Huang, S.Y. & Zou, X. (2006). An iterative knowledge-based scoring function to predict protein-ligand interactions: II. Validation of the scoring function. *J Comput Chem*, Vol.27, No.15, pp. 1876-82

Huang, S.Y. & Zou, X. (2008). An iterative knowledge-based scoring function for protein-protein recognition. *Proteins*, Vol.72, No.2, pp. 557-79

Hutchinson, E.G. & Thornton, J.M. (1996). PROMOTIF--a program to identify and analyze structural motifs in proteins. *Protein Sci*, Vol.5, No.2, pp. 212-20

Irvine, S.W.l.a.U. Membrane Proteins of Known 3D Structure, Available from: http://blanco.biomol.uci.edu/mpstruc/listAll/list

Isralewitz, B., Gao, M. & Schulten, K. (2001). Steered molecular dynamics and mechanical functions of proteins. *Current Opinion in Structural Biology*, Vol.11, No.2, pp. 224-230

Iversen, L.L. (1971). Role of transmitter uptake mechanisms in synaptic neurotransmission. *Br J Pharmacol*, Vol.41, No.4, pp. 571-91

Jabeen, I., Wetwitayaklung, P., Klepsch, F., Parveen, Z., Chiba, P. & Ecker, G.F. (2011). Probing the stereoselectivity of P-glycoprotein-synthesis, biological activity and ligand docking studies of a set of enantiopure benzopyrano[3,4-b][1,4]oxazines. *Chem Commun (Camb)*, Vol.47, No.9, pp. 2586-8

Jardetzky, O. (1966). Simple allosteric model for membrane pumps. *Nature*, Vol.211, No.5052, pp. 969-70

Jiang, F. & Kim, S.H. (1991). "Soft docking": matching of molecular surface cubes. *J Mol Biol*, Vol.219, No.1, pp. 79-102

Jones, G., Willett, P. & Glen, R.C. (1995). Molecular recognition of receptor sites using a genetic algorithm with a description of desolvation. *J Mol Biol*, Vol.245, No.1, pp. 43-53

Jones, P.M. & George, A.M. (2007). Nucleotide-dependent allostery within the ABC transporter ATP-binding cassette: a computational study of the MJ0796 dimer. *J Biol Chem*, Vol.282, No.31, pp. 22793-803

Jones, P.M. & George, A.M. (2009). Opening of the ADP-bound active site in the ABC transporter ATPase dimer: evidence for a constant contact, alternating sites model for the catalytic cycle. *Proteins*, Vol.75, No.2, pp. 387-96

Jorgensen, W.L. & Rives, T. (1988). The OPLS Potential Functions For Proteins - Energy Minimizations For Crystals Of Cyclic-Peptides And Crambin. *Journal of the American Chemical Society*, Vol.110, No.6, pp. 1657-1666

Kandt, C., Ash, W. & Tieleman, D.P. (July 2009). InflateGRO, Available from: http://www.csb.bit.uni-bonn.de/inflategro.html

Kandt, C., Ash, W.L. & Tieleman, D.P. (2007). Setting up and running molecular dynamics simulations of membrane proteins. *Methods*, Vol.41, No.4, pp. 475-488

Kanner, B.I. & Zomot, E. (2008). Sodium-coupled neurotransmitter transporters. *Chem Rev*, Vol.108, No.5, pp. 1654-68

Karplus, M. & McCammon, J.A. (2002). Molecular dynamics simulations of biomolecules. *Nat Struct Mol Biol*, Vol.9, No.9, pp. 646-652

Kitchen, D.B., Decornez, H., Furr, J.R. & Bajorath, J. (2004). Docking and scoring in virtual screening for drug discovery: methods and applications. *Nat Rev Drug Discov*, Vol.3, No.11, pp. 935-49

Klepsch, F., Chiba, P. & Ecker, G.F. (2011). Exhaustive sampling of docking poses reveals binding hypotheses for propafenone type inhibitors of P-glycoprotein. *PLoS Comput Biol*, Vol.7, No.5, pp. e1002036

Klepsch, F., Jabeen, I., Chiba, P. & Ecker, G.F. (2010). Pharmacoinformatic approaches to design natural product type ligands of ABC-transporters. *Curr Pharm Des*, Vol.16, No.15, pp. 1742-52

Knegtel, R.M., Kuntz, I.D. & Oshiro, C.M. (1997). Molecular docking to ensembles of protein structures. *J Mol Biol*, Vol.266, No.2, pp. 424-40

Knutsen, L.J., Andersen, K.E., Lau, J., Lundt, B.F., Henry, R.F., Morton, H.E., Naerum, L., Petersen, H., Stephensen, H., Suzdak, P.D., Swedberg, M.D., Thomsen, C. & Sorensen, P.O. (1999). Synthesis of novel GABA uptake inhibitors. 3. Diaryloxime and diarylvinyl ether derivatives of nipecotic acid and guvacine as anticonvulsant agents. *J Med Chem*, Vol.42, No.18, pp. 3447-62

Kragler, A., Hofner, G. & Wanner, K.T. (2008). Synthesis and biological evaluation of aminomethylphenol derivatives as inhibitors of the murine GABA transporters mGAT1-mGAT4. *European Journal of Medicinal Chemistry*, Vol.43, No.11, pp. 2404-11

Krishnamurthy, H. & Gouaux, E. (2012). X-ray structures of LeuT in substrate-free outward-open and apo inward-open states. *Nature*, doi:10.1038/nature10737 [Epub ahead of print]

Kristensen, A.S., Andersen, J., Jorgensen, T.N., Sorensen, L., Eriksen, J., Loland, C.J., Stromgaard, K. & Gether, U. (2011). SLC6 neurotransmitter transporters: structure, function, and regulation. *Pharmacol Rev*, Vol.63, No.3, pp. 585-640

Kufareva, I., Rueda, M., Katritch, V., Stevens, R.C., Abagyan, R. & participants, G.D. (2011). Status of GPCR modeling and docking as reflected by community-wide GPCR Dock 2010 assessment. *Structure*, Vol.19, No.8, pp. 1108-26

Kuhn, D., Weskamp, N., Hullermeier, E. & Klebe, G. (2007). Functional classification of protein kinase binding sites using Cavbase. *ChemMedChem*, Vol.2, No.10, pp. 1432-47

Kuntz, I.D., Blaney, J.M., Oatley, S.J., Langridge, R. & Ferrin, T.E. (1982). A geometric approach to macromolecule-ligand interactions. *J Mol Biol*, Vol.161, No.2, pp. 269-88

Laskowski, R.A., Macarthur, M.W., Moss, D.S. & Thornton, J.M. (1993). Procheck - a Program to Check the Stereochemical Quality of Protein Structures. *Journal of Applied Crystallography*, Vol.26, 283-291

Leach, A.R. (1994). Ligand docking to proteins with discrete side-chain flexibility. *J Mol Biol*, Vol.235, No.1, pp. 345-56

Lehre, A.C., Rowley, N.M., Zhou, Y., Holmseth, S., Guo, C., Holen, T., Hua, R., Laake, P., Olofsson, A.M., Poblete-Naredo, I., Rusakov, D.A., Madsen, K.K., Clausen, R.P., Schousboe, A., White, H.S. & Danbolt, N.C. (2011). Deletion of the betaine-GABA transporter (BGT1; slc6a12) gene does not affect seizure thresholds of adult mice. *Epilepsy Res*, Vol.95, No.1-2, pp. 70-81

Lesk, A.M. & Chothia, C. (1980). How different amino acid sequences determine similar protein structures: the structure and evolutionary dynamics of the globins. *J Mol Biol*, Vol.136, No.3, pp. 225-70

Lindahl, E. & Sansom, M.S.P. (2008). Membrane proteins: molecular dynamics simulations. *Curr Opin Struct Biol*, Vol.18, No.4, pp. 425-431

Loo, T.W., Bartlett, M.C. & Clarke, D.M. (2003). Simultaneous binding of two different drugs in the binding pocket of the human multidrug resistance P-glycoprotein. *J Biol Chem*, Vol.278, No.41, pp. 39706-10

Loo, T.W., Bartlett, M.C. & Clarke, D.M. (2010). Human P-glycoprotein is active when the two halves are clamped together in the closed conformation. *Biochem Biophys Res Commun*, Vol.395, No.3, pp. 436-40

Loo, T.W. & Clarke, D.M. (1999). The transmembrane domains of the human multidrug resistance P-glycoprotein are sufficient to mediate drug binding and trafficking to the cell surface. *J Biol Chem*, Vol.274, No.35, pp. 24759-65

Loo, T.W. & Clarke, D.M. (2002). Location of the rhodamine-binding site in the human multidrug resistance P-glycoprotein. *J Biol Chem*, Vol.277, No.46, pp. 44332-8

Loo, T.W. & Clarke, D.M. (2008). Mutational analysis of ABC proteins. *Arch Biochem Biophys*, Vol.476, No.1, pp. 51-64

Lu, H. & Schulten, K. (1999). Steered molecular dynamics simulations of force-induced protein domain unfolding. *Proteins: Structure, Function, and Bioinformatics*, Vol.35, No.4, pp. 453-463

Luurtsema, G., Molthoff, C.F., Windhorst, A.D., Smit, J.W., Keizer, H., Boellaard, R., Lammertsma, A.A. & Franssen, E.J. (2003). (R)- and (S)-[11C]verapamil as PET-tracers for measuring P-glycoprotein function: in vitro and in vivo evaluation. *Nucl Med Biol*, Vol.30, No.7, pp. 747-51

Madsen, K.K., White, H.S. & Schousboe, A. (2010). Neuronal and non-neuronal GABA transporters as targets for antiepileptic drugs. *Pharmacol Ther*, Vol.125, No.3, pp. 394-401

Malde, A.K., Zuo, L., Breeze, M., Stroet, M., Poger, D., Nair, P.C., Oostenbrink, C. & Mark, A.E. (2011). An Automated Force Field Topology Builder (ATB) and Repository: Version 1.0. *J Chem Theory Comput*, Vol.7, No.12, pp. 4026-4037

Marti-Renom, M.A., Stuart, A.C., Fiser, A., Sanchez, R., Melo, F. & Sali, A. (2000). Comparative protein structure modeling of genes and genomes. *Annu Rev Biophys Biomol Struct*, Vol.29, 291-325

Matthews, B.W. (2007). Five retracted structure reports: inverted or incorrect? *Protein Sci*, Vol.16, No.6, pp. 1013-6

McCammon, J.A., Gelin, B.R. & Karplus, M. (1977). Dynamics of folded proteins. *Nature*, Vol.267, No.5612, pp. 585-590

Mealey, K.L., Bentjen, S.A., Gay, J.M. & Cantor, G.H. (2001). Ivermectin sensitivity in collies is associated with a deletion mutation of the mdr1 gene. *Pharmacogenetics*, Vol.11, No.8, pp. 727-33

Mehler, E.L., Periole, X., Hassan, S.A. & Weinstein, H. (2002). Key issues in the computational simulation of GPCR function: representation of loop domains. *J Comput Aided Mol Des*, Vol.16, No.11, pp. 841-53

Mizutani, M.Y., Tomioka, N. & Itai, A. (1994). Rational automatic search method for stable docking models of protein and ligand. *J Mol Biol*, Vol.243, No.2, pp. 310-26

Moore, G. (1965). Cramming more components onto integrated circuits *Electronics*, Vol.38, No.8, pp.

Neuhaus, W. & Noe, C.R. (2009). Transport at the Blood-Brain Barrier. Transporters as Drug Carriers. G. F. Ecker and P. Chiba. Weinheim, Wiley-VCH. 1: 263-298

Newby, Z.E.R., O'Connell, J.D., Gruswitz, F., Hays, F.A., Harries, W.E.C., Harwood, I.M., Ho, J.D., Lee, J.K., Savage, D.F., Miercke, L.J.W. & Stroud, R.M. (2009). A general protocol for the crystallization of membrane proteins for X-ray structural investigation. *Nat. Protocols*, Vol.4, No.5, pp. 619-637

Newstead, S., Fowler, P.W., Bilton, P., Carpenter, E.P., Sadler, P.J., Campopiano, D.J., Sansom, M.S. & Iwata, S. (2009). Insights into how nucleotide-binding domains power ABC transport. *Structure*, Vol.17, No.9, pp. 1213-22

Notredame, C., Higgins, D.G. & Heringa, J. (2000). T-Coffee: A novel method for fast and accurate multiple sequence alignment. *J Mol Biol*, Vol.302, No.1, pp. 205-17

Oliveira, A.S., Baptista, A.M. & Soares, C.M. (2011). Conformational changes induced by ATP-hydrolysis in an ABC transporter: a molecular dynamics study of the Sav1866 exporter. *Proteins*, Vol.79, No.6, pp. 1977-90

Olson, A.J., Morris, G.M., Goodsell, D.S., Halliday, R.S., Huey, R., Hart, W.E. & Belew, R.K. (1998). Automated docking using a Lamarckian genetic algorithm and an empirical binding free energy function. *Journal of Computational Chemistry*, Vol.19, No.14, pp. 1639-1662

Omote, H. & Al-Shawi, M.K. (2006). Interaction of transported drugs with the lipid bilayer and P-glycoprotein through a solvation exchange mechanism. *Biophysical Journal*, Vol.90, No.11, pp. 4046-59

Pajeva, I.K., Globisch, C. & Wiese, M. (2009). Combined pharmacophore modeling, docking, and 3D QSAR studies of ABCB1 and ABCC1 transporter inhibitors. *ChemMedChem*, Vol.4, No.11, pp. 1883-96

Pallo, A., Bencsura, A., Heja, L., Beke, T., Perczel, A., Kardos, J. & Simon, A. (2007). Major human gamma-aminobutyrate transporter: in silico prediction of substrate efficacy. *Biochem Biophys Res Commun*, Vol.364, No.4, pp. 952-8

Pallo, A., Simon, A., Bencsura, A., Heja, L. & Kardos, J. (2009). Substrate-Na+ complex formation: coupling mechanism for gamma-aminobutyrate symporters. *Biochem Biophys Res Commun*, Vol.385, No.2, pp. 210-4

Park, S., Kono, H., Wang, W., Boder, E.T. & Saven, J.G. (2005). Progress in the development and application of computational methods for probabilistic protein design. *Comput Chem Eng*, Vol.29, No.3, pp. 407-421

Pearson, W.R. (1990). Rapid and sensitive sequence comparison with FASTP and FASTA. *Methods Enzymol*, Vol.183, 63-98

Penders, B., Horstman, K. & Vos, R. (2007). Proper science in moist biology. *EMBO Rep*, Vol.8, No.7, pp. 613

Pleban, K., Kaiser, D., Kopp, S., Peer, M., Chiba, P. & Ecker, G.F. (2005). Targeting drug-efflux pumps -- a pharmacoinformatic approach. *Acta Biochim Pol*, Vol.52, No.3, pp. 737-40

Pleban, K., Kopp, S., Csaszar, E., Peer, M., Hrebicek, T., Rizzi, A., Ecker, G.F. & Chiba, P. (2005). P-glycoprotein substrate binding domains are located at the transmembrane domain/transmembrane domain interfaces: a combined photoaffinity labeling-protein homology modeling approach. *Mol Pharmacol*, Vol.67, No.2, pp. 365-74

Qu, Q. & Sharom, F.J. (2002). Proximity of bound Hoechst 33342 to the ATPase catalytic sites places the drug binding site of P-glycoprotein within the cytoplasmic membrane leaflet. *Biochemistry*, Vol.41, No.14, pp. 4744-52

Rabindran, S.K., Ross, D.D., Doyle, L.A., Yang, W. & Greenberger, L.M. (2000). Fumitremorgin C reverses multidrug resistance in cells transfected with the breast cancer resistance protein. *Cancer Res*, Vol.60, No.1, pp. 47-50

Rarey, M., Kramer, B., Lengauer, T. & Klebe, G. (1996). A fast flexible docking method using an incremental construction algorithm. *J Mol Biol*, Vol.261, No.3, pp. 470-89

Reyes, C.L. & Chang, G. (2005). Structure of the ABC transporter MsbA in complex with ADP.vanadate and lipopolysaccharide. *Science*, Vol.308, No.5724, pp. 1028-31

Reynolds, C.A., Wade, R.C. & Goodford, P.J. (1989). Identifying targets for bioreductive agents: using GRID to predict selective binding regions of proteins. *J Mol Graph*, Vol.7, No.2, pp. 103-8, 100

Rosenberg, M.F., Velarde, G., Ford, R.C., Martin, C., Berridge, G., Kerr, I.D., Callaghan, R., Schmidlin, A., Wooding, C., Linton, K.J. & Higgins, C.F. (2001). Repacking of the transmembrane domains of P-glycoprotein during the transport ATPase cycle. *EMBO J*, Vol.20, No.20, pp. 5615-25

Saier, M.H., Tran, C.V. & Barabote, R.D. (2006). TCDB: the Transporter Classification Database for membrane transport protein analyses and information. *Nucleic Acids Res*, Vol.34, No.suppl 1, pp. D181-D186

Saier, M.H., Yen, M.R., Noto, K., Tamang, D.G. & Elkan, C. (2009). The Transporter Classification Database: recent advances. *Nucleic Acids Res*, Vol.37, No.suppl 1, pp. D274-D278

Sarker, S., Weissensteiner, R., Steiner, I., Sitte, H.H., Ecker, G.F., Freissmuth, M. & Sucic, S. (2010). The high-affinity binding site for tricyclic antidepressants resides in the outer vestibule of the serotonin transporter. *Mol Pharmacol*, Vol.78, No.6, pp. 1026-35

Schinkel, A.H. & Jonker, J.W. (2003). Mammalian drug efflux transporters of the ATP binding cassette (ABC) family: an overview. *Adv Drug Deliv Rev*, Vol.55, No.1, pp. 3-29

Schlitter, J., Engels, M. & KrÃ¼ger, P. (1994). Targeted molecular dynamics: A new approach for searching pathways of conformational transitions. *Journal of Molecular Graphics*, Vol.12, No.2, pp. 84-89

Schmidt, D., Jiang, Q.-X. & MacKinnon, R. (2006). Phospholipids and the origin of cationic gating charges in voltage sensors. *Nature*, Vol.444, No.7120, pp. 775-779

Schousboe, A., Sarup, A., Larsson, O.M. & White, H.S. (2004). GABA transporters as drug targets for modulation of GABAergic activity. *Biochem Pharmacol*, Vol.68, No.8, pp. 1557-63

Schrauber, H., Eisenhaber, F. & Argos, P. (1993). Rotamers: to be or not to be? An analysis of amino acid side-chain conformations in globular proteins. *J Mol Biol*, Vol.230, No.2, pp. 592-612

Scott, W.R.P., Hünenberger, P.H., Tironi, I.G., Mark, A.E., Billeter, S.R., Fennen, J., Torda, A.E., Huber, T., KrÃ¼ger, P. & van Gunsteren, W.F. (1999). The GROMOS Biomolecular Simulation Program Package. *The Journal of Physical Chemistry A*, Vol.103, No.19, pp. 3596-3607

Seeger, M.A. & van Veen, H.W. (2009). Molecular basis of multidrug transport by ABC transporters. *Biochim Biophys Acta*, Vol.1794, No.5, pp. 725-37

Seigneuret, M. & Garnier-Suillerot, A. (2003). A structural model for the open conformation of the mdr1 P-glycoprotein based on the MsbA crystal structure. *J Biol Chem*, Vol.278, No.32, pp. 30115-24

Shapiro, A.B., Fox, K., Lam, P. & Ling, V. (1999). Stimulation of P-glycoprotein-mediated drug transport by prazosin and progesterone. Evidence for a third drug-binding site. *Eur J Biochem*, Vol.259, No.3, pp. 841-50

Sharom, F.J. (2008). ABC multidrug transporters: structure, function and role in chemoresistance. *Pharmacogenomics*, Vol.9, No.1, pp. 105-27

Sherman, W., Day, T., Jacobson, M.P., Friesner, R.A. & Farid, R. (2006). Novel procedure for modeling ligand/receptor induced fit effects. *J Med Chem*, Vol.49, No.2, pp. 534-53

Shi, L., Quick, M., Zhao, Y., Weinstein, H. & Javitch, J.A. (2008). The mechanism of a neurotransmitter:sodium symporter--inward release of Na+ and substrate is triggered by substrate in a second binding site. *Mol Cell*, Vol.30, No.6, pp. 667-77

Shilling, R.A., Balakrishnan, L., Shahi, S., Venter, H. & van Veen, H.W. (2003). A new dimer interface for an ABC transporter. *Int J Antimicrob Agents*, Vol.22, No.3, pp. 200-4

Singh, S.K., Piscitelli, C.L., Yamashita, A. & Gouaux, E. (2008). A competitive inhibitor traps LeuT in an open-to-out conformation. *Science*, Vol.322, No.5908, pp. 1655-61

Sitte, H.H., Farhan, H. & Javitch, J.A. (2004). Sodium-dependent neurotransmitter transporters: oligomerization as a determinant of transporter function and trafficking. *Mol Interv*, Vol.4, No.1, pp. 38-47

Skovstrup, S., Taboureau, O., Brauner-Osborne, H. & Jorgensen, F.S. (2010). Homology modelling of the GABA transporter and analysis of tiagabine binding. *ChemMedChem*, Vol.5, No.7, pp. 986-1000

Sousa, S.F., Fernandes, P.A. & Ramos, M.J. (2006). Protein-ligand docking: current status and future challenges. *Proteins*, Vol.65, No.1, pp. 15-26

Stenham, D.R., Campbell, J.D., Sansom, M.S., Higgins, C.F., Kerr, I.D. & Linton, K.J. (2003). An atomic detail model for the human ATP binding cassette transporter P-glycoprotein derived from disulfide cross-linking and homology modeling. *FASEB J*, Vol.17, No.15, pp. 2287-9

Stockner, T., de Vries, S.J., Bonvin, A.M., Ecker, G.F. & Chiba, P. (2009). Data-driven homology modelling of P-glycoprotein in the ATP-bound state indicates flexibility of the transmembrane domains. *FEBS J*, Vol.276, No.4, pp. 964-72

Stouten, P.F.W. & Brady, G.P. (2000). Fast prediction and visualization of protein binding pockets with PASS. *Journal of Computer-Aided Molecular Design*, Vol.14, No.4, pp. 383-401

Sucic, S., Dallinger, S., Zdrazil, B., Weissensteiner, R., Jorgensen, T.N., Holy, M., Kudlacek, O., Seidel, S., Cha, J.H., Gether, U., Newman, A.H., Ecker, G.F., Freissmuth, M. & Sitte, H.H. (2010). The N terminus of monoamine transporters is a lever required for the action of amphetamines. *J Biol Chem*, Vol.285, No.14, pp. 10924-38

Szakacs, G., Varadi, A., Ozvegy-Laczka, C. & Sarkadi, B. (2008). The role of ABC transporters in drug absorption, distribution, metabolism, excretion and toxicity (ADME-Tox). *Drug Discov Today*, Vol.13, No.9-10, pp. 379-93

Tanaka, S. & Scheraga, H.A. (1976). Medium- and long-range interaction parameters between amino acids for predicting three-dimensional structures of proteins. *Macromolecules*, Vol.9, No.6, pp. 945-50

Theobald, D.L. & Miller, C. (2010). Membrane transport proteins: surprises in structural sameness. *Nat Struct Mol Biol*, Vol.17, 2–3

Thompson, J.D., Higgins, D.G. & Gibson, T.J. (1994). CLUSTAL W: improving the sensitivity of progressive multiple sequence alignment through sequence weighting, position-specific gap penalties and weight matrix choice. *Nucleic Acids Res*, Vol.22, No.22, pp. 4673-80

Tsuruo, T., Iida, H., Tsukagoshi, S. & Sakurai, Y. (1981). Overcoming of vincristine resistance in P388 leukemia in vivo and in vitro through enhanced cytotoxicity of vincristine and vinblastine by verapamil. *Cancer Res*, Vol.41, No.5, pp. 1967-72

Vandevuer, S., Van Bambeke, F., Tulkens, P.M. & Prevost, M. (2006). Predicting the three-dimensional structure of human P-glycoprotein in absence of ATP by computational techniques embodying crosslinking data: insight into the mechanism of ligand migration and binding sites. *Proteins*, Vol.63, No.3, pp. 466-78

Verdonk, M.L., Cole, J.C., Hartshorn, M.J., Murray, C.W. & Taylor, R.D. (2003). Improved protein-ligand docking using GOLD. *Proteins*, Vol.52, No.4, pp. 609-23

Vriend, G. (1990). WHAT IF: a molecular modeling and drug design program. *J Mol Graph*, Vol.8, No.1, pp. 52-6, 29

Wang, R., Lai, L. & Wang, S. (2002). Further development and validation of empirical scoring functions for structure-based binding affinity prediction. *J Comput Aided Mol Des*, Vol.16, No.1, pp. 11-26

Wang, Y., Shaikh, S.A. & Tajkhorshid, E. (2010). Exploring transmembrane diffusion pathways with molecular dynamics. *Physiology*, Vol.25, No.3, pp. 142-54

Ward, A., Reyes, C.L., Yu, J., Roth, C.B. & Chang, G. (2007). Flexibility in the ABC transporter MsbA: Alternating access with a twist. *Proc Natl Acad Sci U S A*, Vol.104, No.48, pp. 19005-10

Wein, T. & Wanner, K.T. (2009). Generation of a 3D model for human GABA transporter hGAT-1 using molecular modeling and investigation of the binding of GABA. *Journal of Molecular Modeling*, Vol.

Weiner, S.J., Kollman, P.A., Case, D.A., Singh, U.C., Ghio, C., Alagona, G., Profeta, S. & Weiner, P. (1984). A New Force-Field for Molecular Mechanical Simulation of Nucleic-Acids and Proteins. *Journal of the American Chemical Society*, Vol.106, No.3, pp. 765-784

Welch, W., Ruppert, J. & Jain, A.N. (1996). Hammerhead: fast, fully automated docking of flexible ligands to protein binding sites. *Chem Biol*, Vol.3, No.6, pp. 449-62

Wen, P.C. & Tajkhorshid, E. (2008). Dimer opening of the nucleotide binding domains of ABC transporters after ATP hydrolysis. *Biophysical Journal*, Vol.95, No.11, pp. 5100-10

White, K.J., Kiser, P.D., Nichols, D.E. & Barker, E.L. (2006). Engineered zinc-binding sites confirm proximity and orientation of transmembrane helices I and III in the human serotonin transporter. *Protein Sci*, Vol.15, No.10, pp. 2411-22

Willard, L., Ranjan, A., Zhang, H., Monzavi, H., Boyko, R.F., Sykes, B.D. & Wishart, D.S. (2003). VADAR: a web server for quantitative evaluation of protein structure quality. *Nucleic Acids Res*, Vol.31, No.13, pp. 3316-9

Wolf, M.G., Hoefling, M., Aponte-Santamaria, C., Grubmüller, H. & Groenhof, G. (2010). g_membed: Efficient Insertion of a Membrane Protein into an Equilibrated Lipid Bilayer with Minimal Perturbation. *J Comput Chem*, Vol.31, 2169–2174

Yamashita, A., Singh, S.K., Kawate, T., Jin, Y. & Gouaux, E. (2005). Crystal structure of a bacterial homologue of Na+/Cl--dependent neurotransmitter transporters. *Nature*, Vol.437, No.7056, pp. 215-23

Zhao, S., Zhu, K., Li, J. & Friesner, R.A. (2011). Progress in super long loop prediction. *Proteins*, Vol.79, No.10, pp. 2920-35

Zhou, H. & Zhou, Y. (2002). Distance-scaled, finite ideal-gas reference state improves structure-derived potentials of mean force for structure selection and stability prediction. *Protein Sci*, Vol.11, No.11, pp. 2714-26

18

Alternative Perspectives of Enzyme Kinetic Modeling

Ryan Walsh
Chemistry Department, Carleton University, Ottawa
Canada

1. Introduction

The basis of enzyme kinetic modelling was established during the early 1900's when the work of Leonor Michaelis and Maud Menten produced a pseudo-steady state equation linking enzymatic catalytic rate to substrate concentration (Michaelis & Menten, 1913). Building from the Michaelis-Menten equation, other equations used to describe the effects of modifiers of enzymatic activity were developed based on their effect on the catalytic parameters of the Michaelis-Menten equation. Initially, inhibitors affecting the substrate affinity were deemed competitive and inhibitors affecting the reaction rate were labelled non-competitive (McElroy 1947). These equations have persisted as the basis for inhibition studies and can be found in most basic textbooks dealing with the subject of enzyme inhibition. Here the functionality of the competitive and non-competitive equations are examined to support the development of a unified equation for enzymatic activity modulation. From this, a modular approach to pseudo-steady state enzyme kinetic equation building is examined. Finally the assumption that these equations, which stem from the Michaelis-Menten equation, are truly pseudo-steady state is also examined.

2. Pseudo steady state enzyme kinetic

2.1 Michaelis-Menten kinetics

Conventional views on how to handle enzyme kinetic data have remained essentially the same for nearly a century following the proposal of the Michaelis-Menten equation (1913; Equation 1).

$$v = V_{max} \frac{[S]}{[S] + K_M} \tag{1}$$

The Michaelis-Menten equation was a large step forward in our ability to understand how biological systems control chemical processes. This equation linked the rate of enzymatic substrate catalysis to a mass action process relying on the fractional association between the substrate and the enzyme population. That is, the maximum conversion rate of substrate to product (V_{max}) could be directly related to the concentration of the enzyme ([E]) present and the catalytic rate at which individual enzymes converted substrate molecules to product (k_{cat}; Equation 2).

$$V_{max} = k_{cat}[E] \tag{2}$$

The second part of the equation describes the fractional association between the substrate and the enzyme population. Dependent on the Michaelis-Menten constant (K_M; Equation 3), this part of the Michaelis-Menten equation partitions the binding of substrate to the enzyme population relative to the Michaelis-Menten constant.

$$\frac{[S]}{[S] + K_M} \tag{3}$$

At substrate concentrations lower than the Michaelis-Menten constant, also known as the substrate affinity constant, less than half of the enzyme population would be expected to have substrate associated with it (Figure 1).

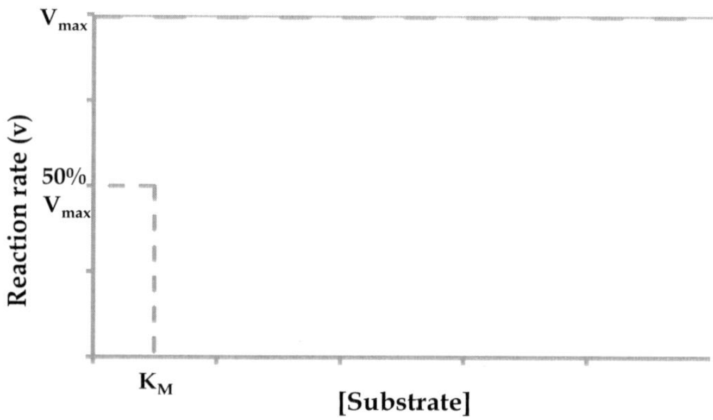

Fig. 1. Rectangular hyperbola plot of the Michaelis-Menten equation relating catalytic rate and substrate concentration.

At a concentration equal to the Michaelis-Menten constant, half of the enzyme population will have substrate associated with it. Therefore, the Michaelis-Menten constant itself is an inflection point. As substrate concentrations exceed the Michaelis-Menten constant, the fraction of the enzyme population interacting with substrate is pushed towards 100%. This term produces the characteristic rectangular hyperbolic profile associated with the Michaelis-Menten equation shown above.

2.2 Linearization of the Michaelis-Menten equation

The introduction of the reciprocal form of the Michaelis-Menten equation (Equation 4) in 1934 (Lineweaver & Burk) made the determination of the kinetic constants (K_M, V_{max}) of the Michaelis-Menten equation much simpler.

$$\frac{1}{v} = \frac{K_M}{V_{max}} \frac{1}{[S]} + \frac{1}{V_{max}} \tag{4}$$

The reciprocal form of the equation produced a straight line with intercept values on the Y axis of $1/V_{max}$ and on the X axis of $-1/K_M$ (Figure 2). This advancement in analysis of the Michaelis-Menten equation allowed for a simplified way of analyzing the effect of compounds that altered the catalytic activity of enzyme systems. Changes in enzymatic activity were observed to result from changes in the substrate affinity or maximum velocity (Lineweaver & Burk 1934) resulting in the definition of inhibitory equations based on their effects on the kinetic constants of the Michaelis-Menten equation.

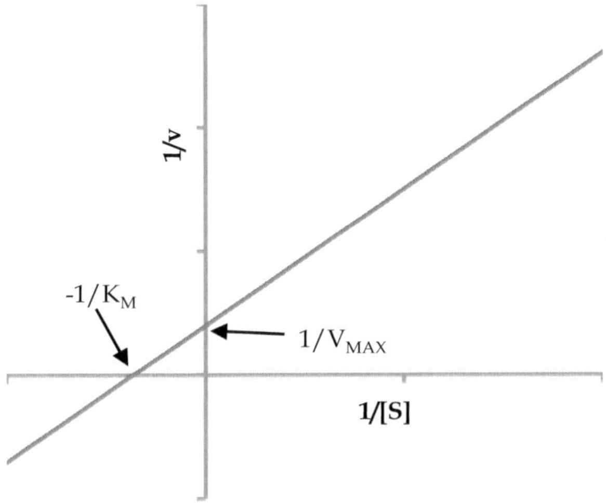

Fig. 2. Double reciprocal plot of the Michaelis-Menten equation indicating how the intercepts provide a simplified way of determining the kinetic constants of the equation.

2.3 Modes of inhibition

By far the most extensively documented form of interactions between modifiers of enzymatic activity and enzymes have been inhibitory, therefore, it is not surprising that the first mathematical models to be defined and accepted in the literature were the competitive (Equation 5) and non-competitive (Equation 6) modes of inhibition (Lineweaver & Burk 1934; McElroy 1947).

$$v = V_{max} \frac{[S]}{[S] + K_M \left(1 + \frac{[I]}{K_i}\right)} \quad (5)$$

$$v = V_{max} \frac{[S]}{([S] + K_M)\left(1 + \frac{[I]}{K_i}\right)} \quad (6)$$

The competitive inhibition (Equation 5) and non-competitive inhibition (Equation 6) equations model different inhibitory processes and are easily identified using Lineweaver-Burk double reciprocal plots (Figure 3). Competitive inhibition has been defined as a direct competition between the substrate and the inhibitor molecule for the active site of the enzyme. As inhibitor concentration is increased, the enzyme's substrate affinity is decreased. However, due to the competitive nature of this interaction, decreases in catalytic activity can always be overcome with sufficient increases in substrate concentration. In contrast, non-competitive inhibition exclusively affects the catalytic velocity of the enzyme population. Shifts in the maximum velocity can be attributed to the inhibitor binding to the enzyme and shutting down its catalytic activity, such that the observed decrease in activity represents the percent of the enzyme population bound by inhibitor.

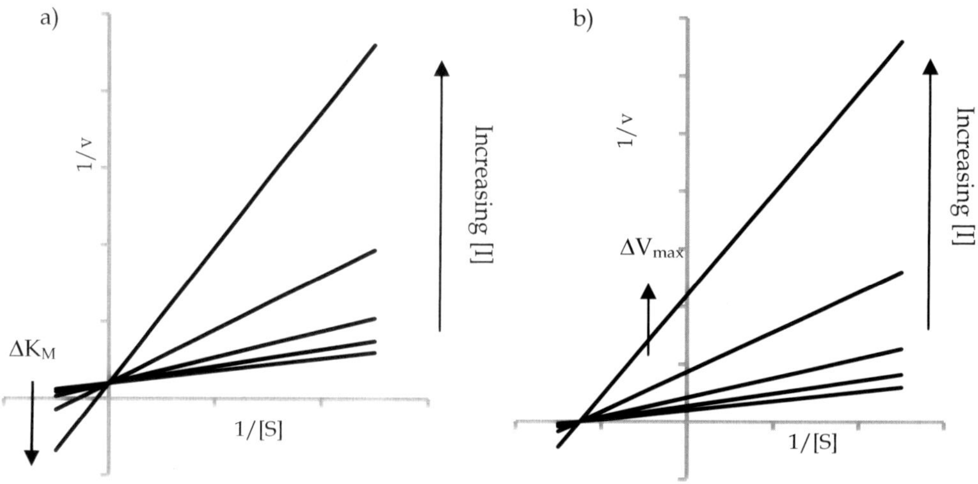

Fig. 3. Double reciprocal plots of a) competitive inhibition, where introduction of the inhibitor produces changes exclusively in the substrate affinity constant (K_M) and b) non-competitive inhibition, where inhibition is observed as a decrease in the maximum velocity of the enzyme catalyzed (V_{max}) reaction.

Both of the competitive and non-competitive inhibition equations can be derived from rate and conservation of mass equations like the Michaelis-Menten equation. The derivation of the competitive (Equation 5) and non-competitive (Equation 6) inhibition equation also results in a similar inhibitory term (Equation 7).

$$\left(1 + \frac{[I]}{K_i}\right) \tag{7}$$

This type of equation derivation, which segregates modes of inhibition based on inhibitory effect on kinetic constants of the Michaelis-Menten equation, has formed the basis for equation derivation in modern enzyme kinetics. However the use of the inhibitory term (Equation 7) found in the competitive (Equation 5) and non-competitive (Equation 6) inhibition equations may be regarded as an incomplete derivation that obscures the relationship between inhibitor binding and kinetic effect (Walsh et al., 2007).

In the competitive inhibition equation (Equation 5), the inhibitory term, as written, directly affects the Michaelis-Menten constant. This might be expected as competitive inhibition exclusively alters substrate affinity. In the non-competitive equation (Equation 6), the inhibitory term is inversely related to the maximum velocity (Equation 8).

$$\frac{V_{max}}{1 + \frac{[I]}{K_i}} \tag{8}$$

A rearrangement of this term (Equations 9-12) demonstrates the similarities of the inhibitory term and the term relating the fractional association between substrate and enzyme population (Equation 3).

$$\frac{V_{max}}{\frac{[I] + K_i}{K_i}} \tag{9}$$

$$\frac{V_{max}}{\frac{[I] + K_i}{[I] + K_i - [I]}} \tag{10}$$

$$\frac{V_{max}}{\frac{1}{1 - \frac{[I]}{[I] + K_i}}} \tag{11}$$

$$V_{max} - V_{max}\frac{[I]}{[I] + K_i} \tag{12}$$

Therefore the inhibitory term of the non-competitive inhibition equation directly equates shutting down of enzymatic activity with the fraction of the enzyme population bound by the inhibitor. This on off analog behaviour provides a simplistic way looking at enzymatic activity and limits the usefulness of this equation for describing anything other than complete inhibition of the enzyme upon inhibitor binding. However, the addition of a governor term (V_{max}-V_{max2}) changes the non-competitive term such that it can be used to account for changes in catalytic activity, other than complete inhibition (Equation 13; Walsh et al., 2007; Walsh et al., 2011a).

$$V_{max} - (V_{max} - V_{max2})\frac{[I]}{[I] + K_i} \tag{13}$$

This rearrangement, or insertion of a governor term, allows for the description of inhibitory effects ranging from just greater than 0% to 100% and has the potential to describe activation as well if the secondary maximum velocity is greater than the initial velocity. It is convenient to classify compounds with the potential to activate as well as inhibit as modifiers, denote here as X (Equation 14).

$$V_{max} - (V_{max} - V_{max2})\frac{[X]}{[X] + K_x} \tag{14}$$

Even without the addition of the governor term to the non-competitive equation, this rearrangement (Equation 9-12) accounts for the rectangular hyperbolic change in maximum velocity produced by the non-competitive inhibition equation (Figure 4). This change is identical to the mass action binding observed between the substrate and the enzyme population in the Michaelis-Menten equation (Figure 1).

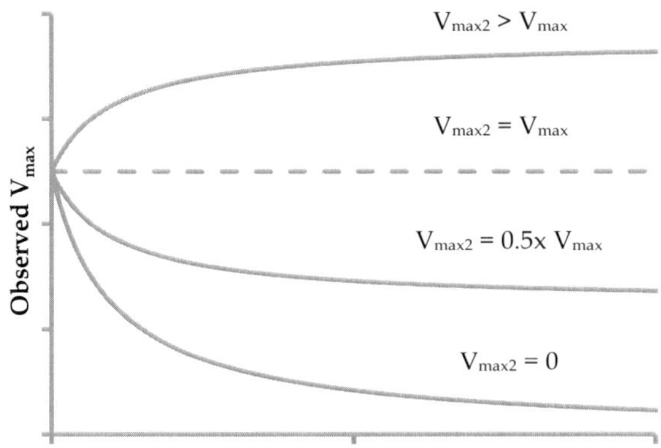

Fig. 4. Rectangular hyperbolic changes in the maximum velocity produced by modifiers. Here the mass action binding between the enzyme population and modifier results in the characteristic shape of the curve but the change in activity depends on the change induced by single binding events between the enzyme and the modifier. For example the four lines represent stimulation ($V_{max2} > V_{max}$), binding without catalytic effect ($V_{max2} = V_{max}$), partial inhibition ($V_{max2} = 0.5x\ V_{max}$) and complete inhibition ($V_{max2} = 0$) as would be observed with the classical non-competitive equation.

With the clear way non-competitive inhibition mimics the kinetics observed with the Michaelis-Menten equation, the manner in which competitive inhibitors affect enzyme activity becomes obscure. This can be demonstrated through the same rearrangement of the inhibitory term which directly affects the substrate affinity (Equations 15-19).

$$K_M\left(1 + \frac{[I]}{K_i}\right) \tag{15}$$

$$K_M\left(\frac{[I] + K_i}{K_i}\right) \tag{16}$$

$$K_M\left(\frac{[I] + K_i}{[I] + K_i - [I]}\right) \tag{17}$$

$$K_M\left(\frac{1}{1-\frac{[I]}{[I]+K_i}}\right) \tag{18}$$

$$\frac{K_M}{1-\frac{[I]}{[I]+K_i}} \tag{19}$$

As can be seen in equation 19, the inhibitory term in the competitive inhibition equation (Equation 5) actually describes a situation where the substrate affinity term is divided by the percent of the enzyme population free of the competitive inhibitor. This implies that modifiers that affect the substrate affinity exclusively produce a linear increase in the substrate affinity with increasing inhibitor concentration (Figure 5). However, as substrate binding specificity and affinity result from three point binding (Ogston, 1948), changes in the ability of an enzyme to bind substrate are more likely to result from inhibitor interactions that shift the enzyme's ability to do this away from its native state. Such perturbations would follow the same mass action mode of interaction as observed with non-competitive inhibition (Equation 6). These changes in substrate affinity would be finite and the overall observable effect would result from individual interactions between inhibitor and enzyme which would shift the binding affinity form that of the native enzyme (K_M) to an affinity produced by the inhibitor (K_{M2}) (Equation 20; Walsh et al., 2007; Walsh et al., 2011a).

$$v = V_{max}\frac{[S]}{[S]+K_M-(K_M-K_{M2})\frac{[I]}{[I]+K_i}} \tag{20}$$

While true competitive inhibition may exist, the criteria for identifying an inhibitor as truly competitive needs to include a linear shift in substrate affinity resulting from increase in inhibitor concentration (Figure 5d; Walsh et al., 2007; Walsh et al., 2011a). This should be examined with global data fitting to confirm the inhibitory effect on substrate affinity.

3. Modular enzyme kinetic equation building

3.1 Unified modifier equation

By recognizing that changes in the substrate affinity and maximum velocity result from stoichiometric interactions between the modifier and the enzyme and that the effects of the modifier can be regulated with a governor term, a single equation for describing these effects can be generated (Equation 21; Walsh et al., 2007).

$$v = \frac{[S]}{[S]+K_{S1}-(K_{S1}-K_{S2})\left(\frac{[X]}{[X]+K_{X1}}\right)} V_{S1}-(V_{S1}-V_{S2})\left(\frac{[X]}{[X]+K_{X1}}\right) \tag{21}$$

Here the maximum velocity term has been abbreviated as V_{S1}, and the substrate affinity term K_{S1}, for simplicity. Of note, the modifier binding constant (K_{X1}) is the same in the term modifying the substrate affinity and the term modifying the maximum velocity. This is in contrast to the mixed non-competitive equation (Equation 22) which has been used to describe similar dual effects on substrate affinity and maximum velocity but requires two separate inhibitor binding constants to accommodate the effects of a single inhibitor.

$$v = V_{max} \frac{[S]}{[S]\left(1 + \frac{[I]}{\alpha K_i}\right) + K_M\left(1 + \frac{[I]}{K_i}\right)} \tag{22}$$

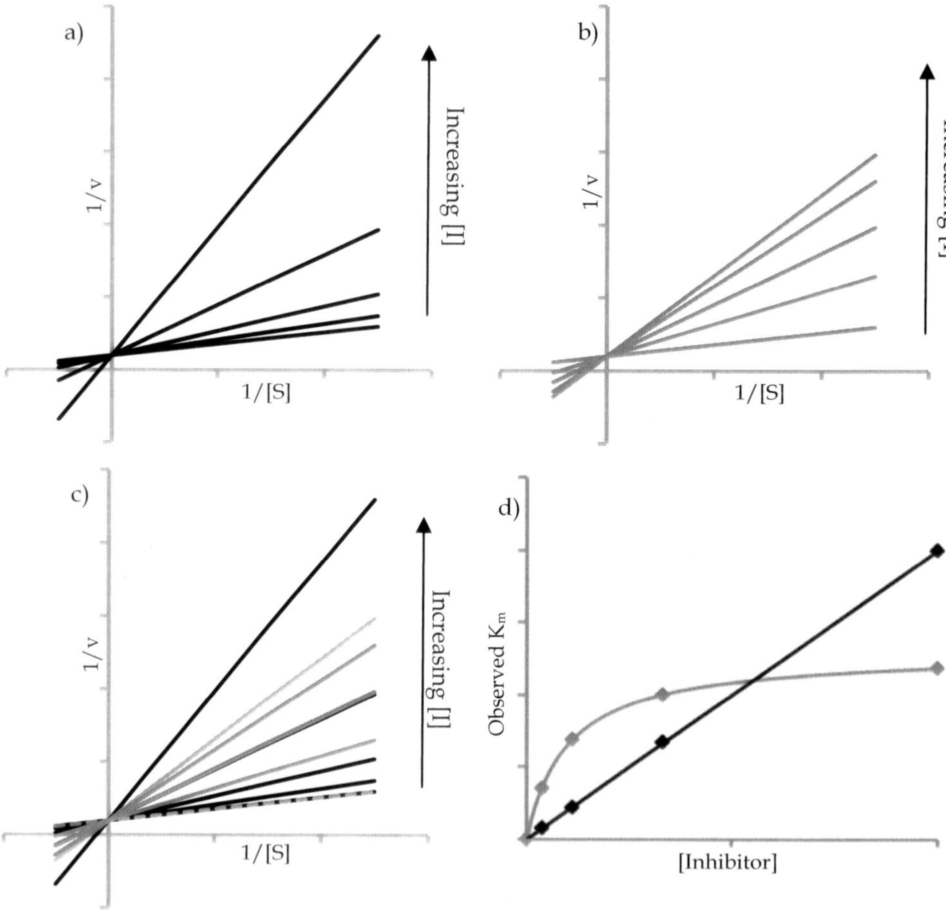

Fig. 5. Double reciprocal plots of the a) competitive inhibition equation (Equation 5), representing a continuous change in substrate affinity with increasing inhibitor concentration, b) Equation 20 representing a hyperbolic change from one substrate affinity to another as the inhibitor binds in a stoichiometric way with the enzyme, c) an overlay of the two plots and d) a plot of the shift in substrate affinity at different concentrations of the inhibitor.

This need for two inhibitor constants and the problems associated with this notation can be attributed to the inverse way in which the inhibitory terms affect the kinetic constants of the Michaelis Menten equation, as outlines in the previous section.

In addition to the unification of binding constants and introduction of governor terms, the format of Equation 21 also represents an improvement over the competitive (Equation 5), non-competitive (Equation 6) and mixed non-competitive (equation 22) equations. This is due to the structure of the modifier term in that they can be expanded in a modular format to include additional modifier effects.

3.2 Modular substrate and modifier term expansion

Cholinesterases are the prime example of enzymes that have been found to be subject to substrate modulation. Specifically, acetylcholinesterase is known to experience substrate inhibition and butyrylcholinesterase is subject to substrate activation. To model these effects, equation 23 (Reiner & Simeon-Rudolf 2000) has been used.

$$v = \frac{V_{S1}[S]}{[S] + K_{S1}} \times \frac{1 + b[S]/K_{SS1}}{1 + [S]/K_{SS1}} \qquad (23)$$

This equation expresses substrate inhibition or activation in the form of a ratio (*b*) with values greater than one indicative of activation and values lower than one indicative of inhibition. This equation, while being able to describe the effects of substrate modulation fairly well, lacks the ability for easy modification so an alternative equation based on a modular expansion of the Michaelis Menten equation was proposed (Equation 24; Walsh et al., 2007).

$$v = \frac{[S]}{[S] + K_{S1}} V_{S1} - \frac{[S]}{[S] + K_{SS1}} V_{S1} + \frac{[S]}{[S] + K_{SS1}} V_{SS1} \qquad (24)$$

This equation is able to produce very similar results to those of equation 23 but is also easily segregated into its components, where the first term relates to reaction rates at lower substrate concentrations, the second term is a transition term that segregates the form of the enzyme present at lower concentrations from the form present at high concentrations and the last term describes the activity of the enzyme at higher substrate concentrations. An example of the expansion used in this equation is depicted in Figure 6, where a theoretical enzyme is affected initially by substrate activation and then by substrate inhibition.

The modular way in which this equation can be expanded (Equation 25) allows for easy integration of modifier terms similar to those found in equation 21 (Walsh et al., 2007).

$$v = \frac{[S]}{[S]+K_{S1}} V_{S1} - \frac{[S]}{[S]+K_{SS1}} V_{S1} + \frac{[S]}{[S]+K_{SS1}} V_{SS1} - \cdots \frac{[S]}{[S]+K_{Sn-1}} V_{Sn-1} - \frac{[S]}{[S]+K_{Sn}} V_{Sn-1} + \frac{[S]}{[S]+K_{Sn}} V_{Sn} \qquad (25)$$

It also demonstrates how the modifier term can also be expanded in a similar modular fashion (Equation 26).

$$V_{S1} - (V_{S1} - V_{S2})\left(\frac{[X]}{[X] + K_{X1}}\right) + (V_{S1} - V_{S2})\left(\frac{[X]}{[X] + K_{X2}}\right) - (V_{S1} - V_{S3})\left(\frac{[X]}{[X] + K_{X2}}\right) \quad (26)$$

This term (Equation 26) is almost identical to equation 24 except that there is an initial catalytic velocity term (V_{S1}). This rate is altered by the high affinity modifier binding term (K_{X1}), shifting the velocity term (V_{S1}) to a new velocity term (V_{S2}). Upon binding of the second modifier molecule (K_{X2}) the velocity shift caused by the single binding event (V_{S2}) disappears and the new velocity term (V_{S3}) resulting from the presence of two modifiers bound to the enzyme replaces it. For example, the modifier homocysteine thiolactone was found to be stimulatory of the non-substrate activated form of human butyrylcholinesterase at lower concentrations but inhibited the enzyme at higher concentrations (Walsh et al., 2007).

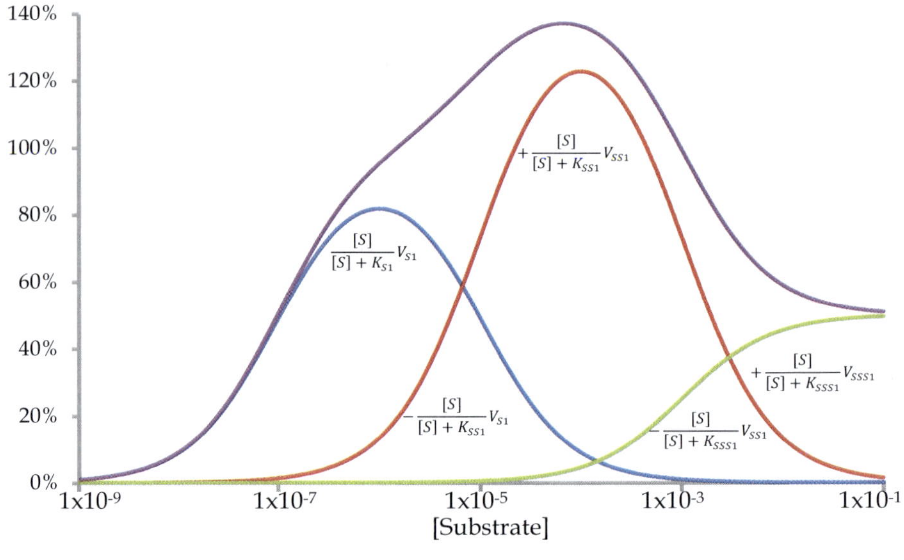

Fig. 6. Modular partitioning of enzymatic states at different concentrations. The purple curve represents the observed enzymatic activity while the other three curves represent the relative contribution to the total activity by the different forms of the enzyme. Blue represents the enzyme found at low substrate concentration where there is no substrate modulation. The red line represents substrate activation produced by secondary substrate molecule binding to the enzyme and the green represents inhibition produced by a tertiary binding event. Reaction rate is reported as values relative to the maximum activity of the enzymatic form not subject to substrate modulation (blue).

The utility of this sort of modular equation building was further expanded in a paper examining the synergistic effects of multiple inhibitors on enzymatic activity (Walsh et al., 2011b). In this example, two inhibitors of human butyrylcholinesterase were examined for their inhibitory effect individually and in combination (Figure 7; Equation 27).

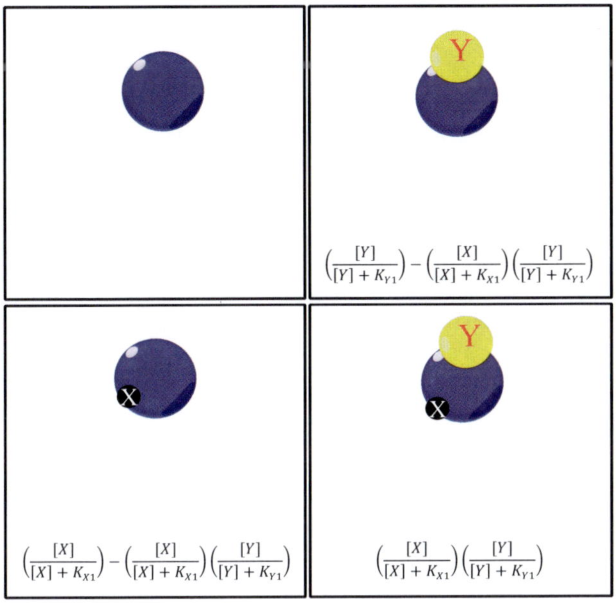

Fig. 7. Schematic representation of an enzyme bound by two inhibitors (X and Y), where the four quadrants represent the whole enzyme population divided into the inhibitor bound fractions that would be present if each inhibitors concentration were equal to its binding constant.

$$V_{S1}-(V_{S1}-V_{SX})\left(\left(\frac{[X]}{[X]+K_{X1}}\right)-\left(\frac{[X]}{[X]+K_{X1}}\right)\left(\frac{[Y]}{[Y]+K_{Y1}}\right)\right)-$$
$$(V_{S1}-V_{SY})\left(\left(\frac{[Y]}{[Y]+K_{Y1}}\right)-\left(\frac{[X]}{[X]+K_{X1}}\right)\left(\frac{[Y]}{[Y]+K_{Y1}}\right)\right)-(V_{S1}-V_{SXY})\left(\frac{[X]}{[X]+K_{X1}}\right)\left(\frac{[Y]}{[Y]+K_{Y1}}\right) \tag{27}$$

Here the inhibitory effect on each catalytic constant was segregated into three effects, the effect that each inhibitor had individually and the effect the two inhibitors had together. Equation 27 uses the example of the non-substrate activated maximum velocity of the enzyme, however the same sort of term was applied to each of the enzymes catalytic constants (Equation 24). The first term denotes the effect the first inhibitor (X) has on the enzyme (V_{S1}-V_{SX}) multiplied by the percent of the enzyme population bound by the inhibitor but subtracting the percent of the population bound by both inhibitors (XY). The second term describes the same process but with the other inhibitor (V_{S1}-V_{SY}). The last term is the effect produced by both inhibitors binding at the same time (V_{S1}-V_{SXY}). Using this strategy, for kinetic equation generation, the effects of galantamine, an inhibitor which predominantly inhibits the non-substrate activated form of butyrylcholinesterase, and citalopram, an inhibitor of both the non-substrate activated form and the substrate activated forms of the enzyme, were modeled individually and together (Rockwood et al., 2011; Walsh et al., 2011b). The modeling of this system suggests a possible mechanism for the clinical benefit observed in the treatment of Alzheimer's disease when these drugs are prescribed together.

4. Pseudo steady state enzyme kinetic equations in time course modelling of substrate hydrolysis

4.1 First order kinetics

The decrease in substrate produced by enzymatic catalysis is exponential in nature and can be described by the first order chemical reactions (Equation 28).

$$A = A_o e^{-kt} \tag{28}$$

The equation describes the breakdown of substrate using the rate constant (k) and Euler's constant (e) to relate the decrease in substrate concentration ($A_o \rightarrow A$) with time (t). Euler's constant raised to the rate constant in this equation represents the fraction of the initial reactant present after the first time interval (k_1, Equation 29-32).

$$A = A_o e^{-k1} \tag{29}$$

$$\frac{A}{A_o} = e^{-k} \tag{30}$$

$$\frac{A}{A_o} = k_1 \tag{31}$$

$$A = A_o {k_1}^t \tag{32}$$

This notation is useful, for it now becomes trivial to define the reduction of substrate in terms of the fraction that is converted to product during each time period ($1\text{-}k_2$, Equation 33).

$$A = A_o(1 - k_2)^t \tag{33}$$

This results in a rate of reaction that is defined relative to the initial concentration of the reactant (Equation 34).

$$A = A_o\left(1 - \frac{v}{A_o}\right)^t \tag{34}$$

This equation can then be used to accommodate the Michaelis-Menten equation, as rates associated with the Michaelis-Menten equation exponentially decrease as substrate is catalyzed to product (Walsh et al., 2010; Equation 35).

$$A = A_o\left(1 - \frac{\frac{[S]}{[S] + K_{S1}} V_{S1}}{A_o}\right)^t \tag{35}$$

The approach was initially used to describe the inhibition of β-galactosidase by imidazole using a global kinetic data fitting approach (Walsh et al., 2010). The open structure of the expression when compared to integral forms of the Michaelis-Menten equation found in the literature allowed for the insertion of modifier terms in the same way outlined in the previous section (Walsh et al., 2010; Equation 36).

$$A = A_o\left(1 - \frac{\dfrac{[S]}{[S] + K_{S1} - (K_{S1} - K_{S2})\left(\dfrac{[X]}{[X] + K_{X1}}\right)} V_{S1} - (V_{S1} - V_{S2})\left(\dfrac{[X]}{[X] + K_{X1}}\right)}{A_o}\right)^t \tag{36}$$

Additionally, global fitting of this equation to the kinetic data was able to confirm that the inhibitor imidazole had an irreversible component to its inhibition of β-galactosidase (Kim et al., 2003) as the simple insertion of modifier terms into equation 35 was unable to describe the effect of the inhibitor on the enzyme. While the hydrolysis of substrate tended towards zero in the absence of imidazole, the introduction of the inhibitor stopped the enzymatic activity in a concentration dependent manner. Therefore it was reasoned that a certain fraction of the inhibitor bound enzyme population was inactivated by this process (Equation 37).

$$k_a \frac{[X]}{[X] + K_{X1}} \tag{37}$$

Therefore a ratio term, defining the ratio between the rate of enzyme irreversible inhibition and the rate of substrate hydrolysis was used to define the fraction of the substrate population that would be hydrolysed before complete enzyme inactivation occurred (Equation 38). An additional term defining the substrate that would persist after the enzyme was also defined (Equation 39). In these terms, equation 21 has been represented as v for simplicity.

$$A_o\left(\frac{\dfrac{v}{A_o}}{\dfrac{v}{A_o} + k_a \dfrac{[X]}{[X] + K_{X1}}}\right) \tag{38}$$

$$A_o\left(\frac{k_a \dfrac{[X]}{[X] + K_{X1}}}{\dfrac{v}{A_o} + k_a \dfrac{[X]}{[X] + K_{X1}}}\right) \tag{39}$$

Inserting these terms into equation 36 produced an equation that was able to model the decrease in substrate concentration with time and take into account the irreversible inhibitory effects of imidazole on β-galactosidase (Walsh et al., 2010; Equation 40).

$$A = A_o\left(\frac{\frac{v}{A_o}}{\frac{v}{A_o}+k_a\frac{[X]}{[X]+K_{X1}}}\right)\left(1-\frac{v}{A_o\left(\frac{\frac{v}{A_o}}{\frac{v}{A_o}+k_a\frac{[X]}{[X]+K_{X1}}}\right)}\right)^t + A_o\left(\frac{k_a\frac{[X]}{[X]+K_{X1}}}{\frac{v}{A_o}+k_a\frac{[X]}{[X]+K_{X1}}}\right) \quad (40)$$

5. Conclusions

5.1 Modular enzyme kinetic equations

The modular method of equation generation discussed here does not necessarily require derivation from initial conservation of mass and rate equations that were used in the generation of classical pseudo steady state enzyme kinetic equations. Rather, by clearly distinguishing between the mass action binding terms and the governor terms, which describe the kinetic effect of modifiers, a general method to characterize the effect of inhibitors and activators on enzymatic activity is suggested (Equation 21). The structure of this modified version of the Michaelis Menten equation allows for its modular expansion to describe multiple substrate binding interactions (Equation 24), multiple modifier binding interactions (Equation 26) and the effects of more than one modifier binding to the same enzyme (Equation 27). The modular way in which these equations can be expanded to describe the bulk kinetic properties associated with enzyme kinetic modeling suggests that they may neglect processes such as modifier and substrate binding order. However there are several possibilities which may result from such processes. For example, an inhibitor may bind to an enzyme only in the absence of the substrate or only in its presence, in both of these instances the inhibition would most likely manifest as a rectangular hyperbolic change in the catalytic constants influencing enzymatic activity. Alternatively if the inhibitor binds both forms of the enzyme, the affinity for each form may be quite different resulting in a term similar to that proposed with equation 26. While there are undoubtedly many more possibilities, as have been outlined in texts such as Enzyme Kinetics by Segel (1993), the derivation of these equations have neglected the division between mass binding and modifier effect proposed here.

This distinction between mass binding and modifier effect combined with the modular equation construction described herein represents a new way of addressing enzyme kinetic modelling which permits the simple adaptation of kinetic models for data analysis. This allows for a simplified comparative global data fitting to discriminate between competing kinetic models using nonlinear regression. A helpful guide to nonlinear data fitting in excel has recently been published in Nature Protocols (Kemmer & Keller, 2010).

5.2 Pseudo-steady state equations in time course modeling

Integral forms of the Michaelis Menten equation have been proposed for use in time course analysis for many years, with more complex mathematical models appearing with time (Russell & Drane, 1992; Goudar et al., 1999). Integral forms of the Michaelis Menten equation however have been found to be limited in their usefulness for time course models which has spurred further research (Liao et al., 2005). Integral forms of the Michaelis Menten equation also predominately model the Michaelis Menten equation and do not deal with modifier interactions. This may be in part due to the problems associated with pseudo-steady state modifier equations, such as lack of governor terms on the effects of modifiers in enzyme systems, as outlined in the first section of this chapter. To attempt to address these issues a new way of using pseudo-steady state equations in time course modeling has been proposed (Walsh et al., 2010). The proposed methodology inserts the pseudo-steady state equations directly into the exponential decay equation (Equation 35) allowing for the same degree of equation flexibility outlined with the methods for modular expansion of pseudo-steady state equations described in section 3.2.

The direct use of so called pseudo-steady state equations in exponential equations relies on several assumptions. Primarily, the development of pseudo-steady state equations has been based on experimental data generated in closed systems. That is, even if preformed in conditions where the rate of substrate hydrolysis is taken as linear or is linearized through the use of tangential slope lines, the observed rates are actually exponentially decreasing. Additionally, single substrate enzymes, which are not subject to conditions that would alter their catalytic activity, such as substrate or product modulation, as catalysts follow first order kinetics in closed systems (Equation 35). Due to this, time course modeling has the advantage of being able to identify a variety of kinetic situations, such as strong substrate activation or inhibition, for which initial rate analysis is not optimal (Shushanyan et.al., 2011). This sort of modeling can also be used to detect the influence of irreversible inhibition as deviation of the exponential curve away from the predicted initial exponential rate in substrate hydrolysis are more apparent with time course models than models using initial rates. For example, in our initial examination of the inhibition of β-galactosidase with imidazole with initial rates the irreversible inhibition of β-galactosidase was not apparent (Walsh et al., 2007), however it became quite apparent using time course models (Walsh et al., 2010).

The ease with which this method allows the integration of pseudo-steady state and time course kinetic equations holds the promise of making time course kinetic modeling a more prominent part of modifier kinetic analysis. Additionally, the modular compilation of kinetic components outlined in this chapter and their application to time course modeling suggest this form of modeling may be particularly useful for in-depth characterization of enzymatically regulated pathways which is directly applicable to systems biology.

6. References

Goudar C.T., Sonnad J.R. & Duggleby R.G. (1999). Parameter estimation using a direct solution of the integrated Michaelis–Menten equation, *Biochim. Biophys. Acta,* 1429, 377–383.

Kemmer G. & Keller S. (2010). Nonlinear least-squares data fitting in Excel spreadsheets. *Nat. Protoc.,* 5, 267-281.

Kim C.S., Ji E.S. & Oh D.K. (2003). Expression and characterization of Kluyveromyces lactis beta-galactosidase in Escherichia coli. *Biotechnol. Lett.,* 20, 1769–1774.

Liao F., Zhu X.Y., Wang Y.M. & Zuo Y.P. (2005). The comparison of the estimation of enzyme kinetic parameters by fitting reaction curve to the integrated Michaelis–

Menten rate equations of different predictor variables. *J. Biochem. Biophys. Methods,* 62, 13–24.

Lineweaver H. & Burk D. (1934). The Determination of Enzyme Dissociation Constants. *J Am Chem Soc.,* 56, 658-666.

McElroy W.D. (1947). The Mechanism of Inhibition of Cellular Activity by Narcotics. *Q Rev Biol.,* 22, 25-58.

Michaelis L. & Menten M.L. (1913). Die Kinetik der Invertinwirkung. *Biochem. Z.,* 49, 333–369.

Ogston A.G. (1948). Interpretation of experiments on metabolic processes, using isotopic tracer elements. *Nature,* 162, 963.

Reiner E. & Simeon-Rudolf V. (2000). Cholinesterase: substrate inhibition and substrate activation. *Pflugers Arch.,* 440, R118-120.

Rockwood K., Walsh R., Martin E. & Darvesh S. (2011). Potentially procholinergic effects of medications commonly used in older adults. *Am J Geriatr Pharmacother.,* 9, 80-87.

Russell R.W. & Drane J.W. (1992). Improved rearrangement of the integrated Michaelis-Menten equation for calculating in vivo kinetics of transport and metabolism. *J Dairy Sci.,* 75, 3455-3464.

Segel I.H. (1993). *Enzyme Kinetics: Behavior and Analysis of Rapid Equilibrium and Steady-State Enzyme Systems,* Wiley, New York.

Shushanyan M., Khoshtariya D.E., Tretyakova T., Makharadze M. & van Eldik R. (2011). Diverse role of conformational dynamics in carboxypeptidase A-driven peptide and ester hydrolyses: Disclosing the "Perfect Induced Fit" and "Protein Local Unfolding" pathways by altering protein stability. *Biopolymers.,* 95, 852-870.

Walsh R., Martin E. & Darvesh S. (2007). A versatile equation to describe reversible enzyme inhibition and activation kinetics: modeling beta-galactosidase and butyrylcholinesterase. *Biochim. Biophys. Acta,* 1770, 733–746.

Walsh R., Martin E. & Darvesh S. (2010). A method to describe enzyme-catalyzed reactions by combining steady state and time course enzyme kinetic parameters. *Biochim. Biophys. Acta,* 1800, 1–5.

Walsh R., Martin E. & Darvesh S. (2011a). Limitations of conventional inhibitor classifications. *Integr Biol.,* DOI: 10.1039/c1ib00053e.

Walsh R., Martin E. & Darvesh S. (2011b). Synergistic inhibition of butyrylcholinesterase by galantamine and citalopram. *Biochim. Biophys. Acta,* 1810, 1230–1235.

Permissions

The contributors of this book come from diverse backgrounds, making this book a truly international effort. This book will bring forth new frontiers with its revolutionizing research information and detailed analysis of the nascent developments around the world.

We would like to thank Dr. Deniz Ekinci, for lending his expertise to make the book truly unique. He has played a crucial role in the development of this book. Without his invaluable contribution this book wouldn't have been possible. He has made vital efforts to compile up to date information on the varied aspects of this subject to make this book a valuable addition to the collection of many professionals and students.

This book was conceptualized with the vision of imparting up-to-date information and advanced data in this field. To ensure the same, a matchless editorial board was set up. Every individual on the board went through rigorous rounds of assessment to prove their worth. After which they invested a large part of their time researching and compiling the most relevant data for our readers. Conferences and sessions were held from time to time between the editorial board and the contributing authors to present the data in the most comprehensible form. The editorial team has worked tirelessly to provide valuable and valid information to help people across the globe.

Every chapter published in this book has been scrutinized by our experts. Their significance has been extensively debated. The topics covered herein carry significant findings which will fuel the growth of the discipline. They may even be implemented as practical applications or may be referred to as a beginning point for another development. Chapters in this book were first published by InTech; hereby published with permission under the Creative Commons Attribution License or equivalent.

The editorial board has been involved in producing this book since its inception. They have spent rigorous hours researching and exploring the diverse topics which have resulted in the successful publishing of this book. They have passed on their knowledge of decades through this book. To expedite this challenging task, the publisher supported the team at every step. A small team of assistant editors was also appointed to further simplify the editing procedure and attain best results for the readers.

Our editorial team has been hand-picked from every corner of the world. Their multi-ethnicity adds dynamic inputs to the discussions which result in innovative outcomes. These outcomes are then further discussed with the researchers and contributors who give their valuable feedback and opinion regarding the same. The feedback is then collaborated with the researches and they are edited in a comprehensive manner to aid the understanding of the subject.

Apart from the editorial board, the designing team has also invested a significant amount of their time in understanding the subject and creating the most relevant covers. They scrutinized every image to scout for the most suitable representation of the subject and create an appropriate cover for the book.

The publishing team has been involved in this book since its early stages. They were actively engaged in every process, be it collecting the data, connecting with the contributors or procuring relevant information. The team has been an ardent support to the editorial, designing and production team. Their endless efforts to recruit the best for this project, has resulted in the accomplishment of this book. They are a veteran in the field of academics and their pool of knowledge is as vast as their experience in printing. Their expertise and guidance has proved useful at every step. Their uncompromising quality standards have made this book an exceptional effort. Their encouragement from time to time has been an inspiration for everyone.

The publisher and the editorial board hope that this book will prove to be a valuable piece of knowledge for researchers, students, practitioners and scholars across the globe.

List of Contributors

Aldo Segura-Cabrera
Laboratorio de Bioinformática, U.A.M. Reynosa Aztlán, Universidad Autónoma de Tamaulipas, Reynosa,
México

Carlos A. García-Pérez
Laboratorio de Bioinformática, Mexico

Mario A. Rodríguez-Pérez and Xianwu Guo
Laboratorio de Biomedicina Molecular, Mexico

Gildardo Rivera
Laboratorio de Biotecnología Ambiental, Mexico

Virgilio Bocanegra-García
Laboratorio de Medicina de Conservación Centro de Biotecnología Genómica, Instituto Politécnico Nacional, Mexico

Mutlu D. Aytemir and G. Karakaya
Hacettepe University, Faculty of Pharmacy, Department of Pharmaceutical Chemistry, Ankara, Turkey

Omar Deeb
Al-Quds University, Faculty of Pharmacy, Jerusalem, Palestine

Rinat Islamov, Tatyana Kustova and Alexander Ilin
Scientific Centre for Anti-Infectious Drugs, Kazakhstan

Laila Mahmoud Mohamed Gad
Faculty of Pharmacy, King Abdulaziz University KAU, Jeddah, Kingdom of Saudi Arabia

Ahmed Kamal, M. Kashi Reddy, Ajay Kumar Srivastava and Y. V. V. Srikanth
Division of Organic Chemistry, CSIR-Indian Institute of Chemical Technology, Hyderabad, India

Tetsuro Kamiya
Gifu Pharmaceutical University, Japan
Gifu University, Japan

Hirokazu Hara and Tetsuo Adachi
Gifu Pharmaceutical University, Japan

Naoki Inagaki
Gifu University, Japan

Halmuthur M. Sampath Kumar and Irfan Hyder
CSIR-Indian Institute of Chemical Technology, Hyderabad, India

Parvinder Pal Singh
CSIR- Indian Institute of Integrative Medicine, Jammu, India

Tomoe Komoriya, Kazuaki Yoshimune and Hideki Kohno
College of Industrial Technology, Nihon University, Nerashino, Chiba

Masahiro Ogawa and Mitsuhiko Moriyama
School of Medicine, Nihon University, Chiyoda-ku, Tokyo, Japan

Yushi Liu
Lovelace Respiratory Research Institute, USA

Joseph S. Verducci
The Ohio State University, USA

Emmanuel M. Papamichael, Panagiota-Yiolanda Stergiou, Athanasios Foukis, Marina Kokkinou and Leonidas G. Theodorou
University of Ioannina, Department of Chemistry, Ioannina, Greece

Demet Coskun and Ahmet Mahli
Department of Anesthesiology and Reanimation, Gazi University Faculty of Medicine, Ankara, Turkey

Vesna Pavelkic and Tanja Brdaric
Institute "Kirilo Savic" Belgrade, Serbia

Kristina Gopcevic
University of Belgrade, School of Medicine, Serbia

Paolo Ruzza
Institute of Biomolecular Chemistry of C.N.R., Italy

Murat Şentürk
Ağrı İbrahim Çeçen University, Turkey

Hüseyin Çavdar
Dumlupınar University, Turkey

Oktay Talaz
Karamanoğlu Mehmetbey University, Turkey

Claudiu T. Supuran
University of Florence, Italy

Shailza Singh and Sonali Shinde
National Centre for Cell Science NCCS Complex, Ganeskhind, Pune University Campus, Pune, India

Andreas Jurik, Freya Klepsch and Barbara Zdrazil
University of Vienna, Department of Medicinal Chemistry, Pharmacoinformatics Research Group, Austria

Ryan Walsh
Chemistry Department, Carleton University, Ottawa, Canada